D1448939

SURVEY
OF
CLINICAL
PEDIATRICS

McGraw-Hill Book Company

A Blakiston Publication

New York   St. Louis   San Francisco
Düsseldorf   Johannesburg   Kuala Lumpur
London   Mexico   Montreal
New Delhi   Panama   Paris   São Paulo
Singapore   Sydney   Tokyo   Toronto

EDWARD WASSERMAN, B.S., M.D.

Professor and Chairman, Department of Pediatrics
New York Medical College
Metropolitan Hospital Center
Director of Pediatrics
Flower and Fifth Avenue Hospitals
New York

LAWRENCE B. SLOBODY, B.S., M.D.

Professor, Department of Pediatrics
New York Medical College
Metropolitan Hospital Center
President, New York Medical College
New York

SIXTH EDITION

SURVEY OF CLINICAL PEDIATRICS

NOTICE

Medicine is an ever-changing science. As new research and clinical experience broaden our knowledge, changes in treatment and drug therapy are required. The authors and the publisher of this work have made every effort to ensure that the drug dosage schedules herein are accurate and in accord with the standards accepted at the time of publication. The reader is advised, however, to check the product information sheet included in the package of each drug he plans to administer to be certain that changes have not been made in the recommended dose or in the contraindications for administration. This recommendation is of particular importance in regard to new or infrequently used drugs.

Library of Congress Cataloging in Publication Data

Wasserman, Edward.
Survey of clinical pediatrics.

In earlier editions Slobody's name appeared first on title pages.
Bibliography: p.
1. Pediatrics. I. Slobody, Lawrence Boris, date joint author. II. Title. [DNLM: 1. Pediatrics. WS100 S634s 1974]
RJ45.W36 1974   618.9'2   73-14561
ISBN 0-07-068430-8

SURVEY OF CLINICAL PEDIATRICS

Copyright © 1955, 1959, 1963, 1968, 1974 by McGraw-Hill, Inc.
All rights reserved.
Copyright 1952 by McGraw-Hill, Inc.
All rights reserved.
Printed in the United States of America. No part of this publication may be reproduced, stored in a retrieval system, or transmitted, in any form or by any means, electronic, mechanical, photocopying, recording, or otherwise, without the prior written permission of the publisher.

2 3 4 5 6 7 8 9 0 K P K P 7 9 8 7 6 5 4

This book was set in Century Expanded by Monotype Composition Company, Inc.
The editors were Paul K. Schneider and Sally Barhydt Mobley; the designer was Anne Canevari Green; and the production supervisor was Leroy A. Young.
Kingsport Press, Inc., was printer and binder.

Dedicated to N.F.W. and E.T.S.

CONTENTS

LIST OF CONTRIBUTORS

Nesrin Bingol, M.D., Assistant Professor, Department of Pediatrics, New York Medical College, Metropolitan Hospital Center; Chief, Section for Genetics.

Harold S. Cole, M.D., Associate Professor, Department of Pediatrics, New York Medical College, Metropolitan Hospital Center; Chief, Section for Metabolic Diseases.

Jack M. Cooperman, Ph.D., Associate Professor, Department of Pediatrics, New York Medical College, Metropolitan Hospital Center.

Magdalena Fuchs, M.D., Assistant Professor, Department of Pediatrics, New York Medical College, Metropolitan Hospital Center; Chief, Section for Growth and Development.

Alta Goalwin, M.D., Clinical Associate Professor, Department of Pediatrics, New York Medical College, Metropolitan Hospital Center; Director, Department of Pediatrics, Jewish Memorial Hospital.

Susan Gordon, M.D., Associate Professor, Department of Pediatrics, New York Medical College, Metropolitan Hospital Center; Chief, Section for Infectious Diseases.

Marvin Green, M.D., Associate Professor, Department of Pediatrics, New York Medical College, Metropolitan Hospital Center; Chief, Section for Neonatology, Metropolitan Hospital; Departmental Poison Control Officer.

Donald Gromisch, M.D., Associate Professor, Department of Pediatrics, New York Medical College, Metropolitan Hospital Center; Chief, Pediatric Service, Metropolitan Hospital.

Peter Immordino, M.D., New London, Connecticut; Former Instructor, Department of Surgery, New York Medical College, Metropolitan Hospital Center.

Silvia Iosub, M.D., Assistant Professor, Department of Pediatrics, New York Medical College, Metropolitan Hospital Center; Chief, Section for Chronic Diseases.

Robert Kahn, M.D., Associate Professor, Department of Pediatrics, New York Medical College, Metropolitan Hospital Center; Chief, Section for Cardiology.

Miriam Lending, M.D., Professor, Department of Pediatrics, New York Medical College, Metropolitan Hospital Center; Chief, Pediatric Service, Flower and Fifth Avenue Hospitals.

A. Leonard Luhby, M.D., Professor, Department of Pediatrics, New York Medical College, Metropolitan Hospital Center; Chief, Section for Hematology.

Anthony Maffia, M.D., Clinical Professor, Department of Pediatrics, New York Medical College, Metropolitan Hospital Center.

David T. Mininberg, M.D., Assistant Professor, Departments of Urology and Pediatrics, New York Medical College, Metropolitan Hospital Center; Chief, Section for Pediatric Urology.

Mario F. Montoya, M.D., Assistant Professor, Department of Pediatrics, New York Medical College, Metropolitan Hospital Center; Chief, Newborn Service, Flower and Fifth Avenue Hospitals.

Eileen Halsey Pike, Ph.D., Associate Professor, Department of Microbiology, New York Medical College.

Arie Ribon, M.D., Assistant Professor, Department of Pediatrics, New York Medical College, Metropolitan Hospital Center; Chief, Section for Allergy and Immunology.

June Schwartz, M.D., Assistant Professor, Department of Pediatrics, New York Medical College, Metropolitan Hospital Center; Chief, Section for Adolescent Medicine.

Arnold Slovis, M.D., Assistant Professor, Department of Pediatrics, New York Medical College, Metropolitan Hospital Center.

Elkan Snyder, Ed.D., Associate Professor, Department of Pediatrics, New York Medical College, Metropolitan Hospital Center; Chief, Section for Learning Disabilities.

Louis Southren, M.D., Professor, Department of Medicine, and Associate Professor, Department of Pediatrics, New York Medical College, Metropolitan Hospital Center; Chief, Section for Endocrinology.

Edward Wasserman, M.D., Professor and Chairman, Department of Pediatrics, New York Medical College, Metropolitan Hospital Center.

Allan B. Weingold, M.D., Professor, Department of Obstetrics-Gynecology, New York Medical College, Metropolitan Hospital Center; Director, Maternal and Child Health.

Jane Wright, M.D., Professor, Department of Surgery, New York Medical College, Metropolitan Hospital Center.

A. Munire Yuceoglu, M.D., Associate Professor, Department of Pediatrics, New York Medical College, Metropolitan Hospital Center; Chief, Section for Nephrology.

PREFACE

Survey of Clinical Pediatrics is designed as just that—a survey of pediatrics—and is not intended to replace the excellent larger and more detailed textbooks that are available to both student and physician. This text focuses on the highlights and relationships of pediatrics. To aid in this focalization and reinforce learning, questions are supplied at the end of each chapter.

The rapid increase in knowledge in the subspecialities necessitates a delineated core of material common to the pediatric generalist and subspecialist. Such core material is not a static body of knowledge, nor is it identical for all pediatric practitioners. The generalist in a large urban area will not be called upon to treat low-birth-weight infants in an intensive care nursery. In many such nurseries the neonatologist does not permit the generalist to practice. In a low-density-population setting the generalist usually is also the neonatologist. Consequently, defining core material requires a personal judgment, and we hope we have achieved a degree of success in this difficult but necessary effort. One technique used to select core material was to have chapters written by generalists with an interest in specific areas of pediatrics.

This edition, the sixth, is the most complete revision of the *Survey of Clinical Pediatrics*. Every topic in the book has been carefully brought up to date. For example, since the last edition, the fetus and its environment have become areas of increased interest to pediatricians. Fetal monitoring, prenatal diagnosis, and genetic counseling are topics of rapidly expanding knowledge. Consequently a new chapter on the fetus has been added. The section on adolescence has been enlarged to reflect the growing realization that this age group has been neglected in the past. The chapter on infectious diseases has been rewritten with increased emphasis placed on viral diseases to present a better balance between viral and other infections. The chapter on respiratory diseases also portrays more accurately the role of viral diseases.

All the material presented has been used with the student in actual work at the bedside, in seminars, and in conference. The integration with the basic sciences, e.g., physiology, pathology, psychology, and biochemistry, has not been presented here in detail but should be constantly kept in mind as the various areas are studied. Finally, comprehensive consideration of the child, mother, and family as a unit—the understanding that physical, mental, emotional, and social aspects are indivisible—requires continual emphasis.

We should like to thank Mrs. Barbara Salamy, Miss Mary Prior, Mrs. Ramona Vega, and Miss Elizabeth Szilagyi for their editorial help.

Edward Wasserman
Lawrence B. Slobody

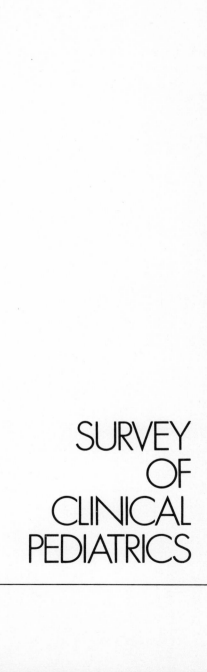

SURVEY
OF
CLINICAL
PEDIATRICS

1 GROWTH AND DEVELOPMENT

Pediatrics is the practice of medicine concerned with the growth and development of the child from conception through adolescence. The objective is to care for the child in disease, but more importantly to help the child to achieve his full potential physically, mentally, emotionally, and socially during the various stages of development and to become ready for productive adulthood. The pediatrician is also becoming increasingly concerned with family counseling and planning and with the preventive and community aspects of medicine.

The study of growth and development is basic to understanding pediatrics, and its importance cannot be overemphasized. For example, the child's stage of development affects the diagnosis, treatment, and course of an illness, and the disease itself can influence development in the near future or later on. Growth and development starts with the fertilization of the ovum. The two are intimately interwoven and cannot be separated, but growth usually is considered an increase in size, and development is considered an acquisition of skills and function.

The life of the child may be divided into the following periods: prenatal, neonatal (first 4 weeks), infancy (1 month to 1 year), preschool or early childhood (1 year to 6 years), prepuberal or late childhood (6 years to 10 years), and adolescence (10 years to 18 years in girls, 12 years to 20 years in boys). Although considerable variation exists in these groups and although the characteristics of one stage blend into the next, the general pattern of each is sufficiently distinctive to require separate evaluation. It is essential to know what is normal within each period and therefore what can be expected as the sum of growth processes at any particular later period.

In order to recognize the abnormal, a thorough knowledge of the normal and its variations are necessary. Data for such evaluation of the individual child have been obtained from studies of large groups of healthy subjects.

The physician is responsible for the supervision of the health of the child. This requires periodic examinations and evaluations of the child's progress and consultations with the child's parents. The rate and progress of growth and development over a period of time give more information than a single evaluation. Marked deviations from the norm that cannot be explained adequately by factors in the history require more special studies such as roentgenograms, laboratory tests, and psychometric examinations. A diagnosis is then made and therapy instituted wherever possible.

FACTORS INFLUENCING GROWTH AND DEVELOPMENT

The normal child has his own schedule of growth and development which falls within the predictable pattern for all normal children. The individual pattern is determined by an interplay of hereditary and environmental factors.

Heredity

1. Race: Orientals tend to be short.
2. Nationality: Scandinavians tend to be taller than Italians.
3. Family: Some families tend to be short.
4. Age: The greatest rates of growth are during fetal life, the first year, and adolescence.
5. Sex: Females mature earlier, starting adolescence at about 10 years of age, while males start at about 12 years.
6. Chromosomal abnormalities: Down's syndrome is associated with short stature.
7. Inborn errors of metabolism: Metabolic errors, e.g., phenylketonuria and galactosemia, affect growth adversely.

Environment

1. External factors
   a. Socioeconomic factors: Poverty is associated with poor nutrition and surroundings.
   b. Physical surroundings: Lack of sunshine and poor hygiene may affect rate of growth.
   c. Season: The greatest increase in height occurs during the spring and the least in the fall, while weight gain is usually greatest in the fall and least in the spring.
   d. Psychologic factors: Interrelationships with parents, teachers, and others may affect growth and development.
2. Exercise and stimulation: Activity promotes growth.
3. Nutrition: Dietary intake, quantitative and qualitative, influences growth and development prenatally and postnatally.
4. Disease: Chronic illnesses and congenital malformations, e.g., chronic nephritis, celiac disease, or congenital heart disease, may cause retardation of physical growth.
5. Endocrine factors: Hormonal imbalance such as occurs in hypothyroidism and hypopituitarism cause retardation of growth.

NORMS IN GROWTH

From birth to adolescence, growth proceeds in biologically predetermined cycles that fall into four distinct periods: (1) a rapid period from birth to 2 years of age, (2) a slow period from 2 years of age to pubescence, (3) a rapid period from pubescence to 15 or 16 years of age, and (4) a sharp deceleration from 15 or 16 years to maturity.

Since the growth of a child proceeds at an individual rate, the studies of individual children will reveal wide variations from the standard or average weight and height tables. However, base lines are essential in the study of the child's growth so that marked deviations can be identified and investigated.

STATISTICAL METHODS

In the evaluation of some measurable aspect of the growth and development of the individual child, e.g., weight, cardiac rate, gross motor performance, red cell count, it is essential to know the normal variations that occur within a group of comparable children, for instance, of the same age or sex. From such data one can estimate the adequacy of the individual child's measurement or performance and, in the case of some of the measurements, it may be possible to predict his future pattern of development.

It is important to know the degree of dispersion of the observations about the mean, the standard deviation. The mean value ±1 standard deviation includes approximately 67 percent of the total number of observations if the observations approximate a normal or bell-shaped curve; ±2 standard deviations includes about 95 percent of the observations; ±3 standard deviations includes about 99.7 percent of the observations. Some measurements, particularly those related to physical growth, are reported as percentiles. In establishing percentiles, the measurements (e.g., the heights of 100 five-year-old boys) are arranged in increasing or decreasing magnitude. The smallest measurement corresponds to the 1st percentile, the greatest measurement to the 100th percentile. If an individual is found to be in the 76th percentile, then 75 percent of comparable children should be shorter than he. If repeated measurements are taken, it is possible to determine whether the percentile position observed at any one time represents the normal growth pattern for that individual or suggests some pathologic condition.

The 40.2-in. 5-year-old is third man from the short end of the line, or in the 3d percentile (see the accompanying chart). Thus, one height measurement compares this boy with his colleagues, and repeated measurements compare him with himself. If he has remained in the 3d percentile at 2, 3, and 4 years of age, he is following a "percentile channel" of a shorter-than-average person who is growing at a normal rate. If past measurements show that he dropped from the 50th percentile at 2 years of age to the 25th at 3 years, to the 10th at 4 years, and to the 3d percentile at 5 years, a pathologic condition should be suspected, even though his height seems acceptable for a 5-year-old boy. Any given physical measurement usually follows a constant percentile channel in the course of healthy growth.

The rules of thumb suggested below are helpful in learning norms for height, weight, etc. Such rules cannot always provide the precise weight and height for a particular age, but the variations are found to fall well within normal limits. (The increased rate of growth of the new generation may make necessary a revision of the norms for weight and height.)

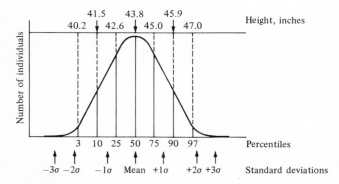

Figure 1-1

WEIGHT

At birth, 7½ lb (3.4 kg) is the average weight; the usual range is from 6 to 9 lb (2.7 to 4.1 kg). The firstborn child is often lighter in weight than subsequent siblings. There is an initial weight loss during the first 3 to 4 days of life, which may be as much as 10 percent of the birth weight. This loss is usually regained by the eighth or ninth day. In the first 5 to 6 months the infant usually gains 6 to 8 oz per week; in the second 6 months, only 3 to 4 oz are gained per week. By the fifth month the birth weight is usually doubled, i.e., 15 lb (6.8 kg). At 1 year of age the birth weight is tripled, i.e., 22 lb (10.0 kg). At 2½ years of age (30 months) the birth weight is quadrupled, i.e., 30 lb (13.6 kg). At 5 years of age the weight at 1 year is doubled, i.e., 44 lb (20.0 kg). At 10 years of age the weight is 10 times the birth weight, i.e., 75 lb (34.1 kg). At 13 to 14 years of age the weight at 1 year is quintupled, i.e., 110 lb (50.0 kg).

Weech has suggested the following helpful mnemonic formulas for average weight at various ages:

3–12 months:	weight = age (month) + 11
1–4 yr:	weight = weight at 1 yr + 2½ lb per 6 months
4–8 yr:	weight = 6 × age (yr) + 12
8–12 yr:	weight = 7 × age (yr) + 5

HEIGHT

Growth of extremities as compared with trunk The progress of growth is cephalo-caudad, so that at birth the head is large, the trunk long, the lower extremities relatively short, with the arms being longer than the legs. The midpoint of the body is ¾ in. above the umbilicus. The extremities grow more rapidly than the trunk. At 2 years of age, the midpoint of the body is slightly below the umbilicus. At 16 years of age, the midpoint is near the symphysis pubis. At about puberty, the trunk and extremities grow at equal rates; after puberty, the trunk grows slightly faster. Linear growth does not cease until maturity is reached, about 18 years of age in girls and 20 in boys.

HEAD

The growth of the head is related to the growth of the brain. Examination of the head in infants is of extreme importance; any deviation from the normal growth may indicate neuromotor disorder or abnormality, for instance, hydrocephaly. Head control should be attained at the age of 3 months.

The posterior fontanel should be closed by 6 to 8 weeks of age, and the anterior fontanel by 16 to 18 months of age. The sutures usually

Table 1-1.   Normal rate of growth*

Age	Increase	Height
Birth		20 in. (50 cm)
First 6 months	1 in./month	26 in. (66 cm)
Second 6 months	½ in./month	30 in. (76 cm)
1–7 yr	3 in./yr	49 in. (124 cm)
8–15 yr	2 in./yr	65 in. (165 cm)

* Weech has suggested the following helpful mnemonic formula to predict height from the ages of 2 to 14 yr: Height (in.) $= 2\frac{1}{2} \times$ age (yr) $+ 30$.

close clinically by 6 to 8 months, but as evidenced by roentgenograms, they are not ossified until maturity.

Measurements of the head

Circumference at birth: 13–14 in. (33.0–35.6 cm)
First year, grows 4 in. ½ in. per month for 4 months, ¼ in. per month for next 8 months: 17–18 in. (43.2–45.7 cm)
Second year, grows 1 in.: 18–19 in. (45.7–48.3 cm)
Third to fifth years, grows ½ in. per yr: 19.5–20.5 in. (49.5–52.1 cm)
Fifth year to puberty, grows ½ in. per 5 yr until maturity; adult size: 20.5–21.7 in. (52.1–55.1 cm)

The facial portion of the head is smaller than the cranial portion at birth. The hair on the scalp may fall out during the early weeks of life and then grow back again; the definitive color of the hair cannot be predicted at birth. The lacrimal glands may produce no tears during the first 2 months of life.

BRAIN

The formation of the central nervous system (CNS) begins very early in intrauterine life. The number of cells within the brain increases linearly until birth and then rather slowly up to about 6 to 12 months of postnatal life. Myelinization starts at about the fourth fetal month. The most active myelin synthesis occurs in the perinatal period, but significant myelinization continues for several years afterward. Proper nutrition is essential for these processes to proceed normally. Interference with cell division and myelin formation during this period may result in permanent deficits in the brain. The brain weighs about 350 Gm at birth and increases rapidly during the first 2 years of life. Thereafter growth is slow, and the adult size is reached at adolescence.

Motor and sensory controls develop from above and proceed downward, so that eye control develops before hand and leg control. Development is related to three functioning levels of the central nervous system—brainstem, archipallium, and neopallium.

The newborn infant functions at brainstem level. Archipallium, which includes part of the temporal lobe, cingulate gyrus, and basal ganglions, supervenes on the brainstem and may be considered responsible for the basic emotions and some primitive motor and sensory control. Neopallium, which includes most of the cerebral hemisphere, has intellectual rather than emotional function and is responsible for skill, discrimination, and fine movements. Clinical application of these developmental patterns is manifold, e.g., changes in physical signs in static brain lesions—upper limb paresis becomes apparent at 5 to 6 months, lower limb at 10 to 12 months; abnormalities of coordination —athetoid and involuntary movements become apparent between 18 to 24 months.

Transient infantile reflexes, e.g., Moro, palmar-grasp, and tonic neck reflexes, normally disappear early in life. Persistence of any of these reflexes is pathologic. The Moro reflex does not return once it disappears, but the palmar-grasp reflex may return if the frontal lobes are damaged. Persistence of the complete tonic neck reflex is associated with damage to the brain. The abdominal reflexes persist even in the presence of congenital or neonatal pyramidal lesions. Plantar reflexes may be physiologically upgoing until the age of 2 years.

Age at time of disappearance of transient infantile reflexes

1 month	2 months	3–4 months
Stepping Cross-extension	Trunk-incurvation Grasp	Tonic neck Placing Moro

SINUSES AND MASTOIDS

The maxillary and ethmoid sinuses are present at birth and may become infected. The sphenoid sinuses may be present at birth but are rarely of clinical importance until 3 to 5 years of age. The frontal sinuses are rarely of clinical significance before 6 to 10 years of age.

The mastoid at birth is a single cell, the antrum. Pneumatization extends from this single cell into the tip of the mastoid by 3 to 4 years of age. The eustachian tube is shorter, straighter, and relatively wider in infants than in adults, so that infection may extend easily from the pharynx to the middle ear and antrum.

DENTITION

Deciduous teeth (milk, or temporary, teeth) are 20 in number, and all are erupted usually by 2½ years of age. The following is the approximate order and time of appearance:

2 lower central incisors: 6–8 months
4 upper incisors: 8–12 months
2 lower lateral incisors: 12–15 months
4 anterior molars: 12–16 months
4 canines: 16–20 months
4 posterior molars: 20–30 months

The approximate number of deciduous teeth is the same as the age in months less 6. For example, at 12 months of age, there are usually six teeth. The number of teeth present, however, should not be considered a milestone of development.

There are 32 permanent teeth. The 6-year molars (first permanent molars) appear first and are most important, since they are the foundations of the dental arch. The following is the approximate order and time of appearance:

4 first molars: 6 years
8 incisors: 7–9 years
8 bicuspids: 10–12 years
4 canines: 11–12 years
4 second molars: 13 years
4 third molars: 17–22 years

Teething (the normal process of tooth eruption) has been implicated as a cause of fever and febrile diseases during infancy. This association is difficult to explain and is not generally accepted. Irritability, ptyalism, and increased desire to suck or chew may occur as a result of teething. No treatment is necessary. Aspirin, teething rings, and picking the infant up more frequently than usual have been suggested to give comfort.

Salivation is sufficient to maintain moisture of the oral mucous membranes in the newborn infant but increases at about 3 months of age, and infants normally drool, failing to swallow the saliva. In older children failure to swallow the saliva that is normally produced may occur because of neurologic damage. Increased salivation (ptyalism) occurs in several conditions, e.g., teething, mouth lesions, diabetes mellitus, acrodynia; following administration of certain drugs; or as a reflex in anticipation of food.

CHEST

At birth the chest is circular, but as the child grows older, the transverse diameter becomes larger than the anterior-posterior diameter, giving an elliptical appearance. At birth the chest circumference is about ½ in. smaller than the head; at 1 year of age the chest is equal to or exceeds the head slightly; thereafter the chest becomes progressively larger than the head.

The abdominal circumference varies with feedings but in general is about the same as that of the chest during the first year.

HEART AND LUNGS

The weight of the heart is about 25 Gm at birth, 45 Gm at 1 year, and 250 Gm at maturity. In the newborn infant, the apex beat is in the 4th intercostal space in, or slightly lateral to, the midclavicular line; by 2 years of age it is usually in the 5th intercostal space in, or just medial to, the midclavicular line. During infancy the heart lies more horizontally in the chest than in later life. After 1 year of age the cardiothoracic ratio should not be more than 50 percent; before then it may be normally as much as 55 percent. Circulation time as determined with fluorescein is slightly less than 5 seconds (umbilical vein to lip) in the newborn; from 1 month to 1 year, the time (arm to lip) is about 7 seconds; this time increases gradually to approximately 11½ seconds at adolescence.

Thoracic walls are thinner and more elastic in infants and young children than in adults. The thinness of the chest walls and the relatively large size of bronchi result in more intense tactile fremitus and a puerile breath sound which is loud and high-pitched and appears to be close to the ear. Diaphragmatic breathing is characteristic of infants and young children, but after 7 years of age the costal element predominates.

THYMUS

The thymus arises as paired evaginations from the 3d and 4th pharyngeal pouches and the corresponding branchial clefts. It plays a role in immunologic competence, probably acting as the original source of lymphoid elements (small lymphocytes) and by secreting thymus-specific factors which affect the function of these cells.

Table 1-2. **Heart and respiratory rates and blood pressure in normal children**

Age	Heart rate, per min	Respiratory rate, per min	Systolic blood pressure, mmHg*
Birth	140	40	60–80
6 months	110	30	90
1 yr	100	28	90
3–4 yr	95	25	100
5–10 yr	90	24	100–110
10–15 yr	85	20	110
Over 15 yr	75–80	16–18	110–120

* The diastolic pressure is usually 30 to 40 mm less than the systolic. The systolic pressure in the lower extremities is approximately 20 to 30 mm higher than in the upper extremities. Cuff width—cuff should cover two-thirds of upper arm—usually, newborn infant, 2.5 cm; 1 month to 1 yr, 5 cm; 1 to 8 yr, 9 cm; 8 yr and up, 12 cm.

The thymus grows rapidly during fetal life, and maximal size relative to body weight occurs during the neonatal period. The weight is very variable. At birth, the average is 10 Gm (range, 3 to 31 Gm). Growth continues through childhood until 12 years, and then involution occurs (see Myasthenia Gravis, p. 534).

In interpreting roentgenograms to determine thymic size, several factors should be considered:

1. Phase of respiration: The shadow is larger during expiration.
2. Position: The shadow is wider if the infant is supine rather than upright.
3. Views: Frontal and lateral views are necessary (a wide thymus is not always a thick one).
4. State of health: Size decreases with stress, infection, or adrenal corticosteroid therapy.

In the frontal view, a notched defect at the junction of wide thymic lobes with the cardiac shadow is characteristic of a thymic mediastinal widening. In the lateral view, displacement and compression of the trachea may be significant; however, it is normal to see partial collapse of the trachea during expiration in infancy.

GASTROINTESTINAL SYSTEM

At first the stomach is in a transverse position; as the child grows older it becomes more upright. It attains the adult shape at about 10 years of age. When measured at the end of expiration, the mean projection of the liver edge below the costal margin in the midclavicular line is approximately 2 cm in the newborn infant, 1.6 cm during the remainder of the first year, 1 cm from 1½ to 10½ years of age, and 0.85 cm from 10½ to 16½ years. The spleen can be palpated in 15 percent of newborn infants and during the remainder of the first year of life and in 10 percent of those 1½ to 10½ years of age. At birth the weight of the spleen is 10 Gm; at 1 year, 25 Gm; at maturity, 150 Gm. The weight of the liver is 150 Gm at birth, 300 Gm at 1 year, and 1,500 Gm at maturity.

GENITOURINARY SYSTEM

The combined weight of both kidneys is about 25 Gm at birth, 65 Gm at 1 year, and 250 Gm at maturity. Before 2 years of age the lower pole of the kidney may be below the iliac crest. The bladder is close to the abdominal wall in infancy and descends into the pelvis in childhood. The frequency of urination in young infants is 10 to 30 times per day. This gradually decreases until at 2½ to 3 years of age the urine can be retained for 6 to 9 hours. The primary sex organs grow very slowly during childhood. During adolescence, they undergo 90 percent of their total development. If the testes are not in the scrotum at birth, they are usually at the external inguinal ring and descend into the scrotum by 2 weeks of age. In the female newborn the labia majora are minimally developed, consequently the labia minora appear prominent. On inspection it is not uncommon to find a mucoid vaginal discharge or, less frequently, distinctly bloody secretions as a result of maternal estrogen withdrawal.

During the newborn period and infancy, there is a structural and functional preponderance of the glomeruli resulting in a glomerulotubular imbalance during this maturational period.

Although there are quantitative functional limitations, qualitative differences are not significant in health when compared to older children or adults. These functional limitations are mainly the result of size and other morphologic characteristics of the organ.

The glomerular filtration rate is low in the newborn (40 to 45 ml per minute per 1.73 sq meters), but the adult rate (120 ml per minute per 1.73 sq meters) is attained at about 2 years of age, which corresponds to the morphologic maturation of the kidney. The low concentrating capacity of the kidney in infancy is probably due to the low rate of urea and electrolyte excretion and the shortness of the loop of Henle.

During the first year of life, bicarbonate threshold is reduced to 21.5 to 22.5 mmoles per liter. This is probably due to nephron heterogenicity or to the low fractional reabsorption of sodium in the proximal tubule. As a result of this, the capacity of the infant to conserve substances such as aminoacids, phosphates, bicarbonates, and glucose are also limited.

OSSEOUS DEVELOPMENT

From birth to maturity there is a definite pattern in the appearance and union of the various centers of ossification. Skeletal age closely parallels chronological age, and therefore, roentgenograms are of great aid in estimating growth and development. The number, size, shape, density, and sharpness of outline of the epiphyseal centers and the fusion between epiphysis and metaphysis are all important for proper evaluation. Different epiphyseal areas give specific information at various chronological ages. At birth and during early infancy, the knee is the most informative. The wrist and hands are good guides at all ages after 6 months. Between the ages of 12 and 18 years the elbow and shoulder regions are also of value for assessment of maturation. There are a number of factors which may either delay or accelerate this process, but the pattern or sequence will not be disturbed. Factors influencing bone maturation include:

1. Race: Negroes have earlier maturation than Caucasians.
2. Sex: Females show an earlier maturation.
3. Prematurity (associated with a delayed maturity).

Table 1-3.   Appearance of ossification centers in the hand and wrist*

Age	Center
First year	Capitate—5 months
	Hamate—6 months
Second year	Distal radius—1 yr 6 months
Fourth year	Triquetrum—3 yr 7 months
Sixth year	Lunate—5 yr 1 month
Seventh year	Navicular—6 yr 11 months
	Lesser multangular—7 yr 0 month
Eighth year	Greater multangular—7 yr 3 months
	Distal ulnar—8 yr 0 month
Twelfth year	Pisiform—11 yr 10 months

NOTE: The metacarpal ossification centers appear from 1 year 11 months to 3 years 2 months in the following order: II, III, IV, V, I.
* Seventy-five percent of all males have the ossification centers as listed in this table; females show earlier maturation.

4. Endocrine disturbances: Hypothyroidism causes a delay, and precocious puberty an acceleration.
5. Poor nutrition (frequently associated with chronic infection or allergic conditions).
6. Disease: Chronic inflammatory conditions, e.g., rheumatoid arthritis may accelerate appearance of centers.

At birth or shortly thereafter 90 percent of full-term male and female infants have five ossification centers—calcaneus, cuboid, proximal tibia, talus, and distal femur.

LABORATORY DATA

The normal changes in the blood count from birth on are considered in detail in Chapter 22, "Blood Disorders."

The normal blood-chemistry, urine, and spinal-fluid findings in childhood are given in Table 1-4.

NORMS IN DEVELOPMENT

Development is an increase in function and maturation. An important feature of normal development is that the sequence is rather constant, even though a normal child may do things somewhat earlier or later than usual. Normal development depends on an intact and functional nervous system. Developmental diagnosis may be considered a form of pediatric clinical neurology, the function of which is to assess and interpret the maturity of the nervous system. The developmental examination should not be considered as a test of intelligence since it has a low predictability in terms of later mental function. However, a developmental examination tends to reflect all aspects of present observable behavior.

Table 1-4.   Normal laboratory data

Blood:

Nonprotein nitrogen	25–40 mg/100 ml
Urea nitrogen	10–15 mg/100 ml
Uric acid	2–6 mg/100 ml
Creatinine	0.4–1.2 mg/100 ml
Creatine	5–7 mg/100 ml
Glucose	60–120 mg/100 ml
Newborn (see p. 644)	
Cholesterol:	
Over 6 yr	150–250 mg/100 ml
Infants	70–125 mg/100 ml
Newborn	50–100 mg/100 ml
Cholesterol esters	60% or more
Bilirubin	0.2–1.0 mg/100 ml
Icterus index	3–5 units
Chlorides (expressed as NaCl):	
Whole blood	450–500 mg/100 ml (70–85 meq/liter)
Serum	585–620 mg/100 ml (100–106 meq/liter)
Sodium—serum	310–330 mg/100 ml (133–143 meq/liter)
Potassium—serum	16–22 mg/100 ml (4.0–5.5 meq/liter)
Phosphorus—serum	3.5–5.0 mg/100 ml (2.0–3.0 meq/liter)
Newborn	May be up to 8 mg/100 ml
Magnesium—serum	2–3 mg/100 ml (1.65–2.5 meq/liter)
Newborn	May be as low as 1.3 meq/liter
Calcium—serum	9–12 mg/100 ml (4.5–6 meq/liter)
Calcium (ionized)—serum	5–5.5 mg/100 ml (2.5–2.8 meq/liter)
Newborn (see p. 235)	
CO_2 content—serum	45–70 vol % (20.3–31.5 meq/liter)
Total protein	6.5–7.5 Gm/100 ml
Serum albumin	4.5–5.5 Gm/100 ml
Serum globulin	1.8–2.7 Gm/100 ml
Alkaline phosphatase:	
Infants	5–10 Bodansky units
Children	3–13 Bodansky units (10–20 King-Armstrong units)
Transaminase:	
Serum glutamic oxalacetic acid:	
Children	5–40 units
Infants	Up to 120 units
Serum glutamic pyruvic acid	5–40 units
Lactic dehydrogenase	30–120 units
Amylase	70–200 Somogyi units
Sedimentation rate:	
Micro	4–10 mm/hr
Westergren	5–20 mm/hr
Coagulation time:	
Capillary	3–4 min
Venous	4–10 min
Bleeding time	1–3 min
Fragility test	0.46–0.30% saline

Table 1-4.   (Continued)

Blood (Continued):
  Prothrombin time (Quick test):
    Plasma   12–15 sec
Urine (see Addis count, p. 480):
  pH   5–7
  Albumin   Negative (occasional trace is often of no
                                      significance)
  Sugar   Negative
  Acetone bodies   Negative
  Specific gravity   1.005–1.030
  Urobilinogen   Positive up to dilution 1:20
  Bilirubin   Negative
  Red blood cells   O–occasional HPF* (centrifuged)
  White blood cells   0–2 HPF* (centrifuged)
  Casts   Absent (a few hyaline casts are often not
                                      significant)

Spinal fluid:†
  Pressure   70–200 mm water
  Cell count   0–10 (chiefly lymphocytes)
  Protein   15–40 mg/100 ml
    Newborn   20–120 mg/100 ml
  Sugar   50–90 mg/100 ml
  Chlorides (expressed as NaCl)   650–750 mg/100 ml (111–128 meq/liter)

* HPF: high-power field.
† Amount in newborn infants ranges from 30 to 60 ml; in a child of 10 yr, there may be up to 200 ml.

Table 1-5 lists some of the important items of motor, adaptive, personal, and social behavior and language during the first 3 years (adapted from Gesell's developmental schedules). Table 1-6 outlines some of the characteristics of fetal growth and development and of development in premature infants.

SENSORY DEVELOPMENT

The infant's first contacts with his environment are made through sensory exploration. Through these experiences he learns to distinguish sounds and objects and to become familiar with them. Impairment of the sensory organs may result in the distortion of reality and may retard normal development.

Vision   The occipital cortex begins to myelinate at about the sixth fetal month. The calcarine portion of the occipital cortex is myelinated at birth. The macula is completely developed shortly after birth; the fovea continues to differentiate to about 16 weeks, and the optic fibers differentiate to about 12 weeks postnatally. The eyeball reaches adult size at 12 to 14 years of age.

Table 1-5. Developmental norms

Age	Motor behavior	Adaptive behavior	Language	Personal and social behavior
Under 4 weeks	1. Makes alternating crawling movements 2. Moves head laterally when placed in a prone position	1. Responds to sound of rattle and bell 2. Regards moving objects momentarily	1. Small, throaty, un-differentiated noises	1. Quiets when picked up 2. Impassive face
4 weeks	1. Tonic neck reflex positions predominate 2. Hands fisted 3. Head sags but can hold head erect for a few seconds	1. Follows moving objects to the midline 2. Shows no interest and drops objects immediately	1. Beginning vocalization such as cooing, gurgling, or grunting	1. Regards face and diminishes activity 2. Responds to speech
16 weeks	1. Symmetrical postures predominate 2. Holds head balanced 3. Head lifted 90° when prone on forearms	1. Follows a slowly moving object well 2. Arms activate on sight of dangling object	1. Laughs aloud 2. Sustained cooing and gurgling	1. Spontaneous social smile 2. Aware of strange situations
28 weeks	1. Sits steadily, leaning forward on hands 2. Bounces actively when placed in a standing position	1. One-hand approach and grasp of toy 2. Bangs and shakes rattle 3. Transfers toys	1. Vocalizes "m-m-m" when crying 2. Makes different vowel sounds (e.g., "ah," "eh")	1. Takes feet to mouth 2. Pats mirror image
40 weeks	1. Sits alone with good coordination 2. Creeps	1. Matches two objects at midline 2. Spontaneously rings bell	1. Says "da-da" or equivalent 2. Responds to name or nickname	1. Responds to social play such as "pat-a-cake" or "peekaboo" 2. Feeds self cracker and holds own bottle

Table 1-5. (Continued)

Age	Motor behavior	Adaptive behavior	Language	Personal and social behavior
	3. Pulls self to standing position	3. Uses thumb and index finger for prehension		
52 weeks	1. Walks with one hand held 2. Stands alone, briefly	1. Tries to build tower of two cubes 2. Attempts to imitate scribble	1. Beginning expressive jargon 2. Gives a toy on request	1. Cooperates in dressing
15 months	1. Toddles 2. Creeps upstairs	1. Builds tower of two cubes 2. Imitates a scribble	1. Says three to five words meaningfully 2. Pats pictures in book 3. Shows shoes on request	1. Points or vocalizes wants 2. Casts objects in play or refusal
18 months	1. Walks, seldom falls 2. Hurls ball 3. Walks upstairs with one hand held	1. Builds a tower of three to four cubes 2. Scribbles spontaneously and imitates a stroke	1. Says 10 words, including name 2. Identifies one common object on picture card 3. Names ball and carries out two directions ("put on table" and "give to mother")	1. Feeds self in part, spills 2. Pulls toy on string 3. Carries or hugs a special toy (e.g., a doll)
2 yr	1. Runs well, no falling 2. Kicks large ball 3. Goes upstairs and downstairs alone	1. Builds tower of six to seven cubes 2. Aligns cubes, imitating train	1. Uses three-word sentences 2. Carries out four directions	1. Pulls on simple garment 2. Domestic mimicry 3. Refers to self by name

Age	Motor	Adaptive	Language	Personal-Social
		3. Imitates vertical and circular strokes		
3 yr	1. Rides tricycle 2. Jumps from bottom step 3. Alternates feet going upstairs	1. Builds tower of 9 to 10 cubes 2. Imitates a three-cube bridge 3. Copies a circle and imitates a cross	1. Gives sex and full name 2. Uses plurals 3. Describes what is happening in a picture book	1. Puts on shoes 2. Unbuttons buttons 3. Feeds self well 4. Understands taking turns
4 yr	1. Walks downstairs one step per tread 2. Stands on one foot for 4–8 sec	1. Copies a cross 2. Repeats four digits 3. Counts three objects with correct pointing	1. Begins to name colors, at least one correctly 2. Understands five prepositional directives ("on," "under," "in back," "in front," "beside")	1. Washes and dries own face 2. Brushes teeth 3. Plays cooperatively with children
5 yr	1. Skips, using feet alternately 2. Stands on one foot for more than 8 sec	1. Copies a square 2. Draws a recognizable man with a head, body, etc. 3. Counts 10 objects accurately	1. Names the primary colors 2. Names coins: pennies, nickels, dimes 3. Asks meaning of words	1. Dresses and undresses self 2. Prints a few letters 3. Plays competitive exercise games

Six years: counts 13 pennies; copies a triangle; differentiates between morning and afternoon and right and left; defines simple objects and knows what they are used for.
Seven years: repeats five digits; copies a diamond; names days of the week; understands basic idea of addition and subtraction.
Eight years: counts backward from 20 to 1; beginning to tell time to quarter hour; participates in group cooperative play following rules; describes similarities and differences between two objects.
Nine years: repeats months in order; makes change out of a quarter; reads on own initiative; does simple division and multiplication.
Ten years: repeats six digits; writes occasional short letters; does simple creative work; uses simple fractions.

Table 1-6. Fetal growth and development

	Weeks of gestation			
	12–14	28–32	32–36	36–40
Growth	Resembles human being Nails form Sex can be determined Three-layered epidermis Palate fused Pancreatic islands Definite shape of lung Heart four-chambered Nasal septum complete	Skin red and wrinkled Eyelids opened Primordia of permanent teeth Testes descend into scrotum Retinal layers complete	Subcutaneous fat Nails complete	Accumulation of fat Downy hair coat is shed
Development	Brief jerky movements Bile secreted Kidney able to secrete Blood formation in marrow begins	Movements meager Breathing shallow and irregular Cry absent or weak	Moro reflex present Movements sustained Muscle tone fair Response to light and sound	Movements active and sustained Lifts head or attempts, in prone position Muscle tone good

Visual responses to appropriate stimuli can be demonstrated in the full-term newborn and the alert premature during the first days of life. Fixation on and following of an object occurs when the object is moved in the range of 45 to 90°. By 2 months an object is followed at an arc of 180°, and by 4 months the infant reaches for objects.

Transient overconvergence (pseudostrabismus) may normally be present in the first few months, but true strabismus should be referred to the ophthalmologist for evaluation as soon as it is discovered.

Visual acuity of 20/20, the normal adult value is reached between the ages of 5 and 6 years.

Speech   Speech implies an understandable, coherent pronunciation of words and an association between words and corresponding objects. The development of speech takes a long time and proceeds at a different rate with each child, tending to be slower and more subject to disruption in boys. Many factors influence this rate of development, for instance, emotional disturbances, lack of adequate socializing experience, overprotection by parents, and physical illness. Parental attitudes which attempt to impose speech training before the child is ready can lead to emotional speech disorders. If speech is delayed beyond 2½ to 3 years of age, psychologic and organic factors should be explored to determine whether the delay is the result of a physiologic developmental lag or of other conditions.

Smell, taste, touch   The sense of smell is slight in the newborn infant, and it develops slowly thereafter; however, the newborn infant can smell milk. Taste is present at birth, and salivation becomes active at the third month. Touch is not highly developed at birth except in the lips and tongue; by the fifth month, localized responses to touch can be observed.

Hearing   After the drainage of amniotic fluid and removal of debris from the middle ear, the newborn infant can respond to sudden or sharp noises. Hearing becomes acute within a few days. At 6 months the infant can often locate the direction of sounds, distinguish familiar voices, and react pleasurably to music. Impairment of hearing may affect speech development.

SLEEP

Each infant has his own sleep pattern. Sleep requirements during the first few months of life are about 18 to 20 hours per day; by 6 months, 16 to 18 hours; by 1 year, 14 to 16 hours; by 2 years, 12 to 14 hours; by 5 years, 10 to 12 hours; by 10 years, 10 hours. Some children require more sleep than others. In addition, some children may require an afternoon nap during the early childhood years.

During early infancy, disturbance of sleep usually results from physical causes, such as hunger, colic, illness, or soiled diaper. However, in a child with organic brain damage or psychosis, sleep pattern may be lacking during this early infancy period. During late infancy and childhood, poor sleep may result from faulty training, e.g., using the bed as a place for punishment; emotional causes, e.g., separation anxiety (which may occur normally at 1 to 2 years of age); or illness. Sleep resistance (which may occur normally, starting at 8 months), nightmares, night terrors, as well as poor sleeping habits, are best managed by correcting the underlying causes and establishing a set routine, for instance, feeding, bathing, and reading a story prior to retiring.

TOILET TRAINING

In toilet training, an automatic function is placed under voluntary control through conditioning and maturation:

1. Through conditioning the infant learns to eliminate when placed on the toilet and to retain urine and stool during the intervening periods.
2. With maturation the child learns to express his needs and assumes a degree of responsibility for them.

Bowel control   Some time after the child has learned to sit with ease and comfort, he can be introduced to the toilet seat for a period of several minutes. The time of his regular daily bowel movement is the time of choice. Children who do not have a regular physiologic rhythm of elimination (or who regularly eliminate at night) are usually not trained early. It may be more profitable with such children to wait until they are capable of understanding through language (about 2 to 3 years of age) what is expected of them.

Bladder control   Usually by 16 to 18 months of age an infant can retain his urine for about 3-hour intervals. At this point he could be placed on the toilet at definite times, e.g., before meals, after rest periods, and at bedtime. As soon as some degree of control is established, pants should be substituted for diapers. Nocturnal control is usually accomplished by 2½ to 3 years of age. Boys may be taught to stand at the toilet when they are about 2½ years old.

Training can be facilitated by watching the warning signs, such as fussing, whimpering, etc. The word "toilet" may be used to associate the word with the act of elimination.

DISCIPLINE

The inculcation of socially desirable values and habits is a necessary step in the development of the child's personality. If the child is to grow into a responsible, conscientious, and dependable adult, he must develop concepts of "right and wrong" and "good and bad," and he must adjust to the moral and ethical standards of society. He must learn to control undesirable patterns of behavior and to assume responsibility for his judgments and actions. Modern concepts of discipline derive from the psychologic viewpoint that limits and restraints are required by the child in order to help him achieve socially acceptable goals of behavior. However, a child learns best to conform in an atmosphere where his creativity, innate potentialities, and emotional needs are recognized and appreciated.

Since maturation involves breaking away from childhood dependency, the child goes through normal phases of rebellion against parental authority. Punishment is necessary at times in order to reinforce controls. It should be related to the act committed and should not be accompanied by a withdrawal of parental love or protection. Since children learn through imitation, an effective means of child training is exemplary parental conduct.

Parents who regularly train their children through scolding or spanking will find that these measures are of no avail in defining the really important disciplinary situations for the child. Demands upon the child can be roughly divided into three categories:

1. Those in which the child has a free choice to accept or not to accept a parent's preference
2. Those in which the parent really prefers the child to obey but in which there is still room for discussion
3. Those in which absolute obedience is required

EMOTIONAL AND SOCIAL DEVELOPMENT

The emotional experiences and reactions of the child strongly affect every aspect of his life—intellectual, physical, and social. The only observable emotional response in the newborn child is a generalized reaction to powerful stimuli, such as the startle response to loud noises. Pleasure and displeasure are the first differentiated emotional responses

Table 1-7. Emotional and social development

Age	Stage of development
1–4 weeks	Emotional reaction on a primitive reflex level; cries when hungry; startle response.
4–8 weeks	Crying becomes differentiated for specific needs (hunger, pain, displeasure).
8–16 weeks	Laughs, smiles in response to another face.
6 months	Cries easily when frustrated; expresses anger through motor activity; amuses self.
7–8 months	Sensitive to strangers; responds emotionally to family members; emotional lability from crying to laughing.

Table 1-7. (Continued)

12 months	Likes to play games that evoke response from others—"shows off"; demands attention by crying or making other sounds. Very labile, experiences and expresses basic emotions of fear, jealousy, affection, and anger. Can adjust well to emotional changes.
15–18 months	Outbursts of temper tantrums and rebellious behavior, but easily distracted; becomes attached to special toys and objects. May throw things or bite.
2 yr	Uses language more frequently to express emotion. Separation anxiety manifests itself. Emotions become more refined; child experiences shyness, pride, and gratification through achievement of new skills. Plays alone contentedly. Tears are related to auditory experiences.
3 yr	Develops interest in group activity, particularly realistic dramatic play. More self-sufficient, less fearful. Outgoing, cooperative. Enjoys and appreciates humor. Resents new siblings, fears the dark, animals, unfamiliar-looking people. Can be introduced to a nursery school experience on a half-day basis.
4 yr	More self-assured, aggressive in play. Pronounced ego development, with distinct "I" feelings. Acts out fears in play situations. Enjoys new language skills.
5 yr	Period of emotional integration and stability. Feelings of strength and self-sufficiency. Cooperative with parents, likes to lead in play. Humorous, enjoys fantasy but is quite realistic.
6 yr	Period of instability as child leaves home and embarks on formal schooling. Reverts to much earlier behavior; emotional outbursts of anger and frustration against parents followed by feelings of remorse and anxiety. Likes to be center of attention, to win at games, and to have all his demands met. Needs reassurance of love and acceptance. Adventurous, pugnacious, and vigorous.
7 yr	Sensitive about sex, avoids self-exposure in front of the opposite sex. A cooperative member of the family group, but at times shows resentment to parental command and self-help activities. Introspective and desires the approbation of his group and his parents.
8 yr	In unsupervised play may become rowdy, dislikes being alone, wants companionship. Segregation of sexes important in choice of playmates and groups. Becomes more resentful of parental authority. Best behavior away from home or when guests are in home. Comic-book reading. Enjoys school. Individual differences are great.
9 yr	Intermediate age between childhood and beginning of adolescence. Better control of himself. Seeks and acquires new forms of independence. Completes task. Looks to future, plans ahead for work and play. Can accept blame. Is truthful and honest. Eating neater, manners observed. Obeys well, as-

Table 1-7. (Continued)

	sumes responsibilities, hero worship. Self-sufficient, self-critical. Reading more realistic.
10 yr	Change of attitude toward sex. Girls are more mature and poised than boys. Power of suggestion for good or evil has influence at this time. Personality traits and abilities become manifest and give fair indication of what he will be like as an adult. Teamwork, fixes rules of play.
11 yr	Girls somewhat behind in physical strength and endurance. Girls apt to be taller. Membership in groups and clubs. Team games are very popular. Shyness increases. More critical of the products of his labor, urge for small jobs after school and during vacation.

and are evoked during the first 2 months, primarily by physical excitation. Emotional patterns become more complex by the end of the first year, by which time five basic responses can be clearly recognized: anger, fear, curiosity, joy, and jealousy. Although norms for emotional adjustment are difficult to establish and may vary in individual children, a child's happiness depends on his emotional adjustment. Healthy adjustment is brought about by:

1. Providing security through affection, acceptance, and approval
2. Understanding the intrinsic behavior pattern of the individual child at different maturational stages and ages and fostering a positive environment that encourages attainment of the child's full potentialities but does not push or force the child beyond his capabilities

When the above conditions are fulfilled, the child develops self-confidence and is able to solve his problems and take his place in society.

Social development is concerned with the child's adjustment to, and identification with, the society in which he lives. Patterns of socialization are developed in the child, first through his early contacts with parents and siblings and later through relationships with his peers in social group situations. Values and standards of adults strongly influence the social behavior of children.

At about 2 years of age, a slow and irregular emancipation from the parents begins and continues through adolescence. The onset of this period of development is manifested in the child by his desire to feed himself, the famous "no-no" to everything, and his attempts to dress himself.

At about 3 years of age, the child likes to be near other children and later learns to play cooperatively with them. Sometimes he wishes to be the leader; at other times, the follower. At nursery school and kindergarten, socialization continues. At school the child wants to learn and enjoys group participation. The teacher is really a parent-substitute.

At about 7 to 8 years of age, the child is more interested in members of the same sex than in those of the opposite sex. He forms groups or joins clubs with the same interests. He looks down upon, and rebels against, adult standards. (Adolescence will be considered separately.)

Emotional and social development depends on an environment which is warm, accepting, and approving and which provides opportunities for satisfaction, achievement, and self-expression.

PSYCHOSEXUAL DEVELOPMENT

Sexual attitudes in the child are almost totally determined by the mores and values that obtain in the environment in which he lives. The sexual taboos and repressions of society have a psychologic impact on the child which, if improperly managed, may often lead to severe conflict and disorder in childhood and in later years. Therefore the pediatrician has a particular responsibility in helping parents to understand and accept the child's sexual curiosity, self-exploration, and mutual exploration with other children.

Infants experience pleasure when diapers are changed or during washing and bathing of the sex organs. At 3 years of age, children begin to verbalize some of their sexual curiosity, particularly at the birth of a new sibling. Parents should be encouraged to answer the child's questions simply and in language that he can understand. Giving the child more information than he can absorb may lead to as much frustration as not giving him enough information. By the time the child has reached puberty, he should have a basic knowledge of the sex organs and their functions. If parents feel unable to provide sex information for their children, the pediatrician can assist by speaking to the child in their presence.

EVALUATION OF THE TOTAL CHILD

There is no test at present that will evaluate the whole, or total, child, including his physical, mental, social, and emotional growth and development.

Periodic inventory and evaluation by the physician, using all available material, are best. The rate of progress, as determined by a comparison of these periodic surveys, is of most value.

For the physical aspects, a comparison with standard height and weight charts. The most commonly used ones are based on the studies of the Harvard School of Public Health and those of Iowa University. Roentgenograms of the ossification centers reveal the skeletal age and progress. The clinician may also want to consider the amount of subcutaneous fat and muscular development. No one type of examination or measurement tells all.

For mental and emotional evaluation, the Denver Developmental and the Gesell tests are helpful in assessing performance and behavior during infancy and early childhood. A number of intelligence tests have been devised for children. Below 3 years of age, the information obtained is less reliable than after that age. Probably the most widely used intelligence test is the Stanford-Binet. For evaluation of emotional progress and disturbance, projective personality tests, such as the Rorschach, may be helpful.

At present, the subjective opinion of the trained physician who uses his clinical judgment and insight into the child, the parents, and their environment, together with all the objective tests and material at his disposal, provides the most reliable evaluation of the total child.

SUDDEN INFANT DEATH SYNDROME (SIDS, Crib Death)

SIDS is defined as sudden death in an infant not known to have a serious disease and whose death remains unexplained after complete autopsy. The incidence is approximately 3 per 1,000, and this syndrome is considered the major cause of death in infants after 1 month of age. The peak incidence is at 2 to 4 months of age. It is rare after 1 year of age. The condition is most common in male, prematurely born infants living in crowded housing and of low socioeconomic status. A history of minor symptoms, e.g., coryzal, or respiratory, is frequently present during the previous 48 hours. There is a seasonal incidence (November through March), and death usually occurs during sleep. The etiology is unknown, but it is thought to be multifactorial depending upon age (instability of the nervous system), infection (failure of the immune system), and sleep (alters response to respiratory and cardiac difficulty, e.g., laryngospasm, cardiac conduction disturbance).

ADOLESCENCE*

Adolescence is the period of transition between childhood and adulthood, a time of rapid growth—second only to the first year of life—and marked physical and physiological changes. It is also the time for emotional and intellectual maturation. Puberty is that stage of adolescence in which the reproductive system has matured, i.e., when the male produces motile sperm and the female ovulates.

There is a wide range of normal age of onset of adolescent growth and development, which often causes fears of abnormality, self-con-

---

* EDITORS' NOTE: The section on Adolescence was prepared by June Schwartz, M.D.

sciousness, and anxiety about body image. Changes can begin at 8 to 10 years and extend to 17 to 19 years. Girls are usually 2 years ahead of boys. The growth spurt starts with increased deposition of subcutaneous fat around the hips and increase in leg length. In girls, this is accompanied by widening of the hips. Then there is increase in trunk length. Increase in muscle mass follows, with broadening of the shoulders in males. In females, growth and muscle development start and stop earlier, and subcutaneous fat deposition continues longer.

Adolescent changes are initiated by the hypothalamus, which stimulates the pituitary to increase production of gonadotropins and growth hormone. At the same time, there is an increase in adrenal androgens in both sexes. Gonadotropins stimulate the growth and development of ovaries and testes; growth hormone stimulates long-bone growth; in the male androgens are responsible for secondary sex characteristics.

Between 12 and 16 years, the growth spurt averages 4 to 12 in. Growth is accelerated during the period of sexual development and decelerates at sexual maturity when sex hormones influence the closing of the epiphyses. By 19 to 20 years most individuals have completed growth.

Although there are differences in age of onset, sexual characteristics usually develop in this order:

Males
1. Increase in size of genitalia
2. Pubic hair
3. Axillary hair, deepening of voice
4. Facial hair
5. Spermatogenesis (true puberty)

Females
1. Broadening of the hips   } Vaginal secretions change from
2. Breast budding   } alkaline to acid pH.
3. Pubic hair
4. Menarche
5. Axillary hair
6. Ovulation (true puberty)

The potential for growth is greatest early in adolescence; therefore the stage of development is important in estimating final height. X-rays of hands and wrists for evidence of epiphyseal closure are helpful aids.

The adolescent has several unique nutritional requirements because of the enormous metabolic increments necessary for growth and activity during this period. There is a tremendous stress on calcium and nitrogen metabolism, and there may be periods of negative balance for these food elements, particularly during disease or because of the frequent food fads and idiosyncrasies of the teen-ager. The adolescent diet should contain 2500 to 3500 Cal per day with at least 15 percent derived from protein (90 to 120 Gm) and sufficient calcium (1 to 1.5 Gm per day). Iron deficiency is prone to develop, especially in menstruating females. The amount, odor, and pH of sweat changes and the sebaceous glands of the skin are stimulated by androgens, producing an oily skin condition which contributes to the development of acne.

Disorders of growth and development that may become apparent at adolescence are delayed puberal development and retarded growth; failure of sexual development; short stature; menstrual disturbances; gynecomastia. Retarded growth is most commonly associated with delayed sexual maturity, often familial, and normal growth is achieved eventually. Poor nutrition, chronic disease, hypothyroidism, and hypopituitarism are other, less frequent causes. Chromosomal aberrations, e.g., gonadal dysgenesis, Klinefelter's syndrome, intersex problems, and pituitary dwarfism may not become apparent until failure of adolescent development is noted.

Benign hypertrophy of the male breast is common in early adolescence and a source of much anxiety. It is usually a unilateral, tender, discoid mass, although it can be bilateral. True gynecomastia, occurring without an endocrine abnormality, is due to end-organ sensitivity to estrogen. More rarely, gynecomastia occurs in endocrine disorders, intersex and chromosomal aberrations, feminizing tumors of the adrenals, cirrhosis, and testicular tumors. (Because of the possibility of testicular neoplasm, it is important to examine the testes carefully when there is gynecomastia.)

Emotional and mental changes are related to the marked physiologic and physical changes. The teen-ager must adapt to changes in his body configuration and developing sexuality. Growing out of childhood, he must learn to control emotions and utilize them constructively. Moving from a situation of dependence toward independence, he must learn to deal with new, strange feelings and drives and develop a capacity for abstract thinking and judgment formation. Problems of personality maturation, identity, education, and vocation are to be solved. The adolescent learns to see himself in relation to others and works toward his own goals while resolving conflicts with diminishing dependence on parents. There is a wide range of normal behavior that would be abnormal in later life—daydreaming, swings of mood, rebellion, regressive behavior. Masturbation, sexual fantasies, and homosexual experience can be part of dealing with developing sexuality, but they often generate guilt and anxieties. Hero worship, "crushes," peer-group activities and fads are part of the need for identifying with others. Conflicts with parents and adult authorities arise in the struggle for identity. The physician must recognize normal variations and be able to differentiate them from anxiety reactions, neuroses and other personality disorders, and schizophrenia.

Anxiety and depression are frequent, and adjustment reactions may take the form of somatic complaints, e.g., recurrent headache, abdominal pain, menstrual cramps; irritability; excessive fatigue;

dizziness; syncopal attacks; insomnia; poor appetite or overeating. Emotional disturbance may be indicated by school failure; withdrawal; acting out, e.g., truancy, delinquency, sexual promiscuity; drug abuse; frequent accidents or suicide attempts. Withdrawal may be the first sign of schizophrenia.

Widespread use of drugs by the young is a major health problem. Drugs may be used for experimentation, rebellion, gaining peer status, escaping reality or life itself by suicide, or to change personality. The latter two indicate severe disturbance. Addiction and personality disorders, both difficult to treat, are found frequently during adolescence. Prevention is most important. Early recognition of emotional disturbance and adjustment reactions and education of children in the appropriate and inappropriate use of drugs will help reduce drug abuse. Physicians, families, community groups, and educators must work together to solve this problem.

The mortality rate is low in adolescence, but it is important to know that accident is the first cause of death. Suicide is fourth. Many of these deaths are related to depression, drug use, or reckless behavior at a time when judgment formation is immature. Safety education, as well as finding and treating the teen-ager with problems, will help reduce the death rate.

Morbidity rates are also low in adolescence, and illness is usually less severe than in other age groups, consequently teen-agers tend to get irregular medical supervision. Care is episodic for trauma, minor respiratory infections, skin disorders, allergies, and menstrual irregularities. Emotional disorders frequently escape attention because the teen-ager does not seek help.

Of menstrual disorders, the most common is primary dysmenorrhea (painful menses not secondary to abnormalities of the genital tract). The cramps, which occur in ovulatory cycles, may be accompanied by vomiting, headache, and dizziness. They are related to labile hormone levels, particularly the action of progesterone on the immature uterus. Irregular contractions and the dilation and constriction of the vessels of the endometrial bed cause the discomfort. Emotional factors mediated through the autonomic nervous system increase the severity of symptoms. Difficulty in accepting the feminine role is said to be important. Treatment consists of reassurance, explaining menstrual physiology, correcting health problems, and aid in solving adjustment problems. Exercise and antispasmodics may help. Dysmenorrhea which is unresponsive to supportive therapy may require treatment with an estrogen-progestogen combination in cyclic therapy. Occasionally a dilatation and curettage will be recommended. Premenstrual tension (fluid retention, tenderness of breasts, abdominal distension, headache, and irritability) which occurs before and on the first day of menses is related to the follicle-stimulating hormone (FSH)/estrogen ratio. When the estrogen level drops, unopposed FSH produces edema. In this condition diuretics and a low salt diet help to relieve symptoms.

Primary amenorrhea (no menses after age 17) is usually constitutional and associated with delayed puberty. Less frequently there may be underdevelopment of the genital tract; systemic disease, e.g., hypothyroidism, hyperthyroidism, liver disorders, malnutrition, anemia, obesity; ovarian infection, e.g., mumps, tuberculosis, pelvic inflammatory disease; or masculinizing tumors of the ovary. Pseudoamenorrhea from an imperforate hymen may cause a pelvic mass, hematocolpos. The most frequent causes of secondary amenorrhea (no menses for more than 3 months after onset) are irregular anovulatory cycles, which are common for 1 to 3 years after menarche; pregnancy; disturbance of the hypothalamic-pituitary-ovarian axis by emotional stress; and any of the causes of primary amenorrhea. Menorrhagia (prolonged menstrual bleeding) and metrorrhagia (frequent menses) are usually associated with anovulatory cycles. Treatment is supportive and includes correction of nutritional deficiencies or anemia if they exist or prescribing hormones if the condition is persistent or severe. Rarely, a dilatation and curettage will be required. Abnormal bleeding may also be associated with systemic disease, e.g., purpura, leukemia, thyroid disease, or rheumatic fever.

Tumors of the female genital tract are rare during adolescence and usually ovarian, the most common being teratomas. Although carcinomas of the cervix are extremely rare in this age group, atypical cells in "Pap" smears done on sexually active girls indicate that routine screening should be done. Tumors of the breast are infrequent, but benign fibroadenoma is the one most commonly found.

Vaginal discharge may be cyclic, physiologic leukorrhea, or caused by infections, e.g., gonorrhea, monilia, trichomonas, nonspecific bacteria.

Pregnancy in unmarried teen-agers is an important problem which can cause conflict in families, social and economic hardship, increased prenatal difficulties, prematurity, and problems of infant care. Contributing factors are rebellion against established mores, need for love and meaningful relationships, use of the body for gratification, and ignorance about consequences of sexual activity. These factors are also involved in the increased exposure of teen-agers to venereal disease. Case finding is most important, and screening for syphilis and gonorrhea should be performed routinely. In solving these problems, parents as well as teen-agers need support and nonjudgmental guidance. Concerned professionals should provide meaningful education in matters of sex, interpersonal relationships, contraception, and protection against venereal disease.

Certain other infections should be considered in adolescence. There is increased susceptibility to infectious mononucleosis and *Mycoplasma pneumoniae* pneumonia. Tuberculosis may occur as a rapidly progressive primary or adult type. Regular tuberculin testing is important in preventing serious morbidity as well as spread of the disease. Mumps infection may involve testes and ovaries and should be prevented by mumps vaccination. Drug addicts are a risk for hepatitis, sepsis, and tetanus. Immunization should not be neglected after childhood.

Acne and obesity are conditions which injure the adolescent's self-image. Treatment of acne should include an explanation of the condition in relation to normal development. Adolescent obesity is complicated by emotional stress and social disadvantage and carries a risk of future cardiovascular disease. Genetic disposition, individual and family eating habits, body type, and the normal increased deposition of fat prior to the growth spurt are influencing factors. Endocrine causes are rare. Management is difficult, but motivation is most important in achieving weight loss. Supportive psychotherapy along with guidance in nutrition and health habits are essential.

In this period of rapid growth, postural abnormalities and backache are rather common. They are usually functional, but structural abnormalities should be ruled out. Because skeletal growth precedes increase in muscle mass, athletic injuries may be more severe in adolescents. Adequate protection and training should be provided in sports. Slipped femoral capital epiphysis should be suspected in adolescence if there is limp or pain in knee or hip. Early diagnosis is important: Osteochondrosis of the tibial tubercle (Osgood-Schlatter disease) is another cause of knee pain and is rather common in the rapidly growing active adolescent male.

Certain conditions may be affected by adolescence. For example, the onset of epilepsy or increased frequency of seizures may be related to both the hormonal changes and the emotional stress of adolescence. The diabetic teen-ager may rebel against his medication and diet at a time when nutritional requirements and activities are increasing and more attention to his disease is required. The teen-ager with heart disease may need reevaluation to determine permissible activity. With any chronic illness or handicap, the patient will need help in achieving realistic goals and in dealing with questions of vocation, marriage, and parenthood. The patient's parents must be considered, and whether the condition is emotional or physical, their anxieties must also be treated.

REVIEW QUESTIONS

Each of the following questions or incomplete statements is followed by several suggested answers or completions. Select the one that is best in each case.

1. In normal development, a child achieves each of the following accomplishments at a different age. The earliest accomplishment is (*a*) drinking from a cup; (*b*) counting to three; (*c*) climbing stairs; (*d*) playing games with other children; (*e*) making a three-word sentence. Select the latest accomplishment.
2. A child is able to ride a tricycle, build a tower of nine cubes, give his sex and full name, and copy a circle. This stage of development is average for (*a*) 5 years old; (*b*) 4 years old; (*c*) 3 years old; (*d*) 2 years old; (*e*) 18 months old.
3. A child is able to walk upstairs with one hand held, hurl a ball, build a tower of three cubes, and say 10 words including his name. This stage of develop-

ment is average for (*a*) 6 years old; (*b*) 5 years old; (*c*) 4 years old; (*d*) 3 years old; (*e*) 2 years old; (*f*) 18 months old.

4. A child can sit alone with good coordination, creep, pull himself to a standing position, spontaneously ring a bell, and respond to social play such as "peek-aboo." This child is at least (*a*) 4 weeks old; (*b*) 16 weeks old; (*c*) 28 weeks old; (*d*) 40 weeks old; (*e*) 52 weeks old; (*f*) 15 months old.

5. A 5-year-old boy, 40.2 in. tall, is in the 3d percentile for his age. A review of his past medical records indicates that he was in the 50th percentile at 2 years of age, the 25th percentile at 3 years of age, and the 10th percentile at 4 years of age. What do these figures indicate?

   Statement 1: A pathologic condition should be suspected even though the boy's height is acceptable for a 5-year-old boy.

   Statement 2: Any given physical measurement usually follows a constant percentile channel in the course of healthy growth.

   Statement 3: Separate norms for boys and girls are necessary because girls are more advanced than boys in osseous development.

   Statement 4: This is the expected rate of linear growth in males. _____

6. The period of most rapid linear growth is (*a*) birth to 2 years of age; (*b*) pubescence to 16 years of age; (*c*) 2 years of age to pubescence; (*d*) 16 years of age to maturity.

7. Head circumference should show the following in the first year of life: (*a*) increase of ¼ in. per month for first 8 months; ½ in. per month for next 4 months; (*b*) increase of ½ in. per month for first 6 months; ⅛ in. per month for next 6 months; (*c*) increase of ½ in. per month for first 4 months; ¼ in. per month for next 8 months.

8. Myelinization of the brain starts about (*a*) second fetal month; (*b*) fourth fetal month; (*c*) sixth fetal month; (*d*) eighth fetal month.

9. Column I is a list of transient infantile reflexes. Column II has ages at which these reflexes usually disappear. Match the items in the two columns. (Items in column II may be used once or several times.)

I		II
Stepping _____		
Grasp _____	(*a*)	1 month
Placing _____	(*b*)	2 months
Tonic neck _____	(*c*)	3 to 4 months
Moro _____		
Trunk incurvation _____		
Cross extension _____		

10. The glomerular filtration rate reaches the adult rate at about (*a*) 6 months; (*b*) 2 years; (*c*) 4 years; (*d*) 6 years.

11. Epiphyseal areas on roentgenograms provide specific information for evaluating growth. X-rays of the knee are helpful (*a*) at birth and during early infancy; (*b*) after 6 months of age until 2 years of age; (*c*) between 12 and 18 years of age; (*d*) only if both knees are visualized.

12. Visual acuity of 20/20 is reached at (*a*) birth; (*b*) 2 to 3 years; (*c*) 3 to 4 years; (*d*) 5 to 6 years.

13. The onset of adolescence in girls (*a*) starts at the same age as in boys; (*b*) starts at an earlier age than in boys; (*c*) starts at a later age than in boys; (*d*) is not influenced by sexuality.

14. Adolescent males develop (*a*) facial hair; (*b*) spermatogenesis; (*c*) pubic hair; (*d*) increase of size of genitalia; (*e*) axillary hair and deepening of the voice. Which of these changes occurs first?

15. Most commonly associated with retarded growth in adolescents is (*a*) menstrual disorders; (*b*) gynecomastia; (*c*) delayed sexual maturity; (*d*) delayed dentition.

16. All the following are seen with increased frequency during adolescence except one: (*a*) rapidly progressive tuberculosis; (*b*) infectious mononucleosis; (*c*) Osgood-Schlatter disease; (*d*) diabetes; (*e*) acne.

2
FEEDING OF INFANTS, CHILDREN, AND ADOLESCENTS

The major clinical pediatric problem during the first few months of life involves the infant's nutrition and the special demands of his metabolic and environmental needs. The caloric requirements are largely provided by breast milk or by cow's (or other species) milk altered in composition to create a nutritional product similar to mother's milk.

In later infancy and childhood, considerable thought and care must be given to patterns of feeding behavior, which often relate to the child's emotional background, and to his physiologic needs in order to provide for growth and physical activity.

NUTRITIONAL REQUIREMENTS

The nutritional requirements of infants and children vary directly with their rate of growth and development. For example, more calories, proteins, and minerals are needed proportionately during early infancy and adolescence than at any other time. A normal child who is offered sufficient food quantitatively (total calories) and qualitatively (individual nutrients), even when he is given the opportunity to select these himself, will usually eat enough to grow and develop properly.

Caloric requirements   Approximately 110 Cal per kg per day (50 Cal per lb) is required in the first year. The 1-year-old requires 1000 Cal per day, and although caloric needs on a calorie per kilogram basis decrease (about 10 Cal per 3-year period), the total requirement increases by 100 Cal for each year of age. (Physically active children may require 100 to 300 Cal more than less active ones.) Ordinarily proteins supply 15 percent, fats 35 percent, and carbohydrates 50 percent of the total calories.

Individual nutrients   *Water* is the most essential element in the diet and is necessary for metabolic transport, regulation of body temperature, ionic equilibrium, and a variety of cellular functions. The water requirements depend on caloric consumption, atmospheric temperature, body temperature, and the specific gravity of the urine; but the average infant requires water in amounts approximating 15 percent of body weight per day, while the older child requires 5 percent. Until the child can communicate his needs, water must be prescribed. For the normal infant, total fluid intake should be 125 to 150 ml per kg per day (50 ml per kg for insensible losses and perspiration, 50 to 70 ml per kg for urine formation, and 25 to 50 ml per kg for necessary reserves). Except in instances of excessive losses, e.g., vomiting, diarrhea, the older child will usually ingest sufficient water to satisfy metabolic requirements.

Proteins are necessary as a source of amino acids for growth and tissue repair; for ions to maintain the acid-base balance; and for vital metabolic groupings, such as hemoglobin, enzymes, hormones, and antibodies. They are also frequently utilized in energy cycles. In the infant, 3 to 4 Gm per kg per day are required, while the older child needs 2 to 2½ Gm per kg per day.

Proteins are derived from milk, meat (the quality or type of meat does not influence the quality of the protein), fish, poultry, cereals, cheese, soybeans, peas, and beans. Small amounts of certain proteins are absorbed unchanged, but normally almost all the dietary protein is broken down to amino acids (little is lost in the stool). Excess amino acids are broken down in the liver and converted to urea, which is excreted by the kidneys. A number of amino acids are essential for new tissue formation, and the lack of any one of these acts as a limiting factor resulting in a negative nitrogen balance.

Carbohydrates are the best source of energy and are also required for production of antibodies and for cellular structure. These substances are broken down by a series of enzymatic reactions to simple sugars and are stored in the liver and muscles as glycogen. The infant has a smaller glycogen reserve than the older child and requires larger starch intake for immediate energy needs. Carbohydrate which is not stored as glycogen or oxidized is converted to fat.

Fats are vital as a source of essential fatty acids in cellular structure, for energy requirements, and for fat-soluble vitamins (A, D, E, and K).

The *minerals sodium* and *potassium* are absorbed from the gastro-intestinal tract and largely excreted through the kidney. They are found in almost all foods. Potassium is primarily found intracellularly, while sodium is found chiefly extracellularly. The requirement of sodium is about 1 Gm per day (infants) to about 3 Gm per day (children); for potassium, the need is 1 to 2 Gm per day (see p. 134).

Calcium requirements vary with total body size and increase during periods of growth. The average breast-fed infant requires 40 mg per kg per day. The requirements rise to 70 mg per kg per day for formula-fed infants, 0.5 Gm per day for the preschool child, 1 Gm at 8 years, and 1.5 Gm for 10- to 18-year-olds. Sources of calcium are milk, milk products, leafy vegetables, clams and fish products not filleted, e.g., canned salmon.

Phosphorus is necessary for skeletal formation and in cellular structure. Intake will usually be adequate (1.5 Gm per day) if the diet contains sufficient amounts of protein and calcium.

Iron is utilized for hemoglobin and myoglobin formation and respiratory enzymes. The premature infant has minimal iron-storage capacity at birth, while the full-term infant's liver stores sufficient iron for about 3 months' need. Iron deficiency may exist in the absence of anemia. The average intake recommended varies from 6 mg per day for the infant to 15 mg for the older child and adolescent. Iron is found in liver and other meat, egg yolk, green vegetables, whole grains, raisins and nuts.

Magnesium is utilized for bone formation, enzyme production, and neuromuscular tissues. The average estimated requirement is 13 mg per kg per day. Cereals, meat, milk, and legumes contain magnesium.

Iodine is essential for thyroxin production. Children require 40 to 100 micrograms per day, while adolescents require 100 to 200 micrograms per day. The chief sources of iodine are iodized salt and seafood.

Fluorides have been shown to be related to hardness of bones and teeth, and there is statistical proof that they prevent dental caries. The use of fluorides in drinking water, 0.7 part per million, during the period of enamel formation has been recommended.

Chlorides are essential to maintain osmotic pressure (composes about two-thirds of the blood plasma anions), acid-base homeostasis, and in the production of gastric hydrochloric acid. Salt, meat, milk, and eggs contain chloride, and the average diet contains many times more than the daily requirement.

Table 2-1.   Comparison of human and cow's milk

	Human milk	Cow's milk
Water	87%	87%
Protein	1.5%	3.5%
Fat	3.5%	3.5%
Sugar	7%	4.5%
Minerals	0.25%	0.75%
Reaction	Alkaline or amphoteric	Acid or amphoteric
Curd	Soft, flocculent	Hard, large
Digestion	More rapid	Less rapid
Calories	20/oz	20/oz

Minerals, e.g., copper, sulfur, are essential to maintain normal metabolism. Others, e.g., molybdenum, manganese, zinc, and cobalt, play important roles in enzyme formation. Still others, e.g., arsenic, are found in trace amounts, and no physiologic need is known.

The source of almost all minerals is the soil which varies considerably from location to location especially for some minerals, e.g., fluoride, iodine. Some members of the vegetable and animal kingdoms and certain organs of animals may contain concentrated amounts of elements, e.g., iron content of liver, but ultimately the soil content is the limiting factor.

Vitamins are necessary for a variety of metabolic needs and will be discussed in Chapter 3.

ESTABLISHMENT AND MAINTENANCE OF MILK INTAKE

During the first 2 to 3 months of life, milk feedings will usually fulfill all the nutritional needs of the infant. Vitamins A, C, and D are started at the second week, and water supplements are supplied as needed. Milk is supplied as preferred through either breast feeding or formula feeding, or through a combination of the two.

BREAST FEEDING

Breast feeding is generally considered to be superior to artificial feeding and should be encouraged by the physician. The mother should be made aware of its advantages and should be given advice about prenatal and perinatal preparation for its use. However, since formula feeding has been greatly refined, it may safely be used in instances where breast feeding is not feasible, and the mother should be shielded from feelings of inadequacy or shame when this becomes necessary.

Advantages

1. Breast milk is a naturally occurring species-specific food.
2. Breast milk has lower curd tension and is therefore more digestible and causes fewer feeding difficulties, such as vomiting, diarrhea, constipation, or allergies.
3. Breast milk is sterile, fresh, less expensive, and more readily available than other milk; it is also always at the proper temperature.
4. Breast milk promotes an intestinal flora which seems to be more effective in absorbing vitamins and food factors.
5. Colustrum contains antibodies (IgA) against various bacteria and viruses. Although the role of such antibodies in preventing disease is not known, it has been reported that breast-fed babies have a lower incidence of infection than do artificially fed infants.
6. Psychologic benefits from breast feedings accrue to the mother and the infant because of the physical closeness. This does not negate the emotional harmony which can exist when artificial feedings are given with care and reason.

Contraindications

Mother
1. Mastitis resulting from fissuring of the nipple or infection of cutaneous origin. Bacteria can be transmitted to the infant through milk intake.
2. Acute infection.
3. Chronic illness: severe diabetes, nephritis, tuberculosis, cardiac disease, chronic anemia, or malnutrition.
4. Postpartum complications: toxemias, hemorrhage, sepsis.
5. Psychiatric and psychologic factors: postpartum psychosis, depressions, and mental illness.

Infant
1. Cleft palate
2. Marked prematurity (less than 4 lb) or weakness
3. Allergy to breast milk

The occurrence of jaundice in a small number of breast-fed neonates due to inhibition of the glucuronyl transferase system by a metabolite of maternal progesterone is not a contraindication to breast feeding, nor is hemolytic disease of the newborn if the infant's condition is satisfactory.

To promote and ensure an adequate supply of breast milk

1. Sucking is the most effective stimulus to lactation. At each feeding one breast alternately should be completely emptied. Supplementary milk feedings should be avoided if possible. Usually a total feeding time of 20 minutes is adequate.

2. A good maternal diet patterned after the mother's usual diet—sufficient calories, minerals, fluids, and vitamins—should be provided.
3. A proper psychologic attitude with freedom from anxiety or fear is very important. This is greatly dependent on the physician's patience with the mother's problems, his continued encouragement and reassurance. For example, the mother should be told not to expect much milk during the first week postpartum. With continued sucking, milk will become more abundant and the infant more satisfied. The nipples may seem retracted and painful at first and the infant may not seem to be satisfied. However, with continued nursing, the nipples become less painful and function better.

At 4 to 6 months of age the infant may be weaned from the breast. Because of possible discomfort to the mother, this should be done slowly, substituting an additional bottle feeding for a breast feeding about every second day until all breast feedings have been replaced. An alternative method is to offer a bottle after each breast feeding, gradually decreasing the feeding time at the breast.

ARTIFICIAL FEEDING

Artificial feeding refers to breast-milk substitutes, which may be derived from cow's milk, soybeans, or meat base. Formulas are usually prepared with evaporated or whole milk, water, and sugar. There are many proprietary milks available. Some are in powdered form, some in concentrated liquids that require addition of sterile water. There are commercial presterilized formulas which require no dilution and are promoted for use while traveling or in instances where preparation of feedings is not feasible.

Evaporated milk provides 40 Cal per oz; whole cow's milk and breast milk, 20 Cal per oz. The proprietary milks are available as 20 Cal per oz or in concentrated form prepared by adding water in specified amounts to provide 20 Cal per oz after dilution. The hypoallergenic milks, e.g., Prosobee, goat's milk, and Nutramigen, when diluted as specified, usually provide 20 Cal per oz or a little less.

Sugar is used in formulas and provides about 120 Cal per oz. Some commonly used sugars are cane sugar, Karo, Cartose (2 tbsp per oz); lactose (3 tbsp per oz); Dextri-Maltose (4 tbsp per oz).

Calculation of formulas   Either the empirical method or the caloric method may be used. The former is very simple and can be demonstrated best by an illustrative case.

An infant 2 months of age, weighing 11 lb (5 kg), requires a formula.

1. Total fluid: the total daily fluid requirements of the infant are 2½ oz per lb (150 ml per kg) or about 28 oz

2. Evaporated milk: weight $\times$ 1 oz $=$ 11 oz, or
   Whole milk: weight $\times$ 2 oz $=$ 22 oz
3. Water $=$ total fluid $-$ evaporated milk, or 17 oz, or
   Water $=$ total fluid $-$ whole milk, or 6 oz
4. Sugar can always be the same—1 oz

Formula as written:

Evaporated milk—11 oz   Whole milk—22 oz
Water—17 oz   or   Water—6 oz
Sugar—1 oz   Sugar—1 oz

   Some physicians prefer larger amounts of sugar and use 1 oz for an infant up to 10 lb (4.6 kg), 1¼ oz up to 12 lb (5.5 kg), and 1½ oz for infants over that weight. Then when cereal and other carbohydrates are given in quantity, they reduce the sugar in the formula to 1 oz.
   The caloric method is also simple. For the same infant weighing 11 lb,

1. Total calories: weight $\times$ 50 Cal $=$ 550 Cal
2. Sugar can always be 1 oz $=$ 120 Cal
3. Total calories $-$ sugar calories $=$ 430 Cal that must be supplied by milk; therefore, if evaporated milk is used, $430 \div 40$ is the number of ounces needed, or approximately 11 oz
4. Total fluid as above, 28 oz, so water again is 17 oz

Formula as written:

Evaporated milk—11 oz
Water—17 oz
Sugar—1 oz

   Five bottles of 5+ oz each should be given, omitting the 2 A.M. feeding—6 A.M., 10 A.M., 2 P.M., 6 P.M., 10 or 11 P.M.

GENERAL SUGGESTIONS

1. In computing the formula, it is unnecessary to use fractions of ounces. The nearest round number is sufficient.
2. Up to 2 months of age, five to six feedings per day are usually given one every 4 hours; 2 to 4 months of age, five feedings; 4 to 6 months of age, four feedings. During the second month, the infant will usually sleep through the 2 A.M. feeding, which indicates that he is ready for only five feedings. At the fourth month, the infant is often ready to discontinue the 10 P.M. feeding. Early in life (first month), some infants, particularly the smaller ones, are more satisfied and happier being fed every 3 hours during the day (seven feedings in 24 hours).

3. A semidemand or reasonably regular time schedule is often recommended for the infant. If the infant is hungry before the scheduled time, he may be fed, but the schedule should not deteriorate into feedings at practically all hours of the day or night.
4. The infant should be allowed to stop feeding when he is satisfied and should not be pressured to finish the bottle.
5. The mother should be in a good mood, comfortable, and enjoying the relationship during the feeding.
6. Ordinarily the total formula should not be more than 32 oz, and usually no more than one can (13 oz) of evaporated milk is used. The maximum amount per feeding is 8 oz. The total fluid requirements for the day need not be supplied entirely by the formula, but may be provided by water, orange juice, etc., which may be offered between feedings.
7. The calculated formula is used on a trial basis and may be modified for the individual infant. The basic criteria are happiness, satiety, and adequate gain in weight. If the infant is hungry and unhappy, the formula may be increased or concentrated. However, overfeeding leading to digestive disturbances should be avoided.
8. Burping or bubbling patterns vary with each infant, and the mother soon learns the infant's eructation needs. Usually this is done midway and at the end of a feeding.
9. At 4 months of age, whole milk is gradually substituted for formula feedings. When the infant is on whole milk, sterilization of bottles is not necessary; thorough scrubbing of bottles, nipples, and utensils with soap or detergent along with sensible hygienic handling of milk will usually suffice.

    Milk-induced enteric blood loss may be a cause of iron deficiency in infancy. The mechanism is unknown, but this relationship to whole cow's milk may be a significant reason to continue the use of heat-treated milk, e.g., evaporated, through the entire first year of life.
10. The infant is usually ready at 12 to 18 months of age to give up the bottle in favor of the cup, although a presleep bottle is often maintained until 2 years of age. While this developmental process should be encouraged by the mother, there is much latitude in timing; at no time should mother or child be chastised for delaying this change.

SUPPLEMENTARY DIET

Vitamins   The use of supplementary vitamin feedings has received perhaps more than its share of recognition. Most normal feedings are adequate as sources of vitamins except for C and D, and many proprietary foods are now being fortified with C and D. Hypervitaminosis A and hypercalcemia from toxic doses of vitamin D (five times the therapeutic dose) have been reported (see Vitamin D Poisoning or Hypervitaminosis D and Idiopathic Hypercalcemia in Chapter 3).

Vitamin C The recommended daily amount is 30 to 80 mg. The best source is orange juice (15 mg per oz), followed by pineapple and tomato juices (8 mg per oz). For an allergic infant, ascorbic acid may be substituted. Usually orange juice diluted with water is introduced at the second week and gradually increased until the infant receives 3 oz of undiluted orange juice.

Vitamin D The recommended daily amount is 400 to 800 units. Most commercial milks contain 400 IU of vitamin D per quart of whole milk or can of evaporated milk. Vitamin D is introduced at the second week and is given until growth is completed.

Vitamin A The recommended daily amount is 1,500 to 5,000 IU which is usually given together with vitamin D.

Water-soluble multivitamin preparations are available in the form of drops, suspensions, chewable tablets, and capsules. These contain vitamins A, C, and D with varying amounts of vitamin B, iron, and sodium fluoride (for prophylaxis of dental caries). The usual dose of 0.6 ml (on a calibrated dropper) will supply the recommended amounts of each vitamin.

Solid foods Solid foods are usually started at 3 months of age, but the trend has been to initiate these at an earlier age, particularly in those infants who are not satisfied by formula feedings alone. Cereal feedings are usually tolerated best at first.

General suggestions
1. Only one food should be added to the diet at a time.
2. A small amount is given at first, 1 tsp perhaps, and increased as desired, usually to as much as 5 level tbsp.
3. It is best to allow an interval of 4 to 5 days between additions of new foods to be sure that there is no intolerance as demonstrated by loose stools or rash.
4. Solids are given usually before the formula at the feeding time.

Age cannot be used as a rigid standard for introduction of solids. Large, rapidly growing infants consuming large quantities of milk yet still hungry may be made content with supplementary cereal or meat before 3 months of age. Small premature infants may not be considered ready until after 3 months of age. Ill infants and those with special problems such as sensitivity to milk may require other modifications. No nutritional or psychologic gain results from early introduction of solids. Solid foods containing iron (requirement, 6 mg) should be introduced early. Commercially prepared cereals contain about 10 mg per oz, an egg yolk about 1 mg, and strained meats about 0.5 mg per tbsp. The following schedule for the introduction of solid foods is suggested:

Second month: precooked cereals, starting with single-grain cereals, e.g., Pablum oatmeal, at 10:00 A.M. Banana flakes are often well tolerated also. A little formula is added to provide the consistency of thin gruel.

Third month: puréed vegetables and strained meats may be begun at 2:00 P.M.

Fourth month: cooked cereals, e.g., Farina, Cream of Wheat, Wheatena. Fruit at 6:00 P.M. Hard-boiled egg yolk may also be introduced at this time. Frequently whole milk is given at this time.

Fifth month: all other foods, including meats and the various combinations, e.g., meats and vegetables.

Sixth to seventh months: hard bread, zwieback, cheese, desserts, and puddings.

Eighth to twelfth months: the 6:00 A.M. bottle is often discontinued and the infant given three meals a day. If desired, an additional bottle may be offered in the midafternoon. Junior (chopped) foods may be begun gradually at 8 months or even earlier. Soups, finely shredded or scraped meats (chicken, beef, lamb, liver, bacon), potatoes and macaroni are added.

Twelfth to eighteenth months: the infant gets three meals a day and four bottles. An adult diet, including fish, whole egg, etc., may be offered.

The tremendous variety of commercial foods now available provides almost all of the above in forms acceptable to almost any age group, economically, hygienically, and tastefully, so that the mother can fix feedings for the infant at any season of the year with a minimum of effort and expense and with no sacrifice of caloric values or nutritional balance.

After the early feeding period, the entire family should be eating the same types of food and, when feasible, at the same table. The child may be permitted to eat as much as he desires from the family diet according to the following basic daily needs:

Milk—1 pt to 1 qt
Meat or fish—one serving
Egg—one daily (in any form)
Vegetables—two servings, one raw and one colored
Fruit—two servings (one citrus if possible)
Butter or oleomargarine—2 tsp or more
Cheese—one serving
Whole-grain or fortified bread and cereals—to meet caloric needs
Iodized salt—small amounts to taste

When these basic needs are not met, supplemental food and vitamins should be prescribed.

The psychologic aspects of feeding are very important, and there is a direct relationship between developmental patterns and feeding behavior. The young infant resists changes in his routines. Thus, a change in the scheduling of his feeding of milk may result in refusal of the bottle. Because of the decrease in the rate of growth at the end of the first year and for many months afterward, the infant's metabolic needs diminish, and there may be a resultant decrease of appetite. If pressures to eat large amounts are applied at this point, poor feeding habits may result and prevail until later years. There may be strange, ritualistic responses later, when the child may object to all round or red or soft food, or food-jag periods when certain foods are constantly demanded. At 5 years and afterward, social influences come into play, and what others eat becomes of great significance. Foods should be prepared and served in an attractive and tasteful fashion. When the child evinces an interest in feeding himself, he should be permitted to do so and given every assistance, despite the hazards of physical damage to his surroundings. Feeding time should be happy and free from pressure. In general, the family that provides a measure of security for the child and has a proper understanding of his developmental patterns will usually avoid feeding problems.

SPECIAL FEEDING PROBLEMS IN DISEASE SYNDROMES

An increasing variety of disease syndromes that relate to nutritional defects have been recognized recently. These fall into two main categories: The first involves malabsorption problems, for example, celiac syndrome, where nutritional intake is quantitatively and selectively adequate, but is inadequately absorbed (see Chapter 17, "Gastrointestinal Diseases"). The other involves inborn errors of metabolism, e.g., phenylketonuria, maple syrup urine disease, where nutritional intake is adequate but where a block exists at some level of metabolism which prevents completion of utilization and often accumulation of toxic levels of metabolites (see Chapter 9, "Immunology and Metabolism").

The nutritional needs during acute illnesses will vary from the normal. Unless contraindicated by the illness, the intake of fluids usually is increased to enhance heat exchange in fevers and to promote liquefaction of secretions in respiratory syndromes. During an acute illness a reduction of total caloric intake is usually insignificant. Some calories can be offered as carbohydrates, which are easily digested and well tolerated.

In the chronically ill child, total caloric expenditures are usually diminished because of lessened activity, and protein needs are increased for replacement of damaged tissues. There may be increased utilization of vitamins and iron in illnesses characterized by weight loss. In the course of certain therapeutic regimens, electrolyte intake may have to be altered, for instance, during long-term administration of adrenal corticosteroids.

CULTURAL ASPECTS OF DIET

When prescribing diets for infants and children and in developing menus in institutions, e.g., schools, hopitals, day-care centers, consideration should be given to the cultural aspects of food acceptance by children of various ethnic and racial backgrounds.

REVIEW QUESTIONS

Each of the following questions or incomplete statements is followed by several suggested answers or completions. Select the one that is best in each case.

1. The daily caloric requirement of a 1-year-old infant is (a) 500 Cal; (b) 750 Cal; (c) 1000 Cal; (d) 1500 Cal; (e) 2000 Cal.
2. A formula containing 22 oz of whole milk, 6 oz of water, and 1 oz of Dextri-Maltose contains (a) 460 Cal; (b) 490 Cal; (c) 560 Cal; (d) 600 Cal.
3. If the formula in question 2 was fed to a 2-month-old infant weighing 11 lb, the caloric intake would be (a) too low; (b) adequate; (c) too high.
4. Advantages of breast feeding include all the following except (a) breast milk is more digestible; (b) breast milk is hypoallergenic; (c) breast milk is sterile; (d) breast feeding is less expensive; (e) breast milk contains more protein than cow's milk; (f) breast milk is less apt to cause enteric blood loss.
5. All the following are contraindications to breast feeding except (a) cleft lip and palate; (b) maternal tuberculosis; (c) breast abscess in the mother; (d) birth weight of 1,000 Gm; (e) hemolytic disease of the newborn.

The following paired phrases each describe two entities that are to be compared quantitatively. In the blanks provided, write the letter A if item (A) is greater than item (B), B if item (B) is greater than item (A), and C if the two items are equal or very nearly equal.

6. ____ (A) Mineral content of human milk
    (B) Mineral content of cow's milk
7. ____ (A) Fat content of human milk
    (B) Fat content of cow's milk
8. ____ (A) Sugar content of human milk
    (B) Sugar content of cow's milk
9. ____ (A) Caloric content of evaporated milk
    (B) Caloric content of cow's milk
10. ____ (A) Amount of milk an infant will take as supplementary feeding
    (B) Amount of milk an infant will take as complementary feeding
11. ____ (A) Calories in a tablespoonful of cane sugar
    (B) Calories in a tablespoonful of corn syrup

The following questions are the matching type. In each blank in column I, insert the letter corresponding to the age in column II at which the item in column I should be introduced into the diet.

Column I lists various constituents of human milk. Column II gives percentages of these constituents. Match the two:

I		II
12. Water ____	(a)	7%
13. Protein ____	(b)	3.5%
14. Fat ____	(c)	0.25%
15. Sugar ____	(d)	87%
16. Minerals ____	(e)	1.5%

17. The most important factor in providing a lunch menu for a group of 6-year-old children is (a) calories; (b) vitamins; (c) cultural aspects; (d) fluid requirements; (e) minerals.

3
VITAMINS AND METABOLISM

A vitamin is an essential organic constituent of the diet that, in minute amounts, aids in maintaining the normal metabolic activities of the body tissues. Vitamin A, thiamine, riboflavin, niacin, vitamins C, D, and K, folic acid, and vitamins B_6 and B_{12} are of particular importance in children. Folic acid and vitamin B_{12} are discussed in Chapter 22, "Blood Disorders."

Full-blown vitamin-deficiency diseases have become rather uncommon, but laboratory and clinical search for early changes reveals that many children are not receiving adequate supplies of vitamins for maximal health. Deficiencies, when present, are usually multiple rather than single, so that, for example, in planning therapy for a thiamine deficiency, it is wise to give such other members of the B complex as riboflavin and niacin in addition to the thiamine.

A well-balanced diet, as described on previous pages, will furnish adequate amounts of the various vitamins. There may be other conditioning factors, however, that will make a particular diet insufficient. A thorough history is therefore helpful in diagnosing vitamin deficiencies. Questions are directed toward obtaining information relative to the following:

1. Qualitatively or quantitatively poor dietary intake for the particular stage of growth and development.
2. Poor absorption: gastroenteritis, celiac syndrome, or vomiting.
3. Increased metabolism or defective utilization: febrile diseases or hyperthyroidism.
4. Increased excretion: for example, following administration of large amounts of intravenous fluids that could wash out the water-soluble vitamins. (Vitamins B and C are water soluble; all the others are fat soluble.)

The above four factors may operate singly or in any combination to produce vitamin deficiencies.

VITAMIN A

Vitamin A is necessary for normal growth of bones and teeth, the integrity of epithelial tissue, and, in the retina, for rhodopsin formation and for cone (color) vision; it is also needed for the production of adrenocortical steroids. Carotene and cryptoxanthin (yellow pigments of fruit and vegetables) are precursors. Fish is a rich source of vitamin A esters. Adequate protein is essential for utilization of vitamin A, which is transported in the blood, to body tissues, bound to albumin.

Clinical features suggesting deficiency   The following may be found singly or in combination:

1. Xerosis of the conjunctiva (minute dry spots in the conjunctiva).
2. Xerosis of the skin (dryness and scaliness of the skin).
3. Keratosis pilaris and papularis of the skin (hard conical elevations around the hair follicles).
4. Night blindness (nyctalopia—subnormal vision in dim light).
5. Xerophthalmia and keratomalacia of the eye are late and irreversible manifestations.
6. Metaplastic changes in the mucosal and glandular tissue of the upper respiratory tract, bronchi, and genitourinary tract.

Laboratory tests

1. The blood test for vitamin A is most reliable. A serum–vitamin A level of 45 international units (IU) per 100 ml probably is the

lower limit for normal infants (average, 50 to 100 IU), and 75 IU for older children. The average carotene level is 50 to 200 micrograms. A modification of the blood test is to give a load or test dose of vitamin A, following which there will be a graduated rise in level of serum vitamin A in normal children but little or no rise in children with deficiency. During acute febrile illnesses, the vitamin A level usually decreases.

2. Scrapings of the mucous membranes of the eye or nose may show cornified epithelium.
3. Biomicroscopy of the conjunctiva of the eye may demonstrate xerosis.

Prophylaxis   The prophylactic dose is 1,500 to 5,000 international (or USP) units of vitamin A per day, depending on the age.

Therapeutic dose   The therapeutic dose is 50,000 units divided into three or four doses per day by mouth. The nonoily preparations are better absorbed.

Carotenemia   Rarely carotene may not be converted to vitamin A at a normal rate, and excessive amounts may appear in the blood. The skin, particularly the palms and soles, may take on an orange-yellow hue, but usually the sclera is spared. Carotenemia may be found in apparently normal children or in those with hyperlipidemia, for example, in diseases of the liver, hypothyroidism, or diabetes. Occasionally the carotenemia is confused with jaundice, but the serum-bilirubin level in carotenemia is normal. (The icterus index is not the preferred test for differential diagnosis because in carotenemia there may be a false elevation.) In treatment, the cartotenemia usually disappears when a diet low in carotene is prescribed.

Vitamin A poisoning, or hypervitaminosis A   Vitamin A poisoning is characterized by a past history of excessive daily dosages (symptoms can occur after a period of several weeks of 10 times the prophylactic dose) of vitamin A in a child from about 15 months to 3 years of age, who presents irritability; pruritus; painful extremities with brawny swelling, which may also occur in the occipital region; pallor; coarse hair; dry skin; and hepatosplenomegaly. (In young infants a bulging fontanel due to increased intracranial pressure may occur in either hypovitaminosis A or hypervitaminosis A.) Roentgenograms reveal periosteal elevation with subperiosteal new bone formation and irregular cortical thickening. The ulnar and metatarsal bones are involved most frequently. Laboratory findings: the serum–vitamin A level is increased to 1,000 or more IU per 100 ml. The treatment is the withdrawal of vitamin A; this results in the rapid subsidence of symptoms, but the roentgenographic changes are slow to disappear. This condition must be differentiated, particularly on roentgenogram, from infantile cortical hyperostosis (see p. 546). Vitamin A in doses of

50,000 IU or more is frequently prescribed for acne vulgaris. The clinical impression that this treatment is beneficial has not been validated, and such dosage may result in intoxication.

VITAMIN B₁ (Thiamine Chloride)

Thiamine chloride (antiberiberi factor), phosphorylated by tissue cells to carboxylase and transketolase, is a coenzyme essential for decarboxylation of pyruvic acid in the Krebs cycle, which supplies energy for all body processes, and is essential for the utilization of pentoses. Sources of vitamin B₁ are meats, especially liver and pork; whole grain or enriched cereals; and legumes.

Clinical features suggesting deficiency   The following may be found singly or in combination:

1.   There may be an enlarged heart with dependent edema and elevated venous pressure. In young infants, acute cardiac failure with pulmonary edema may develop rapidly.
2.   Peripheral neuritis (both motor and sensory) may be present, manifested by loss of strength of the quadriceps, loss of vibratory sense, tenderness of the calves, hyperesthesia of the feet, and diminution or loss of the Achilles-tendon and patellar reflexes.
3.   Early deficiency may be accompanied by vague and nonspecific complaints, such as anorexia, constipation, and those of neurasthenia—nervousness, fatigue, and change in disposition.
4.   In young infants convulsions and coma have occurred. The cranial nerves, primarily the recurrent laryngeal branch of the vagus nerve, may be affected.

Laboratory tests

1.   Decrease of erythrocyte transketolase activity is the earliest sign of thiamine deficiency.

Prophylaxis   The prophylactic dose is 0.5 to 1 mg daily, preferably as part of the diet.

Therapeutic dose   The therapeutic dose is 5 to 10 mg daily—parenterally or by mouth—in divided doses.

VITAMIN B₂ (Riboflavin)

Riboflavin when phosphorylated to flavin mononucleotide and flavin adenine dinucleotide is an essential component of the flavoprotein enzymes and functions as a system together with niacin containing enzymes in tissue oxidation-reduction reactions. It is also important for protein metabolism and cellular respiration. Vitamin B_2 is widely distributed in plant and animal tissues. Milk is the richest source.

Clinical features suggesting deficiency The following may be found singly or in combination:

1. Eye changes: conjunctivitis, corneal vascularization, and keratitis, with possible photophobia, itching, and burning
2. Cheilosis: an inflammation of the mucous membrane or mucocutaneous border of the lip
3. Angular stomatitis (perlèche): a maceration and fissuring at the corners of the mouth
4. Dyssebacia: greasy scales on a reddened base, especially around the nose
5. Magenta-colored tongue, due to glossitis (not a specific indication of riboflavin deficiency)

Laboratory tests

1. Decrease of erythrocyte glutathione reductase activity is the earliest sign of riboflavin deficiency.
2. Measurement of urinary excretion of riboflavin spontaneously or following a test or load dose—excretion of less than 200 micrograms in 4 hours following an oral dose of 5 mg.

Prophylaxis The prophylactic dose is 0.5 to 2 mg daily (depending on the age), preferably as part of the diet.

Therapeutic dose The therapeutic dose is 20 mg orally or parenterally, daily, in divided doses.

NIACIN (Nicotinic Acid)

Niacin (antipellagra factor), the functional group of nicotinamide adenine dinucleotide and dinucleotide phosphate, is concerned with hydrogen transport and is essential for carbohydrate metabolism. Niacin is found in liver, yeast, meat, legumes, and whole-grain and enriched cereals. Hartnup disease is an inborn error of tryptophan metabolism, and the stigmata of niacin deficiency which appear in children with this disease can be treated with niacin. Requirements, as with thiamine, increase with caloric consumption. Tryptophan is a precursor (the body forms 1 mg niacin from 60 mg tryptophan).

Clinical features suggesting deficiency The following may be found singly or in combination:

1. Dermatitis: symmetrical and found particularly over areas exposed to light
2. Encephalopathy: may be manifested by a change in disposition, depression or irritability, poor power of concentration, confusion, and somtimes actual dementia
3. Diarrhea: not infrequent
4. Changes in the tongue and buccal mucosa: redness and edema, followed by congestion and hypertrophy of the papillae of the tongue and subsequently by their fusion and atrophy.

Laboratory tests

1. Measurement of urinary excretion of N-methylnicotinamide spontaneously or following a load or test dose—excretion of less than 500 micrograms in 4 hours following an oral dose of 50 mg.
2. Biomicroscopic examination of the tongue may reveal the changes described above.

Prophylaxis   The prophylactic dose is 10 mg of niacin equivalents daily. Most diets consumed in the United States supply 500 to 1,000 mg tryptophan and about 10 to 15 mg niacin.

Therapeutic dose   The therapeutic dose is 100 mg daily, orally or parenterally, preferably in divided doses.

VITAMIN B$_6$ (Pyridoxine Hydrochloride)

Vitamin B$_6$ as the coenzymes pyridoxal phosphate and pyridoxamine phosphate is concerned with protein metabolism and conversion of tryptophan to niacin and is necessary for utilization of essential fatty acids and decarboxylation and transamination of amino acids. It is essential for hemoglobin, serotonin, and histamine formation. Vitamin B$_6$ is found in meat, especially liver and kidney; whole grains, and soybean.

Deficiency may be induced by isoniazid therapy.

Pyridoxine dependency is a rare condition inherited as an autosomal recessive trait. It may be manifest in utero, and in those cases in which the history of previous sibs is suggestive, large doses of pyridoxine should be given to the mother at term. Infants manifest convulsions which are difficult to control with anticonvulsive therapy. Daily doses of pyridoxine exceeding 10 mg may be required for an indefinite period.

Clinical features suggesting deficiency

1. Usually occurs during early infancy.
2. Irritability and convulsions.

3. Colic, abdominal distension, vomiting, and diarrhea.
4. Skin and mucous-membrane changes similar to those in vitamin B_2 deficiency. (Skin lesions are uncommon during infancy.)

Laboratory tests

1. Urinary excretion of large amounts of xanthurenic acid after tryptophan loading test.
2. Erythrocyte aminotransferase activity is decreased.
3. Microcytic, hypochromic anemia, and lymphocytopenia with normal serum iron level and total iron-binding capacity.

Prophylaxis   The prophylactic dose is 0.2 to 0.5 mg daily.

Therapeutic dose   The therapeutic dose is 5 to 10 mg.

PANTOTHENIC ACID

Pantothenic acid is a component of coenzyme A and takes part in many biosynthetic mechanisms. It is required for antibody synthesis, and the adrenal cortex is an important site of activity. Spontaneous deficiencies have not been observed in man, although it is apparently a vital factor. It is present in all plant and animal tissues and some microorganisms, and this universal distribution makes spontaneous deficiency virtually impossible.

BIOTIN

Biotin is necessary for propionate utilization and functions as the prosthetic group for several carboxylases. Its high potency and intestinal synthesis make spontaneous deficiency improbable. Raw egg white contains a protein, avidin, which binds biotin and prevents its absorption from the intestine.

CHOLINE

Choline functions as a lipotropic agent and is necessary for the synthesis of phospholipids for fat transport. It is also a source of labile methyl groups necessary for amino acid synthesis. In the form of acetylcholine, it functions to transmit nerve impulses across ganglionic synapses. Choline is widely distributed in foodstuffs; a spontaneous deficiency of this vitamin has never been observed.

INOSITOL

Inositol may function as a lipotropic agent, but its role in cellular metabolism has not been elucidated. It is widely distributed in foodstuffs, making a deficiency virtually impossible.

FOLIC ACID

Folic acid is converted in the liver to tetrahydrofolic acid, which functions as a coenzyme for transferring formyl groups. In this role, it is essential for nucleic acid and amino acid synthesis and the formation of deoxyribonucleic acid, necessary for nuclear formation. Deficiency induces maturation arrest in the bone marrow, leading to megaloblastic anemia. Dietary sources include liver, red meats, and green vegetables. Folic acid deficiency may arise from inadequate dietary intake, impaired absorption, excessive demands by tissues or metabolic derangements. Folic acid deficiency is a common element in kwashiorkor, a severe form of malnutrition occurring in tropical and subtropical lands. (Folic acid is discussed further in Chapter 22, "Blood Disorders.")

VITAMIN B_{12} (Cyanocobalamin)

Vitamin B_{12} functions in the formation of protein, nucleoprotein synthesis, transmethylation, and the formation of ribonucleic acid. It is found only in foods of animal origin (meat, milk, and eggs). Deficiency may occur in vegetarians but is usually due to lack of the intrinsic factor in gastric secretion which is necessary for vitamin B_{12} absorption. In a severe deficiency, there may be personality changes, macrocytic anemia, and peripheral neuropathy. (Vitamin B_{12} is discussed further in Chapter 22, "Blood Disorders.")

ASCORBIC ACID (Vitamin C)

Ascorbic acid is a reducing agent and a catalyst in cellular respiration, and it is necessary for carbohydrate utilization and intermediary metabolism of aromatic amino acids. It is important in preserving the integrity of the connective-tissue supporting structures.

Clinical features suggesting deficiency   The following may be found singly or in combination:

1.   Increased capillary fragility: may be manifested by perifollicular petechial hemorrhages, ecchymoses, bleeding from the mucous membranes, and hemorrhages into the joints.

2. Gingival changes: gums may show redness, edema, tenderness, bleeding, thickening, and retraction.
3. Frank scurvy: usually found in infancy from 6 to 18 months of age; characterized by subperiosteal hemorrhages, pain and tenderness over the ends of the long bones (especially about the ankles), marked irritability so that the infant does not want to be moved, pseudoparalysis, the assumption of a squatting or "pithed-frog" position, and occasionally fever.

Laboratory tests

1. Blood-plasma ascorbic acid (reflects recent intake) less than 0.3 mg per 100 ml is considered abnormal. Buffy coat ascorbic acid level (white cell, platelet layer)—normal, 20 to 35 mg per 100 ml —is a better index of tissue concentration.
2. Urinary excretion of ascorbic acid: e.g., excretion in a period of 6 hours of less than 50 mg of a test dose of ascorbic acid (1 Gm orally) suggests a deficiency.
3. Roentgenograms of the bones may reveal distortion of the soft parts from edema or hemorrhage; ground-glass atrophy, especially at the end of the shaft of long bones; "white line of Fraenkel" at the epiphyseal end, due to increased density of the zone of preparatory calcification; ringing of the epiphyseal centers; spurring and epiphyseal separation (epiphyses most often affected— distal femur and tibia and proximal humerus).

Prophylaxis   The prophylactic dose is 50 mg daily.

Therapeutic dose   The therapeutic dose is 500 mg per day, orally or parenterally, preferably in divided doses.

VITAMIN D

Vitamin D exists as D_2 (ergocalciferol) and D_3 (cholecalciferol). The skin contains 7 dehydrocholesterol which, when exposed to ultraviolet rays of the sun, is converted to vitamin D_3. To be physiologically active, vitamin D must be converted in the liver to 25-hydroxycholecalciferol and then in the kidneys to 1,25-dihydroxycholecalciferol. The latter is necessary for

1. Absorption of dietary calcium and phosphate from the intestinal tract
2. Reabsorption of phosphate by renal tubular cells (an interaction with parathyroid hormone)
3. Maintenance of serum-calcium level by mobilizing calcium from bone when the oral intake is inadequate (an interaction with parathyroid hormone)

In deficiency, because the growing parts of the skeleton do not have normal deposition of calcium salts, they may become deformed. In the adult, since endochondral bone growth has ended, only osteomalacia develops.

Clinical features suggesting deficiency   Rickets, found usually from 4 months to 2 years of age, is suggestive of vitamin D deficiency. The earliest sign is craniotabes, which may appear as early as 3 months of age and is a softening and thinning of an area of the skull—commonly occipitoparietal—which indents and rebounds, often with a crackle like that of a ping-pong ball. (Craniotabes may be found normally, particularly in premature infants.) Later there may be frontal bossing; hot-cross-bun skull; late closing of the fontanels; funnel or pigeon breast; Harrison's groove (corresponding to the costal insertions of the diaphragm); rachitic rosary (enlarged costochondral junctions); kyphosis or lordosis of the spine; protuberant abdomen; enlargement of the elbows, knees, ankles, and other bony prominences; and bowlegs.

Laboratory tests

1. Blood-calcium and -phosphorus levels may be normal, but usually the phosphorus level is low. The calcium level is rarely low, but when it is, infantile tetany may result.
2. Alkaline phosphatase concentration is increased.
3. Roentgenograms of the bones—the lower ulna and radius give the best information—may show cupping, spreading, fraying, stippling of the ends of the shafts; spurring (calcified lines extending from the cortex of the shaft down along the side of the proliferating cartilage); and decreased density of the shaft with unusually prominent trabeculae.

Prophylaxis   The prophylactic dose is 400 to 800 USP units daily. (The need for vitamin D can be met by exposure of the skin to sunlight.)

Therapeutic dose   10,000 USP units daily for 6 to 8 weeks. A single-dosage treatment may be given—600,000 USP units over a 24-hour period. Phosphorus levels, if previously depressed, will become normal within 1 week, and x-ray evidence of healing appears by 2 weeks. If no response occurs, a second dose is given; subsequent failure to respond suggests vitamin D–resistant rickets.

Vitamin D poisoning or hypervitaminosis D   Poisoning may produce pallor, malaise, lassitude, polyuria, polydipsia, increased serum-phosphorus level, hypercalcemia with metastatic calcification, calcium crystals and casts in the urine, with eventual renal damage and nitrogenous retention. Hypertension may develop.

Idiopathic hypercalcemia This is probably due to hypersensitivity to vitamin D with excessive calcium absorption, which causes renal damage, developmental failure, and failure to thrive during infancy. Symptoms usually appear between 3 and 7 months of age. A number of cases have an associated supravalvular aortic stenosis.

Clinical features Clinical features include anorexia, vomiting, constipation, hypotonia, hypertension, elflike facies, mental and motor retardation, hypercalcemia, azotemia, and impaired renal function.

Roentgen features Defective osteoidal bone formation, abnormal soft-tissue calcification, and nephrocalcinosis may be noted on x-ray.

Treatment The usual treatment is calcium-free diet (sodium phytate blocks intestinal absorption), restriction of vitamin D, adrenal corticosteroids.

METABOLIC CONDITIONS ASSOCIATED WITH RACHITIC CHANGES IN BONES

Vitamin D deficiency accompanying steatorrhea In celiac syndrome, cystic fibrosis of the pancreas, and atresia of the bile ducts, there is poor absorption of vitamin D and loss of calcium and phosphorus in the feces in the form of soaps. The amount of blood calcium may be diminished, resulting in a tendency toward tetany. The treatment is ultraviolet irradiation, large doses of vitamin D in water-miscible form, and treatment of the underlying condition. The prognosis of the rickets is good although that of the etiologic disease is necessarily guarded.

Renal rickets Renal rickets result from renal insufficiency secondary to chronic glomerulonephritis, recurrent pyelitis, or congenital anomalies of the urinary tract, e.g., polycystic kidneys; or chronic acidosis, e.g., diabetes mellitus with ketosis. There are azotemia, hyperphosphatemia, hypocalcemia, and reduction of serum-bicarbonate level, and dwarfism. Parathyroid activity is stimulated by hyperphosphatemia and hypocalcemia. Histologically there is an osteitis fibrosa, as in hyperparathyroidism. The underlying renal condition must be treated whenever possible. In addition, a low-phosphorous diet and administration of calcium and vitamin D may be helpful. The prognosis is poor.

Renal tubular defects may involve one or more transport mechanisms. The cause of many is not known. They are hereditary or acquired, primary or secondary. Both primary and secondary types may present identical findings and cannot be distinguished on the basis of functional and urinary tests. Therefore, a descriptive rather than an etiologic classification is offered. Several syndromes are described below.

Familial hypophosphatemia and vitamin D–resistant rickets   Familial vitamin D–resistant rickets with hypophosphatemia is a disorder characterized by (1) familial occurrence, the inheritance of the abnormality being a single dose effect of an X-linked gene (X-linked dominant); (2) hypophosphatemia associated with decreased renal tubular reabsorption of inorganic phosphate; (3) rickets in some but not all affected persons, not responsive to physiologic doses of vitamin D; (4) diminished gastrointestinal absorption of calcium in children who have rickets; and (5) an abnormality in the metabolism of vitamin D consisting of decreased conversion of vitamin D to its biologically active metabolite, 1,25-dihydroxycholecaciferol, which could account for the decreased intestinal absorption. Stool-calcium content is high, and the amount of urinary calcium is diminished. The condition usually becomes clinically apparent at 12 to 24 months of age.

Treatment   Vitamin D, 50,000 units daily and increased by increments of 25,000 units daily at monthly intervals is the treatment. Treatment is controlled by determining the blood-calcium level (not to exceed 12 mg per 100 ml) and the urinary calcium (not to exceed 200 mg per day), and by x-rays to indicate evidence of healing. The addition of phosphates to the therapeutic regime may be helpful. The prognosis, in general, is good if treatment is instituted early.

Renal glucosuria   This condition is the result of defective glucose reabsorption in the proximal tubules. It is congenital but usually not discovered until later adult life, and it is not associated with rickets. Inheritance is an autosomal dominant trait. The presence of glucose in the urine with a normal or slightly low serum glucose level establishes the diagnosis. Two types are recognized: in type A, renal plasma threshold and Tm glucose are low; in type B, Tm glucose is normal, but there is a low renal plasma threshold for glucose.

Renal aminoacidurias   Normally amino acids in the glomerular filtrate are almost completely reabsorbed in the proximal tubules. Aminoaciduria in the presence of normal plasma amino acid levels is due to either a specific defect in the reabsorption of one group of amino acids or a nonspecific dysfunction resulting in generalized aminoaciduria.

Renal tubular acidosis (RTA, hyperchloremic acidosis)   This is a condition in which glomerular function is normal or comparatively less impaired than the tubular function. On the basis of underlying pathophysiology renal tubular acidosis can be divided into two forms: (1) proximal renal tubular acidosis caused by a defect in the tubular reabsorption of bicarbonate, and (2) distal renal tubular acidosis, resulting from an inability to establish an adequate gradient of pH between blood and tubular fluid. Clinically urine reaction may be the clue to differentiate these. An alkaline or neutral urine pH, suggests distal RTA whereas slightly acid pH will be in favor of proximal RTA.

Multiple dysfunction of the proximal renal tubules (de Toni-Debré-Fanconi syndrome)   The Fanconi syndrome is a disorder involving multiple functional disturbances of the proximal tubules with glycosuria, phosphaturia, and generalized aminoaciduria. Tabular proteinuria, systemic acidosis, defective sodium and potassium conservation, and inability to concentrate may also be present. The urine pH is 6 or higher. The rate of excretion of titratable acid and ammonium ion is low, and both plasma threshold and Tm of bicarbonate are also low. But a majority of patients are able to excrete adequate hydrogen ions when stimulated with a standard dose of ammonium chloride; therefore, these children have proximal type renal tubular acidosis. They have stunted growth. Therapy is directed toward systemic acidosis and rachitic bone lesions if present.

Hypophosphatasia and rickets   This is a familial disease probably inherited as an autosomal recessive trait and characterized by failure of calcification of bone matrix. There are premature loss of teeth, occasionally premature synostosis of the skull, decreased serum alkaline phosphatase level, and an abnormal metabolite, phosphoethanolamine, in the plasma and urine. Adrenal corticosteroids may be of value.

Cystinuria   This term is applied to a familial disorder of the renal tubule, which fails to reabsorb dibasic amino acids (cystine, arginine, ornithine, lysine). Large amounts of these amino acids are present in the urine, with normal serum levels. Because cystine is insoluble in acid or concentrated urine, cystine stones are formed; they constitute a large part of the urinary stones seen in children. They are radiopaque and occur anywhere in the renal tract. The defect produces no other pathologic change, and it is not related to cystinosis. It is transmitted by a recessive gene; in some families, by an incompletely recessive intermediate gene. In the latter group heterozygotes excrete a slightly elevated cystine content in the urine. The nitroprusside cyanide test is useful as a screening procedure, and a definite diagnosis can be made by paper or column chromatography or by polarography.

Treatment   The urine must not be allowed to become acid and concentrated. Cystine stones may be dissolved by drinking plenty of fluids, especially at night. Penicillamine, 30 mg per kg per day, has been used since it binds cystine in a highly soluble complex. (Cystinuria is to be differentiated from cystinosis—cystine storage disease—in which there is generalized deposition of cystine and an elevated blood level. Involvement of the renal tubules may result in generalized aminoaciduria.)

VITAMIN E (Tocopherol)

Vitamin E is a fat-soluble vitamin whose action is not clearly defined. It is an intracellular fat antioxidant and is necessary to prevent peroxide formation of cell-membrane unsaturated fatty acids. Dietary sources are vegetable oils, cereals, and eggs. Newborn infants, especially premature infants, have low vitamin E tissue levels. Human milk is rich in vitamin E, but cow's milk is low. If newborn infants are fed a formula high in polyunsaturated fatty acids (PUFA) and low in vitamin E, hemolysis of the erythrocytes may occur. To prevent this, 0.6 mg of vitamin E is required for every gram of PUFA. Patients with fat malabsorption require supplementation with vitamin E. The requirements for vitamin E depend upon the PUFA content of the diet.

Laboratory tests

1. Plasma levels below 0.1 mg per 100 ml in the newborn and below 0.5 mg per 100 ml in children and adults indicate vitamin E deficiency.
2. Hemolysis of erythrocytes in dilute peroxide solution may also be observed in vitamin E deficiency.

VITAMIN K

Vitamin K functions as a participant in the formation of prothrombin and other clotting factors (VII, IX, X, and possibly V) in the liver. Its precursor is abundant in food and is converted to the active vitamin in the intestines by bacterial action. Deficiency may be due to inadequate diet; impaired production in the intestines, e.g., following administration of oral antibiotics; impaired intestinal absorption, e.g., celiac syndrome; or treatment with Dicumarol or large doses of salicylates.

Lack of vitamin K may be one of the causes of hemorrhagic disease of the newborn infant (see Chapter 12, "Diseases of the Newborn"). In older children, vitamin K deficiency and hemorrhage may occur after treatment with large doses of salicylates or Dicumarol, in diseases of the liver, or in disorders of intestinal absorption.

Laboratory test   Prothrombin time is prolonged.

Prophylaxis   A dose of 0.2 mg aqueous colloidal suspension of natural vitamin K (Aqua-Mephyton, Konakion) is administered parenterally to the newborn infant. The use of synthetic vitamin K should be discouraged since in infants with a congenital or physiologic deficiency of glucose-6-phosphate dehydrogenase it may cause acute hemolytic anemia and hyperbilirubinemia.

Therapeutic dose   The therapeutic dose is 1 mg parenterally.

MALIGNANT MALNUTRITION

Malignant malnutrition in children (kwashiorkor, protein malnutrition) is a protein deficiency syndrome characterized by impaired growth and development; mental changes, especially irritability and apathy; anorexia; diarrhea; edema; dermatitis ("flaking paint" desquamation); sparse thin hair; weak atrophic muscles; anemia (microcytic and megaloblastic); low serum albumin; lowered activity of many enzymes (alkaline phosphatase, pancreatic enzymes); and frequent infections. Treatment consists of administering fluids and electrolytes to restore losses, antibiotics for infection, gradually introducing an adequate diet beginning with milk and vitamin supplementation for associated deficiencies.

Prognosis   The prognosis is guarded in severe cases. If impairment occurs early enough in life and is severe, physical and mental retardation may be permanent.

MARASMUS

Marasmus is a starvation syndrome occurring when infants consume a diet lacking in sufficient calories. Growth and development ceases and fat layers disappear resulting in loose and wrinkled skin. The infants have distended abdomens, and muscle hypotonia and edema may be present. Treatment is administration of fluids and electrolytes and then an adequate diet with vitamins. In severe or recurrent cases, emotional, physical, and mental retardation may be permanent.

REVIEW QUESTIONS

1. The following are signs of vitamin A deficiency except for one: (*a*) xerosis of the conjunctiva; (*b*) scaliness of the skin; (*c*) hepatosplenomegaly; (*d*) nyctalopia.
2. In differentiating carotenemia from jaundice the preferred test is (*a*) icterus index; (*b*) serum-bilirubin level; (*c*) vitamin A level; (*d*) bile content of urine.
3. In a 2-year-old infant with irritability, painful extremities, pallor, coarse hair, and x-rays revealing periosteal elevation, the most probable diagnosis is (*a*) vitamin A deficiency; (*b*) vitamin C deficiency; (*c*) vitamin D deficiency; (*d*) hypervitaminosis D; (*e*) hypervitaminosis A.
4. The richest source of riboflavin (vitamin B_2) is (*a*) milk; (*b*) fish; (*c*) meat; (*d*) legumes.
5. Dermatitis, encephalopathy, and diarrhea are associated with deficiency of (*a*) pyridoxine; (*b*) niacin; (*c*) biotin; (*d*) folic acid.
6. The vitamin that is essential for hemoglobin, serotonin, and histamine formation is (*a*) B; (*b*) C; (*c*) B_2; (*d*) B_6.

7. Arrest of bone marrow maturation and the production of megaloblastic anemia is due to deficiency of (a) folic acid; (b) iron; (c) biotin; (d) niacin; (e) copper.

8. In vitamin C deficiency a blood plasma-ascorbic acid level less than (a) 0.8 mg; (b) 0.7 mg; (c) 0.5 mg; (d) 0.3 mg per 100 ml is considered abnormal.

9. In rickets the blood phosphorus level is (a) usually low but may be normal; (b) usually high but may be normal; (c) normal; (d) elevated.

10. Renal damage, developmental failure and failure to thrive in a 5-month-old infant is suggestive of (a) hypervitaminosis A; (b) hypervitaminosis D; (c) idiopathic hypercalcemia; (d) rickets.

11. Inheritance as an X-linked trait, decreased renal tubular reabsorption of inorganic phosphate, rickets in some of the affected individuals, and diminished gastrointestinal absorption of calcium in children with rickets is associated with (a) renal aminoaciduria; (b) renal tubular acidosis; (c) familial hypophosphatemia and vitamin D-resistant rickets; (d) hypophosphatasia with rickets.

12. Renal glucosuria is usually recognized (a) at birth; (b) during infancy; (c) during adolescence; (d) in adult life.

13. The de Toni-Debré-Fanconi syndrome is characterized by the following except for one: (a) urine pH lower than 6; (b) phosphaturia; (c) generalized aminoaciduria; (d) glycosuria.

14. Hemolysis of erythrocytes may occur if a premature infant is fed a diet high in polyunsaturated fatty acids and low in (a) vitamin K; (b) vitamin C; (c) vitamin E; (d) folic acid.

15. Prophylactic treatment of vitamin K deficiency at birth is by (a) 2.0 mg of synthetic vitamin K; (b) 0.2 mg of aqueous colloidal suspension of natural vitamin K; (c) either preparation may be used interchangeably.

4
PREVENTIVE PEDIATRICS

The objective of preventive pediatrics is not merely to prevent disease but also to promote the best possible health of the whole, or total, child. Careful consideration should be given to the genetic and environmental background of the infant and child as well as to the physical, mental, behavioral, and social aspects of his life. The physician—obstetrician, general practitioner, and pediatrician—shares with the parent the responsibility for the health supervision of the child from conception through adolescence.

ANTENATAL MEASURES

The following are examples of antenatal measures that may affect the future welfare of the child. Good prenatal care, with particular attention to adequate maternal nutrition and avoidance of unnecessary drugs, has been shown to lower mortality and morbidity of newborn infants. Anticipatory guidance and education of the parents are important and have not been stressed sufficiently. Screening parents and teen-agers prior to childbearing for known inheritable disease, e.g., sickle-cell trait, followed by genetic counseling plays an important role in preventive pediatrics (see p. 151). Intrauterine diagnosis of serious conditions, e.g., Tay-Sachs disease, provides an opportunity for further preventive efforts (see p. 183). The prevention of maternal exposure to the diagnostic and therapeutic use of radiation and to such illnesses as rubella during the first trimester should be emphasized. (Rubella, cytomegalic inclusion disease, toxoplasmosis, mumps, herpes simplex, and varicella early in pregnancy have been implicated as causes of congenital anomalies.) The prophylaxis of congenital syphilis and erythroblastosis fetalis is discussed in Chapters 14 and 22, respectively.

POSTNATAL MEASURES

Periodic medical evaluation   Evaluation is needed at least monthly during the first 6 months and somewhat less frequently during the second 6 months, quarterly during the second year, and semiannually thereafter, to be sure that the child is progressing normally. In this way any deviations from the norm may be recognized early and provisions made for their possible correction. Parents should be told what to expect in the progress of growth and development during the ensuing period.

Nutritional supervision   Diet has been discussed in Chapter 2, "Feeding of Infants and Children," and Chapter 3, "Vitamins and Metabolism."

Active immunizations   The immunizations given during the first 2 years of life are those for pertussis, diphtheria, tetanus, poliomyelitis, rubeola and rubella. Infants who have had febrile convulsions should be given one-tenth to one-fifth the recommended dosage of antigen. Aspirin and phenobarbital may be used prophylactically. Infants who experience significant local or generalized reactions, for example, fever, somnolence, following administration of antigen(s) should be given a decreased volume, i.e., one-tenth to one-fifth the recommended dose of single antigens in subsequent injections. If a convulsion has occurred following administration of DPT, no further injections of pertussis vaccine should be administered, and other immunizations should be completed with single antigens after complete evaluation (risk of exposure, neurologic examination).

Pertussis immunization   Since most of the deaths due to the disease occur in infants under 1 year of age, it is essential to start immunization early. Good antibody response occurs when inoculations are begun at 2 months of age. There is little if any transplacental passage of antibodies. Pertussis immunization should not be repeated if thrombocytopenia occurs after a previous injection of the antigen. Pertussis vaccine is eliminated from the immunization schedule after age 6.

Diphtheria immunization   Infants usually have a congenital passive immunity provided that the mother has had experience with the disease or has been adequately immunized prior to or during pregnancy to provide sufficient antibodies for placental transfer.

Combined preparation (DPT—diphtheria-tetanus toxoid, alum-precipitated or aluminum hydroxide-adsorbed, with pertussis vaccine)   Three injections are given intramuscularly, at 2-month intervals, starting at 2 months of age. A single dose is usually prepared in 0.5 ml, and the total immunizing dosage for pertussis is 12 protective antigenic units.

Recall (booster) injections of a single dose of the combined antigens are given at 18 months and again at 4 to 6 years of age. After that age, combined tetanus and diphtheria toxoids ("adult" type) should be used. Boosters are given at 14 to 16 years, every 10 years thereafter and following exposure. See Tetanus in Chapter 14, "Infectious Diseases," for management of wounds.

For primary immunization against diphtheria and tetanus when the above routine has not been carried out, the following recommendations are made: Under 6 years of age, the routine suggested for infants should be carried out. After 6 years of age, immunization should be carried out using adult-type tetanus and diphtheria toxoids. Two doses are given 4 to 8 weeks apart followed by a booster 1 year later.

Poliomyelitis vaccine   Trivalent oral poliomyelitis vaccine (TOPV) is recommended for immunization of infants, children, and adolescents. Primary immunization of infants requires three doses followed by a fourth dose 1 year later. Children and adolescents require only two doses followed by a third dose 1 year later. Booster doses are given as for tetanus.

Measles vaccine   Active immunization is indicated for all children unless there are specific contraindications. Further attenuated vaccines, e.g., Attenuvax, are given to susceptible people of any age. Primary immunization is recommended after 1 year of age to avoid interference with immunity through residual maternal antibody. A single injection is given. It should be preceded by a tuberculin test. Measles vaccine is also available in combination with rubella or with both rubella and mumps.

Contraindications

1. In pregnancy
2. In leukemia or in lymphoid and other generalized malignancies (In these three situations inactivated vaccine may be given.)
3. In tuberculosis (unless the patient is receiving antituberculous therapy)
4. During therapy which depresses antibody formation, for example, adrenal corticosteroids, irradiation, alkylation agents, and antimetabolites
5. Following use of gamma globulin, blood or serum, administration of live vaccine should be delayed for 8 weeks
6. In diseases in which the mechanism of delayed hypersensitivity is absent

Rubella vaccine   Live vaccine is recommended for children 1 to 14 years of age (see Measles Vaccine, above). Prior to 1 year, persisting maternal antibodies may interfere with development of immunity. Complicating, self-limited arthralgia (common in immunized adults) is rare in children.

Contraindications

1. In pregnancy
2. In leukemia or in lymphoid and other generalized malignancies
3. During therapy which depresses antibody formation

Mumps vaccine   A live attenuated mumps vaccine is available (see p. 283), and it is frequently administered to children (1 to 12 years of age) as part of a triple vaccine (measles-mumps-rubella).

The immunization schedule in Table 4-1 is based on suggestions by the American Academy of Pediatrics.

Passive immunization   Temporary protection may be afforded after exposure to several diseases or as prophylaxis in certain immune deficiency diseases associated with a defect in circulating antibodies. Immune serum globulin (ISG) is valuable for measles and infectious hepatitis (IH). It may be of some value in rubella, chickenpox, and hepatitis (SH). Special immune serum globulin preparations are available for mumps (see p. 283), pertussis, tetanus, vaccinia, and rabies. Antitoxin is available for tetanus, diphtheria, and gas gangrene.

Congenital passive immunity to diseases such as diphtheria, scarlet fever, rubella, rubeola, mumps, influenza, and poliomyelitis may be present during early infancy. It is due to the transplacental transfer of maternal immune bodies to the fetus in mothers who have had these diseases or who have been actively immunized.

Table 4-1. Immunization schedule

Age	Preparation*
2 months	DPT
	OPV
4 months	DPT
	OPV
6 months	DPT
	OPV
12 months	Measles vaccine, singly, in combination with rubella, or with rubella and mumps
1–12 years	Rubella, if not given previously, and mumps as indicated
18 months	DPT
	OPV
4–6 years	DPT
	OPV
14–16 years and every 10 years thereafter	DT (adult type)
	OPV

* Both live and inactivated vaccines should be used with caution in children with egg or dog-dander sensitivity (specific animal sensitivity depends on method of culture of virus) and in those with allergy to antibiotics (depending on addition of specific antibiotics to vaccines).

Special immunization procedures These are important when traveling in foreign countries or where epidemic or endemic disease prevails, such as smallpox, typhoid fever, epidemic typhus, yellow fever, plague, cholera, and Rocky Mountain spotted fever. The immunization schedule for typhoid fever is as follows: For children 10 years and over—two doses, 0.5 ml subcutaneously at a 4-week interval, or three doses at weekly intervals; for children 6 months to 10 years—0.25 ml in the same manner. A recall injection is given every 1 to 3 years, consisting of 0.1 ml intradermally or a single above-mentioned dose, subcutaneously. Paratyphoid vaccines are no longer used.

Smallpox vaccination Children with eczema, pyoderma, or other dermatoses should not be vaccinated. Siblings and close contacts of such children also should not be vaccinated. If it is necessary to immunize a child with eczema, vaccination should be followed by vaccinia-immune globulin, 0.3 ml per kg, intramuscularly, at another site.

The types of reaction are primary vaccinia or "take," major reaction, and equivocal reaction.

A primary vaccinia is characterized by the appearance, on about the fifth day, of a reddish papule that becomes vesicular, with a surrounding erythema. The vesicle is pearly and umbilicated. The height of the reaction is attained in 8 to 14 days, after which there is a gradual fading until about the twenty-first day, when the scab falls off, leaving the pitted scar. There may be accompanying malaise and temperature, most commonly about the ninth day. Rarely, from the third day on, there may be a generalized roseola type of rash, which disappears in 24 hours. (Vaccinia gangrenosa is a rare complication that should be treated with hyperimmune *vaccinia* gamma globulin; there is usually an absence of antibodies, agammaglobulinemia, marked lymphopenia, with no local leukocytic reaction, and lymphadenopathy in the region of the vaccination.)

A major reaction consists of a vesicular or pustular lesion, a definite area of induration or an area of congestion surrounding either a crust or ulcer. This reaction indicates successful revaccination.

An equivocal reaction, as the name implies, fails to reveal any of the above signs of definite evidence of successful immunization. Revaccination with a fresh lot of vaccine is recommended.

Dental prophylaxis   Dental care, even of the deciduous teeth, should be stressed. Improper care of the deciduous teeth may result in defective position and formation of the permanent set. At about 3 years of age there may be one or two visits to the dentist for the primary purpose of establishing rapport between him and the child and teaching him how to brush his teeth properly. These preliminary visits are followed by periodic dental examinations and care. Frequent ingestion between meals of foods high in sugar content promotes the formation of caries and should be avoided.

Some communities are instilling fluorides into their drinking water (1 part per million) in an effort to prevent dental caries. Fluorides are also available in oral form, e.g., Tri-Vi-Flor, containing 0.5 to 1.0 mg fluoride per 0.6 ml, which may be given to infants and children up to the age of 10 in areas where the water supply contains less than 0.7 part per million. The application of fluorides directly to the teeth is also of value in dental prophylaxis.

Other prophylactic measures   Urinalysis should be performed during the first year of life and at least yearly thereafter. Hemoglobin levels should be determined toward the end of the first year and periodically at 2- to 3-year intervals. Visual acuity should be evaluated at various stages of development; in the preschool child there should be an examination following the use of cycloplegics. Hearing, too, should be evaluated as development progresses, and audiometric studies should be made when crude tests, for example, whispered voice or watch sounds, indicate a deficiency.

Prevention of accidents and accidental poisoning   During childhood, after the first year, accidents are the greatest single cause of death. For every fatal injury there are 150 accidents that may produce a minor or major disability. These can be prevented, to a large extent, by proper safeguards through education of the parents and the community. Children who are accident-prone and in whom organic causes, e.g., visual or hearing defects, have been ruled out should be investigated for possible psychologic problems.

Accidents are more often triggered by a chain of events than simply by a single factor. The host etiologic factor and environment combination is a complex situation. Hunger or fatigue; hyperactivity; illness; pregnancy or menstruation of the mother; recent substitution of mother by another person caring for the child; tense relationship between parents; occurrence requiring most of mother's attention; and sudden change of child's environment are events shown statistically to predispose to accidents.

Discussions concerning accident prevention should be an integral part of the periodic medical evaluation. The common causes of injury for each particular developmental stage should be stressed to the parents. For example, during the first year, choking from aspiration of foreign bodies and food, falls, burns, and rarely, suffocation constitute about 85 percent of all fatal injuries; from 1 to 4 years, motor-vehicle accidents, burns, drowning, poisoning, and falls cause about 85 percent of accidental deaths. Special automobile harnesses and car seats are available for infants and young children. Measures for accident prevention should be emphasized to the parents, e.g., during the first year, improperly constructed toys such as those with sharp points or loose small parts, poorly designed playpens, harnesses, and straps should be avoided; later in childhood, flammable fabrics, e.g., cotton and certain synthetics, should be avoided especially in full skirts and flowing sleeves, and poisonous materials should be kept in inaccessible cabinets. Two-thirds of the deaths due to accidental poisoning could be prevented if aspirin, barbiturates, kerosene, lye, lead, and arsenic were made unavailable to small children.

Prevention of accidents to an individual child is based on two principles—protection and education. Until the end of the first year, there must be complete protection by the parents. By the time a child is ready for school he should have been sufficiently educated by virtue of having learned obedience and self-discipline to assume responsibilities for his own safety. In the interim period there is gradually decreasing protection by the parents and increasing education of the child to avoid accidents. The entire process is an integral part of growth and development.

Miscellaneous measures Penicillin is used in the prevention of recurrent rheumatic fever. Tuberculin testing in children will aid in searching out and eradicating tuberculosis. Testing should be performed at the end of the first year, every year thereafter during early childhood, every second year during later childhood, yearly during adolescence, and whenever exposure to tuberculosis is suspected (see p. 312). Children with chronic diseases, e.g., rheumatic heart disease, cardiac insufficiency, bronchopulmonary disease, and neurologic disorders, should be immunized with polyvalent influenza vaccine followed by annual booster doses because these children experience the highest mortality rates. Bacillus Calmette-Guérin vaccine (BCG) is recommended for children who are likely to be exposed to adults with active or recently arrested tuberculosis. (See Tuberculosis, Chapter 14, "Infectious Diseases.") Exposure to excess radiation from roentgenograms and fluoroscopic examinations should be limited to prevent iatrogenic diseases from that source. Exposure of the fetus to radiation must be avoided to prevent developmental anomalies.

Psychologic supervision The optimal emotional and social development of the child may be promoted through

1. Good parent-child relationships in the home and a favorable environment outside the home to help provide security for the child.
2. Teaching the parents the developmental pattern of the child at different stages and ages, so that they may encourage the attainment of his full potentialities but not push him beyond his capabilities.
3. Fostering self-confidence and independence in the child, so that he will be able to meet and solve his own problems and take his place in society.

Preparation for school and development of an acceptable life-style A child's view of life within his family constellation should be complemented by exposure to the experiences of others. Infants, children, and adolescents must be stimulated by nonschool learning, e.g., toys, books, radio, newspapers, parentally supervised television programs; by life situations, e.g., travel (even if limited to a bus ride), trips to the zoo, museum visits, sporting events; by exposure to future career possibilities—many adolescents are either unaware of, feel unprepared to enter, or simply do not know how to go about obtaining training for various professional or job opportunities. The need to provide such exposure to children living in socially and economically depressed environments is especially evident when consideration is given to causes of school failure and antisocial adolescent behavior.

REVIEW QUESTIONS

Each of the following questions or incomplete statements is followed by several suggested answers or completions. Select the one that is best in each case.

1. Children are most apt to be involved in accidents (*a*) immediately after a nap; (*b*) prior to dinner time; (*c*) after lunch; (*d*) before 10 A.M.
2. Primary immunization with the combined diphtheria and tetanus toxoid and pertussis vaccine should be started at (*a*) 2 months; (*b*) 4 months; (*c*) 6 months; (*d*) 9 months.
3. "Adult"-type DT is used for older children and adults because (*a*) heavier individuals require larger doses of antigen; (*b*) fewer reactions occur following its use; (*c*) it does not contain pertussis vaccine; (*d*) it causes a booster effect more promptly.

4. Immunizations for all the following diseases are recommended routinely in the first 2 years of life except for one: (a) pertussis; (b) smallpox; (c) diphtheria; (d) tetanus; (e) poliomyelitis.

5. Infants with a known history of febrile convulsions should receive (a) one-tenth to one-fifth; (b) one-fourth to one-half; (c) three-fourths the recommended dose of DPT.

6. Pertussis vaccine is included in the immunization schedule until the age of (a) 2 years; (b) 3 years; (c) 6 years; (d) 7 years; (e) 10 years; (f) 11 years.

7. The "adult" type of diphtheria and tetanus toxoid should be used after the age of (a) 6 years; (b) 8 years; (c) 10 years; (d) 12 years.

8. If thrombocytopenia occurs after a previous injection of pertussis antigen, then (a) pertussis immunization should not be repeated; (b) the dose should be reduced by 50 percent; (c) the original dose may be repeated; (d) future pertussis immunization should be carried out with adult-type DPT.

9. What is the earliest preferred time at which live attenuated measles vaccine should be given? (a) 3 months; (b) 12 months; (c) 24 months; (d) 36 months; (e) when exposed to rubella.

10. A tuberculin test should be routinely performed prior to immunization for (a) smallpox; (b) pertussis; (c) measles; (d) rubella.

11. Untreated tuberculosis is a contraindication to administration of (a) measles and rubella vaccines; (b) pertussis vaccine; (c) poliomyelitis vaccine.

12. The greatest usefulness of mumps vaccine is in (a) male children over the age of 6 years; (b) female children over the age of 6 years; (c) postpubertal males; (d) postpubertal females.

13. In the following questions, column I lists several diseases; column II lists several agents that are effective in affording temporary protection against these diseases after exposure. Match the items in both columns. (Items in column II may be used more than once, if necessary.)

I		II	
(A)	tetanus _____	(a)	ISG
(B)	diphtheria _____	(b)	IH
(C)	measles _____	(c)	Special immune serum globulin
(D)	mumps _____	(d)	Antitoxin
(E)	pertussis _____		
(F)	infectious hepatitis _____		
(G)	rabies _____		
(H)	vaccinia _____		
(I)	gas gangrene _____		

14. After the first year of life the greatest single cause of death during childhood is (a) meningitis; (b) accidents; (c) Wilms's tumor; (d) leukemia; (e) congenital heart disease.

5 PSYCHOLOGIC PROBLEMS

Psychologic problems in children are caused by damage—e.g., physical handicaps, chronic illness, minimal brain dysfunction—within the organism of the child, by conditions that exist within the environment, or by a combination of both. To determine the root cause or causes is not a simple matter, and frequently consultations from behavior specialists are necessary for both diagnosis and treatment.

Diagnosis should take into account hereditary and constitutional differences, rate of growth, environmental forces, birth history, disease, structure of body, and physiologic functioning. Behavior that is influenced by organic factors creates different psychologic problems—e.g., hyperactivity, perceptual distortion, language disorders—than do behavioral deviations that stem from psychogenic factors—e.g., delinquency, inordinate fears, hysteria, withdrawal. Nevertheless, it is usually an admixture of causes, organic and psychogenic, that create deviant behavior.

The social aspects of variable, regressive, or deviant behavior in children place a burden on the physician to act as agent for the values of the adult world which he represents. When he is asked to suggest treatment of children who manifest behavior problems, he is really being asked by parents to outline a plan of action that will make their child conform to their preconceived notion of behavior.

The determination of what characterizes normal behavior in children is extremely complex. Absolute normality is probably a meaningless phrase. On the other hand, within the cultural bounds of any society, relative normal behavior is measurable. If a child adjusts to the demands of his near environment and if his personality is not too dissimilar from that of children of his age, then relative normality has been achieved.

Normal children usually demonstrate orderly development and maturation in the various components of personality. Personality disorders emerge when there is significant deviation from orderly sequential maturation. Whenever there is extreme variation, be it regression or precocity, abnormal symptomatology emerges. However, the age of the child is important in viewing the behavior. What may be normal for one age group may be abnormal for another, e.g., fantasy and acting out is anticipated in a very young child, whereas some inhibition is expected when a child is of school age. The physician is usually the first person whom parents consult when a child presents symptoms of deviation in behavior. It is incumbent upon the physician therefore to be able to recognize early signs of psychogenic disorders.

Behavior difficulties and psychologic symptoms may arise when the basic security of the child is threatened. Parental rejection, sibling jealousy, and overprotection are some of the underlying factors in emotional insecurity and tension. On the other hand, the origin of the disturbances may be more obscure, for example, as when caused by intrafamily problems such as conflicting parental attitudes or an excessive need to control the child and inhibit his need for developing self-reliance and independence. However, the physician must understand that children differ in their temperaments and that not all children will react the same way when confronted with tension-laden situations.

All children need comforting and reassurance when they have undergone a stressful experience. Sometimes the most primitive measures, such as patting the child or touching him gently, become more soothing than the more advanced techniques of using caressing words. This is particularly true when a child is brought in for "shots" or when a prolonged illness develops. Whenever feasible, parents should be part of the comforting scene.

Although in the following pages each discussion centers about a particular manifestation of maladjustment, e.g., anorexia, masturbation, or thumb-sucking, the treatment of any psychologic problem or psychosomatic illness is successful only when the general personality difficulties and disturbed relationships have been ameliorated. The child should always be evaluated and treated as a total individual.

In addition to thorough physical examination and indicated laboratory tests, separate interviews with the parents and child are necessary to obtain a complete history. This history should include such data as the mental and motor development of the child; habits, e.g., feeding, rest, sleep, elimination, and manipulations of the body; attitudes and interreactions of the child, parents, and other members of the household; the neighborhood situation; and the school situation. Social workers may be of great help in obtaining various aspects of the history.

The physician must then determine whether he can treat the child adequately (not only the presenting symptom), adjusting the environment where necessary. For instance, he can encourage the parents to provide a healthier mental or emotional regimen for the child by replacing such poor attitudes as rejection or overprotection with love, acceptance, and approval. After his evaluation, the pediatrician may find the problem to be sufficiently complex that it can be handled better by the psychiatrist. (The psychotherapeutic agents, discussed in Chapter 6, "Drugs and Treatment," may be helpful as adjuvants to psychologic treatment by the pediatrician or the psychiatrist.)

ORGANIC FACTORS IN BEHAVIOR DISORDERS

Organic diseases may lead to behavior disorders. Cerebral disorders, e.g., hypoxia, postencephalitic syndrome, brain tumor, may directly produce emotional disturbances. Any disease associated with a physical handicap, e.g., cerebral palsy, chronic heart disease, asthma, may affect indirectly the behavioral patterns and psychologic functioning of the child. Intrapersonally, there may be demonstrated feelings of inferiority, frustration, isolation, and anxiety, or irritability. Hyperkinesis and aggressiveness may be demonstrated compensation. Environmentally, the home may be a serious overriding difficulty for the child because parents may be unable to accept the child's handicap; they may feel guilty about the child and thus reject or overprotect him. Further, conflicts between parents may provoke them to use the handicapped child as a means of expressing contempt or exasperation with each other. Siblings, too, frequently display jealousy, regarding the care extended to the handicapped child, and their guilt gets in the way of the child's functioning. The handicapped child in the community is often duped and mocked by his peers and others. When the handicap is not too obvious, the child is expected to perform as well as nonafflicted children. The physician must recognize that the handicapped child and family members require generalized and specific guidance if they are to create the proper kind of environment for the child.

PSYCHOSOMATIC PROBLEMS

Psychosomatic disorders seem to crop up when a child is unable to handle impending danger, e.g., taking a test in school, competing with older children, being asked to do something for which he feels inferior. The result is first anxiety, rage, or loss of control, followed by such fleeting ailments as abdominal pain, nausea, vomiting, breath-holding, and a score of other minor conditions. Usually such a child is seen as being immature.

Children sometimes feign somatic ailments in order to get attention from adults in their world, but occasionally the physician comes across a child who fantasizes illness in a way that real pain exists for him. Scoffing parents or physicians will only aggravate the condition of a truly hypochondriacal child. There is a difference between the conscious make-believe illnesses of children and the hysterical fantasy illness. The latter requires psychologic help.

ANOREXIA

Anorexia is characterized by refusal to eat or fussiness about food. As a possible cause, organic diseases, e.g., tuberculosis, anemia, or chronic infection, should always be ruled out.

In the pathogenesis of psychologic anorexia, the following factors require consideration:

1. The normal, relatively slow weight gain from 1 to 5 years of age, with less need for food; this can be misinterpreted by an anxious parent as anorexia.
2. The normal psychologic development of increasing independence from 1 to 5 years of age, during which period the refusal of food by the child is an avoidance of conforming to parental wishes, an attention-getting maneuver, a means of striking back at being neglected, or the imitation of older children.
3. Oversolicitude and overprotection regarding the child's food, for example, insisting that he can eat certain foods that supposedly are good for him.
4. Failure to permit and encourage normal feeding patterns to develop, e.g., continuing to feed him when he is ready to feed himself.
5. Foods that are prepared uninterestingly and that are presented unattractively.
6. More severe emotional maladjustment that may be involved when security has been imperiled, for instance, in parental rejection of the child, tensions between the parents, parent-child conflicts, or sibling jealousy.

Treatment

1. Organic disease, e.g., anemia, must be treated.
2. The psychogenic factors mentioned above should be corrected.
3. The child's need for security and permissive environment for growth and development and self-reliance should be met in order

to produce good emotional hygiene. (Often it is the parents who are insecure and need help to achieve security.)

4. Vitamin therapy, particularly administration of B complex, may be helpful in preventing or treating a secondary deficiency. Perhaps the major function of vitamin therapy is the relief of parental tension and fear over possible nutritional deficiency in the child who has been eating poorly.

OBESITY

There are individual constitutional differences in body build which sometimes make an accurate diagnosis of obesity difficult. Early in adolescence, following the physiologic spurt in weight, some children are mildly obese, and this corrects itself after puberty. Large weight gains, over short periods of time, always warrant investigation.

All holidays and joyous occasions are usually celebrated by people getting together and eating. Is it any wonder that the child who is obese calls upon eating to compensate for feeling disconsolate? The earliest memories of joy, fun, and feeling part of a group respond to parties at home and being at a table with mounds of food and laughter.

Obesity occurs rarely as a result of organic disease, e.g., endocrinologic disturbance, head injury, encephalitis, brain tumor. Overeating is the usual cause of obesity. If excess caloric intake occurs during critical periods (periods when the fat cells increase in number as well as in size) subsequent weight loss is extremely difficult. In some families, habit and custom foster the overeating, but in the great majority of cases, overeating and obesity are due to psychogenic or emotional factors. Food is frequently a symbolic substitute for love. Psychologically, the child eats for consolation and to escape from a frustrating environmental situation. The consequent obesity makes for further withdrawal, and release is again sought through eating. Withdrawal also promotes inactivity and failure to exercise.

The combined treatment is dietary and psychologic. The diet, although low in calories, should supply all the protein, vitamins, and minerals necessary. The psychologic treatment is the substitution of good for bad emotional hygiene, with relief of the basic anxiety and correction of maladjustment. Drugs, such as amphetamine, and thyroid extract are of no value.

ENURESIS

Enuresis is urinary incontinence, usually nocturnal, past 3 years of age. Children develop bladder control at different ages, some early, some late, and many normal children may not achieve control until $3\frac{1}{2}$ to 4 years of age.

Organic disease, e.g., pyelitis, congenital malformation of the urinary tract, irritation of the genitalia, and spina bifida, should always be ruled out by urinary, urologic, and other indicated examinations.

Enuresis in a physically normal child is usually only one of the manifestations of a psychologic maladjustment. It may have persisted since infancy, come on after an illness, or followed some emotional stress, such as starting school or the arrival of a new sibling. Poor training, for example, insistence on premature toilet training, is a frequent factor. More serious factors are insecurity resulting from jealousy of a sibling, parental rejection, emotional tensions, fears, and resentment against an overprotective environment.

Treatment is directed toward the child and his environment rather than the symptom. The causes are corrected to help provide security, an environment for healthy emotional growth and development, and the fostering of self-confidence and ability to handle problems. It may sometimes be necessary to have the help of a psychiatrist. Tofranil starting with 10 mg for young children and 25 mg for 7-year-olds is effective when given an hour before bedtime. The dosage may be doubled after a week if necessary. Restriction of fluids is of secondary importance. The use of a mechanical apparatus (such as an electric buzzer which starts when the sheet becomes slightly wet, awakens the child, and brings an end to micturition) may be successful in clearing the enuresis and may be generally helpful by increasing the confidence and lessening the secondary anxiety of the child. It is important to convey to parents that children are unable to control enuresis consciously and by willing it. The child's willpower is not as important as the feeling that he is receiving love and affection from his parents.

FINGER-SUCKING

Finger-sucking is normal infant behavior. It should be considered a problem only when carried well past infancy. Thumb-sucking is the most common type. There is a popular misconception that finger-sucking always interferes with tooth and jaw configuration. This is uncommon and occurs mainly when finger-sucking continues after the permanent teeth have begun to erupt. Callus formation may occur on the finger, but this is only a cosmetic problem.

The habit may become established during early infancy, particularly during the teething period. It has been suggested that excessive finger-sucking is partially due to inadequate length of sucking time during feeding. In general, it affords a comforting sensation and is particularly likely to occur at sleeping time and with fatigue, boredom, unhappiness, or insecurity. Finger-sucking may disappear spontaneously by a year; beyond this age, it will often persist until 3 or 4 years of age.

No treatment is needed during infancy, and any active interference, such as the use of restraints or bitter substances, is contraindicated.

A pacifier may be substituted for the thumb if accepted by the infant. Excessive finger-sucking beyond the first few years of life may be suggestive of poor emotional hygiene. This requires further investigation and probably psychologic treatment of the child and his family. The child should not be an object of constant scrutiny by the parents. Diversionary tactics can be employed which provide greater joy to the child than the sucking of the thumb.

TIC

Tics are repetitive, quick, involuntary movements that may last for a brief moment or intermittently come and go. They consist commonly of blinking, clearing the throat, dry coughing, shoulder shrugging, rotating the head to one side, or drawing the corner of the mouth downward. A happy and secure child rarely develops tics. Usually tics appear as a result of tense relationships within the home, internalized conflict relative to the parents' insistence upon specific behavior, sometimes because of overcontrolled feeding patterns. In the extreme form of tic, there may be a sharp outward flinging movement of both arms and legs simultaneously with a barking cry (Gilles de la Tourette disease). Although tics may appear as early as 18 months of age, the most frequent time of onset is the period from 6 years to puberty, when tensions may be generated by necessary socialization and by the child's attempts to become increasingly independent of his parents. A tic is often accompanied by other behavior disorders, e.g., shyness, restlessness, nightmares, vomiting, or nail-biting.

Treatment should be directed toward removing the tension within the environment and the conflicts thus engendered. Home factors, such as coercive or punishing parental attitudes or pressures to excel at school, may be precipitating causes. An overcompetitive school atmosphere may also be responsible. Direct psychotherapy may be required. The total personality structure of the child should be studied to determine the most effective therapy to alleviate the situation. Treatment, including environmental changes, is usually successful. Tics must be differentiated from chorea and neurologic disease causing uncontrolled and purposeless muscular movements.

FEARS AND PHOBIAS

All children demonstrate fear, and it is perfectly normal for them to be frightened when it is justified. Thus they learn to avoid situations that are threatening to them? Fear of the dark, dogs, loud noises, threats of violence, and failure in school are common. They usually are imitations of similar fears residing in parents who serve as their models, albeit the symbols may be different in the adults, and the fears may be masked.

Psychologic problems emerge when children are afraid of everything, i.e., when fear dominates their total perspective; when the effect of fear overrides their judgment and intelligence; when fantasy projections become reality to them. Excessive fear of some particular object or situation which is persistent and without justification is phobic. Phobia is a morbid fear, e.g., fear of falling from heights, fear of being smothered, fear of crowds. Phobias have to be treated by a behavioral specialist, psychologist, or psychiatrist.

All fears are closely connected with immaturity and feelings of insecurity. Obsessive fears (phobias) are so unreasonable that they cannot be eradicated by logic. A physician can help a child by showing him the normalcy of being afraid of a doctor and injections, thus paving the way for the child to self-correct the normal fears that he encounters.

MASTURBATION

Genital manipulation, or masturbation, is normal among children. It usually begins in the last half of the first year of life, soon after the discovery of the genitalia. The disclosure of this pleasant sensation frequently occurs through scratching local irritations and through the touching of genitalia by adults who care for the child. A child can learn about the feelings evoked by pleasurable manipulation before sexual awareness takes place.

Between 3 and 6 years of age, there is an early stirring of sexual feelings as a natural process of growing. It occurs to a degree in all children, and there is a desire to see and touch the genitals. During adolescence sensual feeling may be expressed in "dating," dancing, parties, and erotic daydreams and fantasies.

The majority of children masturbate to some extent in the early years, but the time of onset varies. Frequent masturbation, however, is often a manifestation of anxiety, tenseness, and insecurity. The genitals may be handled without the child's even being aware of people about him. Local irritation of the genital and anal areas is a predisposing factor occasionally. The practice may also be learned from others. In management, it is well to differentiate infrequent masturbation, which is not a behavior problem, from compulsive or uncontrollable masturbation, which is an expression of personality difficulties. The first needs no management except for reassurance to the family; the latter does require help.

In cases of compulsive masturbation, emotional situations that compel the child to this form of consolation and gratification should be corrected. It is necessary also to avoid increasing the sense of guilt in connection with masturbation. The parents should be enlightened about the erroneous conception that masturbation is harmful or may cause insanity. If the child shows concern about it, he should be told that many children masturbate to some extent and that it is harmless.

Interesting pursuits and play that will occupy a child will detract from masturbatory activity. Physicians should in all cases tell parents that their apprehensions about masturbation will cause more damage in relations with children than will actual secret masturbation, but the social implications must be brought to the surface. Open masturbation is frowned upon by society. It is a private venture.

SIBLING RIVALRY

Sibling rivalry is normal and common in families, and usually one child becomes the scapegoat while another is labeled the "instigator." Invariably, the roles are reversed in the attitudes of the parents, and they are unable to see that they unconsciously or subtly arouse the discrimination. It may be difficult to explain the idea to parents, because the parents become defensive and refuse to really see what actually does take place in the household. A simple technique is to suggest that both children involved are in need of guidance and better balance in the pecking order of preference.

Where open rejection exists regarding any child, siblings react with anger because they are unsure about whether they will receive the same type of censure from parents. Nagging, direct derision, and subtle contemptuous retorts by parents, for whatever reason, will exact a toll from the child, and the price that parents have to pay will be great. Stepparents who bring children into the arena of sibling rivalry have to be cautious in developing a setting that makes adjustment possible for two rival groups of children.

LYING—FANTASIES

Young children, usually between 3 and 6 years of age, make up stories about things happening to them that scare the daylights out of their parents. Parents become alarmed when these "lies" appear regularly. Actually, children get rid of their insecurities by manufacturing make-believe stories and telling them to anybody who will listen. This is the way they neutralize their insecurities and fears. Parental fears should be allayed by explaining the normality of this behavior and suggesting that the opportunity be provided for the child to differentiate "real" from "imagined" tales in a number of game situations.

However, a distinction would be drawn between the fantasies expected from young children and a proliferation of fantasies which is used to compensate for every action. If a child is unable to deal with reality in his everyday living, then the fantasy life must be considered extreme enough to warrant specialized behavioral treatment. Older children lie in self-defense, in imitation of adult behavior, to gain admiration, or to gain attention. Pathologic lying that is extensive manifests itself in overall complex verbal productions. Usually a skein of truth is elaborated upon and an "impossible" tale emerges.

TEMPER TANTRUMS

Temper tantrums occur usually from 1 to 4 years of age and are characterized by the child's throwing himself on the floor, kicking, screaming, and holding his breath. (Breath-holding may be so protracted that unconsciousness, followed by spontaneous recovery, ensues.) Organic illnesses, such as convulsions, must be differentiated. Temper tantrums are commonly precipitated by frustration when the child fails to gain his desires; they may be based on sibling jealousy or antagonism between the child and the parent.

Immediate management consists of placing the child in a safe area and leaving him alone for a few minutes. Punishment increases the child's antagonism.

Frequent temper tantrums do not occur in isolation. They combine with other psychologic nuances, e.g., inordinate fear or food avoidance, and have to be treated accordingly. When temper tantrums become all-pervasive and exaggerated, play therapy is indicated to provide a neutral outlet for inner frustrations and hostility.

THE WRONG FRIENDS

Parents regale physicians with the "goodness" of their offspring and the fact that they get into trouble at home, in school, and in the community because they have "the wrong friends." Unfortunately, troubled children seek out troubled friends. They have a need to lean on and add to each others' difficulties even though the basic personality patterns of each of the wrong friends may be different. Physicians can help by suggesting activities that will produce a difference in friends, without resorting to a condemnation of the existing ones.

SCHOOL PLACEMENT

Lack of readiness for school placement can create difficulties and aberrant behavior in children. Expectative levels of parents or teachers that cannot be met because of the immaturity of a child result in psychologic problems that can influence school success in later years. Physicians can be helpful by indicating to a parent that an initial loss of a year in placement from kindergarten to the first grade or retention in a later grade may help the child in future school success.

DIVORCE

A home broken through divorce creates psychologic difficulties in a child for many reasons. The time spent with each parent is not balanced. Loyalty to the parent with whom the child lives is intensified. Sometimes the child feels that he is at fault in breaking up the home. Material things become overemphasized by the parent who lives away from the child. The time spent with the child by the parent who leaves the house eventually becomes a chore, which brings out arguments and hostility between that parent and the child. The absent parent tries to establish rules for the child to follow without being there to implement them. Divorce does not have to be more destructive to the child than the unhappy marriage. The child can be relieved of guilt by the physician. Fears can be allayed by suggesting that the failure of the marriage only shows that adults can fail at things as well as children.

PREPARATION FOR HOSPITALIZATION AND SURGERY

Psychologic preparation of the child for hospitalization and surgery is essential. Children have to be reassured that they will return to their homes shortly after hospitalization. Prior to hospitalization, he should be told in terms he can understand how he will benefit from the procedure and what to expect. For example, if he is to have general anesthesia, he may be told about the mask and the odor. If there will be postoperative pain, as in tonsillectomy, he should be told that there will be a sore feeling in his throat. Knowledge of what to expect will help the child meet the situation adequately. Whenever possible, the procedure should be visually and tactually experienced, e.g., the child should actually hold a mask in his hand, a scent of spray similar to anesthesia should be seen and smelled, the type of room he is to be in should be depicted. Parents should be given sufficient information to answer those questions which the child is certain to ask. Evasion, lying, or excessive reassurance tend to increase the child's feeling of insecurity. The child may be admitted to the hospital 12 to 24 hours prior to elective surgery. He may bring a familiar object, e.g., a toy or a pillow, to help create a tangible tie to the home and add to his security. Allied health professionals, e.g., play therapists and social workers, play a significant role in bridging the gap between physician and patient. If possible, mothers should remain in the hospital for overnight stays, especially with young children. It is helpful for the parent to be present when the child emerges from anesthesia.

Parents should be told that transient behavior changes, e.g., unfounded fears, or regressive behavior, e.g., enuresis or wanting to be fed, may occur following hospitalization.

PREPARATION FOR A NEW BABY

Since many of the emotional problems of childhood stem from sibling rivalry, preparing a child for the advent of a new baby is an important aspect of mental hygiene. Children between 3 to 4 years of age suffer most from sibling jealousy; adolescents experience it least.

Many well-meaning parents begin to involve the young child in the mother's pregnancy long before the birth of the new baby. They expect the child to understand how long the 9-month period will last and to follow each phase as they explain it. Of course, this is beyond the ability of the preschool child. The child should know that the mother is pregnant at the time when the physical manifestations become obvious. He then needs assurance that his own status in the family will not be upset by the newcomer. This is a good time for the father to spend more time with the child, thus helping to wean him from total dependency on the mother.

There should be emphasis on the rewards of being more mature—being more capable of taking care of his own needs, being able to express himself, having his own friends.

If the parents plan to send the child to nursery school, he should be enrolled before he is told about the new baby so that he does not feel thrust out. Nursery school offers the child the opportunity for a world of his own where he can become more self-reliant physically, socially, and emotionally.

If it is necessary to have the child live away from home while the mother is in the hospital, he should be properly prepared. Careful thought should be given to the person in whose custody the child will be while the mother is away. It is better for the child to remain in his own home rather than to move him to unfamiliar surroundings.

ADOPTION

Married couples may adopt children because they are unable to have any of their own or to fill out their desired family complement. Social agencies preferably should be used in the adoption process since they have the experience and professional awareness of how to match a child to a family. Usually, they make every effort to place a healthy child in a home where normal upbringing can be expected. Prospective adoptive parents are informed when an infant or child is handicapped. Adoption during infancy is best for the child because it approximates the relationship between a child and natural parents.

The child of 3 or 4 years of age is aware of environmental changes and may resent them for varying periods even though he is moving to a better home. Adoption in early infancy also involves a risk in that abnormalities and developmental deviations may escape detection. In general, it can be recommended to prospective parents that if possible they select a baby whose background has been carefully investigated and whose physical examination and laboratory tests, e.g., Wassermann, have revealed no abnormalities. Interracial adoptions require lengthy counseling of parents to help them recognize the difficulties involved and to prevent exploitation of the children.

Older children who are adopted may have been through trying emotional experiences and may have developed problems that require special understanding. However, with careful and sympathetic handling by the social worker, foster parents, and the physician, these children and families should work out a happy, normal life. The older child should meet and visit with the adoptive parents and be allowed to take familiar things with him—toys and clothes. His sensitivity about his adopted status may make him interpret discipline or deprivation of any kind as rejection. He needs assurance that he is wanted.

The question of how and when to inform the child that he is adopted always arises. Many feel that it is best to begin to tell the child of his adoption at about 4 years of age. He should know that he has been chosen deliberately and is wanted and that his home is permanent. He may be told of his own nationality and the religious faith of his natural parents. A more detailed explanation may have to be presented at school age, at adolescence, and at early maturity when concern may be expressed about his real family background and heredity. Parents who adopt physically handicapped children should be assisted with particular reference to the additional emotional problems that may arise because of the handicap.

CHILD PLACEMENT

TEMPORARY PLACEMENT

Temporary placement may be indicated when the home atmosphere has become too threatening to the psychic stability or the physical safety of the child. Placement may be either for a short time, because of temporary crisis in the home (mother's illness), or for a longer period, because of a total collapse of the family. Severe emotional breakdown of the child may also indicate the need for separating him from his home environment.

Foster home This is often the best type of temporary placement, particularly if the foster home has been carefully selected and is approved by a social agency. Here, the child has an opportunity to live in a family setting with friendly and understanding adults. Supervision of these homes is usually under the local city departments of welfare and health.

Residential treatment centers The child who is emotionally ill can benefit from a period spent in this kind of setting, where physician, psychiatrist, psychologist, and social worker combine their efforts to rehabilitate the child's total personality.

The pediatrician can guide the family through the period of anxiety involved in the decision to place the child and work with them to help prepare the child for his new environment. It is important to emphasize that relationships between the child and his parents must be maintained throughout the temporary placement period through regular visits, telephone calls, and letters. The child must not feel that he is being abandoned or that his own parents have ceased to love him. Because of the intense situation that leads to placing the child, the help of others may be needed who will work with the parents and the child throughout this period.

MINIMAL BRAIN DYSFUNCTION

Minimal brain dysfunction (MBD) is a complex syndrome characterized by (1) limited alterations of behavior; (2) disturbances in motor and intellectual functioning; (3) learning disabilities. The clinical manifestations cross over between organicity and functionality, e.g., motor coordination, concrete rather than abstract thinking. Gross and localized structural damage are not present in the central nervous system, although higher level and symbolic actions that are sensitive to its integrity are usually demonstrated, e.g., impairment of perceptual and conceptual functioning, disorders of speech and communication, attention and concentration. Electroencephalography is usually of no value in diagnosis. Characteristics of functioning include hyperactivity, a wide scatter on intelligence tests in spite of average or above average IQs, and inability to discriminate appropriately regarding size, position, time, and space. Frequent "soft" equivocal or borderline neurologic indicators are hyperkinesis, poorly coordinated fine motor movements, and mixed laterality. Disorders of motor functioning include delayed motor milestones and general awkwardness. Academic achievement is usually retarded in reading, writing, and drawing. MBD children are usually confused about written instructions and show extreme variability in their performance. Their organization of effort is usually chaotic. Thinking processes are disorganized and can be mistaken for autism. Emotional characteristics include impulsiveness, explosiveness, and loss of control. Social behavior is usually negative and antisocial. Not all the clinical symptoms appear in any one child. Diagnosis should be made by pooling together pediatric, neurologic, psychologic, speech and hearing, and educational findings.

Minimal brain dysfunction may be due to genetic variation (it occurs with much greater frequency in males than females and not uncommonly occurs in several males in the same family), biochemical alterations, perinatal brain insult, illnesses, and environmental factors. Treatment requires early recognition by the pediatrician and consists of providing good management routines at home and special education following the complete evaluation. Psychotherapeutic drugs, e.g., Ritalin or amphetamines, may be of value but should be used only as part of a total management routine. Prognosis is good if special education is combined with counseling when needed and the fears of parents are allayed. Learning problems almost always emerge with children who show minimal brain dysfunction.

DYSLEXIA (Reading Disability)

Reading disabilities in children generally appear when they are beginning school. The child who has difficulty in learning to read feels inadequate as he begins to fail. Soon, his self-image is denigrated, and he develops emotional dysfunction in response to his failure. As the child struggles to keep up with his peers, he usually becomes irritable, aggressive, or defensive. Many times, depending upon other factors, he withdraws and feels rejected.

As much as 10 to 20 percent of elementary school children with normal or above average intelligence fail to progress appropriately in reading. This condition is more frequent in boys than in girls and is often the underlying cause of acting out and behavioral difficulties in the classroom and of school phobias. Treatment should be preceded by a determination of whether the syndrome is primary (dyslexia) or secondary reading disability.

Primary reading disability is characterized by perceptual motor inefficiency, inability to integrate and associate auditory and visual symbols, word substitutions, limited visual and/or auditory memory, and letter reversals. One or more "soft" neurologic signs, e.g., cross laterality, confusion of spatial dimensions, are usually evident upon examination, and in conjunction with a thorough birth and developmental history, minimal brain dysfunction or maturational lag is frequently revealed.

Secondary reading disability is evidenced by the child with adequate neurologic development but with emotional problems which affect school functioning as well as other aspects of social and interpersonal living.

Regardless of cause, feelings of worthlessness and behavioral disturbance are often concomitants of reading disability and thus make unequivocal diagnosis difficult. Treatment should be preceded by a comprehensive evaluation, which should include psychologic and educational testing, neurologic, audiometric, and ophthalmologic examination, and a developmental and school history.

When primary reading disability is diagnosed, treatment consists of corrective educational techniques on an individual or small-group basis. If the problem is secondary reading disability, a course of counseling or psychotherapy is required, followed by corrective education if the child is far enough behind. With some children, psychotherapy should be combined with corrective procedures. Nearly all children will show some improvement with treatment, and the physician should be directly involved with the special education therapist and the psychologist.

DISORDERS OF LANGUAGE, SPEECH, VOICE, AND HEARING

These are considered here because emotional factors are frequently involved as causes or results. Some form of psychotherapy is often necessary, but this is usually decided upon after consultation with the speech therapist or audiologist.

LANGUAGE DISORDERS

Language may be defined as the ability to communicate one's ideas and feelings and in turn to understand the ideas and feelings of others. Communication may be accomplished through gesture, pantomime, etc., but in our society, the means of communication is through the verbal symbol. There are many etiologic factors such as deafness, mental retardation, cerebral palsy, and psychoneuroses which may interfere with language development, but a causal relationship should not be assumed without a complete overall evaluation.

Crying, babbling, voice imitation, understanding what is said, and then the use of language for communication is the order of processes by which children acquire speech, but the process of acquiring speech is different from the manner in which children acquire language. Language is built by the child from the words, thoughts, and ideas that are transmitted to him by peers and adults in his environment. Unless the child can establish some meaning to the words that are heard, language remains an ineffective tool. Language does not always progress at the same pace as general development but parents can stimulate the growth of language in their child, e.g., verbal games, group interaction, exposure to live children's theater, use of the tape recorder. Although the primary goal is the comprehension of language in the child, spontaneous speech should be accepted. With very young children from 2 to 4 years of age the quality of the language is not nearly as important as the expansion of language.

SPEECH DISORDERS

Virtually all children possess the physical-organic equipment that is needed to make the sounds that are required in speech. Considerable variation exists in the onset and speed of speech development. Cleft palate and cleft lip can create pure speech disorders. Impairment of hearing, which prevents auditory perception, will affect the reproduction of sounds in the young child. Enunciation will be faulty because of some physical conditions, e.g., defects of tongue, lips, teeth; deformity of palate, uvula, and larynx. However, most speech disorders are found in combination with language disorders.

If language and speech have not developed in a child by 24 months of age, careful evaluation should be undertaken. The physician is the first person to whom the parents will go to for advice. When specific reasons for the delay of speech are determined, the physician can advise parents what means should be undertaken for rehabilitation. When language and speech therapy are necessary, they should be started in concordance with the age of development. Stuttering and lisping are language and speech problems that have to be dealt with. Children develop gross feelings of inadequacy when their speech disorders are exposed and made fun of by their peers. Speech disorders can be associated with aphasia, mental retardation, emotional disturbance, and cerebral palsy. Baby talk, which is a common complaint of mothers to pediatricians, is not a speech disorder. It is a regressive action that goes along with other psychologic manifestations. It frequently appears with the advent of a new baby in the household. Stuttering is the most frequent speech disorder, but it must be differentiated from the nonfluency which occurs frequently in children between 2 to 4 years of age. If parents visit their tenseness on a child whose speech is nonfluid, it may very well cause an exaggeration similar to stuttering, e.g., tonic and clonic spasms of a pathologic nature. Children become more fluid in speech as their communication skills develop, and language thrives when the emotional climate in the home is valid. When a child exhibits marked hesitancy and nonfluency in speech past 4 years of age, a speech pathologist and psychologist should be used for evaluation and treatment.

VOICE DISORDERS

Voice disorders may be secondary to other impairments such as hearing loss, cleft palate, enlarged adenoids, etc. They may also result from organic impairment of the vocal apparatus itself, as well as misuse of the vocal apparatus. Medical and surgical procedures play a large part in the alleviation of vocal problems, but almost always these must be accompanied by retraining in the use of the voice. Voice disorders are frequently exhibited in the emotionally disturbed or psychotic child. In these instances, some form of psychotherapy along with vocal retraining is essential for complete rehabilitation.

HEARING DISORDERS

In all cases of suspected hearing loss, the cooperation of the otologist and audiologist is mandatory. Early differential diagnosis to determine the cause of the hearing deficiency is basic to efficient rehabilitation procedures. Peripheral hearing loss may involve either conduction or perception of sound or both. The conduction system may be affected by ear malformations, trauma, infections such as otitis media, and diseases of adjacent structures such as the nose and throat. The perception of sound may be affected by prenatal maternal conditions such as rubella or nutritional deficiency. Caution should be exercised in the administration of certain drugs (quinine, streptomycin, neomycin, etc.) to either the pregnant woman or the child since such drugs may cause deafness. Specific brain injury or disease may interfere with the interpretation of sounds and produce symptoms markedly similar to those found in peripheral deafness, and exhaustive study is required before a final diagnosis can be established.

Pure-tone audiometric tests, speech-reception tests, and psychogalvanic skin-resistance audiometric tests are used in the establishment of a diagnosis. Children with congenital or early hearing loss, whether peripheral or not, or children who are unable to interpret sound need direction in almost every aspect of their development and functioning. In such instances, the audiologist, educational therapist, speech pathologist, and psychologist assume major roles.

Mild degrees of hearing loss can go unnoticed for long periods of time and thus interfere with a child's ability to learn, e.g., teachers' instructions and explanations are not comprehended, parental explanations are not fully understood, and learning from peers may be limited. Physicians should pay special attention to even mild impairment of hearing, since a child's personality development and psychologic peculiarities may be intimately tied in with slight hearing loss.

PSYCHOSES

Psychoses in children, no longer rare, are being reported with increasing frequency. More frequent, however, are psychotic reactions, e.g., marked depression following a traumatic incident such as witnessing a horribly violent episode, withdrawal and/or retarded functioning following prolonged separation from the mother at an early age. The incidence in males is two to four times greater than in females.

The organic psychoses may be acute or chronic and may be classified as organic or functional. Their course is determined by the nature of the organic disease process. The acute organic psychoses occur during the course of febrile diseases, drug toxicity, Sydenham's chorea, and convulsive disorders. They are characterized by delirium whose severity and duration follow the severity and duration of the underlying disease. Chronic organic psychoses may be symptomatic of degenerative disease of the brain or of permanent and severe brain injury. Treatment consists of whatever measures are appropriate to the underlying disease. The psychosis will disappear if successful treatment of the organic illness is possible. Various medications such as barbiturates, coal tar, phenothiazine, and bromides may rarely be etiologic factors in producing mental symptoms. In the course of ACTH and adrenal corticosteroid therapy, emotional and even psychotic symptoms can occur. Cessation of the medications will usually result in a return to normal behavior.

CHILDHOOD SCHIZOPHRENIA

Etiology   The cause is unknown, but hereditary and constitutional predisposition, environmental stresses especially in early infancy, and brain disease have been suggested. (Electroencephalographic patterns may be normal or epileptiform, or generally disorganized brain waves may be revealed.)

Clinical features

1. Diminished interest in surroundings and distortions in personal identity and body images.
2. Regression in behavior and interests to those appropriate to an earlier age.

3. Disturbance in motility. This may be characterized by too little movement; too much movement; or unusual motility, such as bizarre gestures, posturing, whirling around in circles, and echopraxia (repetition of observed movements).
4. Disturbance in speech. Speech may be extremely limited or extraordinarily rapid. Made-up words may be used, or odd combinations of actual words may be used in an unexpected manner. There may be echolalia (repetition by the child of what is said to him) at an age when this is no longer normal (after 3 years).
5. Acute disturbance in the mother-and-child relationship, with excessive clinging, marked hostility, or rejection of the child.
6. Alterations in sleep pattern.

Running throughout the behavior pattern is the evidence that thought processes are disturbed. In some children, ideas seem to come completely from within (autistic thinking) and bear little or no relation to the environment.

For the diagnosis of schizophrenia, all the above clinical features should be present, although their severity may vary widely.

INFANTILE AUTISM

Infantile autism usually appears during the first 6 months of life. It is manifest by extreme withdrawal, lack of response to mother, and resistance to environmental changes—"desire for the preservation of sameness." They may appear to be retarded because of their maldevelopment of basic social and intellectual skills. At 3 or 4 years of age, the autistic child may be mute, helpless, and functioning in general on an idiot level. About one-third of autistic children appear to be able to achieve at least a minimal social adjustment, regardless of the kind of treatment they receive.

SYMBIOTIC PSYCHOSIS

In contrast to the autistic infant this one starts out apparently normal and makes a good relationship with his mother. During the second to fourth year of life symptoms appear which are characterized by an inability to separate from the mother. Onset is frequently precipitated by birth of a sibling, hospitalization, or other situations involving mother-child relationship.

Prognosis   The prognosis of childhood psychoses is poor, but in some cases (especially symbiotic psychosis) improvement may be considerable with subsequent good social functioning, although the child may remain apparently shy and have a few peculiar mannerisms. In some there is no improvement; there may even be continued regression in spite of treatment.

BATTERED-CHILD SYNDROME

This term has been applied to children who are subject to severe and frequent injury, physical or emotional, by parents or parent surrogates.

The nature of the injuries and some characteristic features of the history help establish a correct diagnosis. The suspicion of willful trauma is enough justification to report these cases to the authorities. In many states, reporting physicians are protected by statute against legal harassment by parents.

The following clinical features should arouse suspicion:

1. A history of being born out of wedlock or of having one stepparent—often other siblings are well cared for and well nourished.
2. Malnutrition and nutritional anemia.
3. Multiple skin injuries in varying stages of healing from recent ecchymoses to long-healed scars.
4. Painful swelling of one or more extremities.
5. Radiologic evidence of multiple long-bone fractures of diverse age.
6. Radiologic evidence of epiphyseal separation. (When the epiphyseal centers involved are cartilaginous, initial roentgenograms are negative, but subsequent films demonstrate subperiosteal calcification, at times ensheathing the shaft.) Epiphysiolysis may be attributable to yanking or twisting of the extremities.
7. Subdural hematoma with absence of diagnostic evidence of hemorrhagic diathesis or accidental trauma.

Offending parents appear to be earnestly concerned over their child's condition; they are often severely psychiatrically disturbed. The child's physical needs must be met, and a complete evaluation of the family situation should be made before treatment is completed and he is returned to the home.

Though in the past it was thought that most offending adults were socioeconomically deprived, more recent evidence indicates that no stratum of society is immune from sudden outbursts of violent behavior. A concern exists about the subtle difference that may exist between socially acceptable parental administration of physical punishment and uncontrolled acts of violence which constitute "child abuse." We should be equally aware that parental neglect may currently represent a legally acceptable but nonetheless undesirable form of behavior.

REVIEW QUESTIONS

1. Behavior difficulties can arise from (*a*) parental rejection; (*b*) sibling jealousy; (*c*) hypoxia at birth; (*d*) all the above; (*e*) *a* and *b* only.
2. Anorexia can be due to the following: (*a*) chronic infection; (*b*) insistence that

child eat normal amounts of food during an acute illness; (c) individual taste preferences; (d) all the above; (e) a and b only.

3. One of the following statements concerning enuresis is not true: (a) organic disease can be an etiologic factor; (b) premature toilet training can be an etiologic factor; (c) enuresis is frequently found to occur in more than one member of a family; (d) enuresis is urinary incontinence past 5 years of age; (e) diurnal enuresis is more indicative of organic causation than is nocturnal diuresis.

4. Obesity in an adolescent is most difficult to cure if (a) it began at 4 to 5 years of age; (b) it began at the onset of adolescence; (c) the child prefers high-carbohydrate foods; (d) it began in infancy; (e) the child prefers high-fat foods.

5. The most frequent time of onset of tics is (a) 12 to 24 months; (b) 24 to 36 months; (c) 3 to 6 years; (d) 6 years to puberty.

6. The major functional psychosis of childhood is (a) schizophrenia; (b) manic-depressive psychosis; (c) hysterical psychosis; (d) involutional melancholia.

7. Echolalia is considered abnormal after the age (a) 18 months; (b) 24 months; (c) 30 months; (d) 36 months.

8. Childhood schizophrenia is characterized by all the following except (a) bizarre seizures; (b) regression in behavior; (c) spasmus nutans; (d) echopraxia; (e) autistic thinking.

9. A 2-year-old female is brought into the emergency room of a hospital by her mother with the chief complaint that the child has a pain in her right arm of 24 hours' duration. Trauma is denied. Inspection of the child reveals that she is very apprehensive and withdrawn and her skin is covered by numerous healed scars. The mother explains that these are old mosquito bites. The right elbow is swollen and tender, and x-ray reveals fracture of the right elbow as well as a healed fracture of the left radius.

   A diagnosis that should be strongly suspected in the above case is (a) osteogenesis imperfecta; (b) hypervitaminosis D; (c) battered-child syndrome; (d) rickets; (e) accident-prone child.

10. Considering age at onset, which one of the following is apt to occur at the earliest age: (a) school phobia; (b) premature menarche; (c) symbiotic psychosis; (d) tic; (e) Hodgkin's disease.

11. A careful evaluation should be undertaken if language and speech have not developed in an otherwise apparently normal child by (a) 12 months; (b) 24 months; (c) 36 months; (d) 5 years.

12. The most frequent speech disorder in a child past 4 years of age is (a) baby talk; (b) lisping; (c) stuttering; (d) nonfluency.

13. The incidence of psychoses in children is (a) two to four times greater in females than in males; (b) two to four times greater in males than in females; (c) occurs with the same incidence in both sexes.

14. The most frequent age of onset of infantile autism occurs (a) immediately after birth; (b) first year of life; (c) second year of life; (d) at any age that behavior can still revert to the infantile type.

15. Hyperkinesis, poorly coordinated fine motor movements, and mixed laterality are (a) signs of gross organic disturbance; (b) associated most commonly with severe mental retardation; (c) associated most commonly with minimal brain dysfunction; (d) associated most commonly with superior intelligence.

16. A 4-year-old child cannot ride a tricycle, is not welcome in the homes of his friends because he is difficult to manage, falls often, frequently creates situations in which he is unsafe. He has a normal EEG and an IQ of 108. The most

likely diagnosis is (a) cerebral palsy; (b) mild mental retardation; (c) minimal brain dysfunction; (d) normal child; (e) brain tumor.

17. Minimal brain dysfunction occurs (a) more frequently in females than in males; (b) more frequently in males than in females; (c) with the same frequency in both sexes.

18. The incidence of reading disabilities in elementary school children with normal intelligence is (a) 1 to 2 percent; (b) 10 to 20 percent; (c) 30 to 40 percent; (d) over 40 percent.

6
DRUGS AND TREATMENT

GENERAL MEASURES

Rest Children with an acute illness should be kept at rest. Attempts to restrict the child to complete bed rest are often impossible and may be more upsetting to the child and do more harm than permitting some freedom in bed. Occasionally the youngster may refuse to stay in bed in his own room for the entire day but is willing to lie in his parents' bed or on the sofa in another room for part of the day. It is best to keep the temperature (72°F) and humidity (65 percent) of the sickroom constant. Chilling or overheating of the child should be avoided. During convalescence, activities may be resumed gradually. This may be more easily said than done, for it is difficult to restrain the child, once the acute phase has passed.

Occupational activity   Depending on the age of the child, games, records, reading, or watching television, etc., are most helpful in keeping the youngster at rest. The ingenuity of the parents is often taxed severely to hold the child's interest.

Psychologic care   A favorable environment and all the practices of good emotional hygiene are most important to provide security for the child confined to bed. This should receive even more emphasis when the child is hospitalized and separated from his parents (see p. 83).

Diet and fluids   During an acute illness, unless there is some contraindication, such as vomiting, the child may be offered a regular diet. He should be permitted to eat as little as he wishes because it is not necessary to meet nutritive requirements during a short-term illness. Administration of easily tolerated liquids, for example, broth, sweetened tea, diluted fruit juices, carbonated beverages, will compensate for excessive loss of fluid and electrolytes due to fever, increased perspiration, and increased respiratory rate which otherwise predisposes to dehydration and acidosis. It is advisable to forewarn the mother that usually there is a slow return of the normal appetite following an illness.

During chronic illness, an attempt should be made to fulfill nutritive requirements with particular emphasis on protein, vitamin, and mineral needs. At times small frequent feedings are taken better than three large meals. Another aid in fulfilling caloric and protein needs is to fortify the food taken, e.g., serving egg nogs with osterized hard-boiled egg (raw egg is highly allergenic), adding sugar to fruit drinks, and administering oral amino acids.

The psychologic aspects of feeding are of particular importance during an illness. For example, forcing the child to eat may stimulate the development of a psychologic anorexia, which may prove troublesome.

Bowel regulation   Parents are usually concerned about constipation during an illness. They should be reassured that this is temporary and not harmful. If there is no bowel movement for 72 hours or more, a mild cathartic, such as milk of magnesia, is all that is necessary.

ANTIBIOTICS AND CHEMOTHERAPY

Certain principles guide the use of antibacterial agents:

1. Selection of a therapeutic agent on the basis of susceptibility of the causative (if cultured) or probably causative organism (see Table 6-1).
2. Administration of adequate dosages by an effective route for a sufficient period of time to eradicate or control the infection (see Table 6-2).

3. Selection of an appropriate agent that can be administered with the least discomfort and expense to the patient.

Combined therapy (two or more agents that act through different mechanisms) may be indicated in

1. Severe infections: Kanamycin and either penicillin or ampicillin for sepsis in the neonate.
2. Serious infection in which the causative organism is in doubt and while awaiting bacteriologic diagnosis.
3. Infections such as tuberculosis in which a combination of drugs, isoniazid and para-aminosalicylic acid, reduces the occurrence of bacterial resistance to isoniazid.

Mode of action   Antibacterial agents produce their effect by a complex reaction between the host, the drug, and the microorganism. Three sites of action on bacteria have been claimed: (1) cell wall, (2) cell membrane which encloses the cell cytoplasm, (3) cell cytoplasm, in which essential metabolic reactions occur affecting (*a*) ribosomes—kanamycin, gentamicin, chloramphenicol; (*b*) nucleic acid metabolism—griseofulvin; (*c*) intermediary metabolism (reactions producing energy or macromolecular precursors)—sulfonamides. In general, the drugs that act on the wall or membrane are bactericidal and those which interfere with the metabolic processes of the cytoplasm are bacteriostatic. Penicillin and bacitracin probably affect the incorporation of amino acids into the polypeptides of the bacterial cell wall, thus interfering with the formation of this protective covering and rendering such bacterial cells extremely vulnerable to osmotic lysis. Streptomycin, polymyxin, and novobiocin affect the cell membrane by altering its permeability. Streptomycin may also act by inhibiting protein synthesis in the bacterial cell protoplasm, which is the mode of action of chloramphenicol. The tetracyclines also inhibit protein synthesis within the protoplasm, but the exact biochemical effect has not been elucidated. Sulfonamides structurally resemble and replace para-aminobenzoic acid, an integral part of folic acid, which is essential for bacterial growth and multiplication.

Combinations of bactericidal agents may have a synergistic effect against resistant organisms. The final eradication of the invading bacteria must be accomplished by the host's own cellular and humoral defenses.

Certain species of bacteria are naturally sensitive or naturally resistant to particular agents. Resistance may be acquired by repeated passages through patients treated with subcurative doses of antibacterial agents or by change in the bacterial population, where only the more resistant organisms are capable of surviving and multiplying. In addition, certain bacteria are capable of transferring resistance from one organism to another, e.g., pathogenic *E. coli*. In vitro sensitivity testing of the organism with several or all of the antibiotics

Table 6-1. Preferred antimicrobial therapy of specific bacterial pathogens

Organism or disease	Penicillin G	Penicillinase-resistant penicillins	Cephalothin	Ampicillin	Chloramphenicol	Erythromycin	Gentamycin	Kanamycin	Polymyxin or colistimethate	Bacitracin
Klebsiella, Aerobacter species							2	1	2	
Bordetella pertussis				1		2				
Brucella					1 or tetracycline					
Clostridium tetani	1 or tetracycline									2
Corynebacteria diphtheriae	2				3	1				
Diplococcus pneumoniae	1[b]		2			2				
Escherichia coli			3	3			3	1[c]	2 or carbenicillin	
Hemophilus influenzae				1	2	3			3	3
Leptospira species		2[d]								
Listeria monocytogenes	3			1		2 or tetracycline				
Mycobacterium tuberculosis*								3[e]		

Organism										
Neisseria gonorrheae	1				3	2				
Neisseria meningitidis	1			2	3	2				
Proteus vulgaris								1[f]		
Proteus mirabilis			3	1				3		
Pseudomonas							2	3	1 or carbenicillin	
Salmonella paratyphi			3	1	2			3	3	
Salmonella typhosa			3	2	1			3	3	
Shigella			3 or tetracycline	1				3	3	
Staphylococcus aureus		1[g]	2		3		3	2		3
Beta hemolytic streptococcus										
Group A	1		2							
Group B or D	1 or streptomycin						2			
Treponema pallidum	1			2					3	
Rickettsia				2					3	
Mycoplasma pneumoniae						1[h]			3	

Table 6-1. (Continued)

Organism or disease	Penicillin G	Penicillinase-resistant penicillins	Cephalothin	Ampicillin	Chloramphenicol	Erythromycin	Gentamycin	Kanamycin	Polymyxin or colistimethate	Bacitracin
Viruses										
Rheumatic fever (prophylaxis)	1					2 or sulfonamides				

KEY: 1, 2, 3 indicate order of preference and choice. Blanks indicate that a drug is of little value.

* See Tuberculosis, in Chapter 14.
[a] No antibiotic is entirely effective.
[b] Penicillin is the drug of choice. For patients with penicillin sensitivity, use erythromycin in less severe and cephalothin in more severe infections.
[c] In simple urinary tract infections, sulfonamides may be used or nitrofurantoin; in pathogenic *E. coli* infections of the bowel, neomycin or colistinsulfate (nonabsorbable) may be administered.
[d] Tetracycline is the drug of choice.
[e] Isoniazid is the drug of choice, often used in various combinations with PAS or streptomycin. With recent emergence of resistant forms of new drugs such as ethionamide, ethambutol, and rifampin are assuming a more prominent role in therapy.
[f] Carbenicillin has proven effective against most indol-positive proteus species.
[g] Increasing resistance to penicillinase-resistant penicillin has been noted. In life-threatening infections the next drug of choice is cephalothin.
[h] Tetracycline may also be used. Recent evidence indicates no antibiotic has any influence on the course of this infection in infants and children.

Table 6-2. Administration of antibiotics

Antibacterial agent	Dosage*	Interval and mode of administration†	Toxicity and reactions‡
Penicillin G (benzyl), aqueous	25,000–50,000 U/kg/day to obtain blood levels of 0.1–0.5 U/ml	Every 3, 8, or 12 hr I.M. or I.V.	Urticaria and other rashes; serum-sickness-like reaction; anaphylactic shock; glossitis, i.e, blackening of the tongue; moniliasis; diarrhea; fever; thrombophlebitis (if given intravenously)
Penicillin G, aqueous, with procaine	Under 15 kg, 25,000 U/kg/day Over 15 kg, 300,000–600,000 U/day	Every 12–24 hr I.M.	As above, plus allergic reactions from procaine
Penicillin V (phenoxymethyl)	600,000–1,200,000 U/day	Every 6 or 8 hr orally	As above
Benzathine penicillin	600,000–1,200,000 U/day 600,000–1,200,000 U	Every 6 or 8 hr orally Single injection I.M.	As above
Phenethicillin (α-phenoxyethyl)	500,000–2,000,000 U/day	Every 4–6 hr orally	As above plus local pain As above
Methicillin (dimethoxyphenyl)	250–300 mg/kg/day	Every 6 hr I.M. or I.V.	As above, high doses—reversible decrease in renal function, and transient bone marrow depression
Oxacillin	150–200 mg/kg/day; (N) 100–150 mg/kg/day	Every 6 hr orally or intramuscularly	As above
Nafcillin	50 mg/kg/day 50 mg/kg/day	Every 6 hr orally Every 12 hr I.M. or I.V.	As above

Table 6-2. (Continued)

Antibacterial agent	Dosage*	Interval and mode of administration†	Toxicity and reactions‡
Cloxacillin (monohydrate)	50 mg/kg/day	Every 6 hr orally; no other forms available	As above
Dicloxacillin (monohydrate)	50 mg/kg/day	Every 6 hr orally; no other forms available	As above
Ampicillin	100–200 mg/kg/day 25–50 mg/kg/day	Every 6–8 hr orally Every 6 hr I.M. or I.V.	As above
Hetacillin	Same as ampicillin but is more stabile	Same as ampicillin	As above
Carbenicillin	50–100 mg/kg/day; more serious infections, 100–300 mg/kg/day	Every 6 hr I.M. or I.V.	As above
Streptomycin	25–50 mg/kg/day; (N) 15–25 mg/kg/day	Every 6–12 hr I.M.	8th-nerve damage to both vestibular and auditory components, dermatitis, and (rarely) renal damage (if given intravenously)
Lincomycin	30–60 mg/kg/day 10–20 mg/kg/day; (N) not recommended	Every 6 hr Every 8–12 hr I.M. or I.V.	Jaundice and neutropenia, gastrointestinal disturbances, rash, and urticaria
Tetracycline and complexes§	25–50 mg/kg/day 10 mg/kg/day	Every 6–8 hr orally Every 6–12 hr I.M. or I.V. (1 mg/ml)	Nausea, vomiting, diarrhea, dermatitis, pruritus ani, moniliasis, fever, proctitis, colitis, and thrombophlebitis, I.V. may lead to liver toxicity

Drug	Dosage	Route/Schedule	Toxicity
Chloramphenicol (palmitate)	50–100 mg/kg/day; (N) 25 mg/kg/day 50 mg/kg/day; (N) 25 mg/kg/day	Every 6 hr orally Every 12 hr I.M.	As above, plus aplastic anemia (rarely) neurologic reactions such as peripheral neuritis may suppress antibody responses
Chloramphenicol (succinate)	25 mg/kg/day; (N) 15 mg/kg/day	Every 6 hr, either intravenously or subcutaneously as 10% solution	As above
Erythromycin and erythromycin estolate	25–50 mg/kg/day	Every 4 hr, orally ethylsuccinate ester available for parenteral use but irritating and painful. Use another drug if patient too ill to tolerate oral preparation	Gastrointestinal upsets, moniliasis, intrahepatic cholestasis with jaundice with estolate salt; the estolate should not be used parenterally
Gentamicin	7.5 mg/kg/day; (N) 2.0–5.0 mg/kg/day 20–30 mg/kg/day	Every 8–12 hr I.M. Every 8 hr orally for enteric infections	Serious ototoxicity and nephrotoxicity
Polymyxin	10–20 mg/kg/day 3.5–5 mg/kg/day; (P) 1 mg/kg/day	Every 6 hr orally for enteric infections Every 6–8 hr I.M. Every 12 hr I.V.	Toxic nephritis, neurotoxic effects, fever, and urticaria
Nitrofurantoin	5–7 mg/kg/day	Every 6 hr orally	CNS disturbances, rash, intestinal upsets, hemolytic anemias in patients with G6-PD deficiencies, allergic pneumonias

Table 6-2. (Continued)

Antibacterial agent	Dosage*	Interval and mode of administration†	Toxicity and reactions‡
Bacitracin	2,000 U/kg/day	Every 6 hr orally for enteric infections	Toxic nephritis, anorexia, skin rashes, and irritation
Polymixin B	3.5–5 mg/kg/day	Every 8–12 hr I.M.	Paresthesia, ataxia, muscular weakness, nausea, vomiting, nephrotoxic
Colistimethate	5–8 mg/kg/day	As above	As above
Colistin sulfate	15–20 mg/kg/day	Every 6 hr orally for enteric infections (pathogenic E. coli)	As above
Neomycin	100 mg/kg/day; (N) 50 mg/kg/day	Every 4 hr orally for enteric infections (pathogenic E. coli), limit 10 days	Deafness, toxic nephritis, malabsorption syndrome from prolonged administration
Kanamycin	15 mg/kg/day 2.5 mg/ml by slow infusion (P) 7.5 mg/kg/day	Every 12 hr I.M. or I.V. Every 12 hr I.M.	Toxic nephritis, 8th-nerve damage, rash, agranulocytosis, renal toxicity, pain at injection site
Nalidixic acid	50 mg/kg/day	Every 6–12 hr orally	Gastrointestinal upsets, drowsiness, weakness and neurologic disturbances, hallucinations, photosensitivity
Cephalothin and Cephaloridine	30–100 mg/kg/day	Every 6–8 hr I.M. or I.V.	Neutropenia, rash, hives, tenderness and induration locally; cephalothin less irritating but possibly nephrotoxic

| Cephalexin | 125–250 mg/every 6 hr | Orally | |
| Nystatin ¶ | 500,000 U/day | Every 8 hr orally | Gastrointestinal disturbances, usually transitory |

KEY: (P) premature infant; (N) newborn infant—premature and full-term—and anuric children.

* Optimal dosages for children have not been completely established. Such variables as organism sensitivity, virulence, and host resistance markedly influence dosage. Dosages given in this table are general ranges. In the discussion of the various diseases, other dosages may be suggested.

† Antibacterial agents may be used locally, e.g., in eye infections, but avoid use of local antibacterial agent that is to be used systemically as increased incidence of sensitization. Administration by aerosol may be helpful in preventing the spread of infection, e.g., in bronchiectasis.

‡ With the administration of oral antibiotics, milk or acid binders may reduce the incidence of nausea and vomiting. However, in general, with the exception of the estolate salt of erythromycin antibiotics are better absorbed on an empty stomach. Yogurt or acidophilus milk may decrease the incidence of moniliasis. Resistant staphylococcus infections of the gastrointestinal tract may develop following prolonged oral antibiotic administration.

§ Deposition in bones and teeth (causing discoloration if administered between fifth gestational month and 8 years of age) has been noted for all tetracyclines, least for oxytetracycline. This antibiotic is of very little use in the pediatric patient.

¶ Nystatin is effective against a number of yeasts and fungi, including *Candida albicans*. *Candida albicans* infections (moniliasis) may be local—e.g., thrush, pruritus ani, vaginitis—or generalized with sepsis, lung, kidney, and brain involvement.

may be of value as a guide to therapy. (Fever of unknown origin may often be found to be due to an infection with a resistant organism, e.g., staphylococcus, rather than to such conditions as leukemia, hypersensitivity states, etc.)

When toxic and allergic reactions occur, the agent is usually discontinued, except when the danger of the primary disease is greater than that of the reaction. The use of antihistamines or adrenal corticosteroids may lessen such reactions.

USEFUL DRUGS

Most drugs produce their effects by combining with cellular enzymes, cell membranes, or other important cellular subparticles; however, in only a few instances are the precise receptor sites or mechanisms of drug action known.

Potency is influenced by the absorption, distribution, biotransformation, and excretion of a drug.

The chemical reactions concerned with the biotransformation of drugs involve oxidation, reduction or hydrolysis, and conjugation, which take place mainly in the liver microsomes but also in other tissues such as the kidney.

The effect of many drugs is enhanced and their duration of action is prolonged by interference with their enzymatic destruction by liver microsomal enzymes.

Age is an important determinant of microsomal enzyme activity; for example, a newborn infant has decreased ability to metabolize a variety of drugs, and therefore lower drug dosages are required to avoid toxic effects. The newborn infant's low levels of glucuronyl transferase, which conjugates many substances (bilirubin, chloramphenicol, etc.) with glucuronic acid, are a well-known example of his limited ability to break down drugs.

Genetic factors also contribute to the normal variability of drug effects and are responsible for a large number of quantitative and qualitative differences in pharmacologic activity.

Prolonged apnea following the dosage of succinylcholine usually administered is due to inherited pseudocholinesterase (the enzyme which inactivates this drug) deficiency in some patients. Increased susceptibility to hemolysis following administration of drugs such as primaquine is linked directly to the inherited deficiency of an enzyme (G-6-PD) normally found in red blood cells.

When the route of excretion of a drug is impaired, toxic accumulation may occur. For example, using drugs normally excreted by the kidney may present a problem when renal function is reduced to about 25 percent of normal, the point at which the blood urea nitrogen (BUN) rises. In such instances the initial loading dose can safely be given but subsequent dosage should be reduced.

Drugs should be prescribed only for specific indications. Dosages usually cannot be computed from adult doses on the basis of surface area, age, or weight. Infants are often able to take much larger dosages proportionately. (Ideally, there should be a completely new pediatric pharmacology not dependent on adult dosage. In time this will be achieved.) For example, a newborn infant may need $\frac{1}{8}$ gr (8 mg) of phenobarbital or more for sedation.

However, a rule such as Young's,

$$\text{Child dose} = \frac{\text{age} \times \text{adult dose}}{\text{age} + 12}$$

is useful, since it provides a large margin of safety for the initial dose, which can be increased subsequently. A more practical formula is

$$\text{Child dose} = \frac{\text{age} \times \text{adult dose}}{\text{age} + 6}$$

The prescribed dosage is modified by the route of administration, and the extent of the modification varies with the individual drug used. Usually the intravenous dosage is one-fourth to one-third, the subcutaneous dosage is one-half, and the rectal dosage is equal to or twice the oral dosage.

In oral administration, proper psychologic attitudes are helpful. Firmness may be necessary on occasion and will do no harm if the dose is given with speed and good temper. Pleasant-tasting vehicles should be used. If a powder is prescribed, it may be mixed with applesauce, chocolate syrup, jelly, or honey. If part of a tablet is prescribed, e.g., half an aspirin, it may be cut with a razor blade and crushed between two spoons, and then the applesauce or other vehicle added. If a tablet, e.g., Crystoids (hexylresorcinol), is to be swallowed without chewing, it may be embedded within a spoonful of gelatin dessert or ice cream. When the drug comes in capsule form, e.g., ampicillin, it may be opened and the contents mixed as above. A toothpick makes a good spatula.

The individual drugs and their dosages are considered under therapy of the various conditions. Here only a few of the most generally used drugs can be mentioned.

Aspirin (acetylsalicylic acid) is widely used as an antipyretic and analgesic. The dose is 1 gr (0.06 Gm) per year of age up to 5 years and may be repeated as often as every 4 hours if necessary. It is unusual to need single doses greater than 5 gr (0.3 Gm). (Parents should be educated to realize that temperature per se is not to be combated, since it is one of nature's aids against infection. Only when the febrile response is excessive and produces restlessness and discomfort are such drugs as aspirin indicated.)

Phenobarbital is widely used as a sedative. Elixir of phenobarbital has $\frac{1}{4}$ gr (15 mg) per tsp. Infants take $\frac{1}{8}$ to $\frac{1}{4}$ gr (8 to 15 mg) well, and it is rarely necessary to use dosages greater than $\frac{1}{2}$ gr (30 mg) in children.

Codeine or morphine is sometimes combined with aspirin or phenobarbital to enhance their effect. The usual dosages for analgesia of codeine, morphine, meperidine hydrochloride (Demerol), and paregoric are

Codeine phosphate: 3 mg per kg per day or 100 mg m² per 24 hours, orally or subcutaneously
Morphine sulfate: 0.1 to 0.2 mg per kg per dose, subcutaneously
Paregoric (0.4 mg morphine per ml): 0.25 to 0.5 ml per kg per dose, orally
Meperidine hydrochloride (Demerol): 6 mg per kg per day or 175 mg per m² per 24 hours, orally or subcutaneously

ACTH AND ADRENAL CORTICOSTEROIDS

ACTH (adrenocorticotropic hormone of the pituitary gland) and hydrocortisone (17-hydroxycorticosterone), which is the naturally occurring gluconeogenic substance in man, have much the same basic clinical indications and contraindications except that ACTH requires the presence of an intact adrenal cortex. Administration of these substances results in a variety of effects. These include antiallergic effects (perhaps through suppression of antibody formation), depression of mesenchymal tissue reactivity and response to bacterial infection, electrolyte-regulating action, and certain metabolic effects.

ACTH and the adrenal corticosteroids (hydrocortisone or its analogs) may produce a remission or relieve symptoms and signs of a number of inflammatory and allergic disorders while the patient is under treatment. They may be indicated for

1. Replacement therapy
   a. Adrenocortical insufficiency: hydrocortisone either for acute conditions, such as Waterhouse-Friderichsen syndrome; septic shock; or for chronic disorders, such as Addison's disease.
   b. Hypopituitarism: ACTH or hydrocortisone.
   c. Stress situations within 1 to 2 years of prior adrenal corticosteroid therapy
2. Anti-inflammatory effect: rheumatic fever, skin disorders, ocular diseases, croup.
3. Suppression of antibody formation: systemic lupus erythematosus.
4. Diabetogenic effect: hypoglycemia.
5. Calcium excretion: hypercalcemia.
6. Adrenal suppression: adrenocortical hyperplasia (only adrenal corticosteroids).
7. Miscellaneous uses include those conditions where more than one of the above mechanisms may be of equal significance, for example, asthma, celiac disease, idiopathic thrombocytopenic purpura, hemolytic anemia, ulcerative colitis; or those conditions where the effect is unknown, e.g., infantile cortical hyperostosis, leukemia, sarcoidosis.

8. Diagnosis
   a. Adrenocortical reserve: as measured by the response of the adrenal cortex to the administration of ACTH (see p. 649).
   b. Cushing's syndrome (due to hyperplasia of the adrenal cortex): there is a hypersensitivity to ACTH resulting in a greater-than-normal elevation in the level of blood and urinary corticosteroids following administration of ACTH. *Suppression test:* see p. 649 to differentiate adrenocortical hyperplasia from adrenal tumor. *Pituitary-adrenal axis evaluation—Metopirone (SU 4885)* test (see p. 649): normally, 17-hydroxycorticosteroids are derived from hydrocortisone (cortisol). Substance S (11-deoxycortisol) is an immediate precursor of hydrocortisone. SU 4885 blocks 11-carbon hydroxylation; thus substance S cannot be converted to hydrocortisone. A low level of plasma hydrocortisone stimulates secretion of ACTH and more substance S is produced, with a subsequent rise in urinary 17-hydroxycorticosteroids.

Dosage   Optimal dosage has not been established. It is related more to the type and severity of the illness (dosage for replacement therapy is less than for inflammatory diseases) than to age, weight, or surface area. Ordinarily, it is the smallest dosage that will give a therapeutic response.

ACTH   1.5 to 2.0 USP units per kg per day may be given subcutaneously or intramuscularly in divided doses every 6 hours to produce anti-inflammatory effects. Intravenous ACTH is given in one-fifth the intramuscular dosage, in 500 to 800 ml of 5% glucose in distilled water, over a 6- to 8-hour period.

Administration of hydrocortisone or its analogs should not be stopped suddenly at a high-level dosage, but rather should be tapered off, because there may be a period of adrenocortical hypofunction for several days after cessation of administration of hormones. Following withdrawal there may be not only resumption of previous disease activity but also increased activity (rebound effect). This phenomenon is transitory, lasting for several days, after which the disease may resume its previous activity.

Prophylactic administration of antibiotics is advisable as an adjunct to hormone therapy, since hormones lower the body's resistance to bacterial infection and mask the symptoms and signs of infection. Potassium chloride, 1 to 2 Gm daily, or potassium acetate and a low-salt diet are also helpful.

Undesirable side effects and toxicity   In order to effect a remission with hydrocortisone or ACTH, some measure of hyperadrenalism is often induced. Various schedules of interrupted dosage therapy, e.g., alternate day, 3 days per week, have been used to diminish the severity of side effects.

Table 6-3. Dosage for adrenal corticosteroids

Compounds*	Equivalent glucocorticoid effect, mg	Relative potency		Dose	Available form
		Anti-inflammatory	Sodium retention activity		
Cortisone acetate	100	0.8	0.8	5–10 mg/kg	5-, 10-, and 25-mg tablets
Hydrocortisone	80	1.0	1.0	4–8 mg/kg	5-, 10-, and 20-mg tablets
Hydrocortisone hemisuccinate				0.02–0.2 mg/kg/hr by continuous I.V. infusion or 1.0–2 mg/kg may be rapidly infused in a small volume of fluid	100-mg/2 ml vial
Prednisone	20	3.5–4	0.8	1–2 mg/kg	1-, 2.5-, 5-mg tablets
Prednisolone	16	3.5–4	0.8	1–2 mg/kg	1-, 2.5-, 5-mg tablets
Triamcinolone	8	5.0	0	0.5–1 mg/kg	1-, 2-, 4-, 8-, 16-mg tablets
Dexamethasone	2	25.0	0	0.1–0.2 mg/kg	0.25-, 0.5-, 0.75-mg tablets
9-fluorocortisol	0.5	15	125	0.25–0.5 mg/kg	0.1-, 1-mg tablets

* For replacement therapy, the naturally occurring steroid (cortisone) in the dose of 0.7 mg/kg/day is generally used.

Any of the following types of reaction may be produced.

1. Metabolic changes:
   Hypertension
   Hypernatremia
   Hypokalemia
   Increased fat deposition
   Hypochloremic alkalosis
2. Hirsutism
3. Negative nitrogen balance; increased excretion of uric acid, creatinine, and amino acids; growth arrest; osteoporosis
4. Steroid-induced diabetes
5. Hematologic changes
   Lymphopenia
   Eosinopenia
   Polymorphonuclear leukocytosis
   Thrombocytosis leading to thromboembolic phenomena
   Polycytemia
6. Delayed wound healing
7. Tendency to peptic ulcer
8. Psychologic changes and psychotic episodes

Contraindications

1. Hypertension
2. Diabetes
3. Perhaps congestive heart failure. (Adrenal corticosteroids are recommended by some when the heart failure is associated with acute rheumatic fever; if they are used, a low salt intake is necessary.)
4. Viral infection, e.g., varicella.
5. Ulcerations of the gastrointestinal tract (other than ulcerative colitis).
6. Active, untreated infection with the tubercle bacillus.

Psychotherapeutic agents   These agents have been used as adjuncts in therapy for various behavior disorders, hyperactive states, and psychoses in children. They may be classified by their principal pharmacologic action:

I. Central nervous system depressants

	Dosage
A. *Antihistamines*	
Brompheniramine maleate parabromdylamine maleate (Dimetane)	0.5 mg/kg/24 hr divide into 3–4 doses
Chlorpheniramine maleate (Chlor-Trimeton)	0.35 mg/kg/24 hr divide into 3–4 doses

Cyproheptadine hydrochloride (Periactin)	0.25 mg/kg/24 hr divide into 3–4 doses
Dimenhydrinate (Dramamine)	5.0 mg/kg/24 hr divide into 3–4 doses
Diphenhydramine hydrochloride (Benadryl)	5.0 mg/kg/24 hr divide into 3–4 doses

All are central nervous system depressants, cause autonomic imbalance, and gastrointestinal disturbances in addition to individual toxicities. [Hydroxyzine hydrochloride (Atarax), and Hydroxyzine pamoate (Vistaril) are better classified as tranquilizers although these drugs have antihistamine action.]

B.   Skeletal muscle relaxants—nonsedative:
Mephenesin (Tolserol), 175 mg/kg/day divided into 3–5 doses, orally or 1–3 mg/kg in slow intravenous drip (2% solution)

C.   Skeletal relaxants—sedative
Meprobamate (Equanil, Miltown), also classified as tranquilizers, 25 mg/kg/day usually divided into 2 to 3 doses (higher doses may be necessary, e.g., infants, up to 50 to 100 mg/day; 4–8 years of age, 200 mg t.i.d.; older children, 400 mg t.i.d.)
Methocarbaniol (Robaxin), 60 mg/kg/day divided into 4 doses
Chlorzoxazone (Paraflex), 20 mg/kg/day divided into 3 or 4 doses

D.   Sympathetic suppressants—phenothiazine derivatives
1.   Chlorpromazine (Thorazine), 2 mg/kg/day divided into 4 to 6 doses, orally (preferred for tense, agitated, brain-damaged child).
2.   Perphenazine (Trilafon), 1 to 6 years, 4 mg/day; 6 to 12 years, 6 mg/day; over 12 years, 6 to 12 mg/day; or based on weight, 0.06 mg/kg/day. It is given orally in three divided doses.
3.   Prochlorperazine (Compazine), 0.2 to 0.4 mg/kg/day, orally or rectally in three to four divided doses. The intramuscular dosage is one-half the oral dose. (This is a particularly useful drug in the hypoactive, withdrawn, or schizophrenic child. In the pediatric age group extrapyramidal tract involvement is a frequent side effect.)
4.   Trifluoperazine (Stelazine), 0.02 mg/kg/day, orally.

Other tranquilizers
1.   Chlordiazepoxide hydrochloride (Librium): This should not be used in children under 6 years of age or in hyperactive children, where excitement and stimulation may result.
2.   Diazepam (Valium), 0.12–0.8 mg/kg/day orally divided into 3 or 4 doses or 0.04–0.2 mg/kg for I.M. or I.V.

usage (slow administration of I.V. mandatory). This drug is considered contraindicated in infants under 6 months of age, however it has been used to control acute tonic-clonic convulsions in infants.

3. Hydroxyzine hydrochloride (Atarax) and hydroxyzine pamoate (Vistaril), 2 mg/kg/day orally divided into 4 doses.

E. Sympathetic suppressants: Reserpine (Raurine, Serpasil, Reserpoid, and others), 0.02 mg/kg/day in one or two doses orally for tranquilization. (May be used in combination with chlorpromazine.) Also classified as antihypertensive and vasadilator.

II. Central nervous system stimulant: Methylphenidate (Ritalin), 0.75 mg/kg/dose. (May be given orally, intramuscularly, or slowly intravenously.) Effective in the treatment of hyperactive child and for child with minimal brain dysfunction syndrome.

III. Miscellaneous: Amphetamine sulfate (Benzedrine), 0.2 mg/kg/day orally in 3 divided doses or 5 to 20 mg per 24 hours. (May also be given intramuscularly or slowly intravenously.), and dextroamphetamine (Dexedrine), 5 to 30 mg in 24 hours. (Dosage should start with 5 mg and gradually be increased.) These are effective sedatives in the hyperactive brain-damaged infant. Phenylzine (Nardil) and nialamide (Niamid), monoamine-oxidase inhibitors, are given as antidepressants, 75 to 100 mg per 24 hours in 2 to 3 doses.

POISONING*

Among the disorders that children are subject to, poisoning remains one of the most common. This is especially true during the ages of 1 to 4 years, a period when recently acquired locomotor ability and inquisitiveness place children at high risk.

In addition, the problem is complicated by the increasing variety and number of commercial products with intoxicating properties as well as by a widespread tendency for drugs to be used for minor complaints. Partial control of the problem has been accomplished by local poison control centers as well as by the National Clearinghouse for Poison Control Centers which disseminate information, by education carried out at the doctor to parent level, and by safety containerization.

DIAGNOSIS OF OBSCURE POISONING

Whenever diverse symptoms and signs coexist without a history of exposure, poisoning should be considered as a possible diagnosis. Specific clinical signs often suggest the nature of ingested material.

* EDITORS' NOTE: The section on Poisoning was prepared by Marvin Green, M.D.

Clinical features

1. Confusion, convulsions, and coma in sequence are characteristic of many poisons that affect the central nervous system.
2. Hyperpnea, at times severe enough to resemble dyspnea, is characteristic of salicylate poisoning. Auscultation of the lungs will reveal excellent unimpaired transmission of breath sounds.
3. Cyanosis, especially if accompanied by only relatively mild dyspnea, is characteristic of methemoglobin-forming poisons, e.g., aniline dyes, kerosene, and nitrates.
4. Trismus and opisthotonus not only suggest tetanus, but phenothiazines may actually be the cause.
5. Autonomic nervous system symptoms, e.g., flushing of the skin, hyperpyrexia, dry oral mucosa, mydriasis, may indicate poisoning by atropine, antihistamines, or Jimson weed. Others, e.g., hyperhidrosis, diarrhea, vomiting, bradycardia, when associated with absent deep-tendon reflexes, and the confusion-convulsion-coma sequence indicate organic phosphorus esters or mecholyl.
6. Shock may be the principal manifestation of ferrous sulfate or aminophylline intoxication.
7. Odor of the breath is distinctive for alcohol, kerosene, and methyl salicylate.

Laboratory features   Even in the absence of a well-equipped laboratory, some very simple procedures may aid diagnosis.

1. The addition of $FeCl_3$ 10% drop by drop, to a few milliliters of urine may permit detection of salicylates, phenothiazines, antipyrine, and phenolsulfonphthalein. All these compounds produce a purple color. If the color change can be produced in a urine sample that has been previously boiled, the presence of diacetic acid can be ruled out. Though only a small amount of ingested salicylates may produce a positive test and not necessarily indicate intoxication, a positive color reaction on serum accurately indicates the presence of toxic levels in the blood. Phenistix paper strip (Ames) may be substituted for $FeCl_3$.
2. Rapid diagnosis of lead intoxication may be imperative. Urine can easily be tested for the presence of coproporphyrin III. After acidification with a few drops of glacial acetic acid, an equal amount of ether is added. To the etherified portion, an equal volume of 1.5 NHCl is added. Orange fluorescence with a Wood's lamp indicates the presence of coproporphyrin III.

Removal of poisons   All attempts to remove recently ingested poisons must be deferred until such life-threatening events as shock and convulsions are adequately managed.

1. Poisons absorbed through the skin (often extremely lethal and must be removed within minutes): (a) Water-soluble poisons—

prompt removal of contaminated clothing followed by showering or hosing with water; (*b*)Water-insoluble agents, e.g., phenol—liberal application of 10 percent ethyl alcohol. Corrosives should be removed from the eyes by gentle irrigation of the opened eye for a number of minutes.

2. Ingested poison: (*a*) Induction of effective emesis. Syrup of ipecac 15 ml followed by a few ounces of water will usually cause vigorous vomiting in 20 to 30 minutes. The dose may be repeated once if emesis has not occurred by this time. Physicians should recommend that parents keep an ounce of syrup of ipecac in the house in anticipation of poisoning. (*b*) Lavage has been shown to be a less-effective means of removal. Nevertheless, it still is indicated if the effectiveness of emesis is in question. It also permits introduction of a chemical antidote into the stomach. The patient must be adequately immobilized and placed in Trendelenburg's position. Lavage tubing should be of no. 12 to 20 French bore. After aspiration of the gastric contents, small amounts of lavage fluid should be alternately instilled and removed. Prior to removal of the tube, an aqueous suspension of activated charcoal may be administered through the tubing (five to ten times more than the estimated amount of poison ingested). The tube should then be removed with application of continuous negative pressure to prevent pulmonary aspiration of its residual contents.

   Either lavage or emesis is contraindicated in comatose or actively convulsing patients. Emesis is also contraindicated for removal of petroleum distillates or strong corrosive agents. Lavage may be justified if more than 1 ml per kg of petroleum distillate has been ingested. The procedure should then be carried out with a cuffed endotracheal tube in place to minimize the risk of aspiration. Lavage may also be justified for ingestion of corrosives if it is performed within 30 minutes of ingestion.

3. Renal excretion may be enhanced after a poison has been absorbed: This is particularly true for salicylates and long-acting barbiturates if an alkaline urinary pH is maintained.

4. Miscellaneous measures: Peritoneal dialysis, hemodialysis, and exchange transfusion may be employed where the likelihood of lethal intoxication exists. The preferred modality of treatment depends on such factors as plasma protein binding and the pK_a of the intoxicant.

LEAD POISONING

Etiology

1. Ingestion, e.g., high lead content paint from repainted cribs, walls and toys, also from swallowed lead toys, and from food prepared

or served in lead-containing utensils or lead-glazed pottery, or with water obtained from lead pipes.

2. Inhalation of fumes, e.g., from burned battery casings, fumes from leaded gasoline.

Clinical and laboratory features

1. Incidence is highest in children 1 to 3 years of age with a history of pica.
2. Encephalopathy may be manifest by sudden onset of marked irritability, persistent projectile vomiting, followed by severe prolonged convulsions. However, it may begin more insidiously with lethargy, loss of appetite, and loss of recently acquired skills developing over a 1 to 2 month period prior to more fulminating manifestations. Occasionally, a single self-limited convulsion may mark the occurrence of encephalopathy.
3. Abdominal colic and peripheral neuritis are more frequent in older age groups.
4. A lead line (bluish-black and stippled) is found infrequently at the gingival margin.
5. Anemia, hypochromic and microcytic, and basophilic stippling of red blood cells may be present (stippling may be more commonly detected in erythroid cells from the marrow).
6. Urinary lead concentration of 150 micrograms per liter may be found in normal children, but this level is usually indicative of intoxication. Of greater diagnostic value is the enhanced excretion of urinary lead after parenteral administration of calcium versenate. Following three 8-hourly intramuscular doses of 25 mg per kg, urinary lead excretion increases to 500 micrograms per liter.

    Coproporphyrin III in urine is usually associated with high blood-lead levels.

    Urinary Δ aminolevulinic acid levels of above 19 mg per liter are associated with symptoms and signs of intoxication.
7. Blood-lead levels of at least 0.06 mg per 100 Gm blood are found in symptomatic children; however, levels as low as 0.04 mg per 100 Gm blood have been associated with ultrastructural changes in mitochondria of renal tubular cells. Levels of 0.1 mg per 100 Gm blood foreshadow imminent encephalopathy.
8. X-rays may reveal increased density at growing ends of long bones and recently ingested lead-containing plaster in the gastrointestinal tract.

Treatment

1. Removal of lead from the gastrointestinal tract: administer laxatives and enemas prior to starting drug therapy except for management of encephalopathy.

2. Encephalopathy: Treat seizures first; Valium may be given intravenously. Paraldehyde, 0.3–0.6 ml per kg may be diluted with two parts vegetable oil and given rectally three to four times daily. Corticosteroids may be employed to decrease intracranial pressure, but this is of questionable benefit. Mannitol may be a valuable adjunct in decreasing cerebral edema (2 Gm per kg given I.V. over 30 to 60 minutes as a 15 to 20 percent solution).

3. Chelating agents: Removal of lead is instituted only after ability to excrete urine has been ascertained. Give dextrose 10 percent in water I.V. (10 to 20 ml per kg) for 1 to 2 hours; if ineffective, administer mannitol. Maintain urine output at 350 to 500 ml per square meter per 24 hours if encephalopathy exists.

    For children with high blood levels (0.1 mg per 100 Gm) or encephalopathy, use the following regimen:

    a. BAL 4 mg per kg I.M. q. 4 h. for 30 doses. Beginning 4 hours after BAL started, give calcium versenate (20 percent solution) 12.5 mg per kg I.M. q. 4 h. diluted with an equal volume of procaine 0.5 percent for a total of 30 doses.

        For children with blood levels below 0.1 mg per 100 Gm blood, only calcium versenate need be given.

        If elevated blood lead or coproporphyrinuria persists, re-treatment may be carried out in the same manner.

4. Environment: The source of lead must be removed. If the patient is re-exposed to lead in his environment *d*-penicillamine may be given in two divided daily doses totaling 25 mg per kg up to 500 to 750 mg. This may be carried out for 3 to 6 months.

Prognosis

Approximately 25 to 35 percent of those with overt encephalopathy die, while 50 percent of the survivors show marked central nervous system sequelae, e.g., recurrent seizures, severe mental retardation. Milder intoxication without overt encephalopathy may result in more subtle evidence of central nervous system impairment which may first be shown by poor educational performance.

Damage to the kidneys may not be completely reversible. There is evidence that nephrosclerosis may be a sequel to lead intoxication in childhood.

Table 6-4. Treatment of poisoning

Poison	Common source	Specific treatment	Dosage
Unknown		Activated charcoal	Aqueous suspension at least 5 parts to 1 part of poison
Ammonia	Household cleaning agent	See "Lye"	
Aniline	Crayons; diaper dyes; inks	Methylene blue 1% I.V.	1–2 mg/kg. Give slowly, 5 min. May repeat in 30 min
Antihistamines	Allergy therapy; cold remedies	Pentothal sodium 2.5% I.V. for convulsions; Valium 5 mg/ml I.V.; maintain respiration artificially if necessary	1 ml/min 0.5 ml/min up to 1–2 ml
Arsenic	Insecticides; weed killers	Lavage with milk, 10% ferric chloride, or BAL solution 10% BAL I.M.	3.0 mg/kg q. 4 h. 6 first day; same 2d day; 4 doses 3d day; then q. 12 h. × 10 days
Barbiturates	Sedatives	Maintain respiration, artificially if necessary; maintain urinary pH 7.0	Infuse sodium bicarbonate 2 meq/kg during 1st hour and 2–4 meq/kg over next 6–12 hr
Belladonna (atropine, homatropine)	Antispasmodics; eye drops	Lavage, instill activated charcoal; emesis may be ineffective Pentothal sodium 2.5% or Valium 5 mg/ml I.V. for convulsions	5 parts:1 part poison 1 ml/min 0.5 ml/min

118

Benzedrine	Proprietaries used for enuresis; weight-reduction remedies	Pentothal sodium 2.5% I.V. or Valium 5 mg/ml I.V. for convulsions	1 ml/min 0.5 ml/min
Boric acid	Boric acid powders, solutions, and ointments	Peritoneal dialysis, hemodialysis or exchange transfusion may be indicated	
Camphor	Camphorated oils; spirits of camphor	Pentothal sodium 2.5% I.V. or Valium 5 mg/ml I.V. for convulsions	1 ml/min 0.5 ml/min
Carbon monoxide	Automobile exhaust; defective gas appliances; incomplete combustion of organic fuels	Oxygen, transfusions, exchange transfusion, hyperbaric chamber	
Cyanide	Silver polishes; tree sprays; rodenticides; fireworks	1. 3% sodium nitrate followed by 2. 25% sodium thiosulfate I.V.	1. Maximum 10 ml for adolescent; ⅓–⅙ for 2–3-yr-old 2. Maximum 50 ml (5–15 ml for 2–3-yr-old)
DDT	Insecticides	Pentothal sodium 2.5% or Valium 5 mg/ml I.V. for convulsions	1 ml/min 0.5 ml/min
Digitalis	Therapy for heart failure	Gastric lavage with activated charcoal instilled Potassium chloride or acetate orally or subcutaneously Calcium versenate, I.V., may be effective	5 parts:1 part of digitalis 3 meq/kg/24 hr
Formaldehyde	Antiseptics; deodorizing preparations	Ammonium acetate by mouth (forms nontoxic methenamine) Follow by instillation of activated charcoal	3 tsp in 8 oz water 5 parts: 1 part of formaldehyde

Table 6-4. (Continued)

Poison	Common source	Specific treatment	Dosage
Iodine	Tincture of iodine	Lavage with aqueous starch suspension	1 tbsp to 500 ml water
Iron	Therapeutic iron	Induce emesis; follow by instillation of activated charcoal by gavage	5 parts:1 part iron
		Deferoxamine methane sulfonate (Desferal) I.M. if poisoning is severe	0.25–1.0 Gm. Repeat 0.25–0.5 Gm q. 4 h. to a total of 80 mg/kg for 1st 24 hr and 50 mg/kg/day thereafter
Lye	Drainpipe cleaners; household cleansing agents; paint removers; hair-waving solutions	Encourage intake of weak acid Esophageal dilation with catheters is begun on 4th day	
Mercury	Mercurochrome; bichloride of mercury	Lavage with milk or 5% sodium formaldehyde sulfoxalate	See Arsenic
		10% BAL I.M.	
Methadone	Synthetic opioid	Emesis may be ineffective Remove by lavage and instill activated charcoal	
		Nalline or	0.1 mg/kg
		Lorfan I.V. q. 15 min.	0.02 mg/kg
			5 parts:1 part
Methyl alcohol	Varnish and varnish removers; combustibles; as a poison in alcohol	Emesis with syrup of ipecac. Instill 50% ethyl alcohol via gavage tube. Repeat every 2 hr orally or I.V. up to 4 days	1.0–1.5 ml/kg
		Correct acidosis. Hemodialysis if blood methanol more than 50 mg/100 ml	

Poison	Source	Treatment	Dosage
Morphine		*See* Methadone	
Mushrooms (poisonous)		Atropine sulfate I.V. Repeat q. 5–10 min if parasympathomimetic signs persist.	0.05 mg/kg
Nitrates	Well water with high nitrate content	Methylene blue 1% I.V.	1–2 mg/kg slowly over 5 min. Repeat in 30 min
Nicotine	Tobacco; insecticides	After emesis, instill activated charcoal by gavage. Maintain respiration. Atropine sulfate I.V. q. 5–10 min for parasympathomimetic hyperactivity. Try to produce mild signs of atropinism	5 parts:1 part 0.05 mg/kg
Oxalates	Bleaches	Gastric lavage within 30–45 min with dilute lime water. Calcium chloride 5% I.V. Esophageal bouginage (*see* "Lye")	5–20 ml
Petroleum distillates	Kerosene; naphtha; gasoline; lighter fluid	Lavage probably indicated where amount ingested more than 1 ml/kg	
Phenol	Lysol	If seen within 30 min, lavage with olive oil. Instill 15 ml castor oil to hasten intestinal excretion	
Phenothiazines	Antiemetics, tranquilizers	Remove by gastric lavage, with activated charcoal. Benadryl I.V. for extrapyramidal signs	5 parts:1 part of drug
Phosphates (organic)	Insecticides	Atropine sulfate I.V., repeat q. 5–10 min for parasympathomimetic signs. Pralidoxime I.V. in 5% solution over at least a 30-min period.	1–5 mg/kg 0.05 mg/kg 50 mg/kg (up to 2.0 Gm). May repeat q. 12 h.

Table 6-4. (Continued)

Poison	Common source	Specific treatment	Dosage
Phosphorus	Fireworks; rodenticides	Local burn—cupric sulfate 1% Lavage with cupric sulfate 0.2% intravenous fluids and blood for shock (fresh blood may counteract hypoprothrombinemia)	
Salicylates	Aspirin; oil of wintergreen	Composition of I.V. fluids depends on blood pH. Providing blood pH normal or acidemia is present, administer sodium bicarbonate I.V. to alkalinize urine In severe intoxication, hemodialysis, peritoneal dialysis, or exchange transfusion may be indicated	Infuse 2 meq/kg during 1st hr and 2–4 meq/kg over next 6–12 hr
Strychnine	Tonics and cathartics	Control convulsion with pentothal sodium 2.5% I.V. or Valium 5 mg/ml I.V.	1 ml/min 0.5 ml/min up to 1–2 ml
Turpentine	Organic solvents; furniture polishes and waxes; paint thinners	Administer mineral oil and remove by lavage tube or emesis	30–60 ml
Warfarin	Rodenticide	Vitamin K or fresh blood transfusion to control prolonged prothrombin time	

REVIEW QUESTIONS

1. The drug of choice for *H. influenzae* infection is (a) chloramphenicol; (b) ampicillin; (c) erythromycin; (d) bacitracin.

2. The recommended oral dose of ampicillin for infections of moderate severity is (a) 25–50 mg per kg per day; (b) 50–100 mg per kg per day; (c) 100–200 mg per kg per day; (d) 200–400 mg per kg per day.

3. The recommended parenteral dose of kanamycin is (a) 5 mg per kg per day; (b) 10 mg per kg per day; (c) 15 mg per kg per day; (d) 25–50 mg per kg per day.

4. The recommended oral dose of erythromycin is (a) 5 mg per kg per day; (b) 10 mg per kg per day; (c) 15 mg per kg per day; (d) 25–50 mg per kg per day.

5. Undesirable side effects of tetracycline include all the following except (a) diarrhea; (b) staining of teeth; (c) moniliasis; (d) fever; (e) alopecia.

6. All the following drugs may cause auditory disturbances except (a) dihydrostreptomycin; (b) kanamycin; (c) gentamycin; (d) neomycin; (e) bacitracin.

7. All the following drugs may cause renal disturbances except (a) gentamycin; (b) polymixin; (c) bacitracin; (d) kanamycin; (e) lincomycin.

8. All the following may be seen in ACTH toxicity except: (a) hirsutism; (b) psychotic episodes; (c) delayed wound healing; (d) hyperchloremic acidosis; (e) hypernatremia.

9. All the following may be contraindications to treatment with adrenal corticosteroids except for (a) hypertension; (b) rheumatic fever; (c) diabetes; (d) viral infection.

10. Dexedrine used in the treatment of hyperactive children with minimal brain dysfunction syndrome should not exceed (a) 1 mg per kg per 24 hr; (b) 5 mg per kg per 24 hr; (c) 10 mg per kg per 24 hr; (d) 30 mg per kg per 24 hr.

11. All the following substances produce a purple color when $FeCl_3$ 10% is added to urine except for (a) lead; (b) salicylates; (c) antipyrine; (d) phenosulfonphthalein.

7

FLUID AND ELECTROLYTE BALANCE

The fluid and electrolyte homeostasis of the body is maintained by complex physiologic mechanisms. The total body water (TBW) can be divided into two main phases or compartments, extracellular (ECF) and intracellular (ICF). The ECF is subdivided into the blood plasma and interstitial fluid (ISF) which represent 5 and 15 percent of the total body weight respectively. The volumes of ECF and ICF vary with age and sex. Infants have a larger amount of TBW and ECF per unit of body weight than do adults. Changes take place rapidly during the first few months and more slowly during the early years of life.

Electrolyte composition of ECF and ICF differ markedly. The chemical structure of ECF can be precisely determined from the blood plasma, a subcompartment of ECF, readily available for direct analysis.

Table 7-1. Distribution of total body water in
infants and children (percent of body weight)

Age	TBW	ECF
0–1 day	79.0	43.9
1–10 days	74.0	39.7
1–3 months	72.3	32.2
3–6 months	70.1	30.1
6–12 months	60.4	27.0
1–2 years	58.7	25.6
2–3 years	63.5	26.7
3–5 years	62.2	21.4
5–10 years	61.5	22.0
10–16 years	58.0	18.0

The composition of ICF, however, can only be approximated because the fluid within the cells cannot be measured directly.

The composition of ISF except for its lower protein content is similar to that of plasma since they are separated by the capillary membrane which permits free passage of all ions and small molecules.

ECF ELECTROLYTE CONCENTRATION (See Figure 7-1)

The pattern of electrolytes of infants is similar to that of adults; however, there are certain differences. Although mean sodium concentration is the same as in the adult plasma, the range is somewhat greater. The plasma potassium concentration is higher, the average potassium is about 5.0 meq per liter. Calcium and magnesium are similar to those of normal adults. The most striking difference in infants is in the bicarbonate concentration. Average bicarbonate is 20 meq per liter as compared to 24.0 meq per liter in adults, and the difference in the anion concentration is made up by the chloride ion (average chloride is 105 meq per liter). Undetermined anion* concentration is also somewhat increased in infants. Inorganic phosphate is higher than in nongrowing adults. Plasma total protein concentration varies more in normal infants than in adults; accordingly, the valence contributed by protein tends to be more variable.

Regulation of acid-base metabolism   Blood pH is maintained within a rather narrow range 7.35 to 7.45 with a mean pH of 7.4. Variations from 6.8 to 7.7 have been recorded, but these are considered extremes. Two distinct, but interdigitated, mechanisms are responsible for the maintenance and the regulation of the blood pH in normal and pathologic states:

---

* Undetermined anion (UA): the fraction of the plasma anions which is not ordinarily determined in routine clinical chemistry laboratories. It is the difference between the determined cations (Na^+, K^+, Ca^{++}, Mg^{++}) and the usually determined anions (Cl^-, HCO_3^-, and proteinate). UA contains inorganic phosphate, inorganic sulfate, and small concentrations of a number of organic anions.

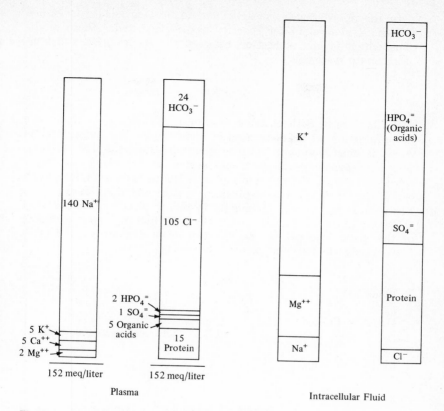

Figure 7-1. Comparison of plasma and intracellular fluid.

1. Buffer mechanism: Buffer in blood or in other compartments of the body fluids may be divided into two groups, the bicarbonate system ($B^+HCO_3^-$) and the nonbicarbonate system—hemoglobin, inorganic and organic phosphate and plasma protein (B^+Buf^-).

    Addition of strong acids (H^+X^-) or base (B^+OH^-) are buffered by both classes of buffers as demonstrated in the following reactions:

    Strong acid added

    $$H^+X^- \;+\; B^+HCO_3^- \;\rightarrow\; H_2CO_3 \;+\; B^+X^-$$

    $$H^+X^- \;+\; B^+Buf^- \;\rightarrow\; H^+Buf^- \;+\; B^+X^-$$

    Strong base added

    $$B^+OH^- \;+\; H_2CO_3 \;\rightarrow\; B^+HCO_3^- \;+\; H_2O$$

    $$B^+OH^- \;+\; H^+Buf^- \;\rightarrow\; B^+Buf^- \;+\; H_2O$$

In the above reactions carbonic acid or bicarbonate is gained or lost. A general buffer reaction takes place under these conditions which is an interaction between the bicarbonate and non-bicarbonate systems:

$$H_2CO_3 \; + \; B^+Buf^- \; \rightarrow \; B^+HCO_3^- \; + \; H^+Buf^-$$

All buffers in both bicarbonate and nonbicarbonate systems are in equilibrium in all body fluid compartments. The buffer system which is most commonly used to determine the acid-base relationship is bicarbonate–carbonic acid system in the blood because it can be accurately quantitated and it is the direct target for physiologic regulation by the respiratory system and the kidneys.

2. Physiologic mechanism, primarily involving renal and respiratory systems: Carbonic acid is one of the principal metabolic products of the body. The pH of the blood depends directly on the ratio between bicarbonate and carbonic acid concentration.

$$\text{Blood pH} = 6.10 + \log \frac{HCO_3^-}{H_2CO_3 + CO_2 \text{ (d)}^*}$$

$$H_2CO_3 + CO_2 \text{ (d)} = P_{CO_2} \times S\dagger$$
$$\text{(Solubility factor constant 0.03 mM/L)}$$

$$pH = 6.10 + \log \frac{HCO_3}{P_{CO_2} \times S}$$

$$\frac{24}{40 \times 0.03} = \frac{24}{1.2} \text{ or } \frac{20}{1}$$

Normally, the HCO_3^- equals 24 meq per liter and the H_2CO_3 equals 1.2 meq per liter. If an approximate 20:1 ratio is preserved between the bicarbonate and carbonic acid, the pH will remain normal, in spite of marked changes in total concentrations of each one.

The importance of this relationship is that if HCO_3^- is reduced, P_{CO_2} can be decreased to maintain the ratio of 20:1. Conversely when the HCO_3 increases, P_{CO_2} can be increased to maintain the normal ratio. This change in P_{CO_2} is accomplished by regulating alveolar ventilation. Alveolar hyperventilation causes a reduction in P_{CO_2}, while alveolar hypoventilation results in an increase.

While the P_{CO_2} is under the control of the respiratory system, the

---

*   Dissolved CO_2.
†   Solubility factor for CO_2 in blood at body temperature is a constant having a value of 0.03 mM gas dissolved per liter of plasma per mmHg P_{CO_2}.

HCO_3^- is regulated by the kidney. The regulation of HCO_3^- concentration in the extracellular fluid (ECF) is achieved by two different mechanisms. First, the kidney will reabsorb less than the filtered HCO_3^- and produce HCO_3^--rich urine in situations where there is a relative excess of HCO_3^- as in acute respiratory alkalosis or an absolute excess of HCO_3^- as is the case of metabolic alkalosis. Secondly, the kidney can synthesize HCO_3^- in conditions with a relative (respiratory acidosis) or absolute (metabolic acidosis) decrease in HCO_3^- concentration. During the production of new HCO_3^- from carbonic acid, hydrogen ion is liberated and must be excreted in the urine in order to "free" the bicarbonate to return to the ECF. Acidification of urine takes place.

In the newborn infant and particularly the premature one, a number of homeostatic mechanisms do not function as efficiently as in the older child. For example, the concentrating power of the kidney during early infancy is less (700 mOsm per liter) than that of the mature kidney (1,400 mOsm per liter). As a result, the newborn infant requires more water to excrete a given amount of solutes than does the child. Consequently, in cases of dehydration, the newborn infant cannot conserve fluid as effectively as an older child by excreting highly concentrated urine. The maintenance of the acid-base balance by the kidney of the newborn infant is also less efficient because of their low excretion rate of ammonium ion in the urine. In addition, young infants excrete very little phosphate in their urine, which limits their capacity to excrete titratable acids, resulting in rapid development and persistence of acidemia in response to only a small additional load of hydrogen ion.

Classification of the altered acid-base metabolism (see Table 7-2)

Metabolic disturbance *Metabolic acidosis* is defined as a state wherein the blood H^+ concentration is increased above normal values. It can be classified into two categories: (1) the gain of strong acid by ECF and (2) the loss of HCO_3^- from ECF.

Metabolic alkalosis is a state in which the H^+ concentration is decreased. It can be the sequence of (1) gain of OH^- by the ECF or (2) secondary to the administration of an excess of exogenous bicarbonate or its precursors.

Respiratory disturbance *Respiratory acidosis* is a primary disorder of the respiratory system which is secondary to the primary increase in the alveolar P_{CO_2}.

Respiratory alkalosis is the opposite of respiratory acidosis and occurs because of decrease in the alveolar P_{CO_2}.

Major pathways in acid-base disturbances can be related to the Henderson-Hasselbach equation as summarized in Figure 7-2.

Table 7-2. Common disturbances of acid-base homeostasis

Type	Etiology	Clinical examples	Compositional changes of the blood				
			pH	HCO₃⁻	P_{CO_2}	BB	BE
Metabolic acidosis	Gain of H⁺ by ECF	Ketone acids (starvation, diabetes) Lactic acid (primary and secondary lactic acidosis)	Low	Low	Low	Low	Low
	Loss of HCO₃⁻ by ECF	Via GI tract (diarrhea) Via kidney (renal tubular acidosis)					
Metabolic alkalosis	Gain of strong base by ECF	Loss of H⁺ Cl⁻ (vomiting) Transfer of H⁺ for K⁺ (hypokalemia)	High	High	High/ normal	High	High
	Gain of exogenous HCO₃⁻ by ECF	Loading with NaHCO₃					
Respiratory acidosis	Alveolar hypoventilation	Intrinsic lung disease (mucoviscidosis, asthma, pulmonary edema) Disease of the chest wall (respiratory muscle paralysis, chest deformity) Disturbances of respiratory center (drugs, head trauma)	Low	High	High	High	High
Respiratory alkalosis	Alveolar hyperventilation	Emotional Stimulation of respiratory center (salicylate, tumor, advanced liver disease)	High	Low	Low	Low	Low

	Acidosis (pH $\downarrow$)		Alkalosis (pH $\uparrow$)	
Metabolic	$\dfrac{HCO_3^-}{H_2CO_3} \downarrow$ =	Total CO$_2$	$\dfrac{HCO_3^-}{H_2CO_3} \uparrow$ =	Total CO$_2$
Respiratory	$\dfrac{HCO_3^-}{H_2CO_3} \uparrow$ =	Total CO$_2$	$\dfrac{HCO_3^-}{H_2CO_3} \downarrow$ =	Total CO$_2$ $\downarrow$

Figure 7-2

As seen in Figure 7-2, total CO_2 determination cannot determine the type of acid-base disturbance because CO_2 is not always decreased in acidosis nor increased in alkalosis; therefore, other acid-base parameters, i.e.; pH, buffer base, base excess,* P_{CO_2}, are needed to identify the nature of the deranged acid-base metabolism.

DEHYDRATION

Dehydration occurs when there is excessive loss of body water. This loss is always accompanied by loss of electrolytes; it may result in no change in the concentration of blood electrolytes (isotonic dehydration), an increase in the concentration of blood electrolytes (hypertonic dehydration), or a decrease in the concentration of blood electrolytes (hypotonic dehydration). Hypertonic dehydration is characterized by marked thirst and cerebral symptoms and has a grave prognosis, particularly if electrolyte solutions are used injudiciously. During periods of dehydration, plasma volume tends to be maintained at the expense of interstitial and intracellular fluid. The recovery phase of dehydration is not complete until there has been proper reconstitution of both intracellular and extracellular water and electrolytes.

Causes in childhood   Inadequate fluid intake, for example, thirsting or excessive loss via

1. Skin: e.g., perspiration during hot weather, fever, burns
2. Gastrointestinal tract: vomiting, diarrhea, fistulas, suctioning
3. Renal: diabetes insipidus, diabetes mellitus, urinary tract infection
4. Lungs: hyperventilation
5. Vascular system: hemorrhage

---

* Buffer base (BB) is the sum of concentrations of whole-blood bicarbonate, plasma proteins, and hemoglobin expressed in milliequivalents per liter. Base Excess (BE) is the base concentration in milliequivalents per liter of whole blood as measured by titration with strong acid to pH 7.4 at a 40 mmHg of P_{CO2} at 37°C. For negative values of base excess, the titration is carried out with strong base. Such negative values are denoted by the term "base deficit."

Clinical features

1. Thirst.
2. The skin, lips, and tongue are dry and the saliva has an increased viscosity.
3. Skin turgor is poor.
4. The fontanel is sunken.
5. The weight is reduced.
6. Urinary output is diminished.
7. Apathy, restlessness, and convulsions may occur.

Laboratory determinations useful in diagnosis and treatment

1. Urinary output is diminished, and the specific gravity is high. BUN may be elevated.
2. Hematocrit reading, red cell count, and plasma-protein level reveal hemoconcentration.
3. CO_2 content is usually low. Chlorides are normal or elevated.

Fluid requirements   The daily requirement may be calculated on a weight-and-age basis from Table 7-3.

Table 7-3.   Daily fluid requirements

Age	Daily requirement, ml/kg	Additional amount for moderate dehydration, ml/kg	Additional amount for severe dehydration, ml/kg
24 hr	0	50	100
1–15 days	60–120*	50	100
16 days–4 months	150	50	100
4–6 months	120	50	100
6–9 months	90	50	100
9–12 months	75	30	60
12–24 months	75	30	50
2–5 years	45	30	50
5–10 years	30	30	50

* Rises gradually.

Fluid requirements may also be calculated on the basis of surface area. This measurement permits the use of a single determinant to calculate fluid requirements regardless of the age and size of the patient. Body surface area can be estimated from body weight alone or from the weight and height (see Figure 7-3).

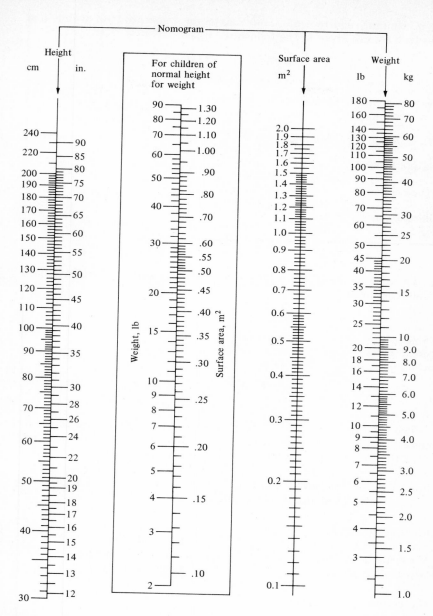

Figure 7-3

Minimum requirements and maximum tolerance for water and electrolytes are given in the following table.

Minimum requirements and maximum tolerance of water and electrolytes per 24 hours

Substance		per m^2
Water, ml	Min.	870
	Max.	4,700
Na and K, meq	Min.	10
	Max.	250
PO_4, meq	Min.	10
	Max.	65
Glucose, Gm	Min.	75
	Max.	300

The average daily water losses in a normal resting infant have been calculated to be:

Urine	700 ml/m^2
Insensible water loss	1,000 ml/m^2
Stool	80 ml/m^2
	1,780 ml/m^2

The average amount of endogenous water produced by the body metabolism (water of oxidation) equals 270 ml per square meter per day; thus the average water expenditure (average daily loss is 1,780 minus endogenous water produced, 270) is approximately 1,500 ml per square meter per day. Figures given below are useful as a guideline in the treatment of children with dehydration.

Fluid requirement
Maintenance   1,500 ml/m^2/24 hr
Moderate dehydration   2,500–3,000 ml/m^2/24 hr
Severe dehydration   3,000–3,600 ml/m^2/24 hr

Electrolyte requirement
Maintenance
   Na^+ 50–75 meq/m^2/24 hr
   K^+ 40–60 meq/m^2/24 hr
Newborn infant (1–7 days)
   Fluid   750 ml/m^2/24 hr
   Na^+ 20 meq/m^2/24 hr
   K^+ 15 meq/m^2/24 hr

TREATMENT OF FLUID AND ELECTROLYTE IMBALANCE

An isolated disturbance of either fluids or electrolytes is seen rarely. More commonly, there is an imbalance of both water and solutes and an alteration in acid-base equilibrium. When treating fluid and electrolyte disturbances, it is also important to determine and treat the underlying disease, e.g., gastroenteritis, diabetes mellitus.

Therapy during the acute phase is aimed at replacing the fluids and electrolytes lost because of the illness and supplying the daily requirements. This phase usually requires 24 to 48 hours and is accomplished by the use of intravenous therapy if disturbances are moderate (rapid loss of more than 5 percent of the body weight as water) or if disturbances are severe (rapid loss of more than 10 percent of the body weight as water). Homeostasis is then preserved by supplying those fluids and electrolytes which are needed for maintenance. This is usually accomplished by a combination of both oral and intravenous therapy. For recovery to be complete all cellular constituents including fat and protein must be replaced. Adequate amounts of some cellular constituents, e.g., calories, iron, cannot be supplied by the intravenous route over an extended period of time. In rare cases, e.g., prolonged coma, in which some oral feedings cannot be taken, it may be necessary to employ gavage feedings or in selected cases hyperalimentation may be used.

Mild dehydration and minimal electrolyte imbalance These conditions are characterized by dryness of mucous membranes and reduced urinary output. Depending on the underlying etiology, the infant may even appear normal. Water, electrolytes, and carbohydrates are supplied orally in the absence of vomiting.

Saline-bicarbonate-sucrose mixture [(1) salt—sodium chloride—½ tsp (2.5 Gm or 43 meq), (2) baking soda—½ tsp (2.5 Gm or 30 meq), (3) cane sugar—10 tsp or 50 Gm, (4) water—1 qt], or commercially available balanced-electrolyte solution may be used orally. (If vomiting has occurred, oral fluids may be withheld for up to a few hours and then started in teaspoonful amounts with gradual increments.)

Moderate and severe disturbances The more severe disturbances are characterized by depression of the fontanel and eyeballs, loss of turgor and dryness of the skin. The child appears acutely ill. Circulatory signs begin with mottling of the skin and cool extremities and progress to tachycardia and circulatory failure (shock). Urinary output diminishes and is accompanied by a rising specific gravity which may fall later to values around 1.010, indicating renal failure. Weight loss as indicated above is perhaps the best single criterion to use in estimating the degree of loss of water and electrolytes.

I.   Blood is drawn for the following laboratory tests:
   A. CO_2
   B.   pH and blood gases
   C.   Hematocrit and hemoglobin
   D.   Plasma-protein concentration
   E.   Sodium, potassium, and chloride levels and BUN
   F.   Blood typing and cross matching

II.   Initial intravenous hydration (see Table 7-4) is begun with isotonic electrolyte solution in 5 percent glucose at a rate of 15 to
   20 ml per kg infused rapidly during approximately 45 to 60
   minutes to restore the circulating volume of blood. Then ⅓ to
   ½ isotonic balanced electrolyte solution is given according to
   the estimated degree of water loss and type of dehydration.
      Of the total daily fluid requirements (see p. 132), 25 percent is
   given during a 3-hour period. The remainder of the calculated
   fluids are given evenly over the period of 21 hours. When the
   clinical condition is improved and urine output indicates adequate renal function, potassium ion is added to the fluid regimen. In hypertonic dehydration the total 24-hour needs are distributed evenly during the entire period. Blood (10 ml per kg)
   may be given to combat shock.

III.   There is always a degree of metabolic acidosis present (blood pH
   below 7.4) with either
   A. CO_2 content below normal (24 meq per liter but above 10
      meq per liter). This degree of acidosis will be corrected by
      the body's homeostatic mechanisms if adequate amounts of
      fluids with balanced electrolytes containing either bicarbon-
      ate or lactate* are administered.
   B. CO_2 content below 10 meq per liter. The correction of this
      degree of acidosis by replacement of base deficit may be
      calculated by the following formula as a guideline to modify
      the bicarbonate concentration in the balanced electrolyte
      solution in these severely acidotic dehydrated infants:

$$24 - CO_2 \text{ meq/L} \times \text{weight in kg} \times 0.7 \text{ (TBW)}$$
$$= \text{Total meq } CO_2 \text{ deficit to be replenished}$$

   This may be calculated as number of ml of buffer, either as
   sodium bicarbonate 5% or ⅙ molar sodium lactate solution.
   If the total volume of calculated fluid of balanced electrolyte solution for the first 24 hours does not contain the
   estimated number of ml of sodium bicarbonate or lactate,
   it is then adjusted to the desired volume of bicarbonate or
   lactate (see Table 7-4).

---

*   Acidosis will be gradually corrected as the normal state of hydration is achieved and excessive
   gastrointestinal losses are decreased.
   The CO_2 content is raised approximately 5 meq per liter by each 20 ml of ⅙ molar sodium lactate
   per kg body weight or 5 meq per liter by each 5 ml 5% $NaHCO_3$ per kg body weight.

Table 7-4. Parenteral solutions (electrolytes listed as meq/L)

Solution	Na	K	Cl	HCO$_3$	Ca	P	Mg
Isotonic saline	154	...	154	...	...	...	...
5% sodium bicarbonate	600	...	...	600	...	...	...
7.5% sodium bicarbonate	900	...	...	900	...	...	...
0.33% saline	56	...	56	...	...	...	...
3% NaCl*	513	...	513	...	...	...	...
Homeolyte #75 (isolyte "M")	40	35	40	20	...	15	...
Homeolyte #48 (isolyte "P")	25	20	22	23	...	3	3
6:2:1*	53	...	34	18	...	...	...
5:2:1 solution‡	58	...	39	19	...	...	...
3:2:1 solution§	77	...	51	26	...	...	...
M/6 Na lactate	167	...	...	167¶	...	...	...
Dextrose-amigen	30	15	22	...	5	30	2
Lactated Ringer's	130	4	109	28	3	...	...
Albumisol	130	...	130	...	...	...	...

* Estimate 2ml of 3% NaCl per meq per liter of Na when raising tonicity of a given solution.
† 6 Parts 10% or 5% D/W, 2 parts isotonic NaCl, 1 part m/6 Na lactate.
‡ 5 Parts 10% or 5% D/W, 2 parts isotonic NaCl, 1 part m/6 Na lactate.
§ 3 Parts 10% or 5% D/W, 2 parts isotonic NaCl, 1 part m/6 Na lactate; 5 ml buffered potassium phosphate solution contains 25.89 meq K.
¶ Lactate as precursor of bicarbonate.

No attempts should be made, however, to correct the acidosis by the rapid infusion of hypertonic bicarbonate solution (5% or 7.5% NaHCO$_3$) except in cases of cardiac and/or respiratory arrests.

IV. If metabolic alkalosis is present (pH is above 7.4 and a CO$_2$ content is greater than 24 meq), it will be corrected by the body's homeostatic mechanism if adequate amounts of fluids and electrolytes are supplied without bicarbonate or its precursors.

After initial hydration, one of the following balanced electrolyte solutions is given according to the type of dehydration the patient presents:

One-third isotonic for normal electrolyte levels (isotonic dehydration)
One-half isotonic for low electrolyte levels (hypotonic dehydration)

Potassium, 2 to 4 meq per kg per day, is added to the therapeutic regimen if urinary output is adequate. Excessive fluid and electrolyte loss, for example, in continued diarrhea, must be replaced by estimating the amount lost and adding it to total requirements.

The treatment of hypernatremic dehydration requires some deviation from the usual therapy of dehydration. Although the principles are the same, slower correction of the state of hydration with normalization of the electrolyte levels are necessary to avoid water intoxication. In this case, a solution is used which contains 30 to 50 meq per liter Na^+, part as chloride and part as bicarbonate or lactate, K^+ (after urinary output is established), 20 to 40 meq per liter as acetate or chloride, and approximately 0.5 Gm calcium gluconate per 12 hours. If shock is not present, the electrolyte deficit should be estimated and added to the calculated volume requirements for 48 hours, and the total solution is then administered evenly over the ensuing 48 hours.

After 24 to 48 hours of therapy, the fluid and electrolytes lost are usually replaced, as evidenced by the disappearance of the clinical features characterizing dehydration and electrolyte imbalance and by more normal results when the laboratory tests are repeated at this time.

In most cases, oral intake will now be sufficient to provide the necessary water, solutes, and calories; if not, the amount of fluid taken orally is subtracted from the total daily requirement and the remainder is supplied by a one-third to one-half isotonic balanced electrolyte solution.

If parenteral therapy is the sole source of nourishment for a prolonged period, it may be advisable to supply some protein in the form of whole blood or protein hydrolysates. Vitamins, particularly water-soluble vitamins (B and C), should also be supplied to replace their loss.

A 7-month-old infant weighing 15 lb with moderate dehydration and acidosis is presented for therapy. The cause is determined and treated whenever possible, e.g., bacterial infection, with the appropriate antibiotic.

1. Specimens are collected for the necessary laboratory tests (see p. 136).
2. If no shock is present, total daily fluid requirement (on the basis of body surface) is 0.36 (SA) $\times$ 3000 ml/m^2 (for moderate dehydration) = 1,080 ml. If continued fluid loss occurs, e.g., in persistent diarrhea or during suctioning via tube in the gastrointestinal tract, it may be necessary to increase the volume of fluid administered by an amount equivalent to the loss.
3. 270 ml ($\frac{1}{4}$ of 1,080) is given as balanced electrolyte solution (see item IV above) during a 3-hour period. (To accomplish this, the solution is administered at a rate of approximately 1 macrodrop per 3 seconds, or 30 drops/min).
4. The remainder of the total daily requirement (1,080 − 270 = 810 ml) is given during a (24 − 3 = 21)-hour period. To accomplish this, the following suggested fluids are administered at a rate of 1 drop per 6 to 7 seconds.

5. Assuming the CO_2 content to be 12 meq per liter, the calculated volume (1,080 ml per 24 hr) of one-third isotonic balanced electrolyte solution will provide 120 ml of $\frac{1}{6}$ molar lactate $= 16$ ml/kg/day, or, if it is $\frac{1}{2}$ isotonic, will provide 180 ml of $\frac{1}{6}$ molar lactate $= 24$ ml/kg/day, which will theoretically raise the CO_2 level by 4 to 6 meq/L at the end of the first 24 hours. Since the body itself has some degree of contribution toward the altered acid-base equilibrium, attempts of rapid correction of the existing CO_2 deficit to near normal levels may cause the overshooting phenomena.

6. The laboratory tests are repeated in 8 to 12 hours and again on the second day. If abnormalities persist, the above procedure is repeated. If the tests indicate normal hydration, electrolyte balance, and normal acid-base homeostasis, the maintenance fluid (see p. 137) is used to complete the second day's fluid requirement. For instance:

   a. Total daily requirement is 2,000 ml/m² $\times$ 0.36 $= 720$ ml (patient gained 1 lb when dehydration was corrected).

   b. If the infant is drinking 1 oz every 3 hours, it could be assumed that in 24 hours he will take 240 ml. Therefore, $720 - 240$ or 480 ml will be given intravenously (a rate of 1 drop per 12 seconds). If after 12 hours the estimated oral intake is incorrect, the rate of the intravenous fluids may be altered to compensate for the difference.

REVIEW QUESTIONS

1. Interstitial fluid (ISF) represents (a) 5 percent; (b) 10 percent; (c) 15 percent; (d) 20 percent of the total body weight.
2. Infants have (a) smaller; (b) larger; (c) the same volume of extracellular fluid (ECF) and total body water (TBW) than adults.
3. In spite of marked changes in total concentration of bicarbonate and carbonic acid, the blood pH will remain normal if an approximate (a) 5:1; (b) 10:1; (c) 15:1; (d) 20:1 ratio is preserved.
4. Alveolar hyperventilation causes (a) a reduction; (b) an increase; (c) no change in P_{CO_2}.
5. In premature infants the concentrating power of the kidney is approximately (a) 500 mOsm per liter; (b) 700 mOsm per liter; (c) 900 mOsm per liter; (d) 1,400 mOsm per liter.
6. The newborn infant requires (a) less; (b) more; (c) the same amount of water to excrete a given amount of solutes than does the older child.
7. Column I lists certain disturbances of body homeostasis. Column II contains some statements about these disturbances. Match the two:

I	II
A. Metabolic acidosis ____	(a) pH high and bicaronate high
B. Metabolic alkalosis ____	(b) pH low and bicarbonate high
C. Respiratory acidosis ____	(c) pH low and bicarbonate low
D. Respiratory alkalosis ____	(d) pH high and bicarbonate low

8. Fluid requirements for maintenance in the pediatric age group are (a) 500 ml/m²/24 hr; (b) 1,000 ml/m²/24 hr; (c) 1,500 ml/m²/24 hr; (d) 2,000 ml/m²/24 hr.

9. The CO_2 content can be raised approximately (a) 1 meq per liter; (b) 3 meq per liter; (c) 5 meq per liter by each 20 ml of ⅙ molar sodium lactate per kg of body weight administered.

10. In the correction of hypernatremic dehydration, fluids must be replaced (a) at a slower rate; (b) at a faster rate; (c) at the same rate as in the therapy of other types of dehydration.

The following questions are the matching type. In each blank in column I, insert the letter corresponding to the word or phrase in column II which is associated most appropriately.

I		II	
11. Normal serum potassium ____		(a)	24 meq per liter
12. Normal serum chloride ____		(b)	150 meq per liter
13. Normal serum sodium ____		(c)	5 meq per liter
14. Normal saline solution ____		(d)	103 meq per liter
15. Normal serum bicarbonate ____		(e)	142 meq per liter

The following paired phrases each describe two entities that are to be compared quantitatively. In the blanks provided, write the letter A if (A) is greater than item (B), B if item (B) is greater than item (A), and C if the items are equal or very nearly equal.

16. ____ (A) Plasma potassium concentration in adults
17. ____ (B) Plasma potassium concentration in children
18. ____ (A) Plasma bicarbonate concentration in adults
19. ____ (B) Plasma bicarbonate concentration in children

8 GENETICS

The development of an individual depends on two sets of interacting influences—genetic factors and environmental experiences. Genetic factors are present at conception and remain unchanged during life with the exception of somatic mutations. Environmental factors are constantly changing. A genetically determined predisposition to a particular disease may occur due to

1. Chromosome abnormality
2. Single mutant gene
3. Multiple mutant genes interacting with environmental factors

Diseases due to chromosome malformations or a single mutant gene are almost entirely genetically determined. Diseases which are partially determined by genetic factors depend on the interaction of many genes with the environment.

Chromosome abnormalities are readily recognizable by karyotyping. Disease due to a single mutant gene is usually recognizable by its simple Mendelian pattern which indicates whether it is an autosomal dominant, autosomal recessive, or X-linked condition. Demonstration of significant genetic predisposition to conditions which are polygenic depend on twin studies and on family studies.

Monozygotic (identical) twins have identical genes, since they are derived from a single zygote which has split during early development. Dizygotic (fraternal) twins are essentially two sibs that happen to be conceived at the same time. They arise when a mother releases two ova within a few days of each other, both being fertilized by different sperms to form separate zygotes.

If monozygotic twins are almost always affected (high concordance rate) but the same sex dizygotic twins are much less often affected (low concordance rate; discordant), the disease is usually determined by genetic factors. If the concordance rate for monozygotic twins is similar to the concordance rate of dizygotic like-sex twins, the disease is not genetically determined.

CHROMOSOMES

There are 23 pairs of chromosomes in man. In metaphase each chromosome divides into two chromatids which are attached to each other by the centromere. When the centromere splits, the two chromatids formed separate and become segregated, one into each daughter cell. The members of a paired chromosome are homologous, complementary in function, and similar in appearance with the exception of X and Y, the sex-determining pair in males. The chromosomes are classified by their total length and the position of the centromere at metaphase. The centromere divides a chromosome into a short arm (p) and a long arm (q). Those with median centromeres are called "metacentric," those with centromeres close to one end are called "submetacentric," and those with terminal centromeres are called "acrocentric." The short arm of acrocentric chromosomes is connected to a small segment (satellite). A constricted portion separates the short arm from the satellite. The autosomes (nonsex chromosomes) are classified into 7 groups, A to G and also numbered from 1 to 22. The twenty-third pair is the sex chromosomes (XX in female, XY in male). The A–G groups are easily recognized morphologically. Distinction within one group is not always possible by light microscopy. Special techniques, e.g., autoradiography and fluorescein-staining, assist in identifying individual chromosomes.

Autoradiography measures the rate at which chromosomes take up tritiated thymidine. It distinguishes one of the X chromosomes in women (late replicating X) and B and D group chromosomes. Fluorescein-staining with quinacrine mustard identifies the Y chromosome, G group chromosomes, and some C group chromosomes.

Chromosome groups

Group	Number	Characteristics
A	1–3	Large with median centromere
B	4–5	Large with submedian centromere
C	6–12 and X	Medium size with submedian centromere (difficult to identify individual members)
D	13–15	Medium size with acrocentric centromere, satellites on end of short arm
E	16–18	Moderately short size with submetacentric centromere
F	19–20	Short size with submetacentric centromere
G	21, 22, and Y	Very short size with acrocentric centromere, satellites on 21 and 22

Description of a karyotype is written in shorthand; first the total number of chromosomes, then the sex chromosomes, and then a description of any anomaly. A normal male is written 46, XY, and a normal female, 46, XX. A female with a single X chromosome (monosomy X) is 45, X; a male with an extra chromosome in G group is 47, XY, G+.

MITOSIS AND MEIOSIS

In mitosis (somatic cell division), the longitudinal separation of each chromosome into two chromatids is followed by cell division. As the cell and nucleus divide, the paired chromatids separate, and one chromatid passes into each daughter cell. The chromatid reconstitutes to a chromosome, and each daughter cell has a complete set of 23 pairs of chromosomes (diploid) as did the original cell.

In meiosis (gamete formation) there are two cell divisions. In the first, the reduction division of primary spermatocyte or oocyte, the chromatids formed do not separate, homologous chromosomes pair together and one member of each homologous chromosome, at random, enters the daughter cell (independent segregation). The 2° spermatocytes (or oocyte) contain 23 unpaired chromosomes (haploid set). During the second division the chromatids separate so that the two gametes formed contain a haploid set of unpaired 23 chromosomes.

In the formation of the ovum one of the daughter cells in each of the two divisions forms a polar body, so that the final product is one ovum with three polar bodies.

During fertilization of the ovum by the sperm, the fusion of their nuclei will result in a set of 23 pairs of chromosomes (diploid).

SEX DETERMINATION

A Y-bearing sperm produces on fertilization an XY zygote (male) and an X-bearing sperm, an XX zygote (female). In a cell nucleus which is not dividing (interphase nucleus), if two X chromosomes are present, one of these is resting (inactive), tightly coiled, and appears as a dark-staining body (Barr body or sex chromatin) at the edge of nucleus. This may be seen in epithelial cells obtained by scraping the inside of the cheek (buccal smear). Cells are scored chromatin negative, implying the presence of only one X chromosome (normal male or gonadal dysgenesis with genotype 45, X) or chromatin positive (normal female or Klinefelter's syndrome with genotype 47, XXY). A buccal smear gives information only about the X chromosomes. The number of Barr bodies seen is one less than the number of X chromosomes present.

Two types of chromosome abnormalities occur.

1. Chromosomal nondysjunction leading to trisomy or monosomy. The most common cause of major chromosome anomalies is an error in meiosis such that one chromosome less or one too many enters a gamete and subsequently the zygote is monosomic or trisomic, respectively.

Individuals with three sex chromosomes are trisomic for the sex chromosomes such as seen in triple X syndrome (47, XXX) or Klinefelter's syndrome (47, XXY). Individuals with one sex chromosome are monosomic for the sex chromosome. This genotype is written XO (or 45, X) and usually causes an early abortion of the fetus; those who survive have Turner's syndrome. YO (or 45, Y) is not compatible with life.

Complete autosomal monosomies are nonviable, but autosomal trisomies are common. In trisomic Down's syndrome there is an extra G chromosome (designated as chromosome 21) 47, XX, G+. In Edwards' syndrome an extra E chromosome (chromosome 18: 47, XX, E18+) is present, and in Patau's syndrome (D_1 trisomy) an extra D chromosome is present (chromosome 13: 47, XX, D13+).

Nondysjunction can also occur at an early mitotic division of the zygote, causing mosaicism, which is the presence of two or more cell lines in an individual derived from a single zygote. In a mosaic condition both cell lines are designated: 45, X/46, XY.

2. Chromosome breaks and translocations causing abnormal chromosome morphology.

Single chromosome breaks are common, but in most instances the raw ends reunite without loss to the chromosome. Simultaneous breaks in a chromosome may lead to the loss of a fragment from short arm (p) or long arm (q) of the chromosome. This is called "deletion." In the cat-cry syndrome there is a deletion of the short arm of the 5th chromosome (46, XY, B5p−). A deleted G22 chromosome is called a Philadelphia chromosome and is frequently present in chronic myelogenous leukemia.

Transverse, instead of longitudinal, breaks at the centromere lead to the formation of two isochromosomes, in one of which both arms of the chromosome correspond to the long arm and in the other, to the short arm, of the original chromosome. An isochromosome of the long arm of the G chromosome is written Gqi. The occurrence of two simultaneous breaks in nonhomologous chromosomes and an exchange of chromosome material leads to two altered chromosomes (reciprocal translocation), but if no genes are lost by the exchange, the translocation is a balanced one. The possessor of a balanced translocation is clinically unaffected, but he may produce children with an unbalanced translocation which manifests itself in a clinical syndrome.

The rate of chromosome anomalies is 1 per 100 live-born infants (divided equally between autosomes and sex chromosomes). Nearly 50 percent of spontaneous abortions occurring in the first trimester reveal a chromosome anomaly. The most common chromosome anomaly is a trisomy of the sex chromosomes.

CLINICAL SYNDROMES DUE TO CHROMOSOME ANOMALIES (See Table 8-1)

Klinefelter's syndrome   One of the most common causes of male hypogonadism occurs in about 1 in 400 male births. The clinical features (see p. 643) do not become obvious until after puberty. These are phenotypic males with a chromatin-positive buccal smear. All cases have at least two X chromosomes and at least one Y chromosome (47, XXY). Clinical variants of the syndrome are the result of sex chromosome mosaicism (XY/XXY or XX/XXY) or of duplication of the sex chromosomes.

XYY syndrome   (see Table 8-1)

Triple X syndrome   The triple X syndrome causes little symptomatology presumably because the third X chromosome is a nonfunctioning one. Intelligence is often reduced, so that it is found five times more often in mentally retarded females.

XXXY syndrome   (see Table 8-1)

Turner's syndrome   (see Table 8-1)

Down's syndrome (mongolism)   (See Chapter 20, "Neurologic Conditions.")   G trisomy is the most common autosomal trisomy. Incidence is 1.8 per 1,000 live births. Frequency of G trisomy is much influenced by maternal age (this is true for most of the trisomies). A woman under the age of 25 has about a 1 in 2,000 chance of having an affected child, while a woman aged 40 or over has a 1 in 100 chance.

Table 8-1. Clinical syndromes due to chromosome abnormalities

Syndrome	Incidence	Type of anomaly	Clinical and laboratory features
Klinefelter's	1:400 male births	47, XXY or variants XY/XXY XX/XXY	One of most common causes of male hypogonadism (see p. 643).
XYY	0.5:100 male births	47, XYY	Phenotypic male, behavioral problems, increased height, elevated plasma testosterone levels.
Triple X	1:1,000 female births	47, XXX	May be mentally retarded, irregular menses, reduced fertility.
XXXY	Unknown	48, XXXY	Retarded, hypertelorism, epicanthus, strabismus, hypoplastic scrotum, small testes, radio-ulnar synostosis, scoliosis, and kyphosis.
Turner's (gonadal dysgenesis)	1:2,500 female births, 5:100 aborted fetuses	45, X or variant XO/XX	Symptomatology is variable (see Gonadal Dysgenesis, Chapter 24, "Endocrine Diseases").
Down's (mongolism)	1.8:1,000 births	47, XX or 47, XY or variant 46	G trisomy is the most common autosomal anomaly (see Down's syndrome, Chapter 20, "Neurologic Conditions").
Edwards' (Trisomy 18)	0.3:1,000 births	47, XX, E18+	Polyhydramnios, small placenta, single umbilical artery, low birth weight, mental retardation, deafness, prominent occiput, low-set malformed ears, small mouth, narrow palatal arch, characteristic position of hand: clenched, index finger overlapping third, fifth over fourth, abnormal dermatoglyphics, skeletal muscle hypoplasia, associated cardiac, gastrointestinal, and renal anomalies.

Syndrome	Incidence	Karyotype	Clinical features
Patau's (Trisomy 13, D1 Trisomy)	0.2:1,000 births	47, XX, D1+ 47, XY, D1+	Incomplete development of forebrain and olfactory and optic nerves, minor motor seizures, mental retardation, microcephaly, wide sagittal suture and fontanels, capillary hemangiomata of forehead, localized scalp defects, microophthalmia, cleft lip and palate, low-set misshapen ears, abnormalities of extremities, cardiac and renal anomalies, persistence of fetal or embryonic hemoglobin.
Cat-cry (cri-du-chat)	Unknown, usually occurs in females	46, XX, 5p− or, less commonly, 46, XY, 5p−	Cry similar to meowing of cat, low birth weight, mental retardation, microcephaly, hypertelorism, epicanthus, low-set abnormally shaped ears, micrognathia, failure to thrive, short stature, large frontal sinuses, premature graying of hair, and seizures.
4p−	Unknown	46, XX, 4p− 46, XY, 5p−	Midline scalp defects, carplike mouth, beaklike nose, hypospadias, and markedly delayed ossification centers.
18q−	Unknown	46, XX, 18q− 46, XY, 18q−	Low birth weight, mental retardation, seizures, dysplasia of the midface, long tapering fingers, abnormal dermatoglyphics.
18p−	Unknown	46, XX, 18p− 46, XY, 18p−	Multiple malformations, but no well-defined syndrome.

147

There is no independent paternal effect. The majority of patients with Down's syndrome have 47 chromosomes and one extra chromosome on G group (designated to be chromosome 21) 47, XX (or XY), G+.

A much smaller group (about 8 percent) have 46 chromosomes. This variant is relatively common among Down's syndrome patients born to mothers under 30. It is usually due to a translocation. There are two main types of translocations, one involving D and G group chromosomes (D/G21 translocation) and the other between G group chromosomes (G/G21 translocation) which could be 21/21 translocation or 21/22 translocation. The majority of translocations occur freshly during gamete formation. Some (about one-fourth) are inherited from normal parents who are phenotypically normal but carriers of balanced translocation. If a parent is the carrier, then he will produce three types of offsprings: (1) normal, (2) phenotypically normal balanced-translocation carrier, (3) mongoloid.

Empirical risks of Down's syndrome for the offspring of parents with D/G translocation may be in the order of 1 in 5 where the mother has the translocation, and 1 in 20 or less where the father has it.

The lower risk for fathers suggests that there is a selection against sperms with an unbalanced chromosome set.

If either parent is a carrier of balanced 21/21 translocation, 100 percent of babies born are expected to be mongoloid.

Nonmongoloid G trisomy is a condition of diverse phenotype in which an extra small acrocentric chromosome is found associated with multiple heterogeneous congenital malformations and mental retardation.

Trisomy 18 syndrome   (Edwards' syndrome) 47, XX (or XY), E18 + is the second most common autosomal trisomy. A majority of infants with trisomy 18 die in infancy, only 10 percent survive the first year.

Recurrence risk for 18 trisomy is low.

Trisomy 13 syndrome   (D_1 trisomy; Patau's syndrome) 47, XX (or XY), D_1 +   About 20 percent of such infants survive the first year. Recurrence risk is considered to be low.

Cat-cry syndrome   (Cri-du-chat syndrome; 5p— syndrome)   This syndrome is caused by a deletion of the short arm of chromosome 5. Approximately one in seven cases is the result of a translocation transmitted from a phenotypically normal parent who has a balanced translocation.

4p— syndrome   Can be differentiated from 5p— syndrome by autoradiographic studies of the chromosomes. Deletion is found in the short arm of the 4th chromosome. Clinically these patients have similar findings as in 5p— syndrome, without characteristic cat cry and severe mental retardation.

18q— syndrome This is a well-defined syndrome which is due to partial deletion of the long arm of chromosome 18. The majority of cases occur de novo, independent of maternal age. The facial dysmorphia is very characteristic.

18p— syndrome (see Table 8-1)

Chromosomal breakage syndromes A tendency to chromosomal breakage and rearrangement in vitro has been found in Bloom's syndrome, Fanconi's anemia, and Louis-Bar syndrome (ataxia-telangectasis). Each of these three conditions is transmitted by an autosomal recessive gene, and each has a tendency to develop neoplasia. Virus infections, ionizing radiation, and drugs can also cause chromosomal breakage.

CHROMOSOME AND GENE MORPHOLOGY

The genetic information in the chromosomes is located in molecules of deoxyribonucleic acid (DNA). These molecules are linked into two strands, loosely attached by their bases (nucleotides) and twisted around each other in the form of a double helix, which forms the backbone of the chromosomes. There are four types of nucleotides; each of them contains a deoxyribose residue, a phosphate group and a purine or pyrimidine base. There are two purines (adenine, guanine) and two pyrimidines (cytosine and thymine). A purine (adenine) is always linked with a pyrimidine (thymine).

DNA has two functions: to reproduce itself and to direct the synthesis of proteins. A gene is a portion of DNA whose function is to produce a polypeptide chain which may combine with other polypeptides to produce biologically active proteins (enzymes). DNA is situated in the nucleus and directs the synthesis of polypeptide chains (transcription) by forming complementary messenger ribonucleic acid (mRNA). RNA nucleic acids are similar to those of DNA except that ribose replaces deoxyribose as the sugar component and uracil replaces thymine. Three consecutive base pairs on mRNA form a triplet code (codon) which are complementary to DNA triplets. Each codon codes for a specific amino acid. mRNA, which is formed along the length of the gene, separates and migrates to the ribosomes in the cytoplasm where proteins are synthesized. mRNA is situated on the several ribosomes and attracts to itself complex small molecules which consist of activated amino acid–transfer RNA (tRNA). The specific amino acid that is coupled with a particular triplet base of tRNA depends on the triplet code. Amino acids line up to form a growing polypeptide chain (translation). mRNA, after producing several molecules of polypeptide, disintegrates.

Mutation is the result of a single base substitution in a structural gene which will reflect itself as one amino-acid substitution in the polypeptide chain. The best evidence for this comes from the "fingerprinting" of abnormal hemoglobins. In sickle-cell hemoglobin (HbS) valine is substituted for glutamic acid in the 6th position of the β-peptide chain. In the mRNA a change of guanine-adenine-adenine code to guanine-uracil-adenine will bring about the glutamic acid to valine substitution.

Diseases due to mutant genes are divided into dominant, recessive, and X-linked. A dominant condition is one in which those who carry the mutant gene on only one member of the chromosome pair (heterozygotes) are clinically affected. A recessive condition is one in which clinically affected individuals are homozygous for the mutant gene concerned, whereas heterozygotes show no significant clinical abnormalities. The basic biochemical defect in the heterozygote (carrier) can be detected by laboratory methods. Some conditions are intermediate in that heterozygotes as well as homozygotes may be clinically affected, though heterozygotes are affected to a lesser degree, e.g., β thalassemia major and minor.

The X-linked conditions are determined by mutant genes on the X chromosome. The Y chromosome has few genes besides the genes determining male sex. Therefore, mutant genes on the X chromosome in males exert their effect on metabolism independent of any homologous gene on the Y chromosome. Females tend to be heterozygous for a mutant gene on the X chromosome, and female homozygotes are uncommon. X-linked conditions may be dominant or recessive.

Dominant conditions: The first case in a family appears sporadically (fresh mutation). Thereafter there is a 1-in-2 risk to the offspring of those affected. When the condition reduces "fitness" to zero, so that the affected individual never has progeny, all cases will be sporadic, i.e., Apert's syndrome (acrocephalosyndactylia). If the fitness is moderately reduced (Marfan's syndrome, neurofibromatosis) or if the onset of the condition is often late in reproductive age (Huntington's chorea), transmissions will often persist through several generations.

Some conditions are dominant with incomplete manifestations (reduced penetrance), and most heterozygotes show some abnormality, but some are normal. This may be recognized when the family members transmit the condition without themselves being clinically affected (skipped generation, e.g., retinoblastoma).

Recessive conditions: The characteristic picture is one in which sibs of the index patient (propositus) are often affected, but parents and other family members, e.g., half-sibs, are not affected. The exact risk to the sibs, where both parents are heterozygous carriers, is one in four. The frequency of affected offspring in first-cousin or other consanguineous marriages is increased. The majority of inheritable enzyme deficiencies are due to a recessive mutant gene.

X-linked conditions: The characteristic family pattern of X-linked conditions (heterozygous mother) is that 50 percent of the sons will be affected and 50 percent of the daughters will be heterozygotes. All the daughters born to an affected male will be carriers and none of his sons will be affected. Hemophilia A and B, Duchenne's muscular dystrophy, Lesch-Nyhan syndrome, glucose-6-phosphate dehydrogenase deficiency are examples of X-linked recessive conditions. X-linked hypophosphatemic rickets is due to an X-linked dominant mutation. No Y-linked diseases are known.

Polygenic inheritance: In many common diseases twin studies and family studies indicate a genetic predisposition. This genetic predisposition depends on genetic variations at several gene loci; e.g., three nonlinked gene loci have been shown to be concerned in the production of different forms of the enzyme, phosphoglucomutase, normally found in red cells. Many common congenital malformations and diseases such as diabetes mellitus are inherited in this manner. The risk to first-degree relatives (sibs and children) is 20- to 30-fold increased over the general population, and a sharp fall-off occurs in the risk to second-degree relatives (aunts, uncles, nieces, and nephews). The recurrence risk is greatly increased if two first-degree relatives are affected.

GENETIC COUNSELING

There are three objectives for genetic counseling:

1. To determine the risk of recurrence in another child, when a malformation or genetically determined disease has occurred.
2. To determine the risk that a particular child may be born with a genetically determined disease, such as galactosemia, cystic fibrosis, pyloric stenosis, so diagnosis and treatment may be instituted promptly.
3. To prevent the birth of children genetically predisposed to serious handicaps.

These objectives could be achieved by detection of heterozygous carriers, e.g., sickle-cell trait, and counseling them or establishing techniques to screen all newborn infants for a homozygous condition, e.g., phenylketonuria.

Techniques, e.g., culturing cells obtained by amniocentesis for detecting chromosome anomalies and some inborn errors of metabolism, early in pregnancy offer the prospect of reducing the frequency of such anomalies at birth by termination of the pregnancy if the fetus is abnormal (see p. 183).

In high-risk pregnancies, e.g., elderly pregnant women, carriers of a balanced translocation, mothers who have previously given birth to a child with a chromosomal malformation, or certain inborn errors of metabolism, amniocentesis at the fourteenth to sixteenth week after conception will aid precise intrauterine diagnosis of the fetus and enable more accurate counseling of the families.

REVIEW QUESTIONS

The following questions are the matching type. In each blank in column I, insert the letter corresponding to the word or phrase in column II which is associated most appropriately.

I	II
1. Haploidy _____	(a) Systematized array of the chromosomes of a single cell prepared either by drawing or photography
2. Diploidy _____	(b) Degree of severity of symptoms due to a gene effect
3. Autosome _____	(c) The frequency with which a gene effect will be manifest even though the gene may be present in more persons
4. Karyotype _____	(d) Normal number of chromosomes in the nucleus of a germ cell
5. Alleles _____	(e) The affected person who first brings the condition to the attention of the medical geneticist
6. Incomplete dominance _____	(f) All the variations of a gene which may be present at a single locus
7. Expressivity _____	(g) Intermediate state in which both genes of a diploid pair have an effect
8. Penetrance _____	(h) Normal number of chromosomes found in the nucleus of a somatic cell
9. Proband _____	(i) A chromosome not specifically concerned with sex differentiation
10. Linkage _____	(j) Populations of cells in the same person with different chromosomal compositions
11. Mosaicism _____	(k) Genes carried on the same chromosome

12. A study of epithelial cells obtained by buccal smear gives information concerning (a) Y chromosomes; (b) X chromosomes; (c) both X and Y chromosomes; (d) autosomes.

13. A deleted G22 chromosome ("Philadelphia") frequently occurs in (a) cat-cry syndrome; (b) Down's syndrome; (c) myelogenous leukemia; (d) congenital hemolytic anemia.

14. The rate of chromosome anomalies is (a) 1 per 10; (b) 1 per 50; (c) 1 per 100; (d) 1 per 1,000 live births.

15. Karyotypes of tissue from spontaneous abortions occurring during the first trimester reveal abnormalities in what percent of cases: (a) 5; (b) 25; (c) 50; (d) 90?

16. A woman over 40 years of age has (a) 1:10; (b) 1:100; (c) 1:1,000 chance of having a child affected with Down's syndrome.

17. Study the following diagrams (Figure 8-1):

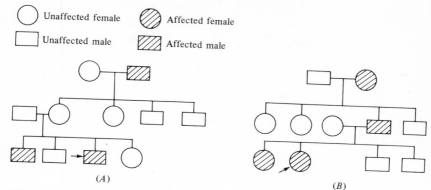

(A)

(B)

Figure 8-1

Proband is marked with an arrow. The mode of inheritance illustrated by the diagram on the left is (a) sex-linked recessive; (b) sex-linked dominant; (c) autosomal recessive; (d) autosomal dominant.

18. All but one of the following diseases are transmitted according to the mode of inheritance illustrated by diagram A in question 17: (a) hemophilia; (b) Hurler's syndrome without corneal clouding; (c) some cases of vitamin D–resistant rickets; (d) vasopressin-resistant diabetes insipidus.

19. The objectives for genetic counseling include the following except (a) permit early recognition and treatment of certain inherited diseases; (b) prevent the birth of children genetically predisposed to serious handicaps; (c) determine the risk that a particular child may be born with a genetically determined disease; (d) prevent the marriage of heterozygous carriers of serious genetic disease.

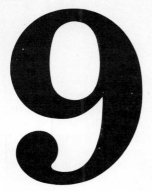

IMMUNOLOGY AND METABOLISM

Syndromes due to inborn errors of metabolism are a group of hereditary diseases (more than 100 are known) which are transmitted by mutant genes from generation to generation and result in certain metabolic defects and clinical symptoms. These defects are not always demonstrable by present routine laboratory means. In many instances the defect is due to an enzyme abnormality that can be detected only by special techniques. Most of the severe disorders are transmitted by an autosomal recessive gene, requiring two heterozygous mates to produce homozygous progeny with the clinical syndrome. Heterozygous carriers may be recognized by special tests.

The most precise diagnosis of metabolic disease is obtained by measurement of the activity of the enzyme involved. The method is limited to disease in which enzyme activity occurs normally in blood cells or skin fibroblasts.

DISORDERS OF PLASMA PROTEINS

Wilson's disease (hepatolenticular degeneration)   Wilson's disease is a hereditary disorder transmitted by an autosomal recessive gene and due to a defect that involves copper metabolism. It is characterized by a chemically low serum-ceruloplasmin (alpha$_2$ globulin) level, a low serum-copper level (normal 25 mg per 100 ml), and an increased level of serum albumin–bound copper. Increased amounts of copper are absorbed from the diet, resulting in accumulation of copper in the liver (causing clinical cirrhosis); brain, especially in the basal ganglions (causing tremor, rigidity, dysarthria, and dysphagia); kidneys (glycosuria, aminoaciduria, phosphaturia, uricosuria); eye, especially the outer margin of the cornea (yellow-green Kayser-Fleischer ring); bone (osteoarthritis, osteomalacia); and fingernails (blue basal lacunae). Clinical onset is from 12 to 20 years of age after copper has had opportunity to accumulate. Treatment consists of decreasing copper intake (deleting liver, mushrooms, and chocolate from diet), rendering ingested copper insoluble (with carboresins), and removing copper already absorbed (with BAL, penicillamine).

Analbuminemia (Bennhold's disease)   Analbuminemia is a genetically determined defect, characterized by extremely low serum-albumin levels. Clinical symptoms are variable; some patients are asymptomatic and some present mild generalized edema. Blood tests, which depend upon serum-protein levels, e.g., erythrocyte sedimentation rate (high), and thymol turbidity, may be abnormal.

Serum liproprotein deficiency   The lipoproteins consist of linked polypeptides and lipids. They have been distinguished from each other by chemical composition, electrophoretic mobility, flotation rates in the ultracentrifuge, density, and metabolic activity. Alpha and beta lipoproteins are differentiated by their respective rates of electrophoretic mobility. Genetic disorders characterized by absence of alpha and beta lipoproteins have been described.

A-alphalipoproteinemia (Tangier disease)   This rare clinical disorder has been identified in two siblings who reside on the island of Tangier off the coast of Virginia. This autosomal recessive disease is apparently the consequence of mating among a highly inbred island population. It is characterized by the virtual absence of alpha lipoproteins in the serum, low serum cholesterol and esters, large, yellow tonsils with a high content of lipids, and the presence of foam cells in the lymph nodes and tonsils but not in the marrow. Lymphadenopathy and hepatosplenomegaly were present in one patient.

A-betalipoproteinemia   See Celiac Syndrome in Chapter 15.

Familial hyperlipoproteinemia   See Inherited Disorders of Lipid Metabolism, Table 9-1, p. 170.

AMINOACIDOPATHY

This term is used to encompass those conditions associated with an increased plasma concentration of amino acids; those conditions due to defective renal tubular absorption of amino acids are classified as aminoacidurias. In both situations hyperaminoaciduria occurs. Aminoaciduria per se is a physiologic phenomenon, and the amounts as well as the types of amino acids will vary with age. In general, amino acids are excreted in greatest amounts in the newborn infant. At least part of the excretion at this age may be due to physiologically deficient tubular function. Perhaps equally important are differences in the metabolism of amino acids that are age-related. Thus, implicit in the diagnosis of aminoacidopathy is the appreciation of quantitatively greater urinary excretion of amino acids in the various disease states.

Phenylketonuria (PKU)   Phenylketonuria is an autosomal recessive disease characterized by a deficiency of phenylalanine hydroxylase, an enzyme in the liver which activates the conversion of phenylalanine to tyrosine. Consequently, certain metabolites (phenylpyruvic acid, phenyllactic acid, and phenylacetic acid, among others) are formed in excess and are excreted in the urine. In addition, phenylalanine apparently competes with tyrosine for available tyrosinase and also inhibits tryptophane metabolism, resulting in deficient production of serotonin.

Mental retardation is related to the retention of phenylalanine and its toxic effect on the brain. Though retardation is generally extreme and most patients have IQs below 50, there are individual exceptions with normal or borderline intellect in spite of high serum-phenylalanine levels. The characteristic musty odor of these patients has been attributed to phenylacetic acid in the urine. Decreased pigmentation of skin, hair, and irises may be related to the competitive inhibition for tyrosinase. Eczema occurs commonly.

Vomiting is a frequent symptom, and in young infants with this condition a mistaken diagnosis of hypertrophic pyloric stenosis may be made.

The heterozygous carrier can be detected by employing loading tests with standard dose of L-phenylalanine. Higher and more sustained serum levels occur than in normal controls. Sensitive enzymatic assays in red blood cells may reveal higher serum levels of phenylalanines in heterozygotes. Lifespan is limited, most untreated patients dying before they reach the age of 40. In many instances early death has been due to unrelated disease.

A low-phenylalanine diet (Lofenolac—Mead Johnson, and Ketonil—Merck Sharp and Dohme) results in clinical improvement. Skin, hair, and iris pigmentation darkens; eczema improves; and neurologic findings revert to normal. Intellectual capacity may be preserved with early institution and maintenance of proper diets. Children on such diets demonstrate not only clinical improvement but also a reversion to normal of serum phenylalanine and its metabolites. Serotonin and tyrosine levels are increased.

In treatment patients must be followed with serum-phenylalanine determinations (desired level is 3 to 8 mg percent). Nutritional deficiency, megaloblastic anemia, convulsions, and death have resulted from too-stringent dietary control.

For dietary management to be most effective, it is imperative that it be initiated soon after birth. Currently in most states testing of the capillary blood of all hospitalized newborn infants is required by law. Since testing is performed early, during the first few days of life before dietary phenylalanine intake has been sufficient to cause high serum levels, a level above 4 mg percent is considered to be a presumptive positive, but only 1 in 20 to 30 infants with this level are true positives.

The drop-by-drop addition of 10 percent ferric chloride to fresh urine will produce a green precipitate indicating the presence of phenylpyruvic acid. Phenistix (Ames) may also be employed for urine testing. Urine tests are of little value before 1 to 2 months of age. By this time, serum-phenylalanine levels of 15 to 20 mg percent are reached, and phenylpyruvic acid appears in the urine.

More effective screening programs should incorporate blood testing in the second week together with follow-up urine testing at 1 to 2 months.

Albinism   This inherited disorder is characterized by the inability to produce melanin. This is the principal pigment in the skin, hair, uveal tract, and retina. The chemical chain of events ultimately resulting in the formation of melanin is interrupted in conversion of tyrosine to dopa and in the conversion of dopa to dopa quinone because of a deficiency of the enzyme tyrosinase.

Universal albinism—absence of skin, hair, and eye pigment—has an autosomal recessive genetic transmission. Localized albinism—pale, depigmented patches of skin and hair is transmitted by autosomal dominant genes. X-linked albinism is localized to the eye. (Occasionally, albino parents give birth to normally pigmented offspring.) These patients have considerable photophobia and in bright light may have pronounced nystagmus. In addition, they are subject to extreme sunburn.

Tyrosinosis   This is an extremely rare disorder resulting from the inability to convert para-hydroxyphenylpyruvic acid to homogentisic acid. It is characterized by early onset of failure to thrive, fever, hepatosplenomegaly, and liver failure. There is a presumed deficiency of the enzyme para-hydroxyphenylpyruvate oxidase. In addition to this enzyme, the reaction normally requires ascorbic acid. The presence of tyrosine and *p*-hydroxyphenylpyruvic acid in the urine of scorbutic patients and premature infants is reversed by the administration of vitamin C. The presence of these compounds in the urine of premature infants is an example of the immature functioning of the enzyme system.

Alkaptonuria   This autosomal recessively inherited metabolic disorder is due to the absence in the liver of the enzyme homogentisic acid oxidase. This enzyme normally converts homogentisic acid to maleylacetoacetic acid. The condition is usually identified by the dark-brown staining of urine-moistened diapers. Though freshly wet diapers are not discolored, characteristic color develops with the passage of time.

This is a so-called no-threshold disorder inasmuch as homogentisic acid is not detected in the blood in spite of the metabolic block enhancing its production. Homogentisic acid is a reducing agent and will give a positive reducing reaction with Benedict's solution. (Glucose oxidase stick tests are negative.)

Though asymptomatic in early life, persons with prolonged deposition of homogentisic acid in cartilage, collagen, tendons, and joints develop ochronosis.

Maple syrup urine disease (branched-chain ketonuria)   This inherited disease is characterized by increased amounts of the branched-chain amino acids leucine, isoleucine, and valine and their keto acids in the blood. These compounds are also found in the urine. Their presence as well as that of the stereoisomer alloisoleucine is believed due to the occurrence of a block in oxidative decarboxylation of the keto acids of the three amino acids. Alloisoleucine is not normally found in plasma; it is believed to be formed from the keto acid of isoleucine.

These patients may have leucine-induced hypoglycemia which, in part, may account for their seizures.

The urine has a characteristic sweet odor closely resembling that of maple syrup. The cause of the odor is not clear. When ferric chloride is added to the urine of these patients, a gray-green color appears.

Patients may demonstrate seizures, spasticity, and opisthotonus; occasionally there may be diffuse flaccidity, coma, and death. Symptoms generally become apparent toward the end of the first week, and death occurs within the first month (see p. 503).

Therapy consists of dietary restriction of the branched-chain amino acids.

Oxalosis   This disorder is characterized by generalized deposition of calcium oxalate crystals throughout the body. Both recessive and dominant kinships have been described.

Though in the strict sense, there is no block in the metabolism of an amino acid with consequent aminoacidemia and aminoaciduria, there is defective conversion of glyoxylic acid to formic acid. Glyoxylic acid is a derivative of glycine.

Patients demonstrate excessive amounts of oxalic acid, glycolic acid, and glyoxylic acid in the urine.

The principal manifestations are those of nephrolithiasis and nephrocalcinosis. Many other organs of the body may demonstrate deposition of oxalate crystals, especially within the walls of arteries and arterioles.

DISORDERS OF THE SULFUR-CONTAINING AMINO ACIDS

Homocystinuria   Homocystinuria is characterized by excessive excretion of homocystine in the urine and at times by high blood levels of methionine.

The majority of patients have demonstrated seizures, fine sparse hair, ectopia lentis, malar flush, osteoporosis, and sticky platelets. Mental retardation is present in half the cases described. The biochemical defect is a deficiency of cystathionin synthetase which condenses homocysteine with serine to form cystathionine. It is transmitted as an autosomal recessive disease. Large doses of vitamin B_6, which induce the enzyme activity, and folate may be helpful.

Cystathioninuria   Cystathioninuria is an autosomal recessive disorder due to abnormal cystathionase formation. Cystathioninuria may occur with neural tumors, in liver diseases or hepatoblastoma, in galactosemia, and phenylketonuria.

Patients usually manifest mental retardation and may have renal calculi. Vitamin B_6 (which acts as a coenzyme) increases the activity of the enzyme and is recommended as a form of therapy.

Hartnup disease   This is a rare hereditary disorder in which there is a defect in the transport of tryptophan by the intestinal mucosa and renal tubules. Aminoaciduria is massive, and plasma aminoacid levels are normal, with the exception of a very low tryptophan level. Poor intestinal absorption of tryptophan results in its bacterial decomposition to indoles and indoxyl derivatives which are absorbed and excreted in the urine—indicanuria.

Cutaneous photosensitivity, a pellegra-like skin rash, and cerebellar ataxia are major manifestations of this disease. The clinical course is variable; remissions may occur spontaneously or in response to nicotinamide.

Indicanuria is commonly observed in bowel stasis (constipation, blind-loop syndrome), in phenylketonuria, and in blue diaper syndrome. This last is a familial disorder characterized by hypercalcemia, nephrocalcinosis, and indicanuria.

Glycinemia with ketosis   This is an autosomal recessive disorder in which glycine is accumulated in the blood and excreted excessively in the urine. Early in infancy, severe recurrent episodes of acidosis and ketonuria occur which cause mental and physical retardation, osteo-porosis, thrombocytopenia, and neutropenia; ketone bodies and ace-tone appear in the urine. The defect is in the conversion of proprionate to methylmalonate.

A diet low in glycine, methionine, threonine, leucine, isoleucine, and valine is effective in preventing acidosis and mental retardation.

DISORDERS OF THE KREBS ORNITHINE–UREA CYCLE

Three disorders associated with defects in the urea cycle have been reported thus far. These are hyperammonemia, citrullinemia, and argininosuccinicacidemia.

Though confirmed clinical examples of each type are unique, these disorders are of interest in that they have increased knowledge of the urea cycle. In spite of enzymatic defects which would be expected to result in diminished urea production, blood urea levels are normal in these disorders. The reasons for this apparent paradox are not clear.

In hyperammonemia there is accumulation of ammonia in the body, and symptoms and signs of ammonia intoxication occur in spite of intact liver function. The associated mental retardation and cerebral atrophy are probably consequent to chronic ammonia intoxication.

Drastic reduction of protein intake can diminish blood ammonia in these patients, but the use of such diets may result in severe malnu-trition.

In citrullinemia, mental retardation and cerebral atrophy also occur. Though blood levels of ammonia may be normal in the fasting state, after the ingestion of protein they may exceed levels found in hepatic failure.

In argininosuccinicacidemia several characteristic features may en-able the clinician to suspect the diagnosis prior to biochemical con-firmation. The most striking of these is unusual hair friability. Hair tends to break above the level of the follicle, a condition known as trichorrhexis nodosa.

Other clinical and laboratory features are mental retardation, sei-zures, and elevated serum-alkaline phosphatase (see p. 13).

Following protein intake, serum ammonia may rise to levels com-mensurate with those in severe hepatotoxicity. However, such signs as trichorrhexis nodosa are probably not attributable to hyperam-monemia.

Dietary restriction of ornithine and citrulline are of no therapeutic value inasmuch as these amino acids can be synthesized in the body.

Histidinemia The discovery of this disease is probably the result of widespread detection programs directed toward phenylketonuria; for as in the latter disorder, the addition of ferric chloride to the urine produces a greenish precipitate. In histidinemia the color change is attributable to the presence of imidazolepyruvic acid.

Mental retardation is not a prominent finding. A large proportion of affected patients have impaired speech. The nature of the impairment is not uniform and thus not diagnostic.

The conversion of histidine to urocanic acid is dependent on the presence of the enzyme histidase in the liver. In its absence histidine is transanimated to imidazolepyruvic acid which, together with histidine, is excreted by the kidneys. Thus histidinemia, histidinuria, and imidazolepyruvicaciduria occur. Histidase is also deficient in the skin, and urocanic acid is absent in the sweat of such patients. Skin biopsies and chemical analysis of sweat may be of diagnostic value.

DISORDERS OF PURINE AND PYRIMIDINE METABOLISM

Orotic aciduria   Orotic acid is an intermediary in the synthesis of pyrimidines. A block due to absence of orotidylic acid pyrophosphorylase and decarboxylase causes this inherited disorder. Megaloblastic anemia which does not respond to folic acid or vitamin B_{12} and orotic acid crystals in the urine are major manifestations. Corticosteroid treatment may be helpful.

Hyperuricemia (gout)   This disorder is transmitted by an autosomal dominant gene with variable penetrance in both sexes. It is six to seven times more common in males than in females. Gout is very rare in children. It is due to reduced activity (90 to 95 percent) of the enzyme hypoxanthine guanine phosphoribosyl transferase (see Lesch-Nyhan disease).

Hyperuricemia (Lesch-Nyhan disease)   This disease is inherited via an X-linked gene. It is characterized by mental retardation, choreoathetoid movements, scissoring position of the legs, and self-mutilation due to uncontrollable aggressive behavior.

Serum uric acid levels are increased (10 mg per 100 ml) and urinary excretion is increased. Gouty tophi appear in older patients. Allopurinol is effective therapeutically. The condition is due to a complete absence of the enzyme hypoxanthine guanine phosphoribosyl transferase, which converts hypoxanthine to its nucleotide inosinic acid. This nucleotide is required for the feedback inhibition of purine synthesis. In its absence, excessive purines are synthesized and excess uric acid, the end product of purine catabolism in man, is excreted.

DISORDERS OF CARBOHYDRATE METABOLISM

Diabetes mellitus   See Chapter 24, "Endocrine Diseases."

Carbohydrate malabsorption syndromes   Deficient intestinal absorption of disaccharides and monosaccharides appears to be genetic in origin, though the exact nature of inherited transmission remains to be clarified.

Disaccharides are normally absorbed into the epithelial cells of the small intestinal mucosa and are hydrolyzed within the cell. No chemical breakdown of these sugars to monosaccharides takes place in the intestinal lumen.

A number of specific clinical entities are recognized with sufficiently common features to help establish the diagnosis of disaccharidase deficiency:

1. The presence of the offending sugar in the diet results in persistent diarrhea and failure to gain weight.
2. Low stool pH (often as low as 4.5 to 5.0) is the result of fermentation of the unabsorbed sugar to lactic acid and other organic acids.
3. Blood-glucose levels following a test load of the offending disaccharide remain unchanged; on the other hand, the introduction of the component monosaccharide results in a significant elevation of blood glucose.

Severe diarrhea (due to any cause) may lead to an inability to hydrolyze disaccharides which in turn prolongs diarrhea if disaccharides are ingested.

Hereditary lactose malabsorption (alactasia) Distinct racial and geographic differences occur in the extent of this disease. It is common among various groups, including American blacks, Jews, and Japanese. Both breast-fed and cow's-milk-fed babies are affected. Symptoms of diarrhea and colic begin within a few days after the introduction of milk feedings.

The high lactic acid content of the stool causes severe excoriation of the buttocks which resists local therapy.

Clinical improvement occurs when the offending sugar is removed from the diet. The enzymatic deficiency apparently is permanent; symptoms will recur upon reintroduction of lactose at any age, though the provocative threshold dose tends to be higher in older patients.

The abatement of symptoms upon removal of lactose and recurrence upon reintroduction should not be misinterpreted as allergy to cow's milk. Diagnosis is confirmed by intraluminal small intestinal biopsy specimens having low or absent lactase content. Lactase is an inducible enzyme whose activity is greatest during infancy and may disappear in adulthood.

Treatment Lactose must be removed from the diet.

Hereditary infantile lactose intolerance Lactose intolerance with lactosemia may be due to diverse pathogenic causes. The absorption of the intact disaccharide molecule into the bloodstream may follow denudation of the lactase-containing intestinal mucosa. Consanguinity in some of the incriminated kinships suggests an autosomal recessive inheritance.

Symptoms generally begin in the neonatal period, though they may also occur after several months of lactose ingestion. In addition to lactosuria, lactosemia occurs. A celiac-like syndrome with severe malnutrition is characteristic.

Renal tubular acidosis occurs with aminoaciduria, proteinuria, as well as lactosuria. Atrophy of the liver and adrenal glands and degeneration of the convoluted tubules have been demonstrated on postmortem examination.

Rapid improvement occurs upon elimination of lactose from the diet.

Malabsorption of sucrose and isomaltose   This inherited disorder is characterized by a lack of intestinal sucrase and isomaltase.

Maltose is also hydrolyzed by these enzymes; consequently hydrolysis of maltose may also be impaired.

Sucrose tolerance tests will fail to show elevation of blood glucose and fructose concentrations. Inasmuch as isomaltose is generally unavailable in sufficient amounts to perform tolerance testing, palatinose, a synthetic disaccharide with a similar alpha-1-6 linkage, may be used as an alternative. The absence of elevation of blood glucose and fructose after testing with palatinose indicates a deficiency of intestinal isomaltase.

Increasing tolerance to the provocative carbohydrates may occur with the passage of time in some patients; in others, the degree of intolerance fails to abate.

The inherited nature of the disorder is certain, but it is not clear whether autosomal recessive or dominant inheritance is operative.

Defective absorption of monosaccharides   Rare examples of defective absorption of monosaccharides have been reported. There is no evidence of deficiency of mucosal disaccharidases. The latter are present, but component monosaccharides diffuse from the mucosa back into the intestinal lumen, where they are fermented to lactic acid. These patients have frequent diarrheal stools with a low pH. Glucose and galactose absorption is defective, while fructose absorption is not impaired. Glucose- and galactose-tolerance testing fails to show elevation of either monosaccharide in the blood.

There is probably a genetic basis for monosaccharide malabsorption.

Essential pentosuria   Characterized by the excretion of the pentose L-xylulose in the urine, it occurs predominately in those of Jewish extraction. The mode of inheritance is through an autosomal recessive gene.

The chief significance of the disorder lies in its possible confusion with diabetes. Both glucose and L-xylulose give a reducing reaction with Benedict's reagent, but only glucose-containing urine will show a positive reaction with glucose oxidase. Paper chromatography is the most convenient method of identifying L-xylulose.

There is a metabolic block in the glucuronic acid oxidation pathway, resulting in the accumulation of L-xylulose in the blood and its consequent excretion by the kidneys. Heterozygotes can be demonstrated by the high blood levels of L-xylulose attained after a loading dose of glucuronolactone.

This disorder is completely asymptomatic and is compatible with normal life expectancy.

Essential fructosuria This disorder is characterized by the excretion of fructose in the urine of asymptomatic individuals. It is due to an autosomal recessive gene.

Fructose, though capable of reducing Benedict's and Fehling's reagents, will not react with glucose oxidase. It can also be distinguished from glucose by the fact that it is fermented by yeast and by its characteristic locus in filter paper chromatography.

Fructose accumulates in the blood of these patients (preliminary to its renal excretion) because of a deficiency of hepatic fructokinase, which is necessary for its conversion to fructose-1-phosphate.

Hereditary fructose intolerance In contrast to essential fructosuria, this is a serious disease. It is characterized by vomiting, severe hypoglycemia, and lowering of serum-phosphorus levels following the intake of fructose or sucrose. If fructose ingestion is not restricted, wasting, hepatomegaly, aminoaciduria, albuminuria, and ultimately death may ensue. Hepatomegaly and renal tubular dysfunction resolve when fructose is eliminated from the diet.

The disease is due to an inherited deficiency of the hepatic enzyme fructose-1-phosphate aldolase. The deficiency state is lifelong.

Hypoglycemia has been attributed to the repressive effect of accumulated hepatic fructose-1-phosphate on glycogenolysis. The exact site of the block in the metabolism of glycogen to glucose has not been elucidated.

Though not without some degree of danger because of the risk of hypoglycemia, an intravenous fructose tolerance test (3 Gm per sq meter) should be performed to establish the diagnosis. More reliable than the serial blood fructose measurements is the marked drop in blood glucose and inorganic phosphorus occurring during the test procedure. If necessary, intravenous glucose may be administered to counteract extreme hypoglycemia.

In most instances the mode of inheritance of this rare disorder is by an autosomal recessive gene. Heterozygote carriers cannot be distinguished by fructose loading tests.

Galactosemia This disease is characterized by cataract formation, hepatosplenomegaly, and mental retardation. It is due to the hepatic deficiency of the enzyme galactose-1-phosphate uridyl transferase, which is necessary for the conversion of galactose-1-phosphate to glucose-1-phosphate. Clinical manifestations are principally the result of the accumulation of galactose-1-phosphate in various organs of the body. Symptoms generally appear within a week or two after the introduction of milk containing lactose. Vomiting and diarrhea occur and are frequently severe enough to cause death from dehydration. As galactose-1-phosphate accumulates in the liver and spleen, portal hypertension, and ultimately cirrhosis develop. Jaundice may accompany the appearance of hepatic enlargement.

In addition to galactosuria, aminoaciduria and albuminuria may occur, reflecting renal tubular damage consequent to the high content of galactose in the renal blood flow.

Brain damage and mental retardation result in part from the deposition of galactose in the brain and in part from hypoglycemia secondary to the repressive effect of galactose on hepatic glycogenolysis.

Clinical manifestations, with the exception of mental retardation, are often completely reversible when galactose is excluded from the diet. Nutramigen and soybean milk are satisfactory substitutes for breast or cow's milk.

Galactose, though capable of reducing Benedict's reagent, will not react with glucose oxidase. The galactose tolerance test should not be performed because of the risk of severe hypoglycemia.

The erythrocytes may be tested for their content of galactose-1-phosphate uridyl transferase. In addition, galactosemic erythrocytes are unable to reduce methylene blue.

The disease is transmitted by an autosomal recessive gene. Heterozygotes may be detected by finding intermediate levels of galactose-1-phosphate uridyl transferase in erythrocytes. It is even possible that heterozygotes may have mild gastrointestinal symptoms upon intake of milk (see p. 184).

Methylmalonic aciduria This hereditary disorder is due to deficiency of an enzyme, methylmalonic CoA isomarase, which converts methylmalonic acid to its isomer, succinic acid.

Methylmalonic acid is excreted excessively in vitamin B_{12} deficiency states. Patients with methylmalonic aciduria resemble infants with hyperglycinuria. Repeated episodes of vomiting and acidosis occur. Mental and physical retardation are characteristic. Vitamin B_{12} is helpful for some patients. (See p. 184.)

Fucosidosis This hereditary disorder is characterized by mental retardation, progressive cerebral degeneration, spasticity, thick skin (resembling the Hurler phenotype). It is due to a deficiency of lysosomal enzyme, γ-fucosidase, in the liver, brain, lung, and kidneys which causes accumulation of a glycolipid, fucose (see p. 184).

GLYCOGEN–STORAGE DISEASES

This group of diseases is characterized by excessive deposition of glycogen in the liver, heart, intestines, skeletal muscles, and kidney. There is defective mobilization of deposits of glycogen from these organs. In a number of instances specific enzymatic defects have also been demonstrated. These are

Cori type 1	Glucose-6-phosphatase
Cori type 2	alpha-1,4-glucosidase (acid maltase)
Cori type 3	Amylo-1,6-glucosidase (debrancher)
Cori type 4	alpha-1,4-glucan 6-glucosyl transferase (brancher)
Cori type 5	Muscle phosphorylase
Cori type 6	Liver phosphorylase
Cori type 7	Muscle phosphoglucomutase
Cori type 8	Liver phosphorylase kinase

Type 1 (hepatorenal glycogenosis—von Gierke's disease)   Type 1 is characterized by hepatomegaly, growth retardation, hypoglycemia, bouts of acidosis, and skin xanthomata.

Hepatomegaly may be present at birth. The liver becomes massive, and this accounts for the pronounced enlargement of the abdomen. The kidneys and intestinal mucosa are also involved.

Laboratory tests

1. Marked hypoglycemia, often unaccompanied by seizures.
2. High and prolonged glucose-tolerance curve.
3. Absent or diminished response in blood glucose to epinephrine or glucagon.
4. Intravenous administration of galactose or fructose normally results in a rise in blood glucose. However, in these patients a rise does not occur.
5. High glycogen content and absence of glucose-6-phosphatase in liver biopsy specimens.
6. Hyperlipemia.
7. Ketonemia, ketonuria, and acidosis.
8. Hyperuricemia. (Clinical gout has been observed.)
9. High serum levels of lactate and pyruvate.
10. Glucosuria and aminoaciduria due to renal tubular involvement.
11. Osteoporosis, attributable to low serum phosphorus and perhaps also to long-standing acidosis. (Alkaline phosphatase is normal.)

Inheritance probably is by an autosomal recessive gene.

Treatment Supportive measures to counteract acidosis and small, frequent carbohydrate meals to maintain blood-glucose levels are useful. Treatment with glucagon and thyroxine has been reported to be successful in elevating blood glucose and decreasing the liver size.

If life can be maintained till at least 4 years of age, the severity of the disease may lessen in spite of the persistence of the enzymatic defect.

Type 2 (generalized glycogenosis—Pompe's disease) Type 2 is characterized by varying degrees of neurologic and muscular (including cardiac) involvement. It probably is transmitted as an autosomal recessive trait.

The disease may be manifested at birth, but usually becomes apparent before 6 months of age. Symptoms include failure to thrive, vomiting, enlargement of the tongue which may suggest cretinism, and muscular weakness and extreme hypotonia. Marked cardiac enlargement occurs, occasionally with an associated apical systolic murmur and changes in the ECG (see p. 406). The liver and spleen are not commonly enlarged. Appropriate staining of leukocytes demonstrates marked glycogen deposition. Blood-glucose levels and responses to epinephrine or glucagon are normal. Acetonuria does not occur.

Diagnosis is dependent on muscle biopsy for assay of glycogen content as well as enzyme analysis (see p. 167). Prognosis is poor, with death occurring before the age of 1 year.

Type 3 (debrancher enzyme deficiency-limit dextrinosis) Type 3 resembles type 1 but is not as severe. Inheritance is by an autosomal recessive gene.

Hypoglycemia may occur; the responses to glucagon and epinephrine are present but deficient. In addition, a hyperglycemic response to intravenous galactose or fructose does occur. Amylo-1,6-glucosidase is deficient in the liver as well as in the skeletal muscles. Prognosis is good.

Type 4 (brancher enzyme deficiency amylopectinosis) Type 4 is a very rare form of glycogenosis with abnormal glycogen deposits in the liver, spleen, and skeletal muscles, but not in the kidneys. Hepatosplenomegaly occurs with cirrhosis of the liver, ascites, and icterus. Glycogen liver deposits appear to resist epinephrine-induced glycogenolysis. Death occurs before 2 years of age. (See p. 167.)

Type 5 (McArdle's disease) Type 5 is due to a deficiency of muscle phosphorylase; hepatic phosphorylase activity is normal. There is increased deposition of glycogen in the muscles, but not in the liver.

These patients are not too disabled, and the deficiency may not affect normal longevity. Patients complain of lack of sustained muscle power. Venous blood draining these muscles shows diminished rather than increased lactate. Electromyograms performed on recently exercised muscles show electrical inactivity. There is a normal hyperglycemic response to glucagon or epinephrine, confirming the presence of hepatic phosphorylase.

The inheritance of this rare disorder is unknown.

Type 6 (Hers' disease) This is a heterogeneous group which may represent several forms of the disease.

Patients show mild hypoglycemia and ketosis. The liver is usually markedly enlarged; on the other hand, skeletal muscles and the heart are not involved. There are mild hypercholesterolemia and lactic acidemia. The response to glucagon and epinephrine is usually deficient.

In addition to deficiency of hepatic phosphorylase, leukocyte phosphorylase is also low. Measurement of this enzyme in leukocytes is a diagnostic substitute for enzyme assay of liver biopsy specimens.

The prognosis is good.

Type 7 Clinically, it is similar to type 5.

Type 8 Clinically, it is similar to type 6.

DISORDERS OF LIPID METABOLISM (See Table 9-1)

DISORDERS OF PIGMENT METABOLISM

PORPHYRIA

Porphyrin is a precursor of heme; the main sites of production are the bone marrow and the liver. Porphyrin is also found in such heme analogs as myoglobin, catalase, and the cytochromes.

Porphyria may occur as a result of ingestion of chemicals, for example, hexachlorobenzene, Sedormid. Other examples of nonhereditary porphyria include

1. The disturbed porphyrin metabolism characteristic of lead poisoning.
2. The excess amounts of the type III isomer excreted in acute rheumatic fever. Quantitatively, they parallel serum-mucoprotein levels as well as the clinical course of the illness.
3. The increased coproporphyrinuria reported in liver damage due to infectious as well as toxic hepatitis.
4. The coproporphyrinuria accompanying acquired hemolytic anemias, which may be due to increased metabolism associated with accelerated hematopoiesis.

Erythropoietic porphyria (congenital or photosensitive porphyria)
This is a rare, autosomal recessive disorder associated with abnormal

Table 9-1. Inherited disorders of lipid metabolism

Disorder	Defect	Inheritance	Clinical and laboratory findings and treatment
Abetalipoproteinemia	Unknown	Autosomal recessive	Steatorrhea, ataxia, acanthocytosis, retinitis pigmentosa, absent serum β lipoprotein. No specific treatment, medium-chain-length triglyceride-enriched diet has been suggested.
"Odor of sweaty feet" syndrome	Acyldehydrogenase deficiency	Autosomal recessive	Dehydration, acidosis, high-pitched cry, seizures, sepsis with pancytopenia and neonatal death. Odor due to butyric and hexanoic acid. No treatment.
Refsum's disease	Deficient degrading of phytanic acid	Autosomal recessive	Ataxia, peripheral polyneuropathy, retinitis pigmentosa, nerve deafness, ichthyosis-like changes, epiphyseal dysplasia increased CSF protein, increased phytanic acid in serum lipids. Special diet has been suggested.
Isovaleric acidemia	Isovaleric acid dehydrogenase	Autosomal recessive	"Sweaty-feet-odor" of body, recurrent acidosis with lethargy or coma precipitated by infection or excessive protein intake, mild retardation, early onset, elevated serum isovaleric acid. Decreased intake of leucine has been suggested.
Sphingomyelin lipidosis (Niemann-Pick disease)	See Diseases Affecting Gray Matter, Chap. 20, "Neurologic Conditions"		
Gaucher's disease	See above		
G_{m2} gangliosidosis, type 1 (Tay-Sachs disease) (See Progres-	Ganglioside G_{m2}-hexosaminidase deficiency	Autosomal recessive, most common in Jews from North-	Developmental regression beginning at 4–6 months, seizures, motor deficit, deafness, enlargement of the head, hypersensitivity to auditory stimuli (early

...sive Degenerative Disease, Chap. 22)		eastern Europe	sign), cherry-red spot of macula, blindness, positive rectal biopsy. Increased central nervous system monosialoganglioside and decreased serum fructose-1-6-diphosphoaldolase. No treatment. Death occurs at 2 to 4 years of age.
Leukodystrophies		See Diseases Affecting White Matter, Chap. 20, "Neurologic Conditions"	
Cerebrotendinous Xanthomatosis	Unknown	Unknown	Cataracts, progressive ataxia, xanthomas in tendons, free cholesterol in xanthoma cells, cholesterol storage in cerebellar and cerebral white matter. No treatment.
G_{m1} gangliosidosis (Generalized gangliosidosis)	β galactosidase deficiency	Autosomal recessive	Retardation, hepatosplenomegaly, bony abnormalities, may have cherry-red spot of macula, increased CNS ganglioside, positive rectal biopsy, Alder-Reilly granules in leukocytes. No treatment. Death occurs before 2 years of age.
Fabry's disease Glycosphingolipid Lipidosis	Ceramide Trihexosidase deficiency	X-linked recessive	Angiomatous skin lesions, severe sharp pain usually in fingers and toes, recurrent fever, paresthesia, cardiac disease, kidney lesions resulting in renal failure in middle age, glycosphingolipid accumulation in CNS and small blood vessels. No specific treatment. Prophylaxis of pain—maintenance Dilantin.

Familial hyperlipoproteinemias types I–V (types III, IV, and V are extremely rare in the pediatric age group)

Type I (familial lipoprotein lipase deficient hyperchylomicronemia)	Lipase	Autosomal recessive (Also types III, IV and V)	Severe abdominal pain, may have hepatosplenomegaly, pancreatitis, xanthomas serum is lactescent due to elevated triglycerides. Low-fat diet with supplemental medium-chain-length triglycerides.

Table 9-1. (Continued)

Disorder	Defect	Inheritance	Clinical and laboratory findings and treatment
Type II (familial hyper-β-lipoproteinemia	Unknown	Autosomal dominant	Xanthomas of tendons, premature coronary. Cerebral and peripheral vascular disease causing death, cholesterol levels are increased and triglycerides are usually normal. Diet high in polyunsaturates and low in polysaturates and cholesterol. Drugs, e.g., cholestyramine combined with nicotinic acid.

porphyrin metabolism in the erythropoietic component of the bone marrow as well as increased urinary excretion of uroporphyrin.

There may be intermittent attacks of hemolytic anemia. The spleen is usually enlarged. Hypertrichosis may be present. In addition to increased urinary excretion of uroporphyrin, there is increased deposition in various structures of the body. Deciduous and permanent teeth may be stained red (erythrodontia). Depositions of porphyrin in normoblasts may be demonstrated as inclusions or by red fluorescence when viewed with Wood's ultraviolet lamp.

A characteristic vesicular or bullous eruption (hydroa aestivale) may appear on exposed areas as a result of exposure to strong sunlight.

Treatment   Treatment includes minimal exposure to sun. Both hemolysis and photosensitivity may be reduced following splenectomy.

HEPATIC PORPHYRIAS

Porphyrias associated with excessive synthesis of porphyrins in the liver may be inherited or acquired. Acquired hepatic porphyria may be associated with such diseases as leukemia, disseminated lupus erythematosus, and Hodgkin's disease.

The inherited forms of hepatic porphyria have not been elucidated, and the sites of enzymatic block in porphyrin metabolism have not been defined. Primarily because of these unknowns, it is difficult to classify what may be a heterogeneous group of inherited disorders.

A tentative classification would include acute intermittent porphyria, porphyria variegata, and porphyria cutanea tarda.

Acute intermittent porphyria   Onset rarely occurs before puberty and may be confused with acute appendicitis or intestinal obstruction. However, other clinical manifestations soon appear: hypertension, tachycardia, neurologic signs of no single pattern, dermal photosensitivity, hyponatremia associated with concentrated urine, and hypersecretion of antidiuretic hormone. Slight fever and leukocytosis may be present at times.

Attacks are of variable duration and may last for days to months. Intervening asymptomatic periods may last for years. Severe attacks may terminate in death due to respiratory paralysis, cachexia, or renal failure.

Though there is great difficulty in detecting asymptomatic kin, available evidence points to transmission by an autosomal dominant gene. Because barbiturates, estrogens, and sulfonamides accentuate acute porphyria, these drugs should be used with extreme caution in asymptomatic kin.

Treatment   Treatment includes avoidance of the above-cited drugs and restrictions on exposure to strong sunlight. Appropriate supportive treatment, for such manifestations as dehydration, hypertension, and uremia, may sometimes be lifesaving.

Porphyria variegata   Cutaneous photosensitivity may be the only manifestation for several years before visceral and neurologic signs appear.

Inheritance is by an autosomal dominant gene. The asymptomatic individual may be detected by measuring the coproporphyrin and protoporphyrin content of the stool.

Treatment   Treatment is the same as for intermittent acute porphyria.

Porphyria cutanea tarda   This is a clinical disorder of porphyrin metabolism which becomes manifest in adult life. It is not clear whether this is a distinct, inheritable form of porphyria. Some cases, on ultimate analysis, may turn out to be acquired porphyria or porphyria variegata. It is probable that a small proportion of cases represents a distinct, inherited form of porphyria.

PRIMARY HEMOCHROMATOSIS

This disease is a hereditary iron-storage disorder. There is excessive hemosiderin deposition in the liver, pancreas, heart, and other organs. It is associated with increased gastrointestinal iron absorption.

The metabolic defect is unknown. The classical triad of hepatic cirrhosis, bronze pigmentation of skin, and diabetes mellitus manifests itself in adulthood. Serum iron levels are normal in childhood. The mode of inheritance is not clear.

THE ZELLWEGER SYNDROME
(Cerebrohepatorenal syndrome)

This is an autosomal, recessive syndrome. Its manifestations include severe hypotonia, multiple minor abnormalities, a characteristic facies which resembles mongolism, psychomotor retardation, and seizures. A defect in iron storage (congenital hemosiderosis) has been identified. The white matter of the brain is sclerotic with severe demyelinization. Death occurs before 6 months of age.

THE IMMUNOLOGIC SYSTEM

Resistance to infection is dependent upon several factors which are maximally effective when they function in a coordinated fashion. The integrity of each mechanism is controlled by different genetic factors.

The immunologic system has three types of function:

1.   Primary function: phagocytosis and inflammatory response. Phago-

cytic cells (polymorphonuclear leukocytes and macrophages) are essential for this function. The opsonin and complement systems together with specific antibodies aid the process of phagocytosis.

2. Secondary function: antigen elimination by (a) elaboration of specific antibodies [gamma M (IgM), gamma A (IgA), gamma G (IgG), gamma E (IgE), gamma D (IgD)], which depends on the presence of plasma cells and thymic-independent lymphocytes (BL) or (b) cell-mediated immunity which requires the presence of thymus-dependent lymphocytes (TL).

3. If the antigen cannot be eliminated by the above two mechanisms, the tertiary response comes into effect. Persistence of the antigen causes four types of interactions. (a) reagin mediated, e.g., penicillin hypersensitivity; (b) cytotoxic injury; (c) antigen antibody (immune complex) injury; (d) delayed hypersensitivity or cell-mediated injury. These responses are not beneficial to the host, and they manifest a disease phenomenon, e.g., autoimmune disorders or penicillin hypersensitivity.

The diagnosis of immune deficiency diseases due to abnormalities of gamma globulin is age-related because the placental transfer and postnatal development of individual gamma globulin proceed at different rates (see p. 195).

Cell-mediated immunity (delayed hypersensitivity) can be tested in vivo (skin testing with candida, trichophyton, or DNCB) or in vitro (lymphocyte-stimulation test or migration-inhibitory factor).

In vivo tests for delayed hypersensitivity measure either prior natural sensitization or de novo sensitization. It is known that over 80 percent of children have delayed hypersensitivity responses to candida, trichophyton, streptokinase, streptodornase. Consequently, these antigens provide a convenient test vehicle for determining delayed hypersensitivity. In addition, if it is known that a patient has had other fungal infections previously or tuberculosis, delayed hypersensitivity reactions to these organisms can also be tested. The de novo sensitization test is performed with dinitrochlorobenzene (DNCB), a substance to which almost all individuals will demonstrate a delayed response when challenged 7 days following initial exposure.

In vitro tests demonstrate the ability of TL to respond to antigens. The lymphocyte-stimulation test is based on the transformation and proliferation responses of normal lymphocytes to in vitro stimulation by either nonspecific stimulants, e.g., phytohemagglutinin, foreign cells, or a specific antigen. The end point of the reaction is measured by blast formation, a mitotic index, or incorporation of radioactive precursors into RNA or DNA.

The migration-inhibition test depends on the release of an effector protein molecule, migration-inhibition factor (MIF), by lymphocytes stimulated by an antigen. The effect of MIF on monocytes in culture is to render them sticky so that their migration from a capillary tube is inhibited.

Table 9-2. Immune deficiency diseases

Disorder	Immunological findings	Clinical manifestation	Genetic transmission	Tests and treatment
Disorders of primary immune function				
1. Familial neutropenia—infantile lethal	Neutropenia	Recurrent, severe, pyogenic infections in early infancy	Autosomal recessive	Low peripheral and bone marrow leukocytes. Supportive treatment
2. Chronic granulomatous disease (CGD)	Intracellular defect of neutrophils—ingest but do not digest bacteria	Infections by bacteria of low virulence, hepatosplenomegaly, microabscesses, death in early childhood	X-linked or autosomal recessive	IgG is elevated, WBC is elevated, quantitative nitroblue tetrozolium (NBT) test, bacteriocidal test. Supportive and antibacterial treatment
3. Chédiak-Higashi syndrome	Defective granulocyte regulation	Oculocutaneous albinism, recurrent pyogenic infectious, death in early childhood with sepsis.	Autosomal recessive	Giant lysosomes in WBC. Supportive treatment
Disorders of secondary immune response				
1. Thymic-independent system				
(a) Congenital agammaglobulinemia (Bruton's disease)	All immunoglobulins are deficient (IgG, IgA, IgM). Normal cell-mediated immunity (delayed hypersensitivity, homograft rejection)	Marked susceptibility to bacterial infections; sprue-like syndrome; absence of adenoids; predisposition to eczema; rheumatoid arthritis, pneumocystis	X-linked recessive	Failure to form antibodies after immunization, e.g., positive Schick test after DPT, isohemagglutinins. Monthly injections of gamma globulin (0.6 ml/kg following double

		Carinii pnemonitis (plasma cell pneumonia)		initial dose) to maintain level of 100 to 300 mg/100 ml
2. Dysgammaglobulinemia, types I-VII	Deficient synthesis of specific immunoglobulin fraction (or different combinations)	Frequent infections in IgG deficiency syndromes	Type 1: X-linked recessive, others ?	Immunoelectrophoresis Treatment—gamma globulin of IgG deficiency exists
3. Wiskott-Aldrich syndrome	Deficiency of one or more immunoglobulins	Eczema, recurrent pyogenic infections, thrombocytopenia	X-linked recessive	Immunoelectrophoresis: IgA depressed, IgM depressed, Supportive and antibacterial treatment
4. Ataxia-telangectasia, Louis-Bar syndrome	(See Ataxia in Childhood, Chap. 22)			
5. Thymic-dependent system (a) Congenital aplasia of thymus (Di George's syndrome)	Absent cell-mediated responses, normal humeral antibodies	Congenital absence of thymus and parathyroids: neonatal tetany, hypocalcemia, increased susceptibility to infections, abnormally shaped ears, hyperterlorism, anomalies of great vessels		Serum calcium decreased, phosphorus elevated Skin testing: 1. in vitro tests: candida, trichophyton, streptokinase-DNCB, antigens skin homografting (failure to reject) 2. in vitro: lymphocyte mitosis stimulation test, macrophage migration test Treatment of neonatal tetany and thymus transplants

Table 9-2. (Continued)

Disorder	Immunological findings	Clinical manifestation	Genetic transmission	Tests and treatment
(b) Thymic dysplasia with normal immunoglobulins (Nezelof's syndrome)	Thymic dysplasia and impaired cell-mediated immunity	Recurrent local and systemic infections; disseminated vaccina severe bullous varicella, p. 265 carinii and bacterial pneumonias	Autosomal recessive	Immunoelectrophoresis: Normal as above with the exception of normal serum calcium. Treatment: thymus transplant
6. Combined deficiency of thymic-dependent and independent systems Thymic dysplasia with agammaglobulinemia (Swiss-type)	Deficiency of humeral and cell-mediated immunity	Early onset of severe bacterial, fungal, and viral infections, oral thrush, intractable diarrhea, and progressive respiratory disease	X-linked recessive or autosomal recessive	Lymphopenia, absent delayed hypersensitivity, defective homograft rejection. Avoid live-virus vaccines Bone marrow grafts may be helpful

REVIEW QUESTIONS

The following questions are of the matching type. In the blank next to the item in column I list the letter of the item in column II with which it is most closely associated:

I	II
1. Wilson's disease ____	(a) Defect in transportation of tryptophan
2. Maple syrup urine disease ____	(b) Deficiency of ceruloplasmin
3. Hartnup's disease ____	(c) Abnormal metabolism of leucine, isoleucine, and valine
4. Galactosemia ____	(d) Hepatorenal form of the disease is the commonest type
5. von Gierke's disease ____	(e) Deficiency of galactose-1-phosphate uridyl transferase
6. mothball poisoning ____	(f) Deficiency of glucose-6-phosphate dehydrogenase
7. phenylketonuria ____	(g) Intelligence usually normal but speech is impaired
8. histidinemia ____	(h) Less pigment in skin, hair, and eyes than in other members of family

9. All the following are examples of disorders associated with protein metabolism except (a) congenital agammaglobulinemia; (b) galactosemia; (c) von Gierke's disease; (d) albinism; (e) alkaptonuria.

10. Coproporphyrinuria (predominantly type III isomer) is often seen in the following conditions except: (a) mongolism; (b) acute rheumatic fever; (c) lupus erythematosus; (d) lead poisoning; (e) poliomyelitis.

11. All the following statements concerning phenylketonuria are true except: (a) phenylalanine cannot be converted to tyrosine in these patients; (b) the patients appear normal at birth; (c) the disease is associated with a characteristic odor of the urine; (d) dietary therapy causes a rise of phenylalanine in the blood; (e) some states have laws requiring PKU screening tests to be done routinely on all newborn infants.

12. Disaccharidase deficiency caused by malabsorption is characterized by all the following except (a) colic; (b) high stool pH; (c) failure to break down the offending disaccharide within the intestinal lumen; (d) inherited condition; (e) occurrence in both breast-fed and artificially fed infants.

13. Many carbohydrate disturbances are symptomatic; which one of the following is asymptomatic: (a) sucrose malabsorption; (b) isomaltose malabsorption; (c) galactosemia; (d) essential fructosuria; (e) monosaccharide malabsorption.

14. All the following are associated with maple syrup urine disease except for one: (a) seizures; (b) leucine-induced hypoglycemia; (c) urine forms green color when treated with ferric chloride; (d) death occurs by the end of the first year.

15. All the following are associated with galactosemia except for one: (a) cataract formation; (b) jaundice; (c) hepatosplenomegaly; (d) mental retardation.

16. The following characterize acute intermittent porphyria except for one: (a) usually occurs in early childhood; (b) hypertension; (c) tachycardia; (d) hypersecretion of antidiuretic hormone.

17. All the following are associated with congenital agammaglobulinemia (Bruton's disease) except for one: (a) positive Schick test after DPT; (b) autosomal recessive trait; (c) marked susceptibility to bacterial infections; (d) all immunoglobulins are deficient.

10

THE FETUS AND FETAL ENVIRON- MENT

FETAL MONITORING

Assessing the status of the fetus in utero has become an objective of increasing importance. The fetus appears to be affected more by factors present antepartum than by those existing acutely during delivery. The appearance of clinically obvious fetal distress as defined by bradycardia and the passage of meconium, in the presence of normal uterine activity and presentation, suggests a preexisting uteroplacental insufficiency. Similarly, the course of neonatal events rests, in great measure, on antepartum factors. Fetal monitoring designed to detect subclinical fetal distress is clearly indicated.

The first step is the identification of the high-risk pregnant patient and the application to that patient of comprehensive prenatal care. A minority of gravidas with a variety of demographic, obstetric, and medical complications account for a significant proportion of unfavorable pregnancy outcomes. The criteria for the selection of high-risk pregnancy are

1. Demographic: teen-age gravida (under 17), elderly gravida (over 36), underweight, overweight, and socioeconomic indigency.
2. Obstetric: grand multiparty, previous operative delivery, previous prolonged labor, previous early fetal loss (repetitive), previous late fetal loss, previous live premature, previous early infant death, and traumatized or anomalous infant.
3. Medical: hypertensive disease, renal disease, diabetes and other endocrine disorders, cardiovascular disease, hereditary disorders, e.g., sickle-cell disease, Rh sensitization, and narcotic addiction.
4. Current pregnancy: toxemia, bleeding, rubella and other teratogens, malnutrition and anemia, multiple pregnancy, and abnormal presentation.

The degree of risk imposed by each complication varies considerably, with relatively low perinatal morbidity and mortality rates associated with maternal obesity, grand multiparity, and previous operative delivery, and higher risk noted with prior poor obstetric history, hypertension, diabetes, and in the elderly gravida. An environment of low socioeconomic life-style characterized by poor nutrition, inadequate housing, unhygienic surroundings, overcrowding, and lack of education is associated with increased morbidity and mortality of both mother and fetus.

The myriad metabolic processes involved in fetoplacental growth are marked by the presence of a number of enzymes, steroids, and other materials in the maternal blood and urine, making them available for simple and serial sampling during the course of pregnancy. In addition, many of these substances are present in the amniotic fluid and can be measured following amniocentesis in order to obtain more direct information about fetal status. The following indices of the fetal environment are being clinically applied.

1. Biochemical: (a) enzymatic: diamine oxidase, heat-stabile alkaline phosphatase, and oxytocinase; (b) nonenzymatic: folic acid and serum copper.
2. Endocrine: estriol, pregnanediol, chorionic gonadotropin, and placental lactogen.
3. Biophysical: ultrasonography, amniocentesis, and amniography.

Of particular use in the management of the complicated obstetrical patient are the assay of urinary estriol, the measurement of fetal head growth by serial biparietal ultrasonography, and the information obtained by amniocentesis.

ENDOCRINE PARAMETERS FOR EVALUATING FETAL STATUS

While estriol is synthesized in the placenta, its immediate precursor, 16 alpha-hydroxy-dehydroepiandesterone, sulfate, is produced by a series of enzymatic processes involving the fetal adrenal gland and liver. In the absence of normal fetal adrenal function, e.g., anencephaly, little or no estriol is produced. Clinically measurable at 1 mg per 24-hour urine specimen at the twentieth week of pregnancy, this hormone is found in increasing quantity through later gestation. Levels of 12 mg per 24 hours are considered normal at term. Levels below 4 mg per 24 hours suggests imminent fetal death in utero. Falling values of greater than 50 percent from previously normal levels are a sign of fetal compromise and call for intensified medical management. This assay has been effective in the reduction of perinatal mortality in diabetic pregnancy, postmaturity, and in hypertensive disorders. In the latter case, normal maternal renal function with clearance of estriol from the plasma must be verified in order to avoid misinterpretation of false-positive low values in the urine.

BIOPHYSICAL PARAMETERS FOR EVALUATING FETAL STATUS

The use of pulsed ultrasound bidimensional scanning is gaining widespread acceptance. These sound waves appear to be nontoxic in in vivo experiments, and they reveal the following data:

1. The gestational sac can be visualized as early as the fifth week of pregnancy.
2. The fetal head, which is first seen at 13 weeks, can be measured for continued growth. A nomogram for the fetal biparietal diameter in normal pregnancy has been established which indicates a growth rate of nearly 2 mm per week.
3. Gestational age can be accurately determined when the expected date of confinement is unknown.
4. In addition to its obvious value in third trimester bleeding, placental localization is extremely important in diagnostic amniocentesis and the avoidance of damage to fetal vessels.

Amniocentesis In the early second trimester of pregnancy, amniotic fluid can be obtained with safety. Viable fetal cells can be grown with regularity, providing tissue cultures for cytogenetic analysis and for the identification of a growing number of inborn errors of metabolism. Those familial metabolic disorders which can be suspected or detected with accuracy during the early stage of pregnancy in order to provide accurate information for genetic counseling are

1. Mucopolysaccharidosis
   Hurler's syndrome

        Hunter's syndrome
        Maroteaux-Lamy syndrome
        Morquio's syndrome
        Sanfilippo's syndrome
        Scheie's syndrome

2. Disorders of lipid metabolism
        Gaucher's disease
        G_{m1} gangliosidosis
        G_{m2} gangliosidosis
          (Tay-Sachs disease)
        Metachromatic leukodystrophy
        Niemann-Pick disease
        Fabry's disease
        Krabbe's disease

3. Amino acid metabolism
        Argininosuccinicaciduria
        Citrullinemia
        Cystinosis
        Homocystinuria
        Hyperammonemia
        Hypervalinemia
        Maple syrup urine disease
        Hyperglycinemia
        Methylmalonic aciduria

4. Carbohydrate metabolism
        Glycogen-storage disease, types II, III, IV
        Galactosemia
        Fucosidosis
        Glucose-6-phosphate dehydrogenase deficiency
        Mannosidosis

5. Other categories
        Acatalasemia
        Chédiak-Higashi syndrome
        Congenital erythropoietic porphyria
        Cystic fibrosis of pancreas
        "I"-cell disease
        Lesch-Nyhan syndrome
        Lysosomal acid phosphatase deficiency
        Marfan's syndrome
        Orotic aciduria
        Trisomies or translocation defects
        Xeroderma pigmentosum

In later pregnancy, amniocentesis is utilized to provide material for the assessment of fetal maturity. The progressive dilution of the amniotic fluid during the last 8 weeks of pregnancy is reflected in decreased osmolarity and in the disappearance of bilirubin, as determined by spectrophotometry. The increasing fetal muscle mass and the progressive development of fetal renal function produces an increasing quantity of creatinine in the amniotic fluid, reaching levels of 2 mg percent and remaining above both fetal and maternal plasma levels. Staining the cells of the amniotic fluid with nile blue sulfate discloses, in the last month of pregnancy, an increasing percentage of lipid containing orange-colored cells. Thin-layer chromatography of the amniotic fluid supernatant with quantitation of phospholipids has been successfully utilized as a specific index of fetal pulmonary maturity. Between the thirty-sixth and thirty-seventh week of pregnancy, a sharp increase in the amount of lecithin is noted reversing the sphyngomyelin: lecithin ratio to a lecithin predominance. Infants born under these conditions have been almost totally without evidence of respiratory distress syndrome. The application of these indices of fetal maturity plus measurement of the biparietal diameter have proved particularly useful in the reduction of iatrogenic prematurity associated with elective repeat cesarean section and induction of labor. The following values are indicative of the fetus of at least 36 weeks' gestation and a predicted birth weight of over 2,500 Gm.

1. Fetal biparietal diameter (ultrasound)—8.7 cm or more
2. Amniotic fluid: bilirubin—absent, osmolarity—less than 250 mOsm, creatinine—greater than 2 mg percent, fetal squamae—greater than 20 percent, and lecithin/sphingomyelin ratio—greater than 2:1.

FETAL HEART RATE AND PATTERN AS AN INDEX OF FETAL STATUS

Intrapartum continuous recording of the fetal heart rate with simultaneous measurement of uterine contractions has added another dimension to fetal monitoring. Fetal heart rate information can be obtained by phonocardiography or electrocardiography, utilizing an electrode attached to the presenting part or through pulsed ultrasound using the Doppler effect. Uterine contractions can be measured quantitatively by external or internal tocodynamometry. These techniques have allowed differentiation of several distinctive patterns of fetal heart rate response during labor. Table 10-1 outlines the alterations in fetal heart rate and their potential clinical significance.

The degree of fetal compromise associated with the various pathologic fetal heart rate alterations can be further defined by fetal scalp sampling. This technique involves the aspiration of fetal scalp capillary blood and the measurement of pH and blood gases with microelectrodes. The highest degree of correlation between these determinations and neonatal condition is provided by measurement of fetal pH. Apgar scores of 4 or less are usually associated with fetal pH values below 7.20.

The primary objective in a program of intrapartum monitoring is to establish the timing and necessity for prompt intervention during the labor process before the appearance of severe clinical fetal distress. A reduction in intrapartum fetal loss and decrease in the incidence

Table 10-1.   Fetal heart rate abnormalities

Type	Rate change	Clinical significance
Baseline tachycardia	Greater than 160/min	Associated with maternal febrile and vascular complications
Baseline bradycardia	Less than 120/min	Associated with maternal hypotension and hypoxia
Acceleration	Over 160/min with contraction	Apparently benign
Deceleration		
Early	Coincident with the onset of contraction; brief 10–40 beat/min decreases with prompt recovery	Benign, appears in late labor due to head compression
Late*	Appears after lag period; drop in rate persists after contraction, slow recovery	Ominous, due to fetal hypoxia (P_{AO_2} less than 20 mm) secondary to uteroplacental insufficiency, e.g., maternal vascular disease, uterine hypertonicity
Variable	Timing, frequency, and configuration of rate decrease is variable and often pronounced but with prompt recovery	Generally benign except when severe and persistent—due to cord compression
Loss of any beat irregularity*	Continuous fixed heart rate	Ominous, due to fetal central nervous system depression and loss of vagal tone frequently produced by analgesics and sedatives

* Significant correlation with low Apgar score.

of morbid neonates can be achieved by the use of these procedures. The pediatrician is provided with invaluable information about the infant soon to be under his care and can effectively prepare for indicated resuscitative efforts and for continuous neonatal intensive care.

THE PLACENTA

DEVELOPMENT AND CIRCULATION

The primitive trophoblast proliferates rapidly after implantation. Three layers appear: the syncytium, the cytotrophoblast, and the mesoblast. The latter provides a supporting structure in which villus vascular elements make their appearance. Electron microscopy reveals that the outer syncytial layer is complex with abundant highly developed microvilli, pinocytotic vesicles, and ribonucleoproteins. After the second week of gestation, islands of red blood cells develop in situ, and vascular channels appear. The villi in contact with the maternal decidua are exposed to a rich blood supply and multiply rapidly, becoming the chorion frondosum or future placenta.

By the fourteenth week, the placenta is a discrete organ. Most of the villi lie free in maternal blood of the intervillous space; anchoring villi are attached to the decidua. Circulation within the intervillous space is dependent upon (1) maternal blood pressure with a resultant gradient between arterial and venous channels and (2) uterine contractions. Arterial blood enters the placenta from the endometrial arteries under a head of pressure. The villi act as baffles, and by their pulsations, resulting from fetal cardiac action, are of great importance in mixing the blood. Eventually the blood disperses laterally and falls back on the multiple orifices of the maternal veins.

IMMUNOLOGIC PROPERTIES

The placenta corresponds to a natural homograft in that it is a transplant of living tissue within the same species; yet it does not normally evoke the usual immune response reaction of homografts resulting in rejection of the graft. Theories proposed to explain its immunologic defense include (1) altered maternal immunocompetence, (2) antigenic immaturity of the fetus, (3) mechanical blockage of antigens, and (4) the uterus as a "privileged site" for tissue graft. A probable explanation lies in the fact that pure trophoblastic tissue is immunologically inert and appears to form a buffer zone between the fetus and the mother.

TRANSFER MECHANISMS

Fetal growth exceeds that of the placenta in the last two trimesters of pregnancy. The placenta adjusts to increasing fetal demands by (1) increasing the surface area of the villi and (2) thinning of the syncytium. Numerous factors influence the rate and type of transfer of substances across the placenta.

1. *Simple diffusion:* Movement of molecules occurs from an area of high concentration to a lower one and is proportional to the concentration gradient. This type of transport involves no work or energy by the membrane and continues only until electrochemical equilibrium is established on both sides of the membrane. Materials of small molecular size such as respiratory gases, electrolytes, water, and nitrogenous end products pass by simple diffusion.
2. *Facilitated transport:* In spite of its obvious influence, the size of the molecule is not necessarily the determining factor in the movement of materials across the placenta. In some cases, there is a speeding up of the process of transfer at a rate in excess of that

predicted if only simple diffusion were involved. This would augment membrane transit without requiring a chemical alteration of the carrier. Glucose and galactose are examples of facilitated transport.

3. *Active transport:* Some compounds cross a membrane against an electrochemical gradient or "uphill." Energy is required, and thus the participation of some enzymatic pathways is inferred. In some instances large molecules such as maternal lipids are broken down into fatty acids before passage and are resynthesized by the fetal liver. Many of the amino acids are transferred to the fetus in this fashion.

4. *Pinocytosis:* Visualization of the ameboid motion of syncytial cells has made tenable the concept of "droplet transfer," or pinocytosis. This mechanism is cited as important in the transfer of large molecules across the placenta whose size precludes their transfer by any other process, e.g., albumins, gamma globulins. It is evident that the various mechanisms operate in accordance with the particular demands of the fetus. Normally certain substances essential for fetal growth occur in higher concentration in the fetal than in the maternal circulation. These include calcium, inorganic phosphorus, free amino acids, nucleic acid, and ascorbic acid.

The concept of a placental barrier has been clearly contradicted by observations demonstrating the presence of fetal blood cells in the maternal circulation and the converse. The various transfer mechanisms, from simple diffusion to cellular migration, occur in both directions across the placenta. For practical purposes, it must be assumed that any pharmacologic agent administered to the mother can be considered as potentially present in the fetal circulation. The drugs in Table 10-2 have demonstrated adverse effects in human or animal studies.

In addition, it is possible that a variety of drugs currently in familiar use are producing congenital malformations when taken in the early months of pregnancy. These consequences may occur only in extremely sensitive individuals and hence do not universally follow the use of the drug. These defects cannot be located epidemiologically because they are obscured by the presence of indistinguishable defects of genetic origin and because the teratogen is inconstant in its effects. Furthermore, animal studies have shown that drugs may disappear from the fetal circulation and be considered as having been rapidly excreted, and yet significant tissue levels may persist in critical organs, e.g., the brain and liver.

ENDOCRINE ASPECTS

In addition to its function as an intrauterine organ of respiration, nutrition, and excretion for the growing fetus, the placenta functions

Table 10-2. Drugs having potential effects on the fetus

Maternal medication	Fetal or neonatal effect
Heroin, morphine, methadone	Neonatal withdrawal
Androgens, progestogens	Masculinization
Anticoagulants	Fetal death, hemorrhage
Phenobarbital	Neonatal withdrawal
Reserpine	Stuffy nose, respiratory obstruction
Antihistamines	Anomalies*
Chloroquine, quinine	Thrombocytopenia
Chloramphenicol	"Grey" syndrome
Streptomycin	Eighth nerve deafness
Sulfonamides	Kernicterus
Tetracycline	Discoloration of teeth, retarded bone growth
Antineoplastics	Anomalies and abortion
Propylthiouracil, iodides	Goiter, mental retardation
Corticosteroids	Cleft palate*
Thiazide diuretics	Thrombocytopenia
Hypoglycemics	Anomalies*
Salicylates	Neonatal bleeding
Thalidomide	Phocomelia, hearing loss
Novobiocin	Hyperbilirubinemia

* Based on laboratory experiments with animals.

as an endocrine gland. The chief purpose of the dramatic changes in endocrine function during pregnancy is to maintain the gestation and to support the fetus in utero until termination of the gestation period. From a practical point of view the fetus and the placenta should be regarded as a single functional endocrine unit.

Chorionic gonadotrophin Human chorionic gonadotrophin is of pure placental origin. Its chemical composition differs from the pituitary gonadotrophins in a single carbohydrate moiety of the glycoprotein molecule. The function of placental gonadotrophin is to prolong the lifespan of the corpus luteum of menstruation during the initial stages of implantation. This hormone is therefore able to induce continuous progesterone secretion until such a time as the placental steroid production is sufficient to replace ovarian sources.

Placental lactogen A growth hormone–like substance possessing lactogenic properties is synthesized solely by the placenta. It is produced by the syncytial trophoblast and is transferred almost exclusively into the maternal circulation. The role of human placental lactogen is a key one in maternal metabolic adjustments promoting utilization of fat stores as fuel and, in turn, increasing maternal capacity for protein and glucose sparing.

Progesterone   All steroid-producing endocrine tissues form this hormone, and it is the major steroid produced by the placental syncytial cells. The functions of progesterone are chiefly the development and maintenance of the decidual bed. In addition, it reduces excitability of the uterus possibly by affecting membrane potentials of myometrial fibers, particularly at the placental site.

Estrogen   After the seventh week of pregnancy there is a gradual rise in urinary excretion of estradiol and estrone, which is not influenced by removal of the fetus. Perfusion experiments with the human placenta indicate the ability of the placenta to synthesize both estradiol and estrone. However, unless special precursors are added to the perfusion media, no estriol is synthesized. Although the site of final production of estriol is in the syncytium, precursors are produced in the fetal adrenal tissue.

   The function of estrogens during pregnancy include stimulation of uterine and breast growth. Estriol excretion by the placenta is apparently a method of metabolism of fetal adrenal steroids. Measurement of this relatively inert estrogen provides a reliable means of assessing fetal well-being.

Relaxin   This nonsteroid hormone appears in the blood of women early in pregnancy and increases gradually to term. It is thought that the placenta may be its source and that its function is to act synergistically with progesterone in a relaxation of pelvic ligaments and connective tissues in various parts of the body.

REVIEW QUESTIONS

1. A number of indices of the fetal environment are being monitored. Levels of a number of enzymes, steroids, and other materials in the maternal blood and urine as well as other tests are being carried out. These include (*a*) diamine oxidase, (*b*) estriol, (*c*) ultrasonograph, (*d*) amniocentesis, (*e*) pregnanediol, (*f*) folic acid, (*g*) serum copper.
   The three most helpful indices are (1) _____, (2) _____, (3) _____.
2. Urinary estriol is synthesized in the placenta and is first clinically measurable in a 24-hour urine specimen at the (*a*) fourth week, (*b*) tenth week, (*c*) twentieth week, (*d*) thirtieth week of pregnancy.
3. The following values of urinary estriol are obtained at term: (*a*) 3 mg per 24 hours, (*b*) 14 mg per 24 hours, (*c*) 20 mg per 24 hours, (*d*) 25 mg per 24 hours. Which is the critical value suggesting imminent fetal death in utero?
4. By use of ultrasound waves, the gestational sac can be visualized as early as (*a*) fifth week, (*b*) seventh week, (*c*) twelfth week, (*d*) twentieth week of pregnancy.
5. By use of ultrasound waves the fetal head can be seen first at (*a*) fifth week, (*b*) seventh week, (*c*) thirteenth week, (*d*) twentieth week of gestation.
6. The biparietal diameter of the fetal head grows at a rate of (*a*) 2 mm, (*b*) 4 mm, (*c*) 6 mm, (*d*) 8 mm per week.

7. Which of the following time intervals is considered the earliest time for safely performing an amniocentesis? (*a*) first trimester, (*b*) early second trimester, (*c*) late second trimester, (*d*) early third trimester.

8. Amniocentesis in the thirty-sixth or thirty-seventh week of pregnancy normally reveals: (*a*) lecithin level lower than the level of sphyngomyelin, (*b*) lecithin level higher than the level of sphyngomyelin, (*c*) lecithin level equal to the level of sphyngomyelin, (*d*) none of the above applies.

9. Column I lists certain characteristics or substances found in amniotic fluid. Column II represents values for these parameters indicative of a fetus with a predicted birth weight of over 2,500 Gm. Match the items in both columns.

I	II
(*A*) Bilirubin (mg) ____	(*a*) Greater than 20 percent
(*B*) Osmolarity (mOsm) ____	(*b*) Greater than 2
(*C*) Creatinine (mg percent) ____	(*c*) Absent
(*D*) Fetal squamae ____	(*d*) Greater than 2:1
(*E*) Lecithin-sphyngomyelin ratio ____	(*e*) Less than 250
	(*f*) Less than 2:1

10. Alterations in fetal heart rate have clinical significance: Column I indicates a variety of fetal heart rates; column II lists possible clinical significance of altered fetal heart rates. Match the items.

I	II
(*A*) Tachycardia—greater than 160 per min ____	(*a*) Benign
	(*b*) Benign; appears in late labor due to head compression
(*B*) Bradycardia—less than 120 per min ____	(*c*) Associated with maternal hypotension and hypoxia
(*C*) Acceleration—over 160 per min with contractions	(*d*) Associated with maternal febrile and vascular complications.
(*D*) Deceleration—early in uterine contraction	

11. A capillary blood pH value of 7.20 is usually associated with (*a*) Apgar score of 8 or more, (*b*) Apgar score of 4 or less, (*c*) unrelated to Apgar score.

12. The placenta is a discrete organ by the (*a*) eighth week, (*b*) fourteenth week, (*c*) twentieth week, (*d*) twenty-eighth week of gestation.

13. In the last two trimesters of pregnancy, one of the following statements is true: (*a*) fetal growth is less than that of the placenta, (*b*) fetal growth is equal to that of the placenta, (*c*) fetal growth exceeds that of the placenta.

14. Numerous substances cross the placenta. In column I are four methods by which substances are transferred. In column II there is a list of some of the substances. Match the two.

I	II
(*A*) Simple diffusion ____	(*a*) Glucose and galactose
(*B*) Facilitated transport ____	(*b*) Amino acids
(*C*) Active transport ____	(*c*) Respiratory gases, electrolytes, water, nitrogenous products.
(*D*) Pinocytosis ____	(*d*) Albumin, gamma globulins

15. Calcium, inorganic phosphorus, free amino acids, nucleic acid, and ascorbic acid all occur in the fetus in (a) lower concentration, (b) equal concentration, (c) higher concentration than in the maternal circulation.

16. Several drugs that are able to cross the placental barrier have been demonstrated to have adverse effects in human or animal studies of the fetus. Column I lists several of these drugs. Column II lists some fetal or neonatal effects of the drugs. Match the items.

I		II	
(A)	Methadone ____	(a)	Kernicterus
(B)	Reserpine ____	(b)	Discoloration of teeth
(C)	Sulfonamides ____	(c)	Stuffy nose and respiratory obstruction
(D)	Tetracyclines ____	(d)	Withdrawal symptoms
(E)	Thiazide diuretics ____	(e)	Thrombocytopenia

17. In its functions as an endocrine gland the placenta produces several important hormones. Column I lists several hormones. Column II lists functions of placental hormones. Match the items.

I		II	
(A)	Chorionic gonadotrophin ____	(a)	Development and maintenance of the decidual bed.
(B)	Placental lactogen ____	(b)	Stimulation of uterine and breast growth
(C)	Progesterone ____	(c)	Acts synergistically with progesterone
(D)	Estrogen ____	(d)	Prolongs lifespan of corpus luteum during initial stages of implantation
(E)	Relaxin ____	(e)	Promotes utilization of fat stores and increases maternal capacity for protein and glucose sparing

11 THE NORMAL NEWBORN INFANT

PHYSIOLOGY OF THE NEWBORN

The "newborn" period is generally considered to be the first month of life. The change from the relatively hypoxic and parasitic intrauterine existence to extrauterine life is profound. The physiologic changes are most marked during the first hours and become less marked as time goes on.

TEMPERATURE CONTROL

Difficulty in heat regulation in the newborn is due to a predisposition to heat loss, not an inability to produce heat. Although the newborn rarely shivers (which in adults increases heat production two- to threefold), he produces heat via basal metabolism, muscular activity, and chemical thermogenesis. Peripheral receptors stimulated by temperature change activate the autonomic nervous system, via the central nervous system, to release norepinephrine. Peripheral vasoconstriction occurs and brown fat (located in the interscapular region, nape of the neck, and around the heart and kidneys) breaks down triglycerides to fatty acid with production of heat. Heat is lost by radiation, evaporation, convection, and conduction. Because of scant subcutaneous fat stores, insulation in the newborn is minimal. The large surface area relative to body size is another cause of increased heat loss, as is being wet with amniotic fluid. A fall of only a few degrees of environmental temperature can double the infant's need for oxygen. In addition, chilling causes increased acidosis and a decreased blood glucose level.

SKIN

Variations in color may be found in the normal newborn infant because of vasomotor instability and sluggishness of the peripheral circulation, e.g., cyanosis of the hands and feet particularly when cool, deep redness or purplish color in the crying infant, and mottling of the skin. Harlequin color change is a sharp division of the body in the midline from forehead to pubis into a red half and a pale half. (This is probably a positional color change, with redness of the dependent side and blanching of the nondependent side.) This change is transient and of no significance and may occur about the third or fourth day. (For discussion of mongolian spots, see p. 691.) The newborn infant is susceptible to staphylococcal infection of the skin.

CIRCULATORY SYSTEM

Circulation changes   (See Fig. 11-1)

Closure of the foramen ovale   Functional closure at birth, anatomic closure at about 4 months of age.

Closure of the ductus arteriosus   Functional closure the first few days of life, anatomic closure at several weeks to 2 months.

Closure of the ductus venosus and umbilical and hypogastric vessels Functional closure shortly after birth, anatomic, by 3 weeks.

The electrocardiogram usually shows a preponderance of the right ventricle (right axis deviation). For a discussion of heart rate and blood pressure, see p. 9.

BLOOD PICTURE

(The cellular changes are described in Chapter 22, "Blood Disorders.")

1. The blood volume is about 85 ml per kg body weight at birth and falls to about 75 ml per kg after the first month of life.

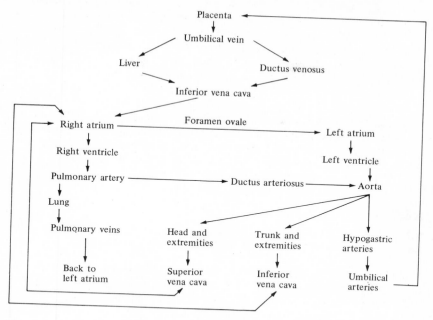

Figure 11-1   Fetal circulation

2. The prothrombin time is normal at birth and prolonged about the second or third day, gradually returning to normal by the sixth or seventh day.
3. The capillary walls are highly resistant to trauma from birth until the fifth week of life, after which time there is no marked change through childhood. Peripheral circulation is sluggish and capillary blood shows a concentration of cells.
4. The blood sugar level is variable. Average values of 55 to 60 mg per 100 ml fall during the first 4 to 6 hours then rise to above-original values by 6 days of age. Normal newborn infants may exhibit very low levels (20 mg per 100 ml) without presenting abnormal clinical findings (see p. 666).
5. The levels of blood proteins are normal at birth, then decrease and are lowest at 2 to 4 months of age, after which they increase to adult levels. The fetus produces albumin and alpha and beta globulins but little gamma globulin (IgM and IgA antibodies may be formed in utero from about 20 weeks' gestation in response to intrauterine infection). Under normal circumstances the full-term neonate is endowed with maternal IgG. Transplacental passage begins between the third and fourth months of intrauterine life. Gamma globulin levels fall during the first month (because of the disappearance of the major component—maternal IgG) and do not begin to rise until 3 months of age; they reach adult levels by the

end of the first year. The newborn infant does not produce IgG until about 2 months of age. The newborn infant synthesizes IgM at birth, and by 1 year he achieves 75 percent of the adult level. IgA is synthesized by about 1 month of age; 75 percent of adult levels are reached by 12 years of age.

6. Wide variation in arterial oxygen saturation is noted at birth (some vigorous infants have no measurable arterial oxygen). However, oxygenation increases rapidly following the onset of respirations, rising to 90 percent saturation within 30 minutes to 3 hours after birth. Varying degrees of metabolic acidosis are present at birth. The derangements in pH are corrected more slowly, but normal acid-base balance is usually attained by 12 hours of age. See Chapter 7, "Fluid and Electrolyte Balance."

RESPIRATORY SYSTEM

Inhibitory mechanisms probably prevent respiration in utero except for an occasional respiratory movement. The onset of extrauterine respiration appears to be initiated by sensory stimuli, e.g., changes in environmental temperature; handling and chemical stimuli, e.g., increased CO_2 tension, hypoxia. The first breath requires extra force to overcome the cohesiveness of the lung surfaces, so that a negative pressure of 15 to 25 cm water may be needed for primary expansion. As the lung expands, the pulmonary vascular resistance decreases, pulmonary blood flow increases, and there is less shunting of blood from the right to the left side of the heart. The fluid filling the potential air spaces is removed by the capillaries and lymphatics as well as by being moved to the upper respiratory tract. Respirations are normally accomplished by the diaphragmatic and abdominal muscles with little thoracic movement. The respiratory rate is 40 to 50 per minute, and the rhythm may be somewhat irregular or periodic during the first week of life. The apices of the lungs expand first, with the periphery and inferior portions expanding last, requiring 2 to 4 days for all areas to be filled with air.

DIGESTIVE SYSTEM   (See p. 10)

1. Anatomically, there are a relatively large intestinal or absorptive area and a plenitude of secreting glands to ensure good digestion. The intestinal muscles are weak and readily permit distention.
2. Rate of food passage: feedings move slowly through the upper gastrointestinal tract. Gastric emptying is largely completed in 2 to 4 hours, but some food occasionally remains in the stomach as long as 7 to 8 hours. Fat and large milk curds delay emptying time. The lower intestinal tract empties rapidly. The total time for passage through the entire tract is usually 14 to 18 hours. The position of the infant affects emptying time of the stomach, which is slower in the horizontal position and more rapid when the in-

fant is in the upright position or on his right side. Air enters the stomach immediately after birth; by 12 hours it fills the small intestines and by 24 hours, the large bowel.

3. Absorption of protein, carbohydrates, and simple sugars is good, but that of fats is somewhat decreased for several weeks after birth.

4. Ferments: hydrochloric acid is present in adequate amounts in the neonate, and all pancreatic and intestinal enzymes except for amylase (which appears after several weeks) are normally present. After the first few days, however, there is a decrease in hydrochloric acid secretion lasting several weeks. Salivary gland secretion is not appreciable until 2 or 3 months of age.

5. Meconium and transitional stools: meconium passage may occur in the first hour but usually occurs by the tenth hour of life. (If it does not occur by 24 hours, obstruction should be suspected.) It consists primarily of a mucopolysaccharide and also of desquamated and swallowed cells, lanugo, vernix, calcium soaps, and bile pigments; it is greenish black in color and disappears by the fourth day. Transitional stools may be seen from the fourth day on into the second week; they are slightly loose and slimy, varying in color from green to yellow.

6. Liver function is immature, with inadequate development of the enzyme systems, e.g., glucuronyl transferase, involved in the conversion of the indirect bilirubin to bilirubin glucuronide (direct bilirubin), the excretable form.

URINARY SYSTEM (See p. 10)

1. Urinary output on the first day is about 15 ml. Urine is produced beginning at 4 months' gestation. Occasionally there is no urination for the first 24 hours (urination may occur and be unobserved at delivery). If after 2 days the newborn infant still has not voided, a complete investigation is indicated. The output increases to 100 to 300 ml by the tenth day.

2. The excretion of uric acid from cellular breakdown is high. The diaper may be stained pink from the urates, and there may be uric acid infarcts in the kidney.

3. Renal function—see Chapter 7, "Fluid and Electrolyte Balance."

GENITAL SYSTEM

Male Erectile tissue is present. The foreskin usually adheres to the glans but does not require treatment, as long as there is no interference with urination. The testes may not be palpable at certain times, but this does not necessarily indicate cryptorchism. If the infant cries or is cold, the testes are frequently drawn back into the inguinal canal. A hydrocele is sometimes present but usually disappears spontaneously in 1 to 4 months.

Female   (See p. 11)

NERVOUS SYSTEM   (See p. 5)

The cerebral cortex participates very little in the function of the central nervous system during the neonatal period. An anencephalic infant with a brainstem and basal ganglions may respond with all the reflex activities of a normal newborn infant. The acquisition of myelin (which progresses in a cephalocaudal direction) and the maturation of neurons at different stages of development in the spinal cord, brainstem, and cerebral hemispheres can be correlated with the emergence and differentiation of various changing neural activities as evidenced by the normal evolution of reflexes and normal patterns of mental and motor development. A thorough knowledge of normal patterns of development is necessary for early detection of neurologic and mental disorders.

Normal reflexes

1. Moro reflex: the most effective way to elicit it is by dropping the head, with the examiner's hand supporting the body behind the shoulders. The patient's back is extended, the arms are extended and abducted, and the hands and fingers held wide open. The arms are then moved as in an embrace. Movements of the legs and hips are inconsistently present. This reflex usually disappears by 3 or 4 months of age.
2. Tonic neck reflex: in the resting state the infant's posture is maintained by flexor tonicity of the arms and legs. Lateral rotation of the head to one side abolishes flexor tone on that side, causing extension of the arm and leg. This reflex is incomplete in the normal newborn infant. Easy elicitation of the full response or its persistence in the late months of infancy is indicative of a motor disorder.
3. Grasp reflexes: when the palm is stimulated by one's finger, the infant grasps and holds it; when the sole of the foot is stimulated from the heel forward, the toes turn downward. This reflex disappears after 3 to 4 months of age.
4. The deep tendon reflexes are present but tire easily.
5. The abdominal reflexes are present.
6. Babinski reflex is present; unsustained ankle clonus (5 to 6 beats) may normally be present until 2 to 4 months of age; this reflex disappears at 10 to 16 months.
7. Chvostek's sign is positive in 50 percent of newborn infants during the first week.
8. The pupils react to light with contraction, but there may be a secondary dilation.
9. Swimming and walking reflexes are present during the first weeks.

10. Rooting, sucking, and swallowing reflexes are important to feeding. (Rooting reflex—when the infant smells milk, he turns his head to find the source, and when the cheek is touched by a smooth object, the mouth turns toward the object and the lips open as if to grasp a nipple.)
11. Stepping response: when the infant is held in an upright position and lowered until the feet touch the table, stepping movements are made.
12. Traction response: the examiner grasps the hands and forearms and pulls the infant gently forward to a sitting position. A normal response shows neck flexion, head control, and shoulder muscle assistance.
13. Placing response: the infant is held in an erect position. Drawing the dorsum of the infant's foot across the lower edge of the table will cause him to flex the knee and hip, followed by extension of the hip.

ENDOCRINE SYSTEM

Pituitary tropic hormones do not pass the placental barrier; thyroid hormone does pass it. The pituitary and thyroid glands are well developed and functioning prior to birth (protein-bound iodine values above 8 micrograms are common at birth). Although cretins do not often show signs of clinical hypothyroidism at birth, retarded bone age and central nervous system damage are already present during the newborn period.

The parathyroid glands probably function normally at birth, although transient depressed parathyroid activity may occur and may be responsible for the high phosphorus and low calcium values observed during the first week of life (see Tetany of the Newborn in Chapter 12).

Fetal adrenal glands are formed by two layers, a large reticular zone (inner layer) and a thin cortical zone (outer layer). These glands do not secrete 17-hydroxycorticosteroids, but adrenal corticosteroids cross the placenta to the fetus in a relatively fixed ratio to the maternal concentration. The reticular zone secretes 19-carbon steroids (androgens). The adrenal glands are proportionately larger in newborn infants than in older children (the weight of both glands is 8 Gm at birth and 5 Gm at 2 weeks of age). Involution of the fetal zone starts immediately after birth, while the cortical layer increases in size. Within the first week of life the infant's adrenal glands begin to form adrenal corticosteroids; thereafter this function is maintained at adult levels.

Plasma levels of 17-ketosteroids obtained from the umbilical cord blood are always considerably above those of the mother. During the first 10 to 14 days of life the urinary output of 17-ketosteroids is 1.2 to 2.5 mg per day, falling to 0.5 mg by the third or fourth week. The newborn infants of mothers who have been given large doses of adrenal corticosteroids during pregnancy may develop adrenal insufficiency.

Maternal estrogens and progesterone pass the placental barrier. The blood levels of estrogen, progesterone, and prolactin in newborn infants are relatively high but fall to zero in a few days. The excretion of pregnanediol (end product of progesterone metabolism) in the urine of the newborn infant gradually decreases during the first week.

Engorgement of the infant's breasts, due to maternal (placental and ovarian) estrogen stimulation, may occur a few days after birth in either sex. The maternal hormone prolactin, from the anterior pituitary, may produce oozing of milk ("witch's milk"). These signs subside spontaneously, and no treatment is indicated.

The islet cells of the pancreas are relatively large, particularly in infants born to diabetic mothers.

There is, rarely, in the offspring of mothers with poorly controlled diabetes, a temporary hyperinsulinism, which could produce hypoglycemia. However, the degree of hypoglycemia appears to have no direct relationship to the severity of the symptoms manifested by the infant (see p. 663).

IMMEDIATE CARE OF THE NEWBORN

The immediate care of the newborn infant after delivery is of great importance. Precautions to prevent infection should be observed during transportation to the nursery and in handling the infant. Gentle handling should be the rule; occasionally excessive zeal or haste may result in unnecessary trauma. The following measures are recommended:

I. Establishment of respiration
    A. The majority of normal infants breathe within a few seconds after delivery. The infant should be kept in a head-down position, and the mucus should be cleaned from the nasopharynx with a soft catheter, preferably before the first breath, to prevent aspiration.
    B. Flicking the heels lightly or gently passing a nasal catheter will frequently initiate a deep breath, followed by a crying episode.
    C. If spontaneous breathing is delayed beyond 1½ minutes, a plastic pharyngeal airway should be inserted and oxygen supplied.
    D. If resuscitation is necessary, the pressure under which the oxygen is delivered must be carefully controlled up to 20 cm H_2O either steadily or in puffs for intervals of 1 to 2 seconds. With some apparatus, e.g., the Krieselman machine, the oxygen is delivered into the posterior pharynx, and the flow is hand-regulated. When the newborn infant takes a

breath, the pressure can be stopped if desired. (Resuscitation is discussed in Chapter 12, "Diseases of the Newborn.")

II. Detection of life-threatening disease
   A. Observation of the rate and rhythm of respiration, palpation of the apex beat, and auscultation of the heart and lungs will provide sufficient information for immediate needs.
   B. Inspection and palpation of the head and back is usually sufficient to rule out gross anomalies of the central nervous system, e.g., meningoencephalocele, anencephaly, of immediate significance.
   C. The skin should be inspected for jaundice or undue cyanosis, which are early signs of danger.
   D. Examination of the upper respiratory tract (choanal atresia), upper gastrointestinal tract (esophageal atresia—usually associated with tracheal fistula), and lower gastrointestinal tract (imperforate anus) can be accomplished by passing a soft catheter.

III. Warmth: a heated crib and warm receiving blanket should be in the delivery room. The infant should immediately be covered and placed in this crib on his side. The foot end of the crib may be elevated 4 to 5 in. to promote drainage of the respiratory tract.

VI. Eye care: as a precaution against gonococcal infection, a few minims of fresh silver nitrate 1% are instilled. (Antibiotics, e.g., penicillin, have also been used.) The silver nitrate should then be washed out with sterile water.

V. Umbilical cord care
   A. Initial care in the delivery room
      1. The cord should be ligated securely.
      2. A cross section of the cord should be closely observed and the number of arteries present recorded. Infants with only one artery show an increased incidence of congenital anomalies, have an increased incidence of low birth weight and an increased mortality rate.
   B. Care in the nursery: infection should be guarded against by cleansing with alcohol and application of neosporin ointment. Triple dye (brilliant green 2.29 Gm, proflorine hemisulfate 1.14 Gm, crystal violet 2.29 Gm, and water 100 ml) applied to the cord and 1 in. of the surrounding tissue daily until the cord separates may be of value. No dressing is necessary.

THE NURSERY

Aseptic technique to prevent infection is most important. Nursery linen should be sterilized by autoclave. Incubators and bassinets should be cleansed scrupulously, and antiseptic solutions should be used for washing. Gas sterilization of a cleaned bassinet is an effective method of care. No dry dusting or cleaning should be allowed in a unit. Temperature of the nursery should be 80 to 85°F with a relative humidity of less than 50 percent. Good nursing care, adequately supervised, is of utmost importance. Careful handwashing before and after handling each infant should be emphasized. Detergents containing hexachlorophene are now suggested for this purpose.

SKIN CARE

Daily baths with soap and water are helpful in preventing infection. (Routine use of total body washing with 3% hexachlorophene is not advised because of possible neurotoxicity. Nevertheless, local application or even total-body use followed by thorough rinsing is indicated as a control measure if there is evidence of staphylococcal infection in a nursery.) When the umbilicus is healed (usually by 2 weeks), tub baths may be given.

TONGUE–TIE

Tongue-tie is caused by a short lingual frenulum. Usually no treatment is required.

FEEDING

1. No feeding is given for the first 4 to 12 hours, then prelacteal feeding—lactose or glucose 5 percent in water every 3 to 4 hours for three feedings. Smaller infants are usually fed every 3 hours.
2. Breast-fed infants, during the second day, are given alternate breasts at 4-hour intervals for 3 to 5 minutes. As the milk supply increases, the duration of the feeding is gradually extended to 20 minutes. Prelacteal feedings may be given between breast feedings to satisfy fluid requirements.
3. Artificially fed infants, presterilized commercially prepared formula available in dilutions of 20 cal per oz is recommended. (These are supplied also with iron.) A formula of evaporated milk, 1 part, and water, 2 parts, with added carbohydrate may also be used, e.g., evaporated milk, 7 oz; water, 14 oz; carbohydrate, 1 oz. Water or glucose 5% in water may be offered between feedings if the infant is awake and crying or restless. The total daily fluid requirement during the first 10 days of life increases gradually from 1 to 2 oz per lb (60 to 120 ml per kg). Thereafter the total daily fluid requirements are 2½ oz per lb (150 ml per kg) through early infancy.

VITAMINS

1. Vitamin K_1 (0.5 to 1.0 mg) given intramuscularly may be used prophylactically at birth to prevent decrease of prothrombin level.
2. Vitamins A, C, and D are routinely begun in the second week (see Chapter 2, "Feeding of Infants, Children, and Adolescents").

ROOMING–IN PLAN

The newborn infant has a crib in the mother's room full time or part of the time. The advantages are said to be improved psychologic integration of father, mother, and child; education of the mother and father in the care of the child; and reduction of cross infection among newborn infants. Mothers must be psychologically and physically able to carry out this program. There is no saving in nursing time with this program if proper education must be supplied.

MULTIPLE BIRTHS

Monozygotic twins occur with the same frequency all over the world—about 3 per 1,000 births. Dizygotic twinning is familial and occurs most commonly among blacks. Twinning is associated with a number of specific problems. In the mother there is a higher incidence of toxemia. Abnormalities of the placenta include a higher incidence of velamentous insertion of the cord and the development of a single amnion (associated with high morbidity and mortality rates). Low birth weight of the infant is common, and fetus-to-fetus transfusion occurs.

REVIEW QUESTIONS

1. The blood volume of a newborn infant, in milliliters per kilogram, is (a) 40; (b) 65; (c) 85; (d) 110; (e) 150.
2. The following statements concerning the newborn infant are true except for one: (a) the newborn produces heat via basal metabolism; (b) the infant has scant subcutaneous fat stores; (c) the infant has a large surface area relative to body size; (d) an increase of a few degrees in environmental temperature can double the infant's need for oxygen.
3. The neonate's IgG level is (a) low at birth and increases until the fourth month of life; (b) normal at birth and decreases until the fourth month of life; (c) there is no change in the newborn infant's IgG level after birth; (d) none of the above is true.
4. IgM is produced normally beginning at (a) 1 month; (b) 3 months; (c) 6 months; (d) 9 months.
5. IgA may be present in the neonate because (a) it crosses the placenta; (b) intrauterine infection occurred; (c) the fetus normally produces it; (d) it is present in witch's milk.
6. All the following affect the onset of extrauterine respiration except for one: (a) environmental temperature changes; (b) chemical stimuli; (c) analgesics given to the mother; (d) IgG level.
7. At birth all pancreatic and gastrointestinal secretions are present in appreciable amounts except: (a) amylase; (b) trypsin; (c) lipase; (d) hydrochloric acid.
8. After birth, air reaches the large intestine: (a) within a few minutes; (b) in 1 to 2 hours; (c) in 6 to 12 hours; (d) in 24 hours; (e) after the first meconium is passed.

9. Urine production begins at (a) 2 months' gestation; (b) 4 months' gestation; (c) 6 months' gestation; (d) birth; (e) the time of adequate fluid intake.

10. A pink-stained diaper in a 48-hour-old male infant probably indicates (a) phenylpyruvic oligophrenia; (b) cystitis; (c) congenital nephritis; (d) urate excretion; (e) hemophilia.

11. Experience with umbilical cords showing only one artery is that the following facts will apply except for one: (a) an increased incidence of congenital anomalies; (b) an increased incidence of low birth weight; (c) an increased incidence of cyanosis; (d) an increased mortality rate.

12. A newborn infant, age 5 minutes, with the following findings—O₂ saturation of 30 percent, Apgar score of 8, respiratory rate of 40 with irregularity, blood sugar level 35 mg per 100 ml—is (a) normal; (b) probably born from a diabetic mother; (c) in respiratory distress; (d) probably low birth weight.

12 DISEASES OF THE NEWBORN

CONGENITAL ANOMALIES

Congenital anomalies are a frequent cause of spontaneous abortion and of death in the neonatal period (see Chapter 10). (With prematurity and birth trauma they constitute the three most common causes of death in the perinatal period.) These malformations can occur in any part of the body and often may interfere with normal function and social acceptance. Severe malformations are said to be apparent in about 3.5 percent of live-born infants; often they are manifested later on: at 5 years of age they are found in about 7.5 percent of children. Minor anomalies occur in about 15 percent of live-born infants.

Etiology

1. Hereditary (*consanguinity:* increased expression of recessive traits, and *sex:* increased incidence of sex-linked recessive traits).

     a.   Gross chromosomal abnormalities: trisomy syndromes.

     b.   Genetic defects: color blindness, sickle-cell disease.

2.   Infections during pregnancy: rubella, toxoplasmosis.

3.   Maternal exposure to large doses of radiation: microcephaly.

4.   Mechanical factors: metatarsus varus or valgus due to fetal position.

5.   Drugs and chemicals: thalidomide (see p. 189).

6.   Nutrition: It is difficult to evaluate whether faulty maternal intake, for instance, hypovitaminosis, hypervitaminosis, or alcoholism, is sufficient to cause an anomaly or whether more direct interference with the developing ovum, for example, advanced age of the mother, is necessary.

7.   Maternal age: Increased maternal age is associated with increased incidence of anomalies, e.g., Down's syndrome.

    Congenital anomalies are frequently multiple. This fact should be considered in making a differential diagnosis. For example, if there is doubt as to whether a child has congenital heart disease, the presence of additional malformations would be suggestive.

    Furthermore, it may be difficult to identify the etiologic agent responsible when anomalies occur, especially if they are single. For example, a congenital cataract may be hereditary or it may be due to rubella infection during the first trimester of pregnancy. When combinations of anomalies are present, as in the rubella syndrome, the etiology is clearer.

    In counseling a couple concerning prospective parenthood or parents of a child with genetically influenced disease, the discussion should include the statistical risk as far as simple Mendelian ratios are concerned; the severity of the disease; the availability of therapy (for example, insulin or oral antidiabetic drugs for diabetes, a galactose-free diet for galactosemia), how anxious the parents are to have children, and whether there are other alternatives, e.g., adoption. In some instances karyotyping the parents may be of value in properly evaluating the risk of producing defective babies. For example, one type (translocation) of Down's syndrome is transmissible. Although it is time-consuming and complex, obtaining medical histories of relatives may provide valuable clues. Ultimately the decision must be made by the parents (see Chapter 8).

    Strenuous efforts should be directed toward the prevention of congenital anomalies. If these fail, early correction of the malformations should be attempted whenever possible.

MENINGOENCEPHALOCELE, OR CRANIUM BIFIDUM

Cranium bifidum is a congenital defect in the skull with protrusion of the meninges alone (meningocele) or of the meninges and brain tissue (meningoencephalocele). The defect usually occurs in the midline most often in the occipital area but rarely in the nasal, nasopharyngeal, or frontal area. There is a fluctuant, pulsating swelling. Pressure on this mass usually makes the infant cry by increasing the intracranial pressure. The mass can be transilluminated more or less, depending on the amount of brain tissue it contains. Convulsions, mental retardation, and hydrocephalus are commonly associated findings. A roentgenogram reveals the defect. Surgery may be successful if there is only a meningocele but does not offer too much hope if a meningoencephalocele is present.

SPINA BIFIDA

Spina bifida is a congenital anomaly in which there is a defective closure of the spinal column. It occurs most often in Caucasians, less frequently in blacks, and least in the Japanese. (The most severe type is a rachischisis in which the neural tube is open and exposed for a number of segments. Paralysis of the lower extremities is always present. Surgical correction of this type is very difficult.) The defect may be anterior, or more commonly, posterior. In either case there may be an associated defect of the central nervous system, e.g., meningocele (involvement of meninges), meningomyelocele (involvement of meninges and spinal cord). In meningomyelocele, neurologic involvement is common, with paralysis of the lower extremities and loss of bowel and bladder sphincter control.

Arnold-Chiari malformation   Arnold-Chiari malformation is a herniation of the cerebellar tonsils and medulla into the upper cervical region due to either a congenital anomaly or postinfectious fibrosis in the region of the foramen magnum. Treatment is surgical removal of the posterior portion of the foramen magnum and the arches of the first four cervical vertebrae to relieve the compression of the inferior lobes of the cerebellum and of the medulla.

Spina bifida occulta   Spina bifida occulta includes all lesions in which fusion defects of the vertebral column are present without protrusion of intraspinal contents to the surface. The defect commonly involves the 5th lumbar and 1st sacral vertebra and is usually of no clinical significance. The overlying skin may reveal a dimple, a tuft of hair, or a small, fatty tissue mass. It is discovered most often when x-rays are obtained for other reasons.

Diastematomyelia   This is an unusual form of spinal bifida occulta in which a midline bony spicule divides the spinal column into two compartments. By transfixing the spinal cord, it may disturb normal growth of the spinal cord and the function of the lower extremities and sphincters. Roentgenograms are diagnostic. Treatment is surgical removal.

CONGENITAL OBSTRUCTION OF THE NASOLACRIMAL DUCT (Dacryostenosis)

Normally, the nasolacrimal duct becomes patent by 3 months of age. Congenital obstruction is a comparatively frequent condition, which is more often unilateral than bilateral. There is tearing from the involved eye or eyes, which is made worse by the cold or wind. It may be complicated by a secondary infection of the tear sac (dacryocystitis), with swelling and redness at the inner corner of the lower lid; pressure on the tear sac will expel pus. There is commonly an associated purulent conjunctivitis.

Medical treatment will usually give good results if started early.

1. Gentle massage is given twice daily over the duct from the eye toward the nose so that drainage may be reestablished.
2. If there is infection (dacryocystitis), local antibiotics, e.g., neosporin ophthalmic drops should be used 5 to 6 times a day.

Surgical treatment (probing of the nasolacrimal duct) is indicated in those cases that do not improve spontaneously during the first 6 to 8 months.

THYROGLOSSAL–DUCT CYST

Thyroglossal-duct cyst may occur anywhere in the course of the descent of the thyroid gland from the foramen cecum at the base of the tongue to the definitive thyroid area. It is usually manifested by a painless cystic movable swelling in the midline of the neck. Rarely it may be located laterally and simulate a branchial-cleft cyst. The cyst may become infected during the course of any upper respiratory infection and rupture, with the formation of a sinus. Treatment is complete surgical removal of both the cyst and the thyroglossal duct.

BRANCHIAL–CLEFT CYST

Branchial-cleft cyst may occur in the remnant of a branchial cleft. It is painless, freely movable, and usually located on the lateral aspect of the neck anterior to the sternocleidomastoid muscle at the middle lower third. It may become secondarily infected. Treatment consists of complete surgical excision when the infection has subsided.

INCLUSION AND RETENTION CYSTS OF THE MOUTH

Epithelial pearls (Epstein's pearls) occur along the median raphe of the palate or near the junction of the hard and soft palates. They are pinhead-sized white bodies which are formed by epithelial inclusions and may occur singly or in groups. They disappear spontaneously in a few weeks.

Inclusion cysts are gray lesions occurring at the gingival margins. They disappear spontaneously in several weeks.

Ranula is a retention cyst of the sublingual salivary glands. They usually disappear spontaneously and rarely require surgery.

CLEFT PALATE AND CLEFT LIP

Congenital cleft palate and cleft lip occur in about 1 of 1,000 deliveries and may be associated with other malformations, e.g., D and E tri-somies. Because it is socially unacceptable, the cleft lip is usually repaired as soon as possible after the baby has reached a weight of at least 4.5 kg (10 lb), if he is in good health, is gaining weight steadily, and is 5 or 6 weeks of age. The cleft palate is corrected when the involved structures are sufficiently developed to permit adequate repair, but not too long after speech develops. Usually this is when the patient weighs at least 9.1 kg (20 lb), is in satisfactory condition, and is approximately 14 months of age. The immediate problems in the infant with a cleft palate are the maintenance of nutrition and pre-vention of infection. Middle-ear and sinus infections are common com-plications. (Hearing should be evaluated because a deficiency is often present.) A large nipple with large holes will usually suffice for feed-ing, although special cleft-palate nipples are available.

A cleft palate may occasionally be associated with a small mandible (micrognathia), in which case the tongue falls backward (glossopto-sis), and difficulty in breathing develops (Pierre Robin syndrome). With micrognathia, the mandibular growth is usually sufficient so that respiratory difficulty is not a problem after the infant reaches 6 to 8 months of age. If respiratory distress is marked early, tube feeding may be useful. If that is not tolerated, gastrostomy may be necessary. Cooperative management by various specialties, including pediatrics, surgery, and otolaryngology, should occur. The tongue can also be sutured forward for short periods of time in some cases. Feeding should be done carefully while the infant is in a prone position.

CONGENITAL HEART DISEASE

See Chapter 16, "Heart Diseases."

CONGENITAL DIAPHRAGMATIC HERNIA

This condition, which may cause cyanosis, is discussed in Chapter 18, "Surgical Conditions of the Abdomen."

CONGENITAL DEFICIENCY OF THE ABDOMINAL MUSCLES ("Prune Belly")

Partial or complete absence of abdominal muscles occurs most com-monly in males in association with obstructive manifestations of the genitourinary tract (enlarged bladder or hydronephrosis), undescended testes, and anomalies of the gastrointestinal tract (malrotation) and legs. Treatment is correction of the genitourinary and gastrointestinal anomalies if possible and abdominal support or plastic repair of abdominal musculature. Prognosis depends on associated anomalies, e.g., hydronephrosis.

CONGENITAL ANOMALIES OF THE UMBILICUS

Anatomically there are three types of navel—normal, amniotic, and skin. The type is determined by the way in which the umbilical cord joins the abdominal skin. In the normal type, the umbilical cord and skin meet at the level of the abdomen, and a concave umbilical scar results. In the amniotic type, the amniotic membrane covers the skin, which does not extend to the base of the cord, resulting in a flat navel. In the skin type, the skin forms a sleeve for the base of the cord, resulting in a protruding skin stump which may require differentiation from umbilical hernia. In the skin navel there is no defect in the abdominal wall and the navel does not change in size with increased intraabdominal pressure.

Granuloma   The umbilicus usually heals within 2 weeks. Mild saprophytic infections may cause a slight discharge and moist granulating tissue at the base as the cord heals. A number of different treatments have been successful, such as frequent application of damp alcohol sponges or the use of bacitracin ointment. Granulations that become exuberant at the base are common. Silver nitrate stick for cauterization is efficacious; its use is repeated when necessary.

Granuloma must be differentiated from a very rare anomaly, umbilical polyp. This is the distal remnant of the omphalomesenteric duct, pinkish red in appearance; it does not respond to cauterization. When an umbilical polyp is palpated, mucus will stick to the finger; the granuloma will feel moist, but nothing remains on the examining finger. Once the diagnosis of umbilical polyp is made, surgery is indicated.

Umbilical hernia   An umbilical hernia forms because of imperfect closure of the umbilical ring. It is most frequent in Negro children, premature infants, and children with hypothyroidism. The hernia protrudes when the infant cries but can be reduced through the fibrous ring. The hernia may include omentum or intestine. Incarceration is rare. Usually no treatment is necessary, and surgery is rarely indicated since almost all defects close spontaneously.

Urachus   Discharge of urine at the umbilicus is due to failure of closure of the allantoic duct, resulting in a patent urachus. Lipiodol or Diodrast may be injected into the tract and visualized on roentgenograms, or methylene blue, given orally or parenterally, may be recovered from the umbilical wound. There is also the cystic form of urachus, with a midline mass in the abdominal wall, which is noted when it becomes infected. Surgery is necessary.

Umbilical fistula   An umbilical sinus that discharges mucus or fluid is suspected of being a Meckel's diverticulum communicating with the navel. Exploration with a probe and Lipiodol or Diodrast may reveal the communication. If fecal material exudes, and there is no history of previous operations or disease that would produce the fistula, the diagnosis is clear.

Omphalocele   Omphalocele is an umbilical eventration of abdominal viscera, which may be a massive defect of the abdominal wall or only a cystic swelling of the umbilical cord. The omphalocele is covered by peritoneal membrane and amnion. It must be operated on immediately. The prognosis, even in large defects, is fair.

Single umbilical artery   The presence of only one umbilical artery is associated with an increased incidence of fetal loss, low birth weight, and congenital anomalies, e.g., gastrointestinal and genitourinary defects. It is encountered in about 1 percent of single births and 7 percent of twin births. The etiology of this condition is unknown.

CONGENITAL OBSTRUCTIONS OF THE GASTRO-INTESTINAL TRACT (See Chapter 18)

Early recognition depends on being alert to any history of obstetric complication, especially breech presentation or polyhydramnios; signs of respiratory distress; production of excessive frothy mucus in the mouth; difficulty in swallowing at the time of the first feeding; emesis of bile-stained fluid; abdominal distension; or failure to pass meconium within the first 24 hours.

Esophageal atresia   The commonest form (85 percent of cases) of esophageal atresia is that in which the upper portion of the esophagus ends blindly near the bifurcation of the trachea and the lower segment forms a fistulous tract between the stomach and trachea at or near the bifurcation, permitting air to enter the stomach. In the second type, both segments are blind; in the third type, the upper segment communicates with the trachea and the lower pouch is blind; in the fourth type, both upper and lower segments communicate with the trachea. (Isolated tracheoesophageal fistula can occur also.)

Clinical features

1. At delivery the nasopharynx of the infant will require a great deal of suctioning, and in the nursery it will be noted that there is an excessive amount of frothy mucus in the mouth and pharynx.
2. A catheter cannot be passed into the stomach.
3. At the first feeding, the child will swallow a few mouthfuls and then overflow, choking and becoming cyanotic and dyspneic.
4. Rales may be heard as evidence of an aspiration pneumonia.
5. Roentgenograms, with a dilute solution of barium for contrast, reveal the obstruction. (Barium should be suctioned out after the

x-ray procedure.) Failure of air to enter the stomach indicates that the lower segment does not communicate with either the upper segment or the trachea.

Treatment   Direct anastomosis, if possible, is the surgical procedure of choice. The prognosis is improved with early diagnosis. Feeding should be withheld if this diagnosis is suspected. Proper preparation, head elevated 45° to prevent aspiration of regurgitated gastric juice, continuous suction proximal to the obstruction, administration of oxygen, antibiotics, and fluids and electrolytes are important.

Other congenital obstructions of the gastrointestinal tract, e.g., diaphragmatic hernia, pyloric stenosis, duodenal atresia, malrotation of the intestine, meconium ileus, congenital megacolon, and anorectal obstructions, are discussed in Chapter 16, "Surgical Conditions of the Abdomen."

CONGENITAL LESIONS OF THE GENITOURINARY TRACT (See Chapter 19)

CONGENITAL LESIONS OF THE EXTREMITIES (See Chapter 21)

NEONATAL HYPOXIA (Apnea Neonatorum, Asphyxia of the Newborn)

Fetal and neonatal hypoxia may occur before, during, or shortly after birth (see Chapter 10). Clinical signs and symptoms will depend to a degree on which system is involved, i.e., the central nervous system or the peripheral chest structures. Respiratory movements are abnormal, e.g., labored, shallow, or irregular, and there is cyanosis. Important guides in assessing the condition of the infant are time of onset of respiration after delivery and heart rate. Severe asphyxia is suggested by bradycardia (fewer than 100 beats per minute), pallor or grayness of the skin (suggesting asphyxia plus shock), flaccidity, and absence of response to sensory stimuli.

Etiologic factors

1. Central origin: respiratory center dysfunction—from conditions causing hypoxia, e.g., preexisting maternal conditions (see p. 181); compression or prolapse of the umbilical cord; cerebral edema or hemorrhage from precipitous delivery, prolonged labor, difficult forceps delivery, or even with normal spontaneous delivery; and congenital malformations of the brain.
2. Peripheral chest structures: inadequate oxygenation of the blood by the lungs caused by conditions such as immaturity of the lungs, aspiration of mucus or amniotic fluid, diaphragmatic hernia, laryn-

geal obstruction, hyaline membrane with resorption atelectasis, congenital heart disease, and tracheoesophageal fistula.

Predisposing factors

1. Prematurity and low birth weight.
2. Maternal toxemia, bleeding, or overdosage with analgesics or anesthesia.
3. Cesarean section—usually because of the pathologic condition necessitating the section.
4. Infants of diabetic mothers may be apneic; they are often large and have electrolyte disturbances. (The gastric contents in infants born by cesarean section or of diabetic mothers may be increased; immediately after delivery, aspiration may be of value and does rule out esophageal atresia.)

The Apgar score for the evaluation of the newborn infant's condition is used most frequently as a guide by obstetricians and pediatricians. A newborn infant is scored in the manner shown in Table 12-1, 1 minute and 5 minutes after complete birth of the baby and subsequently, if so indicated. The score at 1 minute correlates well as a prognosticator of neonatal survival. The score at 5 minutes is a better predictor of subsequent neurologic damage.

A score of 10 would indicate that the infant is in excellent condition, while a score of 0, 1, or 2 persisting for 2 or 3 minutes would indicate a depressed condition and a guarded prognosis.

Another method of scoring, that of Silverman and Andersen, is of particular value for premature infants and is used in the nursery to which the baby has been transferred for further observation (see Table 12-2). It is based on respiratory effort and the presence or absence of retractions. Five types of retraction are noted, each having

Table 12-1. Apgar score

Sign	0	1	2
Heart rate	Absent	Slow (below 100)	Over 100
Respiratory effort	Absent	Slow, irregular	Good, crying
Reflex irritability (response to catheter in nostril tested after oropharynx is cleared)	No response	Grimaces	Cough or sneeze
Muscle tone	Limp	Some flexion of extremities	Active motion
Color	Blue, pale	Body pink, extremities blue	Completely pink

Table 12-2. Silverman-Andersen score

	Observation of retractions			Nares dilatation	Expiratory grunt
Grade	Upper chest	Lower chest	Xiphoid		
0	Rises synchronously with abdomen	No intercostal sinking on inspiration	None	None (no movement of chin)	None heard
1	Lag or minimal sinking as abdomen rises	Just visible sinking of intercostal spaces on inspiration	Just visible	Minimal (chin descends, lips closed)	Heard with stethoscope only
2	"Seesaw" sinking with rising abdomen	Marked sinking of intercostal spaces on inspiration	Marked	Marked (chin descends, lips part)	Heard with naked ear

a scale rating of two points. (The Silverman-Andersen score is in reverse of that used by Apgar.) An infant showing all five types of retraction is rated 10 and is therefore in poor condition with a bad prognosis; an infant with a score of 0 has no respiratory-tract retractions and is in excellent condition.

Prevention   Requires obstetric and pediatric cooperation and care in respect to the causative factors mentioned above.

Treatment   Resuscitation requires provision of a clear airway, warmth, and oxygen. The following steps may be taken in succession until respirations are established:

1. On delivery, the baby should be held in a head-down position while the nasopharynx is cleared, preferably before the first breath. The upper airways are cleared of mucus and detritus by aspiration with a soft plastic catheter. The newborn infant is then loosely wrapped in a warm blanket and placed in a supine position in a heated crib or incubator. If no damage to the central nervous system is suspected or clinically evident, the foot end of the incubator may be elevated 4 to 5 in. to promote drainage of mucus from the respiratory airways. However, the foot end of the crib should not be raised when intracranial damage is suspected, since this may increase intracranial pressure.
2. Stimulation in the form of gentle flicking of the heels may be applied.

3. A small plastic pharyngeal airway is inserted, and oxygen is supplied at a concentration sufficient to prevent cyanosis via a mask at 16 cm water pressure for 1- to 2-second intervals.

4. In the flaccid infant, it may be necessary to clear the airway under direct vision by laryngoscopic suction. This should be done only by a person trained in the procedure. With the laryngoscope still in place, pure oxygen under positive pressure may be given directly through a soft catheter or an endotracheal cannula inserted in the larynx. Administration of oxygen via this route should be intermittent to stimulate the normal respiratory rate and should be continued until spontaneous respirations are established.

5. Rarely, heart sounds are not heard even after the lungs have expanded. Closed-chest cardiac massage should be instituted. Two fingers are placed to the left of the lower sternal border. Light pressure (sufficient to depress the chest about ½ in.) is applied rhythmically about 100 times per minute. Pulmonary ventilation is maintained by supplying positive-pressure oxygen after every three cardiac massage cycles.

6. The infant is transported to the nursery in an incubator or heated crib.

7. Drugs such as caffeine (a central nervous system stimulant) and epinephrine (a cardiac stimulant) are of questionable value. Other stimulants are of no value and may, in fact, be hazardous for the infant since their therapeutic and toxic doses are too close for safe use. Glucose 50%, 2 ml per kg, given intravenously has been used in infants requiring resuscitation and may be of some value. Nalline (*N*-allylmorphine) is of value to counteract narcosis from morphine derivatives given to the mother shortly before delivery (either 10 to 15 mg given intravenously to the mother 5 to 15 minutes prior to delivery or 0.2 mg in 2 ml saline solution injected into the umbilical-cord vein of the newborn infant).

CYANOSIS IN THE NEWBORN

Cyanosis in the newborn infant is most commonly due to direct involvement of the central nervous system, respiratory tract, cardiovascular system, or the blood.

INTRACRANIAL HEMORRHAGE

Etiology The causes of intracranial hemorrhage are birth trauma, hypoxia, and hemorrhagic disease of the newborn. Intracranial hemorrhage is more frequent in premature infants, infants born by cesarean section, infants with breech presentation, infants delivered by mechanical aids other than low forceps, and infants born to toxemic mothers.

Pathologic features   The bleeding may be subdural, which is almost always traumatic in origin and usually occurs in first-born, large babies; subarachnoid, which usually occurs in a premature infant following asphyxia; intraventricular, which usually happens in a spontaneously delivered, probably hypoxic low-birth-weight or premature infant; or intracerebral, which usually occurs in large babies with difficult delivery following both trauma and hypoxia. Severe cases may involve several or all of these areas.

Clinical features   The signs and symptoms may be present at birth or shortly after birth, or they may not appear for several days. Some or all of the following may be present:

1. Somnolence or restlessness.
2. Twitching or convulsions.
3. Tachypnea, dyspnea, irregular respiration, and pallor.
4. Poor feeding, failure to suck properly, forceful vomiting.
5. Shrill cry—the so-called "cerebral cry."
6. Bulging or tense fontanel, if the bleeding has been above the tentorium. There may be undue enlargement of the head.
7. Adder-like protrusion of the tongue—Foote's sign.
8. Eye changes: there may be retinal hemorrhage or edema, ocular palsies, nystagmus, irregular pupils, or absent pupillary reflexes.
9. Moro reflex may be absent; opisthotonos may be present.
10. Paralyses (spastic or flaccid) may appear after several days, the extent depending on the particular localization of the hemorrhage.
11. Bloody spinal fluid, only when the bleeding has occurred about the subarachnoid space; the fluid is often xanthochromic, but slight xanthochromia may be present in normal newborn infants for the first 10 days.

Treatment

1. Warmth.
2. Oxygen.
3. The head may be elevated slightly.
4. The infant should be handled as little as possible.
5. Oral feedings should not be given until the critical period is over, since aspiration may occur easily.
6. Vitamin K is of value only in those rare cases which are associated with vitamin K deficiency.
7. Drugs: e.g., phenobarbital, 4 mg per kg, intramuscularly, Valium (an effective drug but not yet approved for use in the neonate), up to 10 mg, intravenously (slowly), for the control of convulsions.
8. Spinal taps are used by some to relieve the excessive intracranial pressure when there are increasing cyanosis and irregular respirations. Others feel that this lowering of pressure may increase the bleeding and that spinal taps should not be used.

Prognosis The prognosis is guarded, especially when persistent cyanosis and respiratory difficulty are present. Recovery is frequently complete, but some infants have residual permanent cerebral damage, e.g., cerebral palsy or mental retardation.

Early, the clinical features of cerebral edema are indistinguishable from those of cerebral hemorrhage. Cerebral edema may proceed to hemorrhage but usually clears rather promptly with no residua.

Subdural hematoma

Etiology The cause is almost invariably traumatic, occurring in large babies, in primiparas, older mothers, breech deliveries, and difficult forceps deliveries.

Pathogenesis Most commonly falx cerebri or tentorium cerebelli tears result in rupture of small veins which are most commonly supratentorial. There is bleeding into the subdural space, with subsequent breakdown of the red blood cells, producing a relatively hypertonic solution. This draws spinal fluid through the arachnoid into the subdural space and causes progressive enlargement of the hematoma. [The basic mechanism in the formation of subdural fluid secondary to subdural hematoma or bacterial meningitis (see p. 322) may be an effusion through damaged capillary walls.]

Clinical features Subdural hemorrhage may be part of the picture of intracranial hemorrhage of the newborn described in the previous pages. When subdural hematoma is present alone, there may be no characteristic symptoms or signs for several months. Suspicion may be aroused after the third or fourth month by anorexia, poor weight gain, slow development, and vomiting. Later there will be signs of increased intracranial pressure, convulsions, and abnormally enlarging head with a widening of the biparietal diameter. Transillumination of this skull area normally shows only a narrow rim of light (0.5 to 1.5 cm); with subdural hematoma the rim extends 2 to 10 cm.

Laboratory findings Findings from subdural taps are diagnostic. The taps should always be bilateral; 0.5 ml or more of xanthochromic fluid with increased protein is obtained from one or both sides. (Normally only a few drops of clear fluid are obtained.)

Treatment Daily subdural taps removing 10 to 15 ml fluid may be sufficient. In bilateral cases, alternate sides should be tapped each day. If a diminishing amount of fluid occurs each day until no excess fluid is obtained and the patient is asymptomatic, no further treatment may be necessary. If the head size increases and symptoms persist, craniotomy and resection of the capsular membrane and its contents are necessary. The rare infratentorial hematoma requires surgery.

Prognosis   The prognosis is good, if the treatment is begun early and the subdural hematoma has not been associated with other intracranial hemorrhage.

ATELECTASIS

Congenital (primary) atelectasis is the absence of the normal expansion of the lung that occurs after birth. Secondary atelectasis is the result of obstruction after expansion has occurred.

Etiology   The same factors that cause neonatal hypoxia prevent expansion of the lungs. There may be respiratory-center dysfunction because of cerebral injury, obstruction of the bronchi by aspiration of amniotic fluid and mucus, weakness of the respiratory and accessory muscles as in prematurity, and abnormal external pressure.

Histologic features   Varying histologic pictures have been described. There may be areas of expanded lung intermingled with the atelectatic areas. Interalveolar congestion is prominent, and amniotic debris may be present in the bronchioles. Superimposed pneumonia and hemorrhage are not uncommon. Hyaline membrane with resorption atelectasis is discussed separately below.

Clinical features   The clinical features are the same as those described above for neonatal hypoxia and may vary from very mild to severe. The diagnosis of the areas that are involved depends on roentgenograms and on physical examination, which may reveal dullness and diminished breath sounds.

Treatment   The treatment is the same as for neonatal hypoxia, plus antibiotics to prevent secondary infection.

IDIOPATHIC RESPIRATORY DISTRESS SYNDROME (IRDS)

IRDS (hyaline membrane disease, idiopathic respiratory distress syndrome I and II, transient tachypnea of the newborn) is a broad term referring to a neonate with respiratory distress during the first few days of life. A distinction is made between the syndrome in premature infants and term newborn infants.

IRDS of prematurity (type I, hyaline membrane disease)

Etiology   Type I IRDS results from immaturity of the lungs with inability to produce surfactant which acts by decreasing the alveolar surface tension, thus permitting easier expansion of alveoli during normal respiration (see p. 196). This syndrome is seen also in babies born of diabetic mothers.

Clinical and laboratory features

1. Respiratory symptoms develop gradually, usually starting at 2 to 6 hours of age but may be present at birth.
2. There are tachypnea, grunting, flaring of alae nasi, retractions (subcostal followed by intercostal).
3. Lack of activity.
4. Cyanosis, at first peripheral, later generalized.
5. Diminished air exchange, CO_2 retention and inability to absorb O_2, and respiratory acidosis.
6. Hypotension due to hypovolemia and myocardial depression (associated with hypoxia).
7. Decreasing ability to be well oxygenated even in high oxygen environment.
8. Metabolic acidosis ensues (increased production of lactic acid).
9. X-ray early reveals depression of diaphragm and hyperaeration. Later, reticulogranular appearance of the lung fields occurs and an air bronchogram may be observed.

Hyaline membrane disease is a pathologic diagnosis in which the lungs show not only atelectasis and congestion but also a membrane which lines the dilated alveolar ducts and the terminal bronchioles in those portions of the lung which are not collapsed. The principal component of the membrane is fibrin, which derives from the fetal pulmonary tissue.

IRDS II (transient tachypnea of the newborn, neonatal disseminated atelectasis)

Etiology   The cause is unknown, although it has been speculated that there may be a partial deficiency of surfactant. The infants with this syndrome are usually full term.

Clinical and laboratory features

1. The clinical symptoms are similar to those discussed above; however, they are usually milder and the onset may be earlier. Also, treatment with oxygen is more effective.
2. X-rays may reveal increased bronchovascular markings extending from the hilum.

Treatment   Treatment is the same for both types but not as urgent in type II.

1. Infant is best treated in an intensive care nursery.
2. Incubator—oxygen for cyanosis, initially not to exceed 40 percent concentration. If arterial PO_2 is measured, O_2 concentrations may be increased accordingly. Humidity is best at 65 percent.
3. Intravenous fluids—dextrose, 10 percent in water, 65 to 80 ml per kg per 24 hours on the first day. On subsequent days dextrose

5 percent and ¼ normal saline is given increasing the total amount by 10 to 15 ml per kg per day. Electrolytes are added according to needs. Potassium and calcium may also be needed after 48 hours of age. Sodium bicarbonate is added to the fluids for treatment of the acidosis. The amount is calculated by formula given on page 136. A practical rule is to use 2 to 3 meq per kg by slow intravenous "push" infusion or 5 meq per 100 ml intravenous fluid in a continuous infusion.

4. Continued monitoring of blood gases is essential during the period of respiratory distress. The utilization of peripheral veins for intravenous fluid therapy presents problems when prolonged treatment is necessary. Therefore, umbilical artery or vein catheterization is suggested. If an umbilical artery catheter is in place, blood gas monitoring is easier. The umbilical artery catheter should be placed at the junction of the thoracic abdominal aorta or at the level of the diaphragm. A 20 percent complication rate has been reported, but the complications are usually minor, e.g., blanching of extremities. Thromboses, and in some rare cases, gangrene may occur. Umbilical vein catheterization has a lower rate of complications, about 8 percent. The catheter should be placed in the inferior vena cava just below the diaphragm. It should not be in the portal or hepatic veins since serious complications may occur. The hyperosmolar or hypertonic solutions may cause liver damage or produce portal vein thrombosis. An x-ray should always be taken after a catheter is passed to ensure proper placement. The catheter should be removed as soon as the clinical picture improves. It should not be kept in place for more than 7 days.

5. Antibiotics are given while the catheter is in place.

6. Oral feedings should be started when the respiratory distress is significantly improved, not before. Gavage feedings are better tolerated.

7. Ventilatory support with respirators may be necessary when the clinical symptoms increase in severity despite treatment and proper oxygenation cannot be maintained. Various respirators have been used. Recently the type allowing continuous positive pressure is recommended, initially with an endotracheal tube in place.

Prognosis   The prognosis varies. In type I, commonly seen in prematures, the mortality varies from 30 to 50 percent; in type II, the prognosis is usually good.

Oxygen toxicity affecting the eyes and bronchopulmonary system has been reported following treatment of some infants.

I.   Eye—retrolental fibroplasia (see page 248) may occur when PaO_2 levels are maintained over 100 mmHg.

II. Bronchopulmonary system

A.   The Wilson-Mikity syndrome is usually seen in infants of less than 36 weeks' gestation. These infants usually have a history of respiratory distress at birth necessitating oxygen but improving for a week or two before showing signs of recurrence. Some infants have been reported as having no problem initially, but showing signs of respiratory difficulty including cyanosis at a later date. The symptoms increase over a 2- to 6-week period and may persist for several months. On physical examination fine rales, sometimes wheezing, and a grating sandpaper quality of the breath sounds are heard. The x-ray, which is diagnostic, shows bilateral, coarse, streaky infiltrates early; later, small cystic lesions appear in both lungs. These cysts then enlarge and coalesce producing overexpanded hyperlucent lungs. Treatment is supportive.

B. Pulmonary hemorrhage may be seen with bleeding elsewhere or may occur with sepsis. It usually occurs in low-birth-weight babies. Emphysema, atelectasis, or both may be observed on x-ray. X-ray findings vary from massive consolidation to minimal streaky or patchy lesions. The prognosis is grave.

C. With bronchopulmonary dysplasia, interstitial pulmonary fibrosis develops which may be seen on x-ray. Chronic lung disease frequently occurs in these infants.

PNEUMONIA IN THE NEWBORN

Pneumonia is a common cause of death in stillborn and newborn infants, especially premature infants. It may be acquired in utero, either transplacentally or via the maternal genital tract. Pneumonia occurring in utero may result in a stillborn child or one which dies within 2 to 3 days. Postnatally it is frequently secondary to atelectasis or aspiration of vomitus or maternal fecal matter, particularly in premature or debilitated infants. Gram-negative organisms, e.g., *E. coli, Pseudomonas*; staphylococci; and the anaerobic group are the common invading bacteria. Viral pneumonia is now found more frequently in newborn infants. Pneumonia in the newborn infant is usually of the disseminated lobular type, with scanty physical findings. Roentgenograms are most helpful in making the diagnosis. Pneumonia is discussed in detail in Chapter 15, "Respiratory Diseases."

PNEUMOTHORAX

Pneumothorax and air block are discussed in Chapter 15.

OBSTRUCTION TO THE UPPER AIRWAYS

Obstruction to the upper airways, particularly the larynx, is also discussed in Chapter 15. In the newborn infant, it is usually due to any of the following:

1. Aspirated material
2. Congenital laryngeal stridor
3. Congenital anomalies such as a web over the larynx
4. Tumors of the larynx
5. Laryngospasm
6. Choanal atresia (diagnosis established by inability to pass a catheter through the nares)

ACUTE PULMONARY INTERSTITIAL AND MEDIASTINAL EMPHYSEMA (Air Block) AND PNEUMOTHORAX

This condition, which may cause cyanosis and dyspnea, is discussed in Chapter 15.

ADRENAL HEMORRHAGE

Adrenal hemorrhage may be due to trauma or hemorrhagic disease of the newborn infant and occurs more commonly in difficult deliveries. There may be cyanosis, pallor, or severe shock, progressing rapidly to death; the symptoms often resemble those of cerebral hemorrhage. Occasionally in adrenal hemorrhage, an abdominal mass is palpable. If the diagnosis is suspected, hydrocortisone or its analogs, intravenous fluids and electrolytes, and small blood transfusions may be tried. The prognosis is poor.

METHEMOGLOBINEMIA

Methemoglobinemia may be congenital (caused by the absence of coenzyme I within the red blood cell, resulting in failure to convert ferric ion to ferrous ion), or it may be acquired (due to sulfonamides, aniline dyes, and well water containing nitrates or chlorates). Cyanosis is persistent and diffuse, with lack of evidence of respiratory or cardiac distress and no improvement following oxygen administration. The blood is chocolate color, with no change upon oxygenation. Spectroscopy of blood is diagnostic. Treatment is intravenous administration of either methylene blue, 1 to 2 mg per kg, intravenously, or ascorbic acid, 50 mg, orally every 4 hours or 200 mg intramuscularly or intravenously.

JAUNDICE

PHYSIOLOGIC JAUNDICE, OR ICTERUS NEONATORUM

Etiology   In the first few days of life there are an increased destruction of red blood cells and a relatively decreased excretion of bile pigment by the immature liver. [There is inadequate development of the liver enzyme glucuronyltransferase which is involved in the conversion of indirect or free bilirubin to bilirubin glucuronide (direct or conjugated bilirubin), the excretable form.]

Clinical features Jaundice usually appears from the second to the fourth day and disappears from the seventh to the fourteenth day. The liver and spleen are not abnormally enlarged. This jaundice is entirely physiologic and occurs visibly in more than 50 percent of full-term newborn infants and 80 percent of premature infants.

Laboratory data

1. The blood-bilirubin level is increased, but usually not over 10 mg per 100 ml.
2. Bilirubin is found in the stools but not in the urine.
3. Van den Bergh's reaction is indirect.
4. The blood picture is normal for that age.

Treatment None is usually necessary. However, if bilirubin levels rise to above 10 mg per 100 ml, phototherapy may be helpful. (See Phototherapy, Chapter 15.)

SEPSIS

Etiology The organisms found most commonly are *E. coli, Pseudomonas,* and staphylococci. Prolonged rupture of membranes, amnionitis, prematurity, and prolonged and difficult delivery may be predisposing causes. There is a preponderance of males involved.

Clinical features

1. There may be evidence of the local infection that was the source, e.g., omphalitis.
2. There are no characteristic symptoms and signs, but anorexia, failure to gain weight, and restlessness or lethargy are common.
3. Fever may or may not be present; the temperature may even be subnormal or within the normal range but fluctuant.
4. Toxicity is marked in severe infections.
5. The jaundice may become apparent soon after birth or later and can be confused with physiologic jaundice.
6. The liver and spleen are often enlarged.
7. Hemorrhagic phenomena are not uncommon.
8. Sclerema is an occasional late finding.

Laboratory findings

1. A positive blood culture is most important. Several blood cultures should always be made in every obscure illness of the newborn infant.
2. The white blood count may be indicative of infection but is difficult to evaluate because a polymorphonuclear leukocytosis is normally present at this age. In coliform infections leucopenia is

often seen. The red blood cell count may show evidence of a hemolytic anemia.

3. Biphasic van den Bergh's reaction is usual.
4. The amount of urobilinogen is increased in the urine; in the stools, stercobilinogen is present.
5. Sedimentation rate is slow in the newborn infant; during the first few days of life rates of over 5 mm per hour are significantly elevated.
6. C-reactive protein is not transferred across the placenta, therefore a positive value in the newborn infant is indicative of infection.
7. An elevated IgM level may occur in infants born of mothers with infection, e.g., toxoplasmosis, rubella.
8. Examination of urine for pus and microorganisms.
9. Examination of a frozen section of umbilical cord for presence of bacteria, inflammatory cells, and arteritis may suggest infection.
10. Culture and examination for leukocytes of gastric aspirate may be helpful in early identification of infection.
11. Nose and throat cultures.
12. A spinal tap should always be performed because meningitis is a frequent complication.

Treatment

1. Selected antibacterials, depending on the causative organisms for a minimum of 10 days. Initially penicillin or ampicillin and kanamycin is recommended.
2. Fluids and transfusions.
3. Cortisone or adrenocortical extract (aqueous) may be of value.
4. Surgery, if there is a localized abscess.

Prophylaxis

1. Aseptic technique at delivery and in the care of the neonate.
2. Management of premature rupture of membranes.

If there is gross evidence of amnionitis at delivery or if the mother was febrile in labor prior to delivery, the infant should receive a course of antibiotic therapy for 10 days (see above).

A work-up for sepsis including blood culture, nose and throat culture, gastric aspirate culture, urine culture, should be made prior to treatment.

If membranes are ruptured for 12 to 24 hours before delivery but the mother is asymptomatic and the baby is normal, treatment of the baby is not suggested. If the membranes have ruptured over 24 hours prior to delivery, it is probably best to treat the infant with antibiotics for 5 to 7 days. If cultures are negative, treatment is then discontinued. If blood cultures are positive or there is other evidence of infection, treatment for a minimum of 10 days is recommended.

Omphalitis Omphalitis is an inflammation in the umbilical region due to infection with staphylococci, streptococci, colon bacilli, etc. It is characterized by redness around the cord and a moist granulating area at the base of the cord, often with odorous discharge. The newborn infant may appear normal or may be fretful or somnolent and fail to thrive. Sepsis is a common complication and must be prevented. The treatment is to administer the indicated antibacterial drugs, locally and parenterally.

ACUTE INFECTIOUS DIARRHEAS OF THE NEWBORN
(Including Epidemic Diarrheas of the Newborn)

Acute infectious diarrheas of the newborn infant are a heterogeneous group of communicable diseases, with diarrhea as the common outstanding clinical finding. Although isolated cases occur more commonly, outbreaks occur in the nurseries of hospitals with lying-in services, with rapid spread and sometimes high fatality rates. Historically, recognized outbreaks in hospital nurseries were designated "epidemic diarrhea of the newborn."

Etiology This is variable, and some outbreaks have no demonstrable causative organisms. Known enteric pathogens have been implicated such as the salmonella and shigella organisms, certain resistant strains of staphylococci, group D beta-hemolytic streptococci, as well as the *Pseudomonas aeruginosa,* and even fungi (*Candida albicans*). Certain types of *Escherichia coli,* including 0111: B4; 055: B5; 026: B6; 0127: B8, and viruses, particularly ECHO type 18 and adenoviruses, are responsible for most outbreaks.

Contributory factors

1. Overcrowding of nurseries
2. Failure to individualize care of infants in nurseries
3. Lack of cleanliness in the care of infants
4. Lack of aseptic techniques in the preparation of formulas and care of equipment
5. Infection of infant at time of delivery via maternal feces
6. Carriers among nurses and other personnel

Clinical features The incubation periods, clinical features, course, and duration of the primary acute infectious diarrheas of newborn infants will vary from case to case and from one outbreak to another, depending on the underlying etiologic agent. The general features are as follows:

1. Incubation period is usually 2 to 4 days but may be as long as 2 to 3 weeks. (Infants who have been discharged from the hospital may return with diarrhea.)
2. The stage of invasion (preceding the diarrhea) may be several hours or days and is characterized by anorexia, drowsiness, loss of weight, vomiting, distension, change in the character of stools, but usually no elevated temperature.
3. The toxic stage is characterized by rapid dehydration and acidosis; shock; frequent watery stools expelled explosively with no pus, blood, or mucus except in infection with pathogens of the salmonella-shigella groups; scanty urine or none; usually very little fever or at times even subnormal temperatures. Death may supervene rapidly.

Mode of spread   These diseases are usually spread by the fecal-oral route—and less commonly by droplet infection—either directly from infant to infant or indirectly by carriers, e.g., mother or attendant.

Period of communicability   This period is probably as long as symptoms are present among sick infants or a carrier state persists.

Differential diagnosis   This group of diarrheas must be distinguished from acute diarrheas in newborn infants secondary to parenteral infections, e.g., pneumonia and sepsis, or due to improper feeding.

Prognosis   The prognosis is guarded; in severe outbreaks the fatality rate may rise to 50 percent. Relapses are common.

Treatment   Treatment should be continued for 10 to 14 days and consists of the following:

1. Replacement of fluids and electrolytes.
2. Antibiotics as indicated by the infecting organism. Until identification is made the drugs of choice are (*a*) neomycin, 100 mg per kg per day, orally (*b*) colistin, 10 to 15 mg per kg per day, orally.

Control measures

1. The local health department should be notified immediately.
2. The obstetric service and nurseries for newborn infants should be closed.
3. All ill newborn infants should be isolated, and all who have been exposed should be quarantined.
4. All newborn infants who were discharged after exposure should be followed carefully.
5. A careful inspection of the hospital facilities and techniques should be made, e.g., water supply, handling of milk, and formula preparation.

6. All mothers, doctors, nurses, and personnel should be carefully studied as possible sources of the infection.
7. Nasopharyngeal and stool cultures should be taken from infants and personnel. If no other cause is found, a search for a virus infection should be made.
8. Breast feeding should be encouraged because enteropathic *E. coli* infection is rare in such infants.
9. When the outbreak has subsided, the obstetric wards and nurseries should be thoroughly aired, washed, and all equipment sterilized.

MENINGITIS IN THE NEWBORN

Etiology Meningitis in the newborn infant is usually secondary to sepsis but may also result from a contiguous infection, for example, an infected meningocele or otitis media. *E. coli, Aerobacter, Proteus, Pseudomonas,* streptococcus, staphylococcus, and pneumococcus are the most common etiologic organisms.

Clinical features The symptoms and signs are very variable and may not point to the nervous system. There may be any of the following: fever, vomiting, diarrhea, apathy, somnolence or restlessness, convulsions, cyanosis, jaundice, tachypnea, or apnea. Meningeal signs (nuchal rigidity, etc.) are usually not present, but fullness of the fontanel may be present. If there is any possibility of meningitis, it is best to perform a diagnostic spinal tap.

Laboratory findings

1. Spinal-fluid findings are shown in Table 14-6, under the discussion of the meningitides in Chapter 14, "Infectious Diseases."
2. Other findings are similar to those of sepsis of the newborn.

Treatment

1. Correction of fluid and electrolyte imbalance.
2. Until an organism is identified, a combination of kanamycin and either penicillin or ampicillin should be administered. (See Chapter 6, "Drugs and Treatment," for dosage.)

CYTOMEGALIC INCLUSION DISEASE OF INFANCY

This condition may be observed as the generalized visceral form in the newborn infant; the salivary glands may be involved alone, or the condition may occur in association with other diseases, e.g., pulmonary interstitial pneumonia or gastrointestinal conditions. It may produce widespread disturbance in cellular function, particularly in the reticuloendothelial system.

Etiology   The cause is a specific viral infection which may occur in utero. Stillborn infants may show pathologic evidence of the disease, and the condition may be present at birth. The infection is transmitted usually from the mother (who is asymptomatic) across the placenta to the infant. Postnatal infection occurs also in the newborn.

Clinical and laboratory features in newborn infants

1. Jaundice usually at birth or soon thereafter in a premature or low-birth-weight infant with hepatosplenomegaly.
2. Thrombocytopenia and anemia—hemorrhagic manifestations: e.g., showers of petechiae and gross hemorrhage. Bleeding time is prolonged.
3. Central nervous system: meningoencephalitis.
4. Chorioretinitis.
5. Roentgenograms of the skull may show small intracranial calcifications.
6. Stained smears of tissues and fluids, e.g., cerebrospinal, subdural, or the urinary sediment, may be diagnostic by demonstrating the inclusion cells. Virus may be grown from the urine for a number of months.
7. Pathologic study of the salivary glands and various visceral organs, particularly the kidneys, is diagnostic: characteristic nuclear and cytoplasmic inclusion bodies are seen, particularly in the epithelial cells.

Differential diagnosis   This disease should be distinguished from hemolytic disease of the newborn, sepsis, toxoplasmosis, herpes simplex, congenital rubella syndrome, neonatal hepatitis, and syphilis.

Treatment and prognosis   There is no specific therapy; transfusion is indicated for anemia, platelet-rich plasma for thrombocytopenia, and anticonvulsants for seizures. Elevated bilirubin levels may require exchange transfusion. The prognosis is very poor.

Prophylaxis   Aseptic techniques at delivery and in the care of the newborn infant are necessary preventive measures.

HERPES SIMPLEX

See Chapter 14, "Infectious Diseases."

TOXOPLASMOSIS

Etiology   Toxoplasmosis is caused by the protozoan *Toxoplasma gondii*, which is acquired in utero from an inapparent infection in the mother (a parasitemia). With rare exception it occurs only once in the offspring of a given mother; subsequent infants are usually not affected.

Clinical features The infant may be stillborn, born prematurely, or born at term. Signs and symptoms which may be noted either at birth or at several days of age include fever, maculopapular rash, icterus, hepatomegaly, splenomegaly, lymphadenopathy, hydrocephalus or microcephalus, microphthalmia, convulsions, and chorioretinitis. Psychomotor retardation becomes evident as the child matures.

Laboratory findings Intracranial calcification may be seen on x-ray. The parasite may be found in smears or tissue sections, or it may be isolated following inoculation of susceptible animals with affected body fluids. The diagnosis is confirmed by a rising titer of dye-test antibodies (methylene blue test), by hemagglutination inhibition or by complement-fixing antibodies. Cytoplasm-modifying antibodies (methylene blue test) usually appear within 10 to 20 days and last indefinitely as does hemagglutination inhibition. Complement-fixing antibodies usually appear after the acute phase and disappear later. Demonstration that an infant's antibodies are IgM rules out the possibility of passive transfer of such antibodies.

Treatment Treatment is a combination of pyrimethamine (Daraprim), 1 mg per kg per day in two divided doses, and sulfadiazine, 0.15 to 0.2 Gm per kg for a total of 4 weeks. Drug toxicity, e.g., leukopenia, thrombocytopenia, and anemia, can occur especially following administration of Daraprim.

CONGENITAL RUBELLA SYNDROME

If a pregnant woman contracts rubella during the first trimester, the risk of congenital rubella occurring in the infant is about 20 percent. Laboratory-proved rubella in the first 10 weeks of pregnancy is associated with fetal infection in virtually 100 percent of cases. Clinically the newborn infant may be affected in many ways including the following: intrauterine growth retardation, eye defects (cataracts, glaucoma, and retinopathy), cardiac defects (patent ductus arteriosus, pulmonary artery stenosis, coarctation of the aorta), deafness, thrombocytopenic purpura, cerebral defects (retardation, microcephaly, encephalitis leading to cerebral palsy), hepatitis, bone lesions, pneumonitis, and hepatosplenomegaly. Many of the infants continue to excrete the virus for the first 12 to 18 months of life. Immunoglobulin abnormalities including elevated IgM and low IgG and IgA levels have been reported. Congenital rubella must be differentiated from toxoplasmosis, syphilis, cytomegalovirus infection, and herpes type II infection.

Prophylaxis For children there is no prophylaxis. ISG is not effective in preventing rubella viremia, hence there is no evidence that its use is beneficial to the patient. For pregnant women exposed in the first trimester, the following are recommended:

1. Within the week following exposure obtain blood sample and test for rubella hemagglutination inhibition (HI) antibodies. If antibody is present, no risk of infection exists and the patient can be reassured. If antibody is not detectable, therapeutic abortion is advised; if this procedure is declined, then ISG (20 ml) is given and a second blood specimen is obtained 4 weeks later. The HI antibody test should be repeated on the paired sera. The presence of antibody in the second serum would be indicative of rubella infection. Failure to develop antibody would indicate an absence of infection. (If the original blood sample is obtained longer than 1 week after exposure, the presence of HI antibody cannot be assumed to indicate immunity.)
2. There is an alternative method to making a serologic diagnosis of rubella on a single sample of serum. Obtain a blood specimen 2 weeks after the rash appears which may demonstrate IgM rubella virus antibodies. A sizable portion of the initial rubella antibody consists of IgM antibodies which can be detected for 2 to 3 weeks following the illness.

LISTERIA MONOCYTOGENES INFECTIONS

These infections, which are caused by a small gram-positive bacillus often called a "diphtheroid," occur in newborn infants. The infant is infected in utero transplacentally and may die before birth or manifest the infection within the first week or so after birth. The amniotic fluid in infected cases is often brown. At birth there may be cardio-respiratory symptoms; diarrhea and vomiting are frequent. Delayed infection usually presents as a bronchopneumonia. Purulent meningitis is often present. Miliary granulomatous lesions—dark-red or livid papules—may be seen over the skin and in the oropharynx. The diagnosis is confirmed by finding the organism in the stool, urine, or blood of the infant or mother. Most antibiotics, erythromycin in particular, are effective in the treatment.

ERYTHROBLASTOSIS FETALIS

Erythroblastosis fetalis and other hemolytic diseases of the newborn are discussed in Chapter 22, "Blood Disorders."

CONGENITAL OBLITERATION OF THE BILE DUCTS

Etiology This condition results from malformations of the biliary tract, such as stenosis of the common bile duct and absence or atresia of intrahepatic (uncommon), extrahepatic, or common ducts.

Clinical features

1. The onset of jaundice is often early, appearing to be a continuation of physiologic jaundice, although it may not appear until several weeks of age. It becomes progressively worse, but for short periods its intensity may be diminished.
2. There is neither fever nor toxemia.
3. The liver is usually enlarged; the spleen is only slightly enlarged but may become enlarged terminally following the development of cirrhosis and ascites.
4. The nutritional status remains surprisingly good for a long period of time.
5. Vitamin K deficiency may result in hemorrhagic phenomena, and if the infant survives, other fat-soluble-vitamin (A, D, and E) deficiencies often occur.

Laboratory data

1. Stools are characteristically acholic (clay-colored), but there may be slight bile staining in severely jaundiced infants. (In these cases the tissues are saturated with bile, and enough is secreted from the gastrointestinal tract to be detected in the stool.)
2. Urine contains bilirubin, but no urobilinogen.
3. Serum-bilirubin level is elevated, much of which is due to the direct type.
4. Bleeding and clotting times may be prolonged.
5. A sustained increase in activity of serum glutamic oxalacetic transaminase (SGOT) usually occurs. This sustained increase does not occur in hemolytic disease of the newborn or in physiologic jaundice. (Normal peak value in the newborn infant is 120 units.)
6. Rose bengal ^{131}I excretion test reveals less than 10 percent excretion in the stool.

Differential diagnosis All conditions causing prolonged jaundice must be considered. In addition to the various types of obliteration of the bile ducts listed under etiology, the following must be noted:

1. Choledochal cyst—a palpable mass may be present, but final diagnosis may require cholecystography or even laparotomy.
2. Hemolytic disease of the newborn may be followed by an obstructive type of jaundice. Magnesium sulfate or other cholagogues may be helpful in relieving such obstructions.

3. Bile-plug syndrome—cholangiogram may demonstrate the plug or surgery may reveal it.
4. Neonatal giant-cell hepatitis—both types of infectious hepatitis virus (IH; SH) as well as other viruses, e.g., cytomegalic inclusion virus, have been implicated. The finding of Australian antibody may be helpful in identifying hepatitis due to SH virus.
5. Congenital malformation of erythrocytes—hereditary spherocytosis—transmitted as an autosomal dominant trait, hereditary elliptocytosis, autosomal dominant, sickle-cell disease (rarely a problem in the neonate).
6. Hereditary nonspherocytic anemia due to various red cell enzyme deficiencies, e.g., glucose-6-phosphate dehydrogenase, pyruvate kinase, hexokinase hexophosphate isomerase (see p. 578).
7. Galactosemia (see Chapter 9).
8. Syphilis, cytomegalic inclusion disease, toxoplasmosis, and congenital rubella.
9. Congenital familial nonhemolytic jaundice (Crigler-Najjar disease) may be transmitted as an autosomal dominant or recessive trait; both are phenotypically identical (deficiency of glucuronyltransferase). Jaundice appears in the first few days of life, and bilirubin is mostly the indirect type. Kernicterus may occur. Treatment consists of exchange transfusion, phototherapy, and phenobarbital (enzyme induction).
10. Infection, e.g., sepsis, in addition to those listed in item 8.
11. Drugs, e.g., sulfa drugs, vitamin K.
12. Miscellaneous conditions causing jaundice include cystic fibrosis, intestinal obstruction, hypothyroidism, and hypertrophic pyloric stenosis.

Treatment   Usually by 2 to 4 months of age, suggestive laboratory tests and persistent jaundice are sufficient indications to perform a laparotomy. At this time, open biopsy and examination of the extrahepatic system usually permit definitive diagnosis. Surgical correction should be attempted if possible.

Prognosis   Most cases are not amenable to surgical correction. Longevity is greater in children with uncorrectable intrahepatic involvement (10 years or more) than those with uncorrectable extrahepatic anomalies (6 months to 2 years).

POSTMATURITY (Prolonged Gestation)

This syndrome may occur in pregnancies of more than 300 days. Morbidity and mortality are much greater if no pregnancy occurred during the 10-year period preceding the one in question.

Pathogenesis The pathogenesis is unclear because the mechanism of initiation of labor is not understood.

1. Placental dysfunction: the placenta ordinarily ceases to grow just prior to term; there is reduced blood supply to the fetus, with resultant hypoxia, poor nutrition, and relative weight loss. However, the length of the infant is greater than normal.
2. Disappearance of the protective layer of the vernix leads to maceration of the skin.

Clinical features

Mild The skin is dry, cracked, and peeling but unstained. The newborn infants are relatively long, show evidence of recent weight loss in utero, have an "old" look; the muscles are flabby, and there is loss of subcutaneous tissue.

Moderate Clinical features are the same as in the mild form, plus signs of intrauterine hypoxia with liberation of meconium into the amniotic fluid. Placental membranes, umbilical cord, and skin are stained green. Hypoglycemia of the symptomatic type may occur in these infants more often.

Severe The severe form includes infants who have passed through the first two forms in utero; many of these are stillborn. There is a change from the green staining due to meconium to a brilliant yellow or yellow-green staining of the nails, skin, and umbilical cord.

Prophylaxis Interruption of the pregnancy may be indicated if pregnancy goes beyond term.

Treatment Severe cases are treated as described earlier in this chapter under Neonatal Hypoxia.

OTHER INFECTIONS OF THE NEWBORN

OPHTHALMIA NEONATORUM, OR GONORRHEAL OPHTHALMIA

The infant is exposed to gonorrhea during delivery via infected birth passages. The onset is from the second to the fifth day. There are severe redness and swelling of the eyes and a serosanguineous discharge which rapidly becomes purulent and profuse. This may be complicated by corneal ulceration and perforation with panophthalmitis. The diagnosis is confirmed by smear and culture of the eye discharge.

Prophylaxis Prophylaxis is described under Immediate Care of the Newborn, in Chapter 11, "The Normal Newborn Infant." Isolation of infected newborn infants is recommended.

Treatment

1. Penicillin parenterally.
2. Atropine 1 : 1,000, one drop in each eye once a day.
3. If only one eye is involved, the unaffected eye should be protected by positioning the infant and by local hygiene.

INCLUSION BLENORRHEA

This infection is caused by *Chlamydia oculogenitalis*. The organism is found in the cervix and urethra. The onset is usually 5 to 15 days after birth. There is a purulent discharge and a cobblestone appearance of the palpebral conjunctiva, with the lower lid usually more involved than the upper. Scrapings from the conjunctiva reveal inclusion bodies. Sulfonamides or tetracycline give excellent results (see p. 291).

NONSPECIFIC CONJUNCTIVITIS

Various forms may be caused by staphylococcus, pneumococcus, streptococcus, *E. coli,* or other organisms. Smears and cultures demonstrate the causative organism. The indicated antibiotics are used in therapy. In mild cases, local administration may suffice; in severe cases, parenteral therapy may be necessary.

THRUSH OF THE NEWBORN (Oral Moniliasis)

Thrush is caused by a *Candida albicans* infection from the mother's vagina during delivery or from contamination in the nursery or formula room. Thrush may be seen in healthy newborn infants. (At any other period of life it may be seen following administration of certain drugs, e.g., steroids, immunosuppressive agents, oral antibiotics; in debilitated and dehydrated children; associated with a number of endocrine disorders, e.g., diabetes mellitus, hypoparathyroidism, and in various blood dyscrasias.) There are white patches, pinhead size or larger, on the mucous membranes of the mouth and tongue, which, on removal, leave tiny bleeding areas. Milk particles are occasionally confused with thrush but are easily removed. Topical applications of aqueous gentian violet 1% once or twice a day, not to exceed 4 or 5 days (longer use may result in ulcerations), are helpful. Mycostatin orally, 100,000 units four times a day for 7 days, is recommended. Sterilization techniques in formula preparation should be reevaluated, and nipples used by babies with thrush should be treated separately. Monilial dermatitis, particularly in the diaper region, is an occasional sequela of thrush.

METABOLIC DISTURBANCES IN THE NEWBORN

TETANY OF THE NEWBORN

Etiology   Tetany of the newborn, in contrast to tetany in the older infant or child, is not related to vitamin D deficiency. The relatively high level of phosphates (six times the phosphate level in human milk) in artificial feedings (tetany is very rare in breast-fed infants) and the poor kidney function of the newborn infant may lead to hyperphosphatemia and hypocalcemia. There may also be a transient hypoparathyroidism, especially in infants born of hyperparathyroid mothers. It is the hypocalcemia which produces the tetany. Tetany of the newborn has been found not infrequently in infants born to mothers with a history of diabetes mellitus or toxemia as well as following difficult delivery and postmaturity.

Clinical features   The onset occurs during the first few days of life in those cases associated with the specific pathologic conditions listed above. In the classic type onset occurs during the first few weeks of life with marked hyperirritability, which may be manifested by twitching, tremors, or convulsions simulating meningitis. There may be laryngospasm or carpopedal spasm (Chvostek's sign may be normally present in the newborn). Often hyperpyrexia, subcutaneous edema, and vomiting are prominent.

Laboratory findings   Blood-calcium level is usually below 8 mg per 100 ml; there is hyperphosphatemia, with levels usually above 7 mg per 100 ml; and the phosphatase level is normal.

Treatment   The immediate treatment is to give calcium (see section on treatment under Infantile Tetany in Chapter 20, "Neurologic Conditions").

Prophylaxis   Artificial feedings should not have a relatively high phosphate content.

NEONATAL HYPOGLYCEMIA
(See Chapter 24, "Endocrine Diseases")

DEHYDRATION FEVER

Dehydration fever (inanition fever or transitory fever) is usually seen on the second, third, or fourth day of life and may reach 103 to 104°F (39.4 to 40.0°C). The newborn infant is otherwise normal. The explanation that it is due to dehydration is not entirely satisfactory, since there is not always complete correlation with weight loss or fluid intake. However, giving fluids by mouth and parenterally rapidly results in a normal temperature.

TRANSITORY EDEMA

Transitory edema may be localized or generalized and may occur in the newborn infant either at birth or within the first few days. It may be traumatic in origin, in which case it will be localized at the presenting part. The incidence and severity are increased by hypoxia during labor or at birth. It is more often seen in premature infants and infants of diabetic mothers. There have been many suggestions as to etiology. However, there is no adequate explanation at present for this phenomenon. The edema is of short duration, and no treatment is needed. It must be differentiated from hydrops fetalis, which is the severest form of erythroblastosis fetalis (see Chapter 22, "Blood Disorders"). Rarely there may be a persistent congenital lymphedema, particularly of the lower extremities, which may be familial (Milroy's disease). Congenital nephrosis (microcystic disease of the kidney) may also cause persistent generalized edema in the newborn infant. Turner's syndrome may cause edema of the distal portion of the extremities.

HEMORRHAGIC DISEASE OF THE NEWBORN

Etiology   The causation of hemorrhagic disease is not entirely clear, and no gross coagulation defect exists. It occurs almost exclusively in breast-fed infants. The normal newborn is hypoprothrombinemic at birth. There is a fall during the second and third days of life. It then rises and approaches or reaches normal by 10 days. (In addition to the hypoprothrombinemia, a deficiency of factors VII, IX, and X probably contribute to this condition.)

Clinical features

1.   There is spontaneous hemorrhage from any site, or hemorrhage may follow slight trauma. Typically there are petechiae and ecchymoses in the skin and mucous membranes, beginning on the second or third day of life.
2.   The brain and meninges are the most dangerous locations. (Intracranial hemorrhage has already been discussed.)
3.   Umbilical-cord bleeding, bloody vomitus, and melena are not uncommon. In melena and bloody vomitus, the fetal hemoglobin is resistant to alkali denaturation and a pink color remains, differentiating it from ingested maternal blood, which becomes yellow-brown with addition of the alkali (NaOH 1%)—Apt test.

Laboratory data

1. The prothrombin time is usually increased.
2. The coagulation time is often prolonged, but the bleeding time and clot-retraction time are normal.
3. The platelet count is normal, and if there is extensive hemorrhage, anemia and leukocytosis are found.

Prophylaxis   The administration of vitamin K to the mother reduces the incidence of hemorrhagic disease in the newborn infant. It may also be given to the infant (Vitamin K_1—0.25 to 0.5 mg, parenterally).

Treatment   Vitamin K, 1 mg, is given intramuscularly or intravenously and within several hours corrects a prolonged prothrombin time. If bleeding does not decrease strikingly in 4 to 6 hours, the dose may be repeated. If bleeding is severe, an infusion of fresh plasma will correct the hemorrhagic defect immediately. For severe anemia, a whole blood or packed red cell transfusion may be employed.

SKIN AND MUCOUS MEMBRANE HEMORRHAGE

This may be found in the following conditions:

1. Physiologic bleeding from the vagina.
2. Umbilical-cord bleeding from an inadequately tied stump.
3. Erythroblastosis fetalis (hemolytic disease of the newborn).
4. Sepsis.
5. Hemorrhagic disease of the newborn.
6. Very rare causes include syphilis, leukemia, thrombocytopenic purpura, and hemophilia.

CONDITIONS FOLLOWING TRAUMA

CAPUT SUCCEDANEUM

Caput succedaneum is a swelling of the scalp caused by edema in those tissues of the scalp which are presenting during labor. The edema is situated beneath the aponeurosis external to the periosteum. It is present at birth and is a diffuse, compressible, movable swelling that crosses the suture lines. No treatment is necessary, as it clears in 48 to 72 hours.

CEPHALHEMATOMA

Cephalhematoma is a subperiosteal extravasation of blood, probably caused by the trauma of delivery. It may be single or multiple, varies in size, and does not cross the suture lines. The following areas are usually involved: parietal, biparietal ("devil's horns"), and occipital. As it organizes, a hard border is felt around a very soft center, which may give the impression of a skull defect, but roentgenogram shows none; occasionally, a thin linear fracture of the bone underlying the hematoma may occur. Treatment is unnecessary. Cephalhematomas should not be incised; even the very large ones clear in a few months, usually without any residuals. Rarely, a calcified area may remain.

CHEMICAL CONJUNCTIVITIS

This is due to irritation from the silver nitrate instilled at birth, which may not have been freshly prepared or completely washed out after instillation. In the first day or two after birth there are edema, redness, and discharge. The smear and culture are sterile. The only treatment necessary is sterile water irrigations to keep the eyes clean.

FACIAL PARALYSIS

This is usually due to compression by forceps or some other compression of the facial nerve, e.g., against the mother's pelvis, which produces a peripheral paralysis—the forehead cannot be wrinkled, the face is smooth, the eyelid is partially open, the mouth droops, and when the infant cries the involved side of the face becomes more evident.

There is a very rare nonobstetric type of central facial paralysis that is probably caused by a nuclear agenesis and cannot be treated; in this condition other nerves are involved, particularly the 6th nerve.

The prognosis in the peripheral facial paralysis is usually good, and no treatment is necessary. However, when the nerve has been severed and there is no recovery after 2 to 3 months, an operative procedure may be considered. When there is associated facial and cranial asymmetry that is permanent and not due to molding, the nerve atrophy is caused by long-standing antepartum compression, and the prognosis is poor cosmetically.

BRACHIAL PALSY

Brachial palsy is due to injury of the brachial plexus. It occurs in vertex presentations due to excessive lateral traction of the neck in attempting to deliver the anterior shoulder or in breech presentations during disengagement of a nuchal arm.

Clinical features   *Duchenne-Erb type*   The newborn infant cannot abduct the arm, rotate the arm externally, or supinate the forearm, Moro reflex is absent on the affected side, the power of the forearm and hand is preserved, and the biceps reflex is absent. Paralysis of the diaphragm may be present on the ipsilateral side due to injury of the adjacent phrenic nerve (4th cervical root). Such infants may show dyspnea and cyanosis.

Klumpke's type   In this more rare type of brachial palsy, there are flail hand, paralyzed triceps, and Horner's syndrome (ptosis of the lid and miosis).

Treatment   In the Duchenne-Erb type of paralysis, the infant's sleeve may be pinned to the crib mattress above the head. If there is a palsy of the Klumpke's type, the hand may be padded and an airplane splint used with the forearm at a right angle. Physical therapy is helpful. If the paralysis persists beyond 2 to 3 months, there has been a laceration of the nerve, and neuroplasty should be considered. Unfortunately, no treatment is likely to achieve much benefit if the nerve has been completely separated.

PARALYSIS OF THE PHRENIC NERVE

Paralysis of the phrenic nerve is sometimes associated with brachial palsy and is characterized by cyanosis, dyspnea, and elevated diaphragm on the affected side. Seesaw movements of the leaves of the diaphragm during respiration are seen on fluoroscopic examination. The treatment consists of oxygen for the cyanosis, gavage feeding, and antibiotics to help prevent pneumonia. Prognosis is usually good.

FRACTURE OF THE CLAVICLE

Fracture of the clavicle is characterized by inability to move the arm on the affected side (absence of Moro reflex) and crepitus over the fracture site. Roentgenogram reveals the exact location of the fracture. The treatment is to immobilize the arm and shoulder on the affected side.

TORTICOLLIS

Torticollis (hematoma of the sternocleidomastoid muscle, wryneck) in the newborn infant may be caused by injury to, or circulatory stasis of, the sternocleidomastoid muscle and is commonly unilateral. It is not known whether pathologically it is an organized hematoma or a fibroma. Usually at 1 to 2 weeks of age a mass is felt in the middle of the muscle. The head is pulled down toward the clavicle on the same side, with the chin tilted in the opposite direction. The conservative treatment is rest, manipulation, and exercise to produce overextension of the sternocleidomastoid muscle. If these measures fail, surgery may be indicated to remove the mass.

INFANTS BORN OF DRUG ADDICTS

Considerable variation in the clinical course occurs from infant to infant. There is probably a direct relationship between the duration of maternal addiction and maternal dosage and the severity of symptoms in the neonate. Heroin and methadone are the most common offenders. About half of such infants weigh less than 2,500 Gm at birth, and about half of those are low weight for gestational age. Approximately half the babies born to addicted mothers require treatment. Signs usually appear within 48 to 72 hours and consist of irritability, tremors, vomiting, high-pitched cry, sneezing, hypertonicity and hyperactivity, respiratory distress, fever, diarrhea, sweating, and rarely, convulsions. Infants showing a progressive increase in the severity of signs should be treated. Various drugs have been used successfully. Chlorpromazine, 2.2 mg per kg per day in four divided doses, either parenterally or orally is effective. The dosage is reduced stepwise every 2 to 3 days depending upon clinical improvement. Treatment may be required for as long as 40 days. After discharge, placement of the infant in a suitable environment is a major problem. It may be necessary to remove the infant from the natural mother.

REVIEW QUESTIONS

1. Severe congenital anomalies occur in (*a*) 1.5 percent; (*b*) 3.5 percent; (*c*) 5.5 percent; (*d*) 10 percent of live-born infants.
2. In cases of spina bifida it is important to evaluate (*a*) competence of the anal sphincter; (*b*) vibratory sensation of the legs; (*c*) ability to walk; (*d*) superficial abdominal reflexes.
3. The following statements concerning congenital deficiency of the abdominal muscles are true except for one: (*a*) most common in males; (*b*) associated with obstructive manifestations of the urinary tract; (*c*) associated with anomalies of the ovaries; (*d*) associated with anomalies of the gastrointestinal tract.
4. The following is the treatment of choice for umbilical hernia: (*a*) taping; (*b*) surgery; (*c*) judicious observation; (*d*) prevent crying since this worsens the condition.
5. In the commonest form of esophageal atresia (*a*) the upper and lower segments of the esophagus end blindly; (*b*) the upper portion of the esophagus ends near the bifurcation of the trachea and the lower segment forms a fistulous tract between the stomach and the trachea; (*c*) the upper segment communicates with the trachea and the lower pouch is blind; (*d*) both upper and lower segments communicate with the trachea.
6. A newborn infant is observed to require frequent nasopharyngeal suctioning because of mucus. A diagnosis that should be suspected is (*a*) hyaline membrane disease; (*b*) tracheoesophageal fistula; (*c*) bronchopneumonia; (*d*) pharyngitis.
7. All the following are diagnostic signs of asphyxia in the newborn infant except for one: (*a*) tachycardia; (*b*) pallor or grayness; (*c*) flaccidity; (*d*) absence of response to sensory stimuli; (*e*) bradycardia.
8. Early signs of possible congenital obstruction of the gastrointestinal tract include all but one of the following: (*a*) polyhydramnios; (*b*) respiratory distress; (*c*) bile-stained emesis; (*d*) failure to pass meconium within 12 hours of age; (*e*) having a sib with mucoviscidosis.

9. An infant obtains an Apgar score of 9. One of the following statements is not true: (*a*) baby has a heart rate of 130; (*b*) baby is in poor condition; (*c*) baby has good muscle tone and is active; (*d*) baby has peripheral cyanosis.

10. All the following statements concerning idiopathic respiratory distress syndrome are true except for one: (*a*) inability to produce surfactant; (*b*) respiratory symptoms may be present at birth or develop gradually at 2 to 6 hours of age; (*c*) increased activity and restlessness; (*d*) x-ray early reveals depression of the diaphragm and hyperaeration of the lungs.

11. The following statements concerning transient tachypnea of the newborn are true except for one: (*a*) usually occurs in full-term infants; (*b*) may reveal increase in bronchovascular markings on x-ray; (*c*) usually caused by infection; (*d*) treatment with oxygen is usually effective.

12. Subdural hematoma occurs most often in (*a*) low-birth-weight infant; (*b*) large baby; (*c*) *H. influenza* meningitis of newborn; (*d*) infant, second in order in sibship.

13. Wilson-Mikity syndrome is seen most often in (*a*) full-term infants; (*b*) low-birth-weight infants; (*c*) postmature infants; (*d*) infants with respiratory-tract anomalies.

14. The following statements concerning sepsis in the newborn are true except for one: (*a*) jaundice may become apparent at birth or shortly after; (*b*) temperature may be subnormal; (*c*) biphasic van den Bergh's reaction is usual; (*d*) white blood count of 15,000 per cu mm is significant.

15. A normal baby is born to an asymptomatic mother whose membranes ruptured 15 hours before delivery. Treatment of choice for the baby is (*a*) antibiotics for 5 to 7 days; (*b*) perform a blood culture and spinal tap; (*c*) no treatment is indicated.

16. The following statements concerning cytomegalic inclusion disease of infancy are true except for one: (*a*) bleeding time is prolonged; (*b*) chorioretinitis is associated with this condition; (*c*) the mother is symptomatic; (*d*) no specific treatment.

17. If a pregnant woman contracts rubella (proven by laboratory tests) during the first 10 weeks of pregnancy, the risk of congenital rubella occurring in the infant is (*a*) 5 percent; (*b*) 20 percent; (*c*) 50 percent; (*d*) virtually 100 percent.

18. The most significant clinical sign observed in babies having withdrawal symptoms due to maternal heroin addiction is (*a*) hyperactivity; (*b*) drowsiness; (*c*) poor feeding; (*d*) convulsions.

19. All the following are associated with neonatal narcotic withdrawal except for one: (*a*) jaundice; (*b*) respiratory distress; (*c*) vomiting or diarrhea; (*d*) sweating; (*e*) convulsions.

13

LOW-BIRTH-WEIGHT INFANT

Any infant born alive who weighs 2,500 Gm (5½ lb) or less is considered in the broad category of low-birth-weight infant. Infants are to be considered premature if the gestation period is less than 37 weeks completed. About two-thirds of low-birth-weight neonates are premature; the remainder are small for date as a result of retarded intrauterine growth. Some infants may be both premature and small for date (see Figures 13-1 and 13-2). Morbidity and mortality rates are increased for the low-birth-weight infant.

Physical criteria for estimation of gestational age are listed in Table 13-1.

Neurologic evaluation is utilized to evaluate gestational age. Maturation of the nervous system correlates better with gestational age

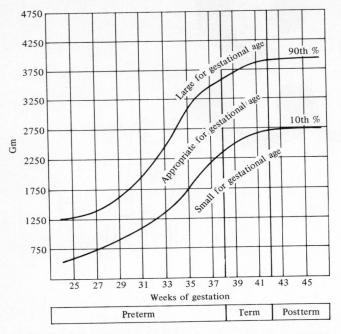

Figure 13-1 Weight-gestational age charts. University of Colorado Medical Center classification of newborns by birth weight and gestational age. (From L. O. Lubchenco, "Neonatal Mortality Rate: Its Relationships to Birth Weight and Gestation Age," *Journal of Pediatrics*, in press.)

Table 13-1. Gestational age (physical criteria)

	36 weeks or less	37–38 weeks	39 weeks or more
Sole creases	Only anterior transverse crease	Occasionally other creases on anterior ⅔	Sole covered with creases
Breast nodule diameter	2 mm	4 mm	7 mm
Ear lobe	Pliable, no cartilage	Some cartilage	Stiffened by thick cartilage
Scalp hair	Fine and fuzzy	Fine and fuzzy	Coarse and silky
Genitals Male	Testes in lower canal, small scrotum with few rugae		Testes pendulous, full scrotum, many rugae
Female	Prominent labia minora	Intermediate	Labia majora prominent

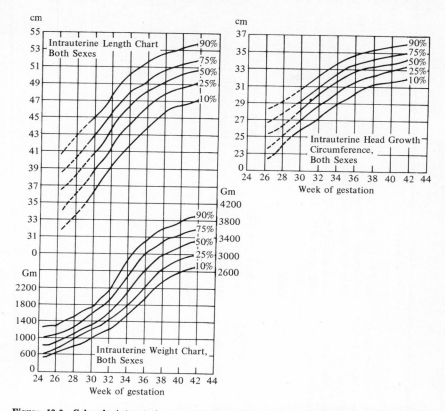

Figure 13-2 Colorado intrauterine growth charts. (From L. O. Lubchenco et al., "Intrauterine Growth in Length and Head Circumference as Estimated from Live Births at Gestational Ages from 26 to 42 Weeks," *Pediatrics,* **37:403, 1966.)**

than with weight. Examination is made best after 48 hours of age. However, even then findings may be variable and are not conclusive.

Criteria for estimation of gestational age as obtained from neurologic examination are listed in Table 13-2.

OTHER CLINICAL, ROENTGENOLOGIC, AND PATHOLOGIC FEATURES OF LOW BIRTH WEIGHT

1. Apgar scores are lower than in full-sized infants.
2. The skin is thin and wrinkled; there is a minimal amount of subcutaneous tissue. The premature has an abundance of lanugo.
3. The head appears relatively large, but the circumference is less than 33 cm (13 in.), with a characteristic wizened facies.
4. Short apneic episodes of 5- to 10-second duration alternating with rapid deep respirations for similar intervals often occur. Such

Table 13-2. Gestational age (neurologic criteria)

	28 weeks	32 weeks	36 weeks	40 weeks
Posture supine	Head turned to side, extremities extended and abducted, hypotonic	Head turned to side, upper extremities extended, lower flexed and abducted	Head frequently in line with trunk, extremities flexed but easily extended	Head strongly in line with the trunk, extremities strongly flexed
Posture prone	Pelvis flat on the table, knees alongside of the abdomen	Pelvis flat on the table, knees along the side of abdomen	Pelvis somewhat off the table, knees under the abdomen	Pelvis high off the table, knees under the abdomen
Sucking reflex	Weak or absent	Present	Good	Vigorous
Rooting reflex	Slow with long latency period	More rapid, good	Brisk, very good	Brisk, very good
Moro reflex	Weak, not always elicited	Reproducible and good	Reproducible and good	Reproducible and good
Grasp reflex	Present but weak	Present but cannot lift body	Strong and can lift body	Strong and can lift body
Cry	Absent or feeble	Weak to good	Good	Vigorous

periodic breathing usually occurs in the waking state and is not accompanied by cyanosis.

5. The initial weight loss is often greater and the regain is not so rapid as in full-term infants.

6. Of the six ossification centers (calcaneus, cuboid, talus, proximal tibia, head of the humerus, and distal femur) usually present at birth in the full-term infant, two (distal femur and proximal tibia) may be absent.

7. Intrauterine growth retardation results in certain organs being large for the weight of the infant, i.e., brain, heart, spleen; others tend to be comparatively small, i.e., lungs, liver, thymus, adrenals. The structural complexity of the brain and kidney is greater than expected from the infant's weight, and there is less extramedullary hematopoiesis.

COMPLICATIONS OF LOW BIRTH WEIGHT

The physiologic and anatomic predisposing factors are

1. Respiratory tract: A weak gag and cough reflex and an immature respiratory center require stronger afferent stimuli for response. Incompletely developed alveoli, a deficiency of the secretion in normal alveolar cells of a material (surfactant) that lowers surface tension, reduced vascularity of the pulmonary capillaries, sparse pulmonary elastic tissue, poor muscle tone and weak movements of the intercostal muscles and diaphragm plus softness and pliability of the bones cause easier collapse of the thoracic cage by the negative intrathoracic pressure necessary to fill the alveoli. The presence of larger amounts of fetal hemoglobin probably plays a role in the high affinity for oxygen of the neonate's blood which releases oxygen less readily to tissues. These factors then produce hypoxia and acidosis which can increase pulmonary vascular resistance and increase shunting of blood via a functionally patent ductus arteriosus and foramen ovale. All the above predispose to the development of respiratory distress syndrome.

2. Circulatory system: Cyanosis (generalized) is commonly due to ventilatory deficiency. Right-to-left shunts (often transient)— patent ductus, foramen ovale, and atelectasis—contribute to failure of oxygen to relieve the cyanosis. Hypoxemia results in bradycardia after an initial tachycardia, and together with hypervolemia (high hematocrits occur in intrauterine growth retardation) or hypovolemia (fetal blood loss) tend to produce shock. Increased capillary fragility predisposes to hemorrhage, particularly cerebral and pulmonary. Increased capillary permeability and hyperbilirubinemia when coupled with hypoxia and acidosis may result in brain damage at levels of bilirubin generally not considered to be dangerous.

    Phototherapy using a high-intensity light is helpful in lowering serum bilirubin concentrations in newborn infants. Bilirubin undergoes gradual decomposition, and the nontoxic degradation products are rapidly excreted from the body in bile and urine. This therapy is particularly helpful in preventing a rise in bilirubin in low-birth-weight infants, thus reducing the need for exchange transfusion. The consensus of opinion suggests its use in these infants when the indirect bilirubin reaches 8 to 10 mg per 100 ml.

The photodestruction of bilirubin occurs gradually so one cannot rely on it if the bilirubin is rising rapidly as in acute hemolytic disease. However, it may be of use in mild Rh and ABO hemolytic disease where the rise in bilirubin is slow or in such cases following an exchange transfusion to reduce the need for a repeat exchange.

The eyes should be protected by shields while the therapy is used. This therapy does not influence the amount of hemolysis and subsequent anemia.

3. Gastrointestinal tract: Hepatic immaturity predisposes the premature infant to develop increased bilirubinemia with jaundice (inadequate amount of glucuronyl transferase for glucuronate conjugation of free bilirubin), hypoglycemia, hypoproteinemia and edema, and hypoprothrombinemia with possible hemorrhage. The premature infant handles fat less well than the full-term infant.

4. Urinary system: The decreased renal function (glomerular and tubular) predisposes to dehydration and acidosis. Glomeruli and their nephrons continue to develop after birth even in the full-term infant. There is diminished ability to concentrate urine and osmotic diuresis is limited. Urea clearance and clearance of various electrolytes are diminished so that conditions affecting fluid and electrolyte balance, e.g., vomiting, diarrhea, infection, cause more profound disturbances than in the full-sized infant.

5. Temperature control: The faulty control of body temperature is associated with hypothermia and hyperthermia. This lability is the result of inadequate function of the sweating mechanism, inability to shiver, diminished body insulation due to paucity of subcutaneous fat, large surface area in proportion to the body weight, and low total heat production due to body inactivity and poor muscular development.

6. Deficiencies: The inadequate antenatal storage of minerals (e.g., iron, calcium, phosphorus), vitamins (A and D), and immune substances makes the premature infant particularly subject to rickets, anemia, and infections. There is also an increased demand for vitamin C which activates parahydroxyphenylpyruvate oxidase necessary for the metabolism of tyrosine. Susceptibility to infection is increased—the bacteriostatic and bactericidal activity of the blood is diminished, and leukocytes have less phagocytic ability. The amount of gamma globulin is deficient, and ability to produce antibodies is decreased.

Retrolental fibroplasia is a disease not fully understood which occurs most frequently in small premature infants. High arterial oxygen tension is a potent contributory factor in the production of retrolental fibroplasia probably through an affect on the developing vasculature. The eye of the infant is not fully vascularized until several weeks after birth. This condition is usually noted in the first few months of life and may involve either one eye or both eyes. The stages in the development of retrolental fibroplasia are spasm, dilatation and tortuosity of retinal vessels, edema and hemorrhage, localized retinal detachment, and partial to complete occlusion of the pupil by an opaque vascularized membrane behind the lens, resulting in loss of vision. The pathologic process may spontaneously arrest during any of the early stages, with the eye returning to normal. The treatment of retrolental fibroplasia has been unsatisfactory. To prevent its occurrence, oxygen should be given only for cyanosis and generally not at greater than 40 percent concentration during the neonatal period. If cyanosis persists and the condition indicates, the oxygen concentration may be increased above 40 percent. Arterial PO_2 should be measured so as to maintain levels below 100 mmHg and preferably between 50 to 70 mmHg.

PROGNOSIS AND CAUSES OF DEATH

In general, the survival rate is directly proportional to the weight of the infant at birth and the duration of gestation. A 4-lb infant usually has a better chance for survival than one weighing 2 lb. Also, the prognosis improves as the period of gestation is lengthened—the product of a 36-week period of gestation should have a better chance for survival than that from a 30-week period. The poorest prognosis occurs in the infant who is both premature and of low birth weight, that is, an infant who is premature and weighs less than is anticipated for the calculated gestational period.

In addition, the groups that have the highest mortality rates also produce survivors with the largest number of handicaps. Congenital abnormalities are most common in small-for-gestational-age babies as compared to full-sized or even premature babies. Somewhat less than 10 percent of infants born in the nation are low birth weight, and about two-thirds of the infant mortality stems from this group.

Prematurity is the leading primary cause of neonatal deaths. Most of these deaths occur in the first 24 hours, fewer in the second 24 hours, and fewest after that. During the first 48 hours, respiratory failure is the most common precipitating factor; later, infection becomes more frequent as the immediate cause of death.

On postmortem examination, there may not be sufficient evidence to account for the death. As our knowledge increases, biochemical and other studies will probably reveal in such cases an immaturity of physiologic function, incompatible with life. Hypoxia, intracranial hemorrhage (especially intraventricular), hyaline membrane with resorption atelectasis, pneumonia and other infections, congenital malformations, and blood dyscrasias may all be found as the main or contributing factors in mortality.

PREVENTION OF LOW BIRTH WEIGHT

In general, promoting optimal health from birth through the child-bearing age will provide the next generation with the best opportunity for being born at term. Optimal health includes having concerned parents, adequate housing, hygienic surroundings, good nutrition, adequate education, and freedom from or appropriate treatment for serious illness and chronic disease. In addition, good obstetric and neonatal care will reduce morbidity and mortality.

CONDITIONS LEADING TO LOW–BIRTH–WEIGHT INFANTS

Maternal (See p. 182)

Fetal

1. Congenital malformations of the fetus, erythroblastosis fetalis and other blood incompatibilities
2. Chromosomal abnormalities
3. Infections

General or constitutional, i.e., genetic   The most common genetic condition is defective ova, possibly of hereditary origin, which results in habitual abortions or habitual prematurity.

Placental

1. Premature rupture of the membranes
2. Premature separation of the placenta and placenta previa
3. Placental insufficiency: infarcts, etc.

Socioeconomic   Mothers in low socioeconomic groups deliver prematurely more often than those in higher groups. The reason for this is not known.

In the majority of cases, no cause can be found.

PROPHYLACTIC TREATMENT OF LOW–BIRTH–WEIGHT INFANTS

Treatment requires cooperation between obstetrician and pediatrician in instituting specific measures to prevent or relieve the complications of low birth weight.

1. Obstetric care with special attention to diet, correction of anemia, prevention of infection, and appropriate treatment of complications of pregnancy, e.g., toxemia, pyelitis. (The use of drugs other than those necessary for specific treatments should be avoided.)
2. Hypoxia may be prevented by the avoidance of excessive analgesia and general (inhalation and intravenous) anesthesia, by gentle manipulations at delivery, and by proper resuscitation.
3. Hemorrhage may be prevented by proper maternal diet, vitamin K prior to delivery or to the newborn infant after delivery (0.5 to 1 mg is sufficient), and proper obstetric care at delivery.
4. Proper provision of warmth (by incubator or heated crib) in the delivery room, in transit from the delivery room to the nursery, and in the nursery.
5. Minimal handling and then only by specially trained personnel.

TREATMENT OF THE LOW–BIRTH–WEIGHT INFANT

Maintenance of heat

1. The infant should be put in a heated incubator immediately after delivery and not removed unless absolutely necessary.
2. The temperature of the nursery should be about 75 to 80°F (24 to 26.7°C) and that of the incubator 90.5 to 96°F (32.5 to 35.5°C). The smaller infants, weighing less than 1,500 Gm, usually require the higher temperatures.
3. There should be frequent checking of the temperature of the incubator, and the infant's temperature should be watched carefully until it has stabilized to 96 to 97°F, with no more than a 1.5 to 2° variation during the day.
4. Control of humidity is also important. A relative humidity of 50 to 65 percent is recommended.

Maintenance of respiration

1. There should be resuscitation equipment in the delivery room and in the nursery, with personnel trained in its use.
2. Proper methods of resuscitation should be practiced in the treatment of asphyxia. Frequent gentle suctioning of the pharynx should be done by the nurse during the first 24 hours.
3. Oxygen should be given only for the relief of cyanosis.
4. The infant should be observed closely for apnea, cyanosis, and stridor, particularly during the first few days. Respiratory distress is indicated by a significant increase in respiratory rate and by the degree of retraction. A chest roentgenogram should be made if distress is present. (Portable films are satisfactory in most instances.)

At the time of resuscitation in the delivery room, if there is evidence of respiratory failure, sodium bicarbonate (2 to 3 meq per kg by slow intravenous "push" infusion) may be given empirically to combat acidosis. However, if the Apgar score remains below 6 at 5 minutes, in spite of an established adequate airway and appropriate body temperature, and respiratory distress continues, e.g., grunting, retractions, tachypnea, monitored specific treatment should be instituted. An umbilical (artery) catheter is inserted; fluids (glucose 10% in water) and medication, e.g., additional sodium bicarbonate, antibiotics are administered and blood drawn for gas analysis.

The use of a respirator (one allowing continuous positive pressure) to assist ventilation is suggested if respiration fails. Prolonged use of positive-pressure oxygen especially in small prematures may result in deterioration of pulmonary function. (Wilson-Mikity syndrome is the severest form of this condition.) Arterial oxygen tension is best kept between 60 to 100 mmHg pressure.

5. The infant should be in a supine position with a small towel rolled and placed under the shoulders to raise the chest to a level slightly higher than the abdomen.

Prevention of infection   Asepsis is essential, and the following are helpful:

1. A separate unit for low-birth-weight infants—space requirements are 30 sq ft per infant.
2. Separate nursing staff trained in the care of such infants.
3. Running water in the nursery and frequent washing of hands.
4. Individual care of infants, with use of individual supplies—thermometer and equipment—and proper draping of the scale for weighing.
5. Isolation facilities are important.
6. Fresh air from outside the nursery; dust control; use of disinfectants for washing—an effective means of cleaning is by dry vacuuming for dust removal followed by use of wet vacuum pick-up machine.
7. Care of incubators and bassinets includes scrubbing with disinfectant solutions between cases. Gas sterilization of the previously cleaned incubator is the method of choice. Antiseptic surface sprays may also be used after cleansing. Filters on isolettes should be changed frequently (every 2 to 3 weeks). Oxygen tubing should be autoclaved, porthole sleeves removed and washed, and the humidity chamber washed and the water changed between cases. Infants kept in the intensive care nursery for an extended period should be transferred to a clean incubator weekly.
8. Routine prophylactic use of antibiotics is not necessary. Infection leading to pneumonitis and sepsis may occur following prematurely ruptured membranes, prolonged labor, hypoxia, and fetal distress.

In such cases antibiotics may be given to the mother to prevent bacterial contamination of amniotic fluid, fetal membranes, placenta, and fetus.

Proper feeding The important aspects of feeding are the avoidance of fatigue and the aspiration of food. Well-trained nursery personnel are essential. Early feeding (4 to 8 hours of age) is the more accepted routine for the low-birth-weight infant. Early feeding minimizes hypoglycemia, hyperbilirubinemia, and excess catabolism of the small newborn. Infants over 1,250 Gm who do not have respiratory difficulty are fed by nipple. In smaller or more immature infants, feeding by gavage tube inserted through the nose into the stomach is utilized. These tubes may be left in place for 3 to 5 days before replacement by a similar tube in the other nostril.

The amount allowed (2 to 10 ml) varies with the size and clinical appearance of the infant. Glucose 10 percent in water is used initially for two to three feedings. If tolerated well, formula is started. Feedings are given every 3 hours with a gradual increase by 1 to 2 ml per feeding as tolerated. In the very small infant occasionally feeding at 2-hour intervals is indicated. The water requirement of 60 to 80 ml per kg per day is made up by intravenous fluids until the oral intake is sufficient (150 ml per kg per day by 7 to 10 days). After glucose in water feedings, a formula allowing adequate caloric intake is offered. The calorie intake should reach 120 Cal per kg per day by 7 to 10 days, if possible. Current formulas for prematures have some reduction of fat content and electrolyte load. The protein is adjusted to reach 4 Gm per kg per day. Iron-enriched formulas are suggested after feedings are established. When the infant's weight reaches 4½ to 5 lb he may be placed on the vitamin- and iron-enriched formula used in full-term neonates. Feedings are then given every 4 hours.

Hyperalimentation using either peripheral or central (jugular) veins has been suggested for use in smaller infants with complications, i.e., intractable diarrhea. A high-amino-acid, medium-chain triglyceride solution with dextrose 10 percent is used (Aminogen). This solution is hyperosmolar, so it is started as a dilute solution and increased gradually by progressive increments.

Many of the prepared formulas currently available contain adequate vitamin content. If not, at the beginning of the second week, a water-miscible vitamin preparation that contains at least 50-mg ascorbic acid, 400 units of vitamin D, and 3,000 units of vitamin A per dose should be given daily. (The requirement and utilization of iron are described in Chapter 22, "Blood Disorders," under Anemia of Prematurity.)

CRITERIA FOR DISCHARGE FROM HOSPITAL

1. Weight should be a minimum of 5 lb (2,270 Gm).
2. There should be a record of regular weight gain, and the infant's general condition should be good.

3. The home conditions and the parents' ability to care for the baby should have been evaluated and found satisfactory.

PREPARATION FOR DISCHARGE AND CARE AFTER DISCHARGE

1. The teaching of parents should begin while the infant is in the hospital. Mothers should participate in the feeding and care of their infants prior to discharge, and there should be proper preparation of the home before the baby is discharged.
2. There should be continued help to the parents in the home immediately after the baby is discharged (this may be provided by the public health nurse).
3. There should be a plan for medical supervision.

REVIEW QUESTIONS

1. The following statements concerning low-birth-weight infants are true except for one: (a) about two-thirds of such babies are premature; (b) periodic breathing associated with cyanosis is seen normally; (c) initial weight loss is often greater than in full-term infants; (d) ossification of the distal femoral epiphysis is usually absent.
2. The use of high-intensity light in low-birth-weight infants is usually ordered when the indirect bilirubin reaches: (a) 5 to 7 mg per 100 ml; (b) 8 to 10 mg per 100 ml; (c) 15 to 20 mg per 100 ml.
3. The following except one are criteria for an infant of 36 weeks' gestation: (a) good sucking reflex; (b) Moro reflex is reproducible and good; (c) grasp reflex is weak; (d) extremities are held in a flexed position.
4. Intrauterine growth retardation results in (a) a spleen large for weight of the infant; (b) a thymus small for weight of the infant; (c) increased extramedullary hematopoiesis for weight of the infant; (d) complexity of the kidney greater than expected from weight of the infant.
5. The following statements concerning prognosis for low-birth-weight infants are true except for one: (a) prognosis improves as the period of gestation is lengthened; (b) the poorest prognosis occurs in an infant who is both premature and low birth weight; (c) postmortem examination always reveals the cause of the death; (d) prematurity is the leading primary cause of neonatal deaths.
6. Prevention of low birth weight is best accomplished by (a) permitting the gravida to gain weight in an unrestricted fashion; (b) use of intravenous alcohol to stop premature labor; (c) promoting optimal health in population; (d) preventing toxemia of pregnancy.
7. The temperature of the incubator for a low-birth-weight infant should be (a) 75 to 80°F; (b) 80 to 84.5°F; (c) 85 to 90°F; (d) 90.5 to 96°F.
8. Low-birth-weight infants are prone to develop the following except one: (a) hypochromic anemia; (b) rickets; (c) infection; (d) obesity; (e) mental retardation.
9. Proper feeding of the low-birth-weight infant includes all the following except for one: (a) initial feeding at 4 to 8 hours of age; (b) gavage-tube feeding for all low-birth-weight infants; (c) glucose 10% in water is used initially for two

to three feedings; (*d*) caloric intake should reach 120 Cal per kg per day by 7 to 10 days.

10. If there is regular weight gain and the infant's general condition is good, a low-birth-weight infant may be discharged from the hospital when his weight reaches: (*a*) 5 lb; (*b*) 5½ lb; (*c*) 6 lb; (*d*) 6½ lb.

14 INFECTIOUS DISEASES

Infectious diseases may be classified as to etiologic agent: viral, chlamydial, rickettsial, bacterial, mycotic, protozoan, helminthic, etc. (Some of the infectious diseases are discussed in other sections; for example, infectious hepatitis is treated in Chapter 17, "Gastrointestinal Diseases.")

VIRAL INFECTIONS

Viruses are classified into two major groups:

1. DNA viruses. Basic characteristic is their DNA genome.
2. RNA viruses. Basic characteristic is their RNA genome. (See Table 14-1 for classification.)

Table 14-1.   Classification of viruses important to man

Major group	Subgroups	Diseases and/or systems involved
DNA	Papovavirus group 1. Papillomavirus 2. Polyomavirus	1. Verruca (warts) 2. Progressive multifocal leukoencephalopathy
	Adenovirus group 31 types pathogenic for man	1. Mucous membranes, particularly Respiratory tract—URI (adenopharyngeal conjunctival fever Eye—epidemic keratoconjunctivitis GI tract—diarrheal disease 2. Lymphoid tissue—adenitis
	Herpesvirus group 1. Herpes simplex viruses a. Type I	1. a. Meningoencephalitis Gingivostomatitis Eczema herpeticum Dendritic ulcer of the cornea Vulvovaginitis in young children Herpes labialis Traumatic herpes
	b. Type II	b. Herpes progenitalis Congenital herpes
	2. Varicella zoster virus	2. Chickenpox Herpes zoster
	3. Epstein-Barr virus	3. Infectious mononucleosis Burkitt's lymphoma
	4. Cytomegalovirus	4. Cytomegalic inclusion disease—congenital and acquired
	Poxvirus group 1. Variola virus 2. Vaccinia virus	Chiefly pathogenic for skin 1. Smallpox 2. Local vaccinia reactions Generalized vaccinia Vaccinia necrosum (gangrenosa) Eczema vaccinatum Vaccinia encephalitis
	3. Molluscum contagiosum virus	3. Molluscum contagiosum
	4. Animal pox viruses	4. Man may sometimes develop cowpox or monkeypox
RNA	Picorna virus group 1. Rhinoviruses (90 isolated) 2. Coxsackie viruses a. Type A—23 types	1. URI (Common cold) 2. a. Herpangina Hand-foot-mouth disease Aseptic meningitis URI Cardiac disorders—adults and children

Major group	Subgroups	Diseases and/or systems involved
	b. Type B—6 types	Parotitis Summer minor illness Summer exanthem *b.* Pleurodynia Aseptic meningitis Neonatal disease including myocarditis and pericarditis or simply anorexia, fever, and lethargy Other cardiac disorders—adults and children URI Orchitis
	3. Echo viruses—over 30 types	3. Aseptic meningitis Summer exanthem Diarrheal disease in infants "Boston exanthem" Vaginitis and cervicitis
	4. Polioviruses—3 types	4. Abortive polio—URI or GI disorder Nonparalytic polio (aseptic meningitis) Paralytic polio—lower motor neuron damage Bulbar polio—brainstem involvement
Diplornovirus group Reoviruses		1. URI Febrile illness Diarrhea

Myxovirus group	1. Paramyxoviruses
	  a. Parainfluenza virus—4 types
	  b. Respiratory synctial virus
	  c. Measles virus
	  d. Mumps virus
	2. Orthomyxoviruses Influenza virus—types A (A₁, A₂), B and C
		1. *a.* Croup, pneumonia
		  b. Bronchiolitis, pneumonia, URI
		  c. Measles, SSPE
		  d. Mumps
		2. Influenza

Rhabdovirus group Rabies virus Oncornavirus group (leukoviruses)		Rabies Leukemia and sarcoma viruses of mice, cats, and fowl—may be significant for man
Coronavirus group "IBV-like" virus Arenovirus group 1. LCM virus 2. Lasa virus		URI, bronchitis 1. Lymphocytic choriomeningitis 2. Lasa fever

Major group	Subgroups	Diseases and/or systems involved
	3. Machupo virus	3. South American hemorrhagic fevers
	4. Junin virus	4. South American hemorrhagic fevers
	Togavirus group	
	1. Alphaviruses (group A arboviruses)	
	a. Rubella virus	1. *a.* German measles
	b. Equine encephalitis viruses	*b.* Encephalitis
	c. Sindbis virus	*c.* Undifferentiated febrile illness or hemorrhagic fever
	d. Chikungunya virus	*d.* Undifferentiated febrile illness or hemorrhagic fever
	2. Flavoviruses (group B arboviruses)	
	a. Yellow fever virus	*a.* Yellow fever
	b. Hemorrhagic fever viruses	*b.* Encephalitis and hemorrhagic fevers
	c. Japanese B virus	*c.* Encephalitis and hemorrhagic fevers
	d. St. Louis encephalitis virus	*d.* Encephalitis and hemorrhagic fevers
	e. Dengue viruses	*e.* Breakbone (Dengue) fever

MEASLES (Rubeola)

Etiology   Virus.

Mode of transmission   Rubeola is spread usually by droplet infection or contact with secretion from the patient's nose, throat, or eyes.

Incubation period   The disease develops in 10 to 12 days.

Prodromal period (catarrhal stage)   There is a prodrome usually of 3 to 5 days' duration with fever, malaise, cough, conjunctivitis, and coryza. The characteristic Koplik's spots are found toward the end of the prodomal period. These minute white patches of hyperplastic endothelial tissue, surrounded by small areas of erythema, are located most often on the buccal mucous membrane adjacent to the first lower molar teeth. There may also be punctate red areas over the hard palate (enanthem). The blood count shows a leukopenia with a lymphocytic predominance. Early in the course of the illness, scrapings from the nasal mucous membrane may show large multinucleated cells (Warthin-Finkeldey cells) containing inclusion bodies.

Eruptive period An erythematous, maculopapular eruption, appearing behind the ears and then spreading rapidly over the face, neck, arms, and upper trunk, appears 24 to 48 hours after the Koplik's spots. The severity of the disease is related to the extent, intensity, and confluence of the rash. There are usually areas of normal skin between the eruptive areas. The constitutional symptoms and cough subside gradually after the rash has reached its maximum. The rash reaches the lower extremities on the third day and then fades in the order of appearance. Upper respiratory involvement including bronchitis is an integral part of the disease.

Period of convalescence The rash fades, leaving areas of "staining" or increased pigmentation, and there may be fine, branny desquamation. Complications occur most frequently in this period.

Complications Otitis media, cervical lymphadenitis (usually due to β hemolytic streptococci), croup, and pneumonia are not uncommon. Pneumonia may be:

Interstitial—due to the measles virus and most likely representing an inability of the host to produce specific measles antibodies (Hecht's giant-cell pneumonia).

Bronchopneumonia—due to secondary invading bacteria, particularly pneumococcus, staphylococcus, *H. influenza,* and streptococcus.

Children with tuberculosis occasionally have an activation of the tubercular process, and there is a diminished reaction to the tuberculin test lasting 4 to 6 weeks.

Encephalitis is a complication that occurs in about 1 in 1,000 cases. It may appear at any time but generally does after the rash has reached its height. It is characterized by hyperpyrexia, convulsions, and lethargy or coma. The spinal fluid shows a moderate increase in number of cells, predominately lymphocytes. The glucose level is usually normal, but the protein level may be increased. The prognosis is guarded (mortality rate is about 10 percent). In those patients who recover, over 30 percent have residual behavior or motor disturbances.

Subacute sclerosing panencephalitis (SSPE, Dawson's encephalitis) appears to be caused by the measles virus. The disease manifests itself in children and young adults by progressive mental deterioration, myoclonic jerks, and an abnormal EEG.

Prophylaxis ISG usually confers complete temporary immunity if administered in sufficient amount within the first few days after exposure has occurred. When given later or in smaller dosage, ISG can modify an attack of measles (this modified measles generally results in a permanent immunity). The usual dosage for prevention is 0.25 ml per kg; for modification 0.04 ml per kg, to be followed in 2 months by active immunization. If the exposed susceptible child is known to have an impaired immune mechanism, ISG 20 to 30 ml is given. An alternative method of caring for exposed susceptibles would be to give Edmonston B live measles vaccine and ISG 0.02 ml per kg at separate sites.

Modified measles   The incubation period is prolonged and may be as long as 21 days. Few Koplik's spots are seen. Fever is low-grade, and symptoms are mild. The rash is sparse and coryza slight. Complications are rare.

Atypical measles   This may occur in children previously vaccinated with inactivated vaccine and subsequently exposed to the natural virus. It is manifested by fever, edema of the extremities, a maculopapular vesicular, urticarial, or hemorrhagic rash centrifugal in distribution, pneumonia, and toxicity. It has also been reported in children who have received live vaccine.

Treatment   In uncomplicated cases, the general measures discussed in Chapter 6, "Drugs and Treatment," are used. No specific treatment is available.

In cases complicated by otitis media, cervical adenitis, or bronchopneumonia, there is a good response to appropriate antibiotics; however these should not be used prophylactically to prevent infections. Large amounts of ISG (0.6 ml per kg) may be of great benefit for the patients with giant-cell pneumonia. Encephalitis and SSPE can only be treated with supportive measures; ISG is of no value, but corticosteroids may be helpful.

GERMAN MEASLES (Rubella)

Etiology   The cause is a virus.

Mode of transmission   Rubella is spread as in measles.

Incubation period   The disease develops in 14 to 21 days.

Prodomal period   There are either no signs and symptoms or those of mild nasopharyngitis; but postauricular, posterior cervical, and suboccipital adenitis is characteristic. There is either a low-grade fever or none.

Eruptive period   The eruption appears after the onset of adenopathy. It is apt to appear first on the face, spreading rapidly over the entire body, in 2 to 3 hours, involving the head, arms, trunk, and to a lesser extent, the legs. There are pink maculopapules, which, though very numerous, do not tend to form the blotchy confluent patches or irregular outlines that are found in rubeola, but tend to blend as they grow older, to form a diffuse erythematous eruption. The rash thus resembles measles the first day and scarlet fever the second day and fades on the third day (kaleidoscopic rash). An enanthem may be present, with very few petechiae scattered over the surface of the soft palate (Forchheimer's spots).

Complications   Rubella is usually an uncomplicated, self-limiting disease. Thrombocytopenia and encephalitis are rare. Neuritis and arthritis are extremely rare but may occur in older children or adults, who require only symptomatic treatment.

Congenital rubella syndrome   See Chapter 12, "Diseases of the Newborn."

Differential diagnosis   The differential diagnosis from rubeola; ECHO viruses types 9 and 16; Coxsackie viruses types A-9, A-16, and B-5; exanthem subitum; and scarlet fever is found in Tables 14-2 and 14-3. A very similar eruption may occur in infectious mononucleosis, in which there is usually a greater degree of malaise and fever and a more marked and generalized lymphadenopathy. Morphologic study of the blood, the mono-spot test, and the sheep heterophil agglutination test (Paul-Bunnell) are diagnostic for infectious mononucleosis. The latter test should be verified by guinea pig kidney, and beef red cell adsorption tests.

Treatment   No specific treatment is available or required, as rubella is generally a mild disease, with few complications or sequelae. Congenital rubella requires symptomatic and corrective treatment.

EXANTHEM SUBITUM (Roseola Infantum)

Etiology   It is probably a specific virus.

Mode of transmission   The transmission is not definitely known; it is probably by droplet infection from healthy persons who harbor the virus.

Incubation period   Roseola probably develops over 10 to 14 days.

Prodromal period   It usually occurs in the 6-month to 3-year age group. There is a sudden onset, with fever rising as high as 105 to 106°F (40.6 to 41.1°C) without apparent cause. The temperature spikes, and the fever lasts 3 to 4 days. Convulsions may occur at the onset, and there may be marked irritability or drowsiness. The anterior fontanel is often bulging. Suboccipital adenopathy is usually present. A characteristic type of periorbital edema has been described. Occasionally there is a moderate pharyngitis and coryza by the third day. The blood picture is characterized by leukopenia with a lymphocytic and monocytic predominance, although there may be leukocytosis on the first day.

Exanthem   An exanthem appears shortly before or after the temperature reaches normal, on about the third or fourth day. It is an erythematous macular or maculopapular rash starting first on the trunk and spreading rapidly to the arms and neck, with minimal involvement of the legs and face, and fades within 24 to 48 hours. There is no desquamation or staining.

Treatment   There is no specific treatment, and the prognosis is excellent.

ERYTHEMA INFECTIOSUM (Fifth Disease)

Etiology   It is probably virus caused.

Mode of transmission   The disease is presumably spread by droplet infection.

Incubation period   It probably develops in 6 to 14 days.

Clinical features and course   The disease usually occurs in the 2- to 12-year age group. The characteristic feature is the appearance of a rash which erupts in three stages. It first appears on the face as an intense erythema, warm but not tender to the touch, especially on the cheeks (the "slapped face" appearance); there is a circumoral pallor. The rash fades rapidly from the cheeks in 1 to 4 days. A day or two after its appearance on the face, a symmetrical rose-red maculopapular rash appears on the extensor surfaces of the extremities, spreading in a day or two to the trunk and buttocks (the "slapped buttocks" appearance). The rash disappears in 3 to 6 days but may reappear as an evanescent rash after a variable period of time, particularly if the skin is irritated. As the rash progresses, initial lesions on arms and thighs fade centrally, leaving a characteristic lacelike network. Generally there are very minimal or no constitutional symptoms and no complications. The white cell count is within normal limits, but in some cases an eosinophilia may be present.

Prognosis   The prognosis is excellent.

Treatment   There is none indicated.

CHICKENPOX (Varicella)

Etiology   The varicella zoster virus (V-2 virus) is the causative agent.

Mode of transmission   Varicella is spread by direct droplet, or indirect contact within a limited time and space.

Incubation period   It develops in 14 to 16 days with a range of 10 to 21 days.

Prodromal period   Fever, malaise, and anorexia may precede the rash by 24 hours. Rarely there is an atypical prodromal eruption which may be scarlatiniform or morbilliform.

Eruptive stage   The lesions appear in the following order: macular, papular, vesicular, and pustular. The erythematous papules quickly develop into "teardrop" vesicles which in 24 hours become filled with cloudy fluid. The crops of scattered vesicles erupt for 3 to 4 days, starting first on the trunk and spreading rapidly to the face, shoulders, and finally, the extremities. The rash is heaviest on the trunk, thus giving it a centripetal distribution. Different stages and sizes of the lesions are present at the same time and in the same vicinity. The vesicular lesions are very pruritic. At the termination of the eruption these lesions become crusted. (Crusts of chickenpox are noninfectious, in contrast to those of smallpox, which are infectious.) The mucous membranes of the mouth, vagina, urethra, and rectum are often involved. The oral lesions may be found prior to the skin eruption. In severe cases fever may last 3 to 4 days. Rare forms of chickenpox include (1) hemorrhagic varicella (malignant varicella), which occurs usually in patients receiving corticosteroids, patients on immunosuppressive therapy, those with leukemia and other malignancies, or children with immunologic disorders (particularly with loss of delayed hypersensitivity). (2) Varicella neonatorum is usually a benign disease except in those infants with congenital varicella (those whose mothers developed varicella just before or just after birth). In this latter group there is about 20 percent mortality rate, largely due to widespread visceral involvement. (3) Varicella in the adult tends to be a more severe disease with greater constitutional reaction. About 15 percent of adults develop varicella pneumonia, which is potentially fatal.

Differential diagnosis   Differentiation from smallpox is most important (see Table 14-3). In herpes zoster, the eruption has a neural distribution and is painful. In impetigo contagiosum, the vesicles become pustular, form crusts, and become irregularly confluent. They usually appear first about the nose and mouth; in adolescent males, the beard area is most frequently involved. The lesions do not appear in crops and are present only in those areas which may be reached by the

Table 14-2. Diagnostic features of common papulo vesicular diseases

Disease	Incubation period (days)	Prodromal features	Eruption	Other diagnostic features	Laboratory tests
Chickenpox (varicella)	14–16 (10–21) range	0–1 day of fever, anorexia, headache, malaise	Rapid evolution of macules to papules, vesicles, crusts; all stages simultaneously present; lesions superficial, unilocular and nonumbilicated; centripetal distribution; appear in crops	Lesions on scalp and mucous membranes, crusts noninfectious, generalized lymphadenopathy	Specific complement fixation and virus neutralization in tissue culture
Smallpox (variola)	8–12 (7–8) range	1–5 days of fever, severe headache, malaise, chills, backache, prostration	Slow evolution of macules to papules, vesicles, pustules, crusts; all lesions in same stage; lesions deepseated, multilocular, and umbilicated, distribution centrifugal	Toxicity, mucous membrane lesions, especially mouth and throat, crusts infectious	Virus isolation on chorioallantoic membranes of chick embryos, complement fixation
Herpes zoster		Sensitivity, itching, pain along course of affected nerve	Erythema and vesicles scattered along dermatone of affected nerve; unilateral	Regional adenopathy, lack of constitutional signs, neuralgia in adults	Specific complement fixation and neutralization
Hand, foot, and mouth disease	3–5	1–2 days of fever, malaise	Papules and vesicles scattered all over the body especially interdigitally on the dorsum of the hands, feet, and on the palms and soles, also perianally	Caused by Coxsackie A–16 primarily—also reportedly caused by A–4, A–5, A–10. Lesions on mucous membranes of mouth, particularly mucosa and tongue, less on palate, gums, and lips	Virus isolation from throat washings or stool
Impetigo (a) contagiosa	2–5	None	(a) At first, vesicular then confluent, rapidly progresses to pustular and crusting; honey-colored crusts;	(a) If severe, fever and malaise, commonly involves nasolabial area; (b) commonly involves lower abdomen; no mucous-membrane lesions in either	Bacterial cultures of lesions
(b) bullosa			(b) Vesicles or pustules, cloudy bullae, discrete small areola of erythema, no crusts		
Molluscum contagiosum		None	Scattered, discrete, waxy, firm and small pustules with central umbilication, no surrounding areola, substance easily extruded; not on palms or soles	No enanthem, no constitutional symptoms	Characteristic cytoplasmic inclusion bodies
Eczema herpeticum and eczema vaccinatum		None	Vesiculopustular lesions in area of eczema or other chronic skin lesions; umbilicated lesions in eczema vaccinatum	Severe constitutional symptoms including fever and toxicity	Herpes simplex virus isolated in tissue culture; vaccinia virus isolated on chorioallantoic membrane of chick embryo
Rickettsialpox	7–10, up to 14	Papule at site of mite bite—vesicle—eschar 1 week after papule, fever, chills, muscle pains last 3–4 days	Papulovesicular lesions, generalized but spares palms and soles; small vesicles superimposed on papules; most do not form crusts	Regional adenopathy, occasional splenomegaly	WBC low, complement fixation, negative Weil-Felix

Table 14-3. Diagnostic features of common maculopapular diseases

Disease	Incubation period (days)	Prodromal features	Eruption	Other diagnostic features	Laboratory tests
Measles (rubeola)	10–12 (7–14) range	3–5 days of fever, coryza, conjunctivitis, and cough; Koplik's spots appear 1 or 2 days before exanthem	Maculopapular, coalescent and purplish-red; begins on head and neck, spreads downward; in 5 to 6 days rash brownish, desquamating	Koplik's spots on buccal mucosa; enanthem on palate; toxic fever drops when rash full-blown	WBC low; complement fixation and virus neutralization in tissue culture; HI antibody
German measles (rubella)	14–21 (up to 25)	Little or no prodrome; may have mild fever, 1–2 days of rhinitis and pharyngitis and lymphadenopathy	Maculopapular, pink; begins on head and neck, spreads downward, fades in 3 days; no desquamation; kaleidoscopic (morbilliform 1st day, scarletiniform 2d day, fades 3d day)	Lymphadenopathy, post-auricular and/or occipital; afebrile, not toxic	WBC normal or low; virus neutralization in tissue culture; HI antibody
Scarlet fever	2–5 (up to 7)	½–2 days of malaise, sore throat, fever, vomiting	Generalized, punctate, orange-red; prominent on neck, in axilla, groin, skin folds, spares face; circumoral pallor; sheetlike desquamation particularly involves hands and feet	Strawberry tongue, exudative tonsillitis, malar flush, Pastia's sign	Group A β-hemolytic streptococci cultures from throat; antistreptolysin O titer rise
Exanthem subitum (roseola infantum)	10–14 (up to 17)	3–4 days of high fever. Begins abruptly with fever and often a convulsion	As fever falls by crisis, pink maculopapules appear on chest and trunk, spreads to face; fades in 1–3 days	Occipital adenopathy (small), 6-mo–3-yr age group	WBC low
Fifth disease (erythema infectiosum)	6–14	None	Red, flushed cheeks; circumoral pallor, rose maculopapules on extremities; lacy appearance on fading; fades in 3–6 days	"Slapped-face" appearance. 2- to 12-year age group. Rash tends to reappear	Eosinophilia may be present
Meningococcemia	2–5	Hours of fever, vomiting, headache	Maculopapules, petechiae, purpuric spots	Meningeal signs, toxic, confused	Cultures of blood, cerebro-spinal fluid
Rocky Mountain spotted fever	2–12	3–4 days of fever, chills, severe headaches	Maculopapules, petechiae, distribution centrifugal	History of tick bite	Agglutination (OX19, OX2), complement fixation
Typhus fever	8–12 (7–14)	3–4 days of fever, chills, severe headaches	Maculopapules, petechiae, distribution centripetal	Endemic area, lice	Agglutination (OX19), complement fixation
Infectious mononucleosis	9–14	Fever, adenopathy, sore throat	Maculopapular rash resembling rubella, rarely papulovesicular	Splenomegaly, exudative tonsillitis, occasional jaundice, marked cervical adenopathy	Atypical lymphs in blood smears (at least 10%); heterophile agglutination

267

Table 14-3. Continued

Disease	Incubation period (days)	Prodromal features	Eruption	Other diagnostic features	Laboratory tests
Enterovirus infections (ECHO, Coxsackie) (Summer exanthem)	2–5	1–2 days of fever, malaise; sometimes abrupt onset, fever 102–105°F, abdominal and muscle pain, vomiting and diarrhea	Maculopapular rash resembling rubella, rarely papulovesicular, discrete sometimes coalescent	Aseptic meningitis; enanthem on faucial pillars, uvula, posterior pharynx and soft palate and may be associated with pleurodyina, pericarditis or myocarditis, particularly common in summer and fall	Virus isolation from pharynx, stool, or CSF; CF titer rise
Drug eruption		Occasional fever	Maculopapular rash resembling rubella, rarely papulovesicular; occasionally erythema multiforme with "iris" and "target" lesions	Edema of mucous membranes. May have lesions of conjunctivae and mouth Stevens-Johnson syndrome	Eosinophilia

patient's contaminated fingers. There is an absence of constitutional symptoms. Vesicular eruptions occasionally caused by ECHO 9 and Coxsackie A-4, 5, 9, 16, and B-3 viruses may present difficulties in differential diagnosis. Eczema herpeticum, eczema vaccinatum, and rickettsialpox may also be difficult to differentiate.

Complications

1. Encephalitis is rare and often manifests itself as cerebellar ataxia. The pathologic picture is similar to other postinfectious encephalitides.
2. Bacterial infections include (*a*) secondary infections of the lesions (staphylococcus, β streptococci), (*b*) otitis media, (*c*) pneumonia, (*d*) septicemia, (*e*) suppurative arthritis, and (*f*) osteomyelitis.
3. Postvaricella acute glomerulonephritis has been reported.
4. Exacerbation of primary tuberculosis and diminished reaction to tuberculin lasting about 10 days.

Prevention There is no prevention for the normal child. Zoster Immune Globulin (ZIG) is available on specific request from the Center for Disease Control (CDC) for the high-risk child (i.e., those on steroids or immunosuppressants, those with leukemia and other malignancies, and those with immunologic disorders, particularly with loss of delayed hypersensitivity). ISG (0.6 to 1.2 ml per kg) may be used for high-risk patients when ZIG is not available.

Treatment Pruritus is relieved locally by starch baths, calamine lotion, or baking-soda pastes, and systematically by antihistamine by mouth. (For the high-risk child drugs not yet proved include idoxuridine (IDU), cytosine arabinoside (Ara-C), or adenine arabinoside (Ara-A).)

Public health aspects Probably no effort should be made to prevent the disease in childhood except in those high-risk cases as previously mentioned or in their adult associates, since the disease in this group tends to be more severe.

HERPES ZOSTER

Etiology The agent is the V-Z virus. Zoster represents a local reactivation of a latent infection. Varicella and zoster are different clinical manifestations caused by the same virus.

Mode of transmission Zoster is spread by droplet infection. Susceptible exposed individuals may develop chickenpox. It is not as contagious as varicella.

Prodromal period   The prodrome is usually 1 to 3 days in duration, with generalized malaise and fever. There may be no symptoms. Burning or itching along the nerve route may occur, but this is unusual in children.

Eruptive stage   Papules appear which rapidly progress to form vesicles and then dry with scab formation in 5 to 10 days. The lesions are unilateral and are distributed along the course of a nerve. Most commonly the thoracic spinal, the 5th cranial, or the 7th cranial nerves are involved. Localized lymphadenopathy is present. In children, pain and tenderness are not so prominent as in adults. The disease is self-limited, usually lasting several weeks.

Complications   When the 5th cranial nerve is involved there may be damage to the cornea. Peripheral paralysis is a rare complication. In the Ramsay Hunt syndrome (involvement of the geniculate ganglion), there are vesicles in the external auditory canal, facial paralysis, sensory loss of taste in the anterior two-thirds of the tongue, and occasionally loss of hearing and disturbance of equilibrium.

Treatment   There is no specific therapy, only symptomatic relief of pain.

HERPES SIMPLEX INFECTION (Herpes Virus Hominus)

Two types of herpes virus are distinguished by biologic and antigenic differences. Type 1 commonly infects the oral mucosa; type 2 commonly infects the genitalia and the neonate. Infections are primary or recurrent. Primary infection infrequently results in illness, but if it does, its usual manifestation is acute gingivostomatitis in the preschool child. Less-frequent forms of primary infection are vulvovaginitis, meningoencephalitis, keratoconjunctivitis, and traumatic herpes. Disseminated herpetic infection of the neonate is variable in outcome, ranging from mild to fatal. Three routes of transmission are postulated for the neonate: transplacental (rare), ascension from the vulva or cervix, and contact during passage through the birth canal (most common). Recurrent herpes is characterized by lesions usually at the mucocutaneous junction of the lip (fever blisters, cold sores) or genitalia which reappear with stress, fever, cold, etc.

See Table 14-4 for laboratory findings.

HERPETIC GINGIVOSTOMATITIS (Vincent's Stomatitis)

Etiology   The disease is caused by the herpes simplex virus.

Table 14-4. Laboratory diagnosis of viral, chlamydial, and rickettsial diseases

Disease	Human specimens to be tested	TC or animals to be inoculated	Route	Tissue to be harvested for passage	Positive result in test system: signs and pathology	Type of test	Source of virus or antigen
				Arthropod-borne			
Encephalitides: California St. Louis Japanese B						Nt in mice or TC	Mouse brain or TC
						CF	Mouse brain or TC
Western equine							
Eastern equine						Hi	Infant mouse brain
Venezuelan Russian spring/ summer West Nile fever Bwamba, etc.	Brain, blood	Mice	Intracerebral	Brain	Encephalitis		
Yellow fever	Blood, viscera	Monkeys Mice	Intraperitoneal Intracerebral	Viscera Brain	Hepatic necrosis Encephalitis	Nt	Mouse brain
Dengue	Blood	Mice (difficult)	Intracerebral	Brain	Encephalomyelitis	Nt, CF	Mouse brain
Sandfly fever	Blood	Infant mice	Intracerebral	Brain	Encephalomyelitis	Nt, CF	Mouse brain
Colorado tick fever	Blood	Hamsters Mice	Intraperitoneal Intracerebral	Brain Brain	Encephalitis Encephalitis	Nt CF	Mouse brain Mouse brain
				Neurotropic, non-arthropod-borne			
Poliomyelitis	Spinal cord, feces, throat swabbings	TC		Fluid of infected culture	Cytopathic effect	Nt, CF	TC
Rabies	Brain	Mice	Intracerebral	Brain	Encephalitis, Negri inclusion bodies in cytoplasm	IF	

Table 14-4. Continued

Disease	Primary isolation of virus					Diagnostic serologic tests	
	Human specimens to be tested	TC or animals to be inoculated	Route	Tissue to be harvested for passage	Positive result in test system: signs and pathology	Type of test	Source of virus or antigen
Lymphocytic choriomeningitis	Brain, blood, spinal fluid	Mice	Intracerebral	Brain	Encephalitis and choroiditis	Nt	Mouse brain
		Guinea pig	Intraperitoneal	Spleen	Death with pneumonia, focal infiltration in liver	CF	Guinea pig spleen
Human papovavirus	Brain	TC			Cytopathic effect	HI	TC
Measles	Brain	Direct exam (or cocultivation in tissue culture)				IF	
Dermotropic							
Variola	Skin lesions, vesicle fluid, blood	Embryonated egg	CAM	CAM	Pocks on membrane, cytoplasmic inclusion bodies	CF, HI, ID	Vesicle fluid or crusts from patient against standard serum for rapid results
Vaccinia	Skin lesions, vesicle fluid	Embryonated egg	CAM	CAM	Pocks on membrane	CF	CAM, rabbit skin or testicle, or mouse brain
		Rabbit	Intracutaneous	Skin	Skin lesion, cytoplasmic inclusion bodies	Nt in eggs, rabbits, mice; HI	
Varicella	Vesicle fluid	TC		Cells of infected culture	Intranuclear inclusions in skin lesions and in TC	CF, Nt	TC
Zoster	Vesicle fluid	TC		Cells of infected culture	Intranuclear inclusions	CF	TC
Measles	Nasopharyngeal secretions, blood	TC		TC fluid	Multinuclear giant cells and intranuclear inclusions	CF, Nt	TC
Rubella	Nasopharyngeal secretions, blood, amniotic fluid	TC		TC fluid	Interference, or cytopathic effect	Nt, CF, HI, IF, ID	TC

Disease	Specimens	Isolation host	Route	Material tested	Pathologic changes	Serologic tests	Other
Congenital rubella syndrome	Throat swab, urine, feces, spinal fluid, blood, bone marrow, conjunctival swab	TC		TC fluid	Interference, or cytopathic effect	Nt, CF, HI, IF	TC
Exanthem subitum	Blood	Monkeys	Intravenous	Blood	Experimental exanthem		
Herpes simplex	Skin lesions, brain	Mouse (newborn), Embryonated egg, TC	Intracerebral, CAM	Brain, Allantoic fluid, Fluid	Encephalitis / Pocks } Intranuclear inclusion bodies; Cytopathic effect	Nt in mice, eggs, or TC; CF; CF	Mouse brain, allantoic fluid; Allantoic fluid; TC

Respiratory and parotid

Disease	Specimens	Isolation host	Route	Material tested	Pathologic changes	Serologic tests	Other
Influenza A, Influenza B, Influenza C	Nasal washings, lung	Eggs, Ferrets, mice, TC	Amniotic and allantoic sacs, Intranasal	Embryonic fluids, Lung, Fluid phase	Hemagglutinin produced, Pneumonitis, Cytopathic effect, hemadsorption	HI; CF; Nt in eggs, mice, or TC	Allantoic fluid; Allantoic fluid; Allantoic fluid, mouse lung, TC
Parainfluenza		TC			Hemadsorption	Nt, CF	TC
Respiratory syncytial (RS) infection		TC			Multinucleate giant cells with cytoplasmic inclusions	Nt, CF	TC
Common cold (rhinovirus group)	Nasopharyngeal washings, swabs	TC		TC fluid	Cytopathic effect	Nt	TC
Mumps	Saliva, spinal fluid, urine	Monkeys, Eggs, TC	Parotid gland, Amniotic and yolk sacs	Parotid gland, Amniotic fluid yolk sac, Fluid phase	Parotitis, Hemagglutinin produced, Cytopathic effect	CF; HI; Nt in TC	Amniotic fluid, Monkey parotid gland, TC
Adenovirus group	Pharyngeal washings, stool	TC		TC fluid and cells	Cytopathic effect	CF, Nt, HI	TC

Table 14-4. Continued

Disease	Human specimens to be tested	Primary isolation of virus				Diagnostic serologic tests	
		TC or animals to be inoculated	Route	Tissue to be harvested for passage	Positive result in test system: signs and pathology	Type of test	Source of virus or antigen
Hepatic							
Infectious hepatitis (type A)	Blood, feces	(No satisfactory experimental system.)					
Serum hepatitis (type B)	Blood, feces, urine	(No satisfactory experimental system.)				CIE, CF, ID, RIA	Serum, feces, urine
Miscellaneous							
Coxsackie infection	Feces, throat washings, spinal fluid	Infant mice	Subcutaneous	Muscle	Paralysis with myositis with certain types, encephalitis, stomatitis; pancreatitis	Nt in infant mice or TC	Mouse muscle
		TC		TC fluid	Cytopathic effect	Nt, CF, HI	TC
ECHO virus infection	Feces, throat swabbings, spinal fluid	TC		TC fluid	Cytopathic effect	Nt, CF, HI	TC
Reovirus infection	Feces, throat swabbings	TC		TC fluid	Cytopathic effect	Nt, CF, HI	TC
Molluscum contagiosum	Skin lesions	(No satisfactory experimental animal. Characteristic cytoplasmic inclusion bodies. Elementary bodies can be seen in the electron microscope.)					
Verrucae (warts)	Skin lesions	(No satisfactory experimental animal. Electron-microscopic examination of warts shows elementary bodies.)					
Epidemic keratoconjunctivitis	Conjunctivas	TC		TC cells and fluid	Cytopathic effect	Nt test for adenovirus 8	TC
Cytomegalic (inclusion) disease	Oral swabs, urine, various organs	TC		TC fluid and cells	Cytopathic effect, inclusion bodies	Nt, CF	TC

Chlamydiae

Disease	Specimen	Culture/Inoculation	Route	Material examined	Findings	Serology	
Psittacosis	Blood, sputum, lung tissue	Mice, Yolk sac, Embryonated egg	Intranasal, Intraabdominal, Intracerebral	Viscera, Brain, Yolk sac suspension	Typical basophilic inclusion bodies	CF	Mouse brain, Mouse viscera
Lymphogranuloma venereum	Pus	Mice yolk sac, TC	Intracerebral	Brain, Yolk sac suspension, TC cells	Frei Test—Cytopathic effect of intradermal test on patient—antigen preparation from infected yolk sac, control from noninfected yolk sac, positive test 7 mm or greater of induration reaching maximum at 4 days		
Tric Agents 1. Trachoma 2. Inclusion conjunctivitis (blenorrhea)	Eye discharge (1 and 2), Cervical swab (female) / Urethral swab (male) (2)	TC, Yolk sac of embryonated egg		TC cells, Yolk sac suspension	Intracytoplasmic inclusion bodies	CF, IF	Conjunctiva epithelial cells

Rickettsiae

Disease	Specimen	Culture/Inoculation	Route	Material examined	Findings	Serology	
Rocky Mountain spotted fever	Blood	Guinea pigs, Embryonated egg	Intraperitoneal, Yolk sacs	Viscera, scrotum, Yolk sac suspension	Fever, scrotal swelling, hemorrhagic necrosis, death; Antigen product	CF, OX19, OX2	Yolk sac suspension
Rickettsialpox	Blood	Guinea pigs, Embryonated egg	Intraperitneal, Yolk sacs	Viscera, scrotum, Yolk sac suspension	As above	CF, Weil-Felix negative	Yolk sac suspension

Table 14-4. Continued

Disease	Human specimens to be tested	Primary isolation of virus				Diagnostic serologic tests	
		TC or animals to be inoculated	Route	Tissue to be harvested for passage	Positive result in test system: signs and pathology	Type of test	Source of virus or antigen
Typhus fever (epidemic and endemic)	Blood	Guinea pigs Embryonated egg	Intraperitoneal Yolk sacs	Viscera, scrotum, Yolk sac suspension	As above	CF OX19	
Scrub typhus	Blood	Guinea pigs Embryonated egg Mice	Intraperitoneal Yolk sacs Intraperitoneal	Viscera, scrotum Yolk sac suspension Peritoneal exudate	Fever, scrotal swelling, hemorrhagic necrosis, death Antigen product Organisms seen on smear	CF OXK	
Q fever	Blood	Guinea pigs Embryonated egg	Intraperitoneal Yolk sacs	Viscera, scrotum Yolk sac suspension	Fever, scrotal swelling, hemorrhagic necrosis, death Antigen product	CF Weil-Felix negative	

KEY: (TC, tissue culture. Nt, neutralization. CF, complement fixation. HI, hemagglutination inhibition. CAM, chorioallantoic membrane. ID, immunodiffusion. IF, immunofluorescence. CIE ,counterimmunoelectrophoresis. RIA, radioimmunoassay)

Incubation period   Incubation is from 2 to 12 days, usually 4.

Prodromal period   There may be an acute onset, with high fever (103 to 104°F—39.4 to 40.0°C) and soreness of the mouth. Frequently the onset is insidious, with irritability preceding the eruption of the oral lesions.

Eruption   The gums are red, and there are vesicular lesions on the mucous membranes and tongue. The vesicles quickly rupture, leaving small ulcerations, which become covered by grayish-white plaques. A fetid odor from the mouth is characteristic. Occasionally there is bleeding of the gums.

Other clinical features   Quite constantly there is submaxillary lymphadenopathy. Food is refused, and dehydration and acidosis may follow. The illness is self-limiting, usually lasting about 10 days.

Laboratory findings   See Table 14-4, Laboratory Diagnosis of Viral, Chlamydial, and Rickettsial Diseases.

Treatment   The treatment of keratoconjunctivitis is local application of idoxuridine (IDU). In meningoencephalitis, parenteral IDU has been tried with variable success.

ECZEMA HERPETICUM AND ECZEMA VACCINATUM

Eczema herpeticum (Kaposi's varicelliform eruption) is a herpes simplex virus infection in children with eczema. Eczema vaccinatum is a secondary involvement of an eczema with the vaccinia virus, contracted either from vaccination or from contact with a newly vaccinated child.

Clinical features

1. These conditions occur in children with eczema or other chronic skin disorders.
2. There is a generalized vesiculopustular rash, which appears quite suddenly.
3. The condition is very toxic in both instances, and the patients have high temperatures.
4. Secondary bacterial infection may occur.

Differential diagnosis   Kaposi's varicelliform eruption and eczema vaccinatum can be differentiated only by history and by laboratory studies that demonstrate the virus or its antibodies. (A third condition that may be difficult to differentiate is generalized vaccinia, which occurs 9 to 14 days after vaccination and not necessarily in a child with eczema.)

Treatment

1. The fluid and electrolyte balance should be maintained.
2. In cases of eczema vaccinatum, vaccinia hyperimmune globulin (VIG) is of value. In severe cases methisazone should also be given.
3. Chemotherapy and antibiotics may be indicated for the control of complicated pyogenic infection.

Prognosis   The prognosis is guarded.

LYMPHOCYTIC CHORIOMENINGITIS (LCM)

Etiology   The disease is caused by a virus.

Mode of transmission   An animal reservoir exists in infected house and field mice. Transmission is by ingestion or inhalation of food or dust contaminated by feces, urine, or nasopharyngeal secretions of infected mice. Transmission by insects or from man to man is questionable.

Incubation period   It probably develops in 8 to 21 days.

Clinical features

1. A grippelike illness may precede the onset of the meningeal signs and symptoms, or there may be a sudden onset.
2. There is usually a mild course which lasts 5 to 15 days. Occasionally the course is severe and even fatal.

Diagnosis   Diagnosis is by laboratory findings (see Table 14-4).

Treatment   No specific treatment is available.

RABIES

Etiology   The causative agent is a virus.

Mode of transmission   Rabies is spread by the bite of a rabid animal, including dogs, bats, skunks, foxes, cattle, cats, squirrels, chipmunks, rats, and mice.

Incubation period   It develops in 10 to 40 days; rarely, up to 1 year.

Clinical features

1. The onset occurs several weeks to several months after the victim has been bitten. If the bite is on the head or neck, the incubation period is usually short.

2. For 1 to 2 days there may be numbness and tingling of the involved skin area.
3. This is followed by either irritability and excitation or depression.
4. Muscle spasm, particularly of the throat, may occur at the mere sight of food or water (hydrophobia), and there is increased salivation.
5. Temperature is elevated to 102 to 104°F (38.9 to 40.0°C).
6. Finally there are convulsions, paralysis, coma, and death.

Diagnostic tests

1. Recovery of virus from saliva or tissues of the infected person
2. Demonstration of Negri bodies in brain nerve cells

Prophylaxis   The spread of rabies is controlled by proper care and control of dogs and other domestic animals.

Treatment

1. Locally, the wound should be scrubbed and flushed with water and then washed with soap or detergent, followed by application of antiseptic solution, e.g., Povidone-iodine solution.
2. The animal should be impounded and observed for 10 days for evidence of rabies.
3. Frequently it is very difficult to decide whether or not to use the specific therapy since it is associated with some risk and is of limited effectiveness. Such factors as prevalence of rabies in the area, whether or not the animal was provoked to bite, and the species of animal involved will influence the decision. The victim should be given specific treatment immediately if the dog is unknown, rabid, or suspected to be rabid, or if the bite is about the head and neck.

    Passive immunization is started with hyperimmune rabies serum (1,000 units per 40 lb). Part of the serum should be used to infiltrate the wound. (Since only horse serum is available, a careful history should be obtained and a sensitivity test performed before administration.) The wound should be left open; antitetanus prophylaxis is also indicated.

    Active immunization is started concomitantly using duck embryo vaccine subcutaneously (alternating the site—abdominal wall, thighs, and back). In mild exposure, single injections are given for 14 days; in severe exposure, double dose or two separate injections are given daily for 7 days, and thereafter single injections for an additional 7 days. Recall injections should follow in 10 and 20 days. Fever, nausea, and headache contraindicate further injections. Such reactions usually precede encephalitis, which is an infrequent complication. Experimental tissue culture attenuated live virus vaccine is presently undergoing field trials.

4. Once the disease has developed, vaccines are of no value. The patient should be given sedatives and kept in a dark, quiet room.

Prognosis   The prognosis is poor.

MUMPS (Epidemic Parotitis)

Etiology   Mumps is caused by a virus, specifically the myxovirus group.

Mode of transmission   Mumps is spread as in measles.

Incubation period   The incubation period is 14 to 21 days, with an average of 18 days.

Prodromal period   There may be a prodrome which lasts 1 to 2 days, with fever, anorexia, headache, vomiting, and generalized muscle aches and pains. The temperature usually rises to 102 to 103°F (38.9 to 39.4°C) as the salivary-gland involvement becomes apparent. The white cell count shows a lymphocytic predominance, but the total count may be within normal limits or slightly elevated.

Salivary glands

Parotid glands   The involvement may be unilateral at the onset but often becomes bilateral. There is a brawny, painful, tender swelling, with the lobe of the ear in the center of the swelling. The ear is pushed outward. There may be trismus and dysphagia. Edema and injection of the buccal orifice of Stensen's duct may be noted. The parotid swelling reaches its maximum in about 3 days and then slowly subsides.

Submaxillary glands   These glands may be involved alone, occasionally with the sublinguals, but most often with the parotids.

Laboratory findings   A presumptive test is elevation of serum amylase. Confirmatory tests include:

1. Recovery of virus from saliva, mouth washings, or cerebrospinal fluid early in the course of meningoencephalitis.
2. Fourfold increase in complement-fixing (CF) or hemagglutination inhibition (HI) antibody titer in convalescent serum.
3. Virus neutralization test (this test is the most indicative of susceptibility or immunity to the virus).
4. The skin-test antigen is not very reliable.

Complications

Mumps meningoencephalitis This complication may occur before, after, or without parotid swelling. Most cases are very mild, with few symptoms or none. Patients often complain only of headache, occasionally severe; there may be vomiting, irritability or lethargy, and elevated temperature. The signs of meningeal irritation may or may not be present. Rarely there is paresis of the bladder, myelitis, or rapidly ascending transverse myelitis (Landry's paralysis) necessitating the use of a respirator.

The spinal-fluid pressure is increased, with a lymphocytosis (10 to 1,500 cells) protein is increased; sugar level is usually normal but rarely is low; and the serum CF and HI tests are positive, with a rising titer when repeated in 2 weeks.

Treatment for the meningoencephalitis is not specific. Lumbar puncture may be used to relieve increased intracranial pressure.

Epididymoorchitis This is rarely found before puberty. It may appear during the first 8 days of mumps. The onset is accompanied by chills, recurrence of fever, and marked tender swelling of one or both testicles. The pain may be referred over the course of the spermatic cord and is very severe because of the lack of elasticity of the tunica albuginea, which does not permit the inflamed testicle to swell. Pressure necrosis of the testicles may lead to atrophy. Since the orchitis is usually unilateral, infertility is not a frequent sequela.

Adrenal corticosteroids for 5 to 7 days may be helpful in severe orchitis. Ice bags are applied locally, and codeine is given for the relief of pain.

Oophoritis This complication may or may not be accompanied by parotid swelling. There are lower abdominal pain and tenderness. As a rule, this complication occurs only in adult or adolescent females. The involved ovary may be palpably swollen and tender on bimanual examination. Oophoritis does not result in infertility, because the ovary is not confined in a fibrous envelope. In treatment, adrenal corticosteroids may be helpful; ice bags and codeine are used for the relief of pain.

Mumps pancreatitis There are fever, epigastric pain, severe vomiting, and abdominal distension. Levels of serum and urinary amylase may be elevated but are not diagnostic since inflammation of the salivary glands may induce these rises; serum-lipase studies are more significant of pancreatic involvement. In treatment, nothing is given by mouth for 24 to 48 hours, but fluids and electrolytes are given intravenously to prevent dehydration and acidosis. Acute pancreatitis may also be caused by trauma, acute infection, or obstruction of the duct by roundworms.

Other rare complications include myocarditis, pericarditis, arthritis, hepatitis, and unilateral nerve deafness.

Differential diagnosis   Mumps must be differentiated from cervical adenitis; mixed tumor of parotid; suppurative parotitis; recurrent nonsuppurative parotitis (recurrent episodes of parotid swelling, unilateral or bilateral, of unknown etiology but possibly due to allergy, onset about 2 to 3 years of age, with no constitutional signs and usually subsiding at adolescence); calculus in Stensen's duct, which may be visualized on roentgenograms and is clinically manifested by a swelling of the parotid gland following ingestion of food; Mikulicz's disease, which is a bilateral, painless enlargement of the parotid and lacrimal glands, accompanied by dryness of the mouth and an absence of tears (this is probably a uveoparotid sarcoidosis).

Treatment   Only the general measures previously discussed are necessary.

Public health aspects   Probably no attempt at prevention should be made in children, since the severe complications occur most frequently in adults. Mumps immune globulin (MIG) is available, but protection after its administration is questionable.

PICORNAVIRUSES (Enteroviruses and Rhinoviruses)

Poliomyelitis, Coxsackie, and ECHO viruses as well as rhinoviruses share common properties such as similar seasonal incidence and epidemiologic pattern and size. They share the ability to produce the clinical syndrome of viral meningitis. Certain ECHO and Coxsackie agents can even produce paralytic disease.

COXSACKIE VIRUS INFECTIONS

There are two groups of Coxsackie viruses: Group A with 23 immunologic types and group B with 6 immunologic types. The incubation period ranges from 2 to 14 days.

Group A viruses produce the following syndromes:

1. Herpangina is characterized by typical lesions in the pharynx, anterior pillars, and tonsillar fauces that are vesicular and surrounded by an areola. They persist for 2 or 3 days and then rupture, leaving a whitish-gray ulcer. There are associated constitutional symptoms, e.g., anorexia, malaise, and high fever.
2. Hand, foot, and mouth disease is characterized by vesicular lesions in the oral cavity and on the extremities (A-16, occasionally A-5).

3. Lymphonodular pharyngitis is associated with fever and small yellowish-white nodules on the anterior pillars and posterior pharynx (A-10).

Group B viruses cause:

1. Epidemic myalgia, or pleurodynia (Bornholm's disease), is characterized by an abrupt onset, severe pain in chest, abdomen, and shoulders, a brief but often recrudescent febrile course, and complete recovery. The highest incidence of the disease occurs in summer and early fall.
2. Myocarditis occurring in infants.
3. Myocarditis and pericarditis occurring in older age groups (to be differentiated from rheumatic fever and other forms of myocarditis).

Group A or B viruses may be responsible for the following illnesses:

1. Acute respiratory illness ranging from URI to pneumonia.
2. Nonspecific febrile illness with or without rash. The rash may be maculopapular or vesicular.
3. Aseptic meningitis and paralytic diseases, resembling poliomyelitis.

Diagnosis depends on isolation of the Coxsackie virus and demonstration of a definite rise in complement-fixing and neutralizing antibodies.

Treatment   There is no specific treatment.

ECHO VIRUS INFECTIONS

There may be respiratory, intestinal, skin, mucous membrane, and neurologic manifestations of varying degree, depending on the offending strain of virus.

Etiology   Over 30 serologically different antigenic strains of ECHO (Enteric Cytopathogenic Human Orphan, E) viruses have been recognized. ECHO viruses 2, 3, 4, 5, 6, 7, 9, 11, 14, 16, 17, 18, 20, and 30 have been particularly implicated in outbreaks among infants and children. Types 3, 4, 6, 9, 11, 14, 16, and 18 have frequently occurred in epidemic form. It is most likely that other types, although usually sporadic, may also appear in outbreaks. Like all enteroviruses, ECHO virus disease is most prevalent in the summer and early fall in temperate zones.

Incubation period   Incubation is about 3 to 5 days but may be longer.

Clinical features

1. Nonspecific febrile illness with or without rash; many types have been associated with this syndrome. Types 4, 6, 9, and 16 have frequently been associated with a maculopapular rash and occasionally petechiae (particularly type 9). Type 9 outbreaks have been common including the following clinical syndrome; fever, coryza exudative tonsillitis with a rash appearing during the febrile phase, and an enanthem consisting of small yellow and gray-white lesions on the buccal mucosa or tonsillar pillars. The rash consists of 1- to 3-mm pink macules or maculopapules that appear first on the face or face and neck and spread to the shoulders and chest in 6 to 12 hr. At times it involves the entire body. It lasts from 1 to 10 days, is seldom pruritic, deepens to a pink tan, and does not desquamate. At times it is petechial. Conjunctivitis may also be present. E16 may cause the syndrome known as Boston exanthem which is striking in its similarity to roseola infantum; i.e., the rash appears when the fever subsides. Patients, however, are usually older children and adults who also complain of sore throat, headache, and abdominal pain. The fever is lower than in roseola and there is little constitutional reaction. An enanthem consisting of raised red and yellow-white lesions on the soft palate, fauces, and uvula were found in about 50 percent of the cases in one outbreak. The rash in this syndrome consists also of pink and salmon-pink discrete macules or maculopapules about 1 cm in size appearing first on the face, chest, and back and sometimes spreading over the entire body including the soles of the feet. It lasts 2 to 4 days.

2. Neurologic syndromes
   a. Aseptic meningitis. Types 3, 4, 6, 9, 11, 14, 16, 25, and 30 have been associated with epidemics of aseptic meningitis, 2 and 5 with sporadic cases. Of all these, types 4, 6, and 9 have been the most frequently involved. The E9 infection often mimics meningococcemia, i.e., petechial rash and meningitis.
   b. Encephalitis has been associated with several of the above types, particularly E9. It has been manifest as an acute cerebellar ataxia with nystagmus, vertigo, falling, and loss of balance. Patients with choreiform movements, facial weakness, and grimacing have also been described.
   c. Paralytic disease resembling poliomyelitis. Epidemics of E6 and sometimes E9 have been associated with mild, transient muscle weakness and mild paralysis. Residual or permanent paralysis is extremely rare. An occasional death has occurred due to neurologic disease caused by E2, 6, 9, and 11.

3. Enteritis. E18 has caused an epidemic of diarrhea in a newborn nursery, and other types have been associated with outbreaks of diarrhea—particularly types 11, 14, and 17.

4. Other clinical syndromes.

a. E20 has been responsible for a febrile disease with both upper respiratory tract and gastrointestinal symptoms.
b. E4 has been associated with vaginitis and cervicitis.
c. ECHO virus may also cause upper and lower respiratory tract illness (without gastrointestinal symptoms), pleurodynia, myocarditis, and herpangina. All these are rare.

Diagnosis Diagnosis is made by recovery of the virus from throat and rectal swabs, stool and cerebrospinal fluid (CSF), and serologic evidence. However, in order to establish the etiologic association of ECHO virus with a disease syndrome the following criteria are needed: (1) a much higher recovery rate of the virus must be obtained from patients with the disease than from healthy individuals of the same age and socioeconomic level living in the same area at the same time as the patient. (2) Antibodies against the virus must develop during the course of the disease. If the same clinical syndrome can be caused by other known agents, then virologic or serologic evidence must be negative for concurrent infection with such agents. (3) The virus must be isolated in significant concentration from body fluids or tissues manifesting lesions, i.e., CSF in cases of aseptic meningitis.

Treatment There is no specific treatment.

Prognosis There is generally complete recovery with a rare mortality in neurologic cases.

POLIOMYELITIS

Classification

1. Nonspecific febrile illness (abortive poliomyelitis)
2. Nonparalytic aseptic meningitis
3. Spinal paralytic
4. Bulbar
5. Spinobulbar paralytic (signs and symptoms are as in both spinal and bulbar)

Etiology There are three groups of virus: type 1 (Brunhilde), type 2 (Lansing), and type 3 (Leon); there is no cross immunity.

Mode of transmission Transmission is probably by direct contact with nasopharyngeal secretion or fecal excretions from persons harboring the virus.

Incubation period Poliomyelitis develops in 7 to 14 days.

Clinical features   Manifestations of the disease vary from those of a mild nonspecific febrile illness which lasts 24 to 48 hours; to nonparalytic aseptic meningitis syndrome, where signs of meningeal irritation predominate; to paralytic disease affecting the anterior horn cells and presenting with flaccid paralysis of the muscles, to the life-threatening form, where the motor nuclei and the vital centers of the medulla oblongata are involved, resulting in interference with cardiorespiratory function, deglutition, and phonation.

Laboratory findings   The spinal fluid is increased in amount and pressure. Cytologic examination shows 20 to over 1,000 cells, usually 50 to 300 cells. Though polymorphonuclear neutrophils may predominate in the earliest stages, they are soon replaced by lymphocytes. The number and type of cells bear no relation to the severity of the illness. In 5 to 10 percent of cases there is no increase in number of cells. Chemical analysis shows increased amount of protein (over 40 mg per 100 ml); the sugar and chloride levels are normal. The complement-fixation and neutralization tests for serum antibodies are diagnostic, and the virus may be isolated from the stool and grown on tissue cultures. Complement-fixation test is usually positive 7 days after the onset (see Table 14-4).

Treatment   Treatment is supportive depending on the severity of the disease. Physical therapy and rehabilitation should be started early. When the muscles of respiration are involved, artificial ventilation is mandatory. There should be complete muscle testing prior to discharge from hospital and again 1 month later.

RHINOVIRUSES (See Table 14-1)

INFECTIOUS NEURONITIS (Landry-Guillain-Barré Syndrome)

Etiology   The etiology is unknown, but the disease is possibly viral, allergic, or a mycoplasma infection.

Clinical features

1.   An upper respiratory infection usually precedes the onset.
2.   There may be a symmetrical ascending paralysis which may be accompanied by sensory changes.
3.   There are usually no cranial nerves involved, except possibly the facial.
4.   The course is chronic, with the eventual return of muscular power.

Diagnosis   The spinal fluid shows a marked increase of protein, but there is little or no increase in cells (albuminocytologic dissociation).

Prognosis   The prognosis is good.

Treatment There is no specific treatment. Adrenal corticosteroids may be tried.

LABORATORY DIAGNOSIS OF VIRAL INFECTION

Five types of laboratory procedures are regularly available for the diagnosis of viral, chlamydial, and rickettsial disease.

1. Isolation and identification of the agent. This is done through animal inoculation, chick embryo inoculation, and tissue culture.
2. Measurement of antibodies developing during the course of the infection. These are serologic tests based on the manner by which the antibody reacts with the antigen. They consist of (*a*) neutralization test, (*b*) hemagglutination inhibition test, and (*c*) complement-fixation test. All detect specific antibodies. Paired sera are used in these determinations, the first taken during the early phase of the disease (the acute serum) and the second one taken 2 to 3 weeks later (the convalescent serum). At least a fourfold rise in titer is diagnostic of an acute infection. If only a single serum specimen (usually acute or early convalescence) is available a 2-ME sensitivity test may be helpful (2-ME removes the IgM antibody). A significant fall in antibody titer after treatment with 2-ME in an acute phase serum is of presumptive diagnostic value.
3. Histologic examination of infected tissue, i.e., identification of type-specific giant cells and inclusion bodies.
4. Detection of viral antigens in lesions by (*a*) the immunofluorescence test (fluorescent-antibody test) using fluorescein-labeled antibodies and (*b*) the immunodiffusion test. Here the antigen and antibody are allowed to diffuse toward each other in a semisolid medium forming a line of precipitate at the zone of optimal proportions. The appearance of a precipitation line indicates the presence of an antigen. This technique has been used to demonstrate the antigen of hepatitis, HBAg. The passive hemagglutination test, the counter-immunoelectrophoresis test and the radioimmune assay test are also used to detect the HBAg and other viruses.
5. Electron-microscopic examination of vesicular fluids or tissue extracts treated with negative and positive stains to identify and count DNA and RNA virus particles.

CHLAMYDIAL (Bedsonial) DISEASES

1. Psittacosis (Ornithosis) is discussed in Chapter 15, "Respiratory Diseases."
2. Lymphogranuloma (Lymphopathia) venereum is not particularly a pediatric problem but may occur in adolescents who are sexually active (one of the venereal diseases). It is characterized clinically by the following: (*a*) primary lesion—vesicle and subsequent ulcer —is usually asymptomatic and goes unnoticed; (*b*) enlargement

of the lymph nodes (It is usually the inguinal nodes which are tender, adherent to each other and to the overlying skin, and often suppurate, with the formation of sinus tracts.) ; (c) mild systemic symptoms; (d) complications, rectal stricture; (e) diagnosis, see table 14-4. Treatment is sulfonamides, penicillin, or tetracycline.

3. TRIC Agents (see Chapter 12, "Diseases of the Newborn").
   a. Trachoma
   b. Inclusion conjunctivitis (blenorrhea)
4. Cat-scratch disease (benign inoculation lymphoreticulosis) is a nonbacterial, regional lymphadenitis presumably due to a bedsonia belonging to the psittacosis-lymphogranuloma group. There is usually a history of a cat scratch, bite, or contact, but cases have occurred following a skin injury from slivers, thorns, or porcupine quills. The incubation period varies from 7 to 14 days, from inoculation to primary lesion; possibly this may be as short as 2 days. The site of the scratch becomes inflamed and may develop into a red papule or an indolent ulcer without evidence of lymphangitis. Regional lymph nodes, most commonly axillary, cervical, or inguinal, are involved, after 2 to 3 weeks becoming tender but movable, with redness, heat, and swelling of the overlying skin. Suppuration and sterile pus may develop. Constitutional symptoms including fever are mild or absent. Transient skin eruptions have been described. Blood counts fail to show a leukocytic response, but the sedimentation rate is moderately elevated. Cultures from the nodes are sterile. An intradermal test using so-called "cat-scratch antigen" is positive in 48 hours (a papule of ½ to 1 cm in diameter or an area of erythema of 1½ to 6 cm in diameter) in almost all cases. The antigen is prepared from pus of a known case treated by heating to 58°C and adding 0.5 percent phenol. This test material is not available commercially. Biopsy will reveal a granulomatous lesion. Differential diagnosis includes tuberculosis, tularemia, Boeck's sarcoid, brucellosis, infectious mononucleosis, Hodgkin's disease, lymphogranuloma venereum, and pasteurellosis (infection with *Pasteurella multocida*) from the bite of a cat. Tetracyclines appear to shorten the course of the disease.

In the oculoglandular form of cat-scratch disease there are ocular granuloma and preauricular adenopathy. Surgical excision of the primary ocular lesion seems to shorten the course of the disease.

RICKETTSIAL INFECTIONS

RICKETTSIALPOX

Etiology   The causative agent is *Rickettsia akari*.

Mode of transmission   The disease is spread by rodent mites.

Incubation period   Rickettsialpox develops in 7 to 10 days.

Prodromal period At the site of the mite's bite a papule develops, which later becomes a vesicle. This goes on to form an eschar. The local lymph glands are tender and large. About 1 week after the formation of the papule, a spiking temperature, chills, and muscle pains develop.

Eruptive stage Three or four days later there is a generalized papulovesicular eruption, usually not found on the palms and soles. The lesions progress to form crusts. The disease is self-limiting, and no complications have been described.

Laboratory findings Laboratory findings include leukopenia, positive complement-fixation test (cross reaction with Rocky Mountain spotted fever), and isolation of causative microorganism from the blood. The Weil-Felix reaction is negative in rickettsialpox, differentiating it from other rickettsial infections.

Treatment The tetracycline drugs and chloramphenicol are of value.

EPIDEMIC TYPHUS

Etiology The agent is *Rickettsia prowazeki*.

Mode of transmission Typhus is spread by body lice (a reservoir exists in man).

Incubation period It develops usually in 7 to 14 days, most commonly 12 days.

Clinical features

1. Onset is abrupt, with malaise, headache, chilly sensations, and generalized aches and pains.
2. Temperature becomes elevated to 102 to 104°F (38.9 to 40.0°C) by the third day of the illness and remains at that level until the death or recovery of the patient.
3. A generalized macular or maculopapular eruption appears usually between the fourth and seventh days of the disease. It begins on the face and spreads in the course of 1 or 2 days over the entire body, except the palms and soles, which are involved only in gravely ill patients. The rash has a centripetal distribution.
4. The second and third weeks of illness constitute the critical period. Increasing prostration may develop. There is mental dullness, which may progress to stupor, delirium, or coma.
5. Uremia and myocarditis may develop. Death may occur from renal insufficiency and myocardial failure.

Laboratory findings There is usually a moderate leukopenia during the first week of the illness, rising titers of type-specific complement-fixation, and Weil-Felix reaction (agglutinins for *Proteus vulgaris* OX-19). Isolation of rickettsia by inoculation into guinea pigs.

Treatment Treatment consists of chloramphenicol or a tetracycline and delousing of child with DDT 5%.

Course If the patient recovers, there are no serious complications. It may take 2 or 3 months to regain full strength and activity.

ENDEMIC TYPHUS

Endemic typhus is sporadic and caused by *Rickettsia mooseri*. A reservoir exists in small rodents; the vector is the rat flea. The signs and symptoms are the same as in epidemic typhus except that they are milder and of shorter duration. There is a positive Weil-Felix reaction (OX19) as in epidemic typhus. Type-specific complement-fixation tests can differentiate the two. The rickettsia may be isolated by guinea pig inoculation.

ROCKY MOUNTAIN SPOTTED FEVER (Tick-borne Typhus)

Etiology *Rickettsia rickettsii* is the causative agent.

Mode of transmission The disease is spread by ticks (a reservoir exists in wild rodents and dogs).

Incubation period The incubation period is 3 to 12 days.

Prodromal period The prodrome comprises fever, chills, muscle pains, headaches, and occasionally nosebleed.

Eruptive stages Three days after the onset a rash appears on the ankles, soles, palms and wrists and spreads toward the trunk. The lesions are bright erythematous maculopapules centrifugal in distribution, which tend to become hemorrhagic. There is a spiking temperature, which lasts about 2 to 3 weeks and terminates by lysis. There is usually a mild to moderate leukocytosis. In fulminating cases coma usually precedes death, which commonly occurs about the second week of the disease.

Laboratory findings There are rising titers in neutralization, complement-fixation (cross reaction with rickettsialpox), and Weil-Felix reactions (OX19 and OX2 strains) are weakly positive.

Complications If the patient survives, complications are uncommon, but recovery is slow.

Prevention Active immunization may be used in areas where the disease is prevalent (Cox yolk-sac vaccine, 1 ml subcutaneously at intervals of 5 to 7 days, for three injections).

Treatment Chloramphenicol and tetracycline should be given.

Q FEVER

Etiology Q fever is caused by *Rickettsia burnetii (Coxiella burnetii)*.

Mode of transmission Q fever is spread by ingestion of raw milk from infected animals, tick bites, inhalation of dust contaminated by manure containing the organism, and direct contact with infected animals.

Incubation period It develops in 14 to 26 days.

Clinical and laboratory features There are no characteristic clinical features. Temperature rises suddenly and lasts about 1 week. Malaise, anorexia, and headache are often present. Pneumonitis occurs frequently, with a patchy infiltration seen on roentgenograms. The specific rickettsia can be isolated from blood, sputum, spinal fluid, and urine by inoculation into guinea pigs, mice, and chick embryos. There are rising agglutination and complement-fixation titers. Absence of a rash and no cross agglutination with *Proteus vulgaris* OX19 distinguish this infection from other rickettsial diseases.

Diagnosis Diagnosis is by isolation of *R. burnetii* from the blood or sputum and specific serologic tests, i.e., complement-fixation.

Treatment Chloramphenicol or tetracycline should be given.

Prognosis The prognosis is good.

BACTERIAL INFECTIONS

STREPTOCOCCAL INFECTIONS (Scarlet Fever, Streptococcal Sore Throat, Erysipelas)

A wide variety of disorders may be caused by the group A beta-hemolytic streptococci. The clinical symptoms will vary, depending on the portal of entry, pathway of spread, and site of localization of the infection, and the presence or absence of the erythrogenic toxin responsible for the rash.

The main entities induced by group A hemolytic streptococci are listed above, but they may also cause such infections as sepsis, peritonitis, osteomyelitis, otitis media, and mastoiditis. The same principles of care of the individual and control of the streptococcus apply to all.

Etiology   The causative agent is group A beta-hemolytic streptococci (*Streptococcus pyogenes*); various distinct serologic types (about 40). (There are at least five types of erythrogenic toxin and three immunologically distinct groups.) The most common serologic variety of toxin, however, is produced by about 75 percent of strains. Thus, although it is possible to have scarlet fever more than once, it is distinctly unusual. Hemolytic streptococci of groups B, C, D, and G have been identified occasionally.

Incubation period   Incubation is short, usually 2 to 5 days.

Mode of transmission   It is spread by direct contact (droplet infection from an active case or carrier); indirect contact through objects handled; explosive outbreaks may follow ingestion of contaminated milk, ice cream, or other food.

Pathogenesis   The site of the primary infection is usually the pharynx, where the organism multiplies and produces a potent soluble toxin; after absorption into the bloodstream, the toxin produces constitutional symptoms, such as fever, headache, vomiting, rapid pulse, and an eruption of the skin.

Prodromal period   There is a characteristic triad of fever, sore throat, and vomiting. The onset is sudden, with a temperature of 101 to 104°F (38.3 to 40°C), and the pulse rate is increased out of proportion to the temperature.

Exanthem   The rash in scarlet fever will depend on the erythrogenic toxin-producing qualities of the offending streptococcus and whether the patient has an immunity to the toxin. If the patient is immune to the toxin, no rash will occur. Similarly, if the organism is a weak toxin producer, no rash will occur.

The rash is diffuse, finely papular, and bright red, and it blanches on pressure. It resembles gooseflesh on a sunburn. It appears 12 to 72 hours after the onset of the triad. The rash starts about the neck, axillae, and groin, being most intense over pressure areas and areas of warmth and appearing later on the trunk and extremities. There is circumoral pallor, with minimal eruption on the face or nose. The rash fades in 3 to 7 days. Pastia's sign is commonly seen—deeply injected, hyperemic transverse lines in the flexor creases, e.g., elbow, inguinal, which do not blanch on pressure. The Rumpel-Leede sign is frequently found—with the application of a tourniquet on the upper arm, petechiae are produced distally. Desquamation following the rash is most marked in the axillae, fingertips, groins, and at the base of the nails and is proportional to the intensity of the rash.

Additional clinical features The throat is deeply injected, often beefy, and petechiae are scattered over the soft palate and uvula. A mucopurulent exudate may occasionally be distributed over the tonsils and posterior pharynx. Often there is a prominent cervical adenitis. On the first 2 days, the tongue is coated grayish white, with prominent papillae (white strawberry tongue). By the third to fourth day the coating desquamates and leaves a beefy red tongue with swollen papillae (raspberry tongue or red strawberry tongue). The constitutional symptoms subside after the eruption has reached its peak.

Laboratory findings Leukocytosis of 10,000 to 20,000, with 75 to 90 percent polymorphonuclear neutrophils, occurs at the onset. After the fourth day of the rash 4 to 20 percent eosinophils may be found. The throat cultures usually yield hemolytic streptococci. There are rising antistreptolysin O serum titers during convalescence. (A clinical condition resembling scarlet fever but due to a staphylococcus, coagulase-positive, does occur.)

Complications Otitis media, cervical adenitis, and sinusitis are the most common complications and may be seen during or after the acute phase. A transient toxic nephritis, manifested by albuminuria and casts, is seen in a majority of cases during the acute stage. Acute toxic carditis is a rare complication, found early in the disease. Acute glomerulonephritis and rheumatic carditis occur on a basis of sensitivity to the streptococcus. Their onset is usually in the second or third week. Urinalysis should be made weekly from the second to the fourth week to detect subclinical cases of acute glomerulonephritis. Bronchopneumonia is rather uncommon. Other rare complications are septicemia, meningitis, metastatic abscesses of the viscera, and septic arthritis.

Treatment Penicillin in adequate dosage is the treatment of choice. Optimum treatment eradicates the streptococci from the site of infection, prevents septic complications (otitis media, mastoiditis, bronchopneumonia, empyema, osteomyelitis, etc.), and greatly reduces second-phase complications (rheumatic fever and perhaps acute glomerulonephritis). Treatment should be continued for at least 10 days regardless of apparent clinical recovery.

Dosage schedules Any of the following may be used:

1. Benzathine penicillin G. For patients weighing less than 60 lb, one intramuscular injection of 600,000 units; for patients weighing over 60 lb, one intramuscular injection of 900,000 to 1,200,000 units.
2. Procaine penicillin with 2% aluminum monostearate, intramuscularly, 300,000 to 600,000 units every third day for three injections.

3. Oral penicillin V, 400,000 units (250 mg) three or four times daily for 10 days.
4. For patients allergic to penicillin, erythromycin may be substituted.

Immunity   Immunity to streptococci is type-specific and long lasting.

Public health aspects   The patient should be isolated for 1 day after treatment is begun. Contacts should be carefully examined (particularly the throat) for any evidence of disease, and a throat culture should be taken. Those who have manifestations of a respiratory tract infection or beta-hemolytic streptococci in their cultures should be treated in accordance with one of the above regimens. If observation of contacts is not possible treatment should be given.

WHOOPING COUGH (Pertussis)

Etiology   The disease is caused by *Bordetella pertussis.*

Mode of transmission   Pertussis is spread in the same way as measles.

Incubation period   Incubation is 5 to 21 days, averaging about 10 days.

Catarrhal period   The cough is mild at the onset and is apt to be more frequent at night. In the ensuing 10 days, it becomes progressively more intense, spasmodic, and diurnal. There are coryza, sneezing, and sometimes hoarseness. Injection of the pharynx and a low-grade temperature are often present. This is the period of greatest communicability. (Six weeks after onset of symptoms, the patient is considered noninfectious.)

Spasmodic, or paroxysmal, stage   Near the end of the second week the cough becomes markedly aggravated. In the typical severe paroxysm, a series of explosive efforts occurs, followed by vomiting or by coughing up or swallowing of large amounts of thick, tenacious, mucoid sputum. The paroxysms may be initiated by eating, inhalation of smoke, sudden changes in temperature, gentle external compression of the trachea, or gagging. Varying degrees of cyanosis may occur during a paroxysm. Very young infants often have prolonged periods of apnea following such an episode. The characteristic inspiratory whoop is frequently absent in infants under 1 year of age.

Additional clinical features are sweating, distension of the neck and scalp veins, mental confusion and exhaustion which may follow paroxysms; epistaxis and subconjunctival hemorrhages also occur. Edema of the lower eyelids may be found. Coarse inspiratory rales scattered throughout both lung fields are heard on auscultation.

Convalescent period The cough paroxysms become less severe and less frequent about the fourth week. The chest findings become minimal. Intercurrent respiratory infection, however, may cause a recurrence of the whoop and paroxysms.

Differential diagnosis Diagnosis is sometimes difficult in infants who do not have the typical cough. In children who have had prophylactic injections there may be an atypical course and a mild cough. The isolation of the organism is the only way of making an absolute diagnosis in these cases.

The pertussis syndrome, i.e., paroxysm of cough with or without a whoop and a high white blood cell count with an absolute lymphocytosis, may also be caused by certain adenoviruses, particularly type 2 (see Chapter 13). *Bordetella bronchoseptic, H. influenza, Mycoplasma pneumoniae,* and other viral pneumonias are often mistaken for pertussis because of a prolonged course and persistent cough which is often paroxysmal. *Bordetella parapertussis* may cause the syndrome of parapertussis. The incubation period is 6 to 15 days. Clinically the disease is indistinguishable from mild pertussis. The differential diagnosis can be made only from nasopharyngeal culture or cough plate. There is no cross immunity, and active immunization against pertussis gives no immunity to parapertussis. Complications are rare, and the prognosis is good. Other entities to consider in the differential diagnosis are tuberculosis (tracheobronchial nodes), mucoviscidosis, aspirated foreign body, or Loeffler's pneumonia.

Laboratory findings

1. There is an absolute lymphocytosis ranging from 15,000 to 45,000 per cu mm, occasionally even higher. Absence of lymphocytosis does not exclude the diagnosis, particularly in young infants.
2. The best way to grow the organism is to culture the nasopharynx by means of a special technique. A flexible wire swab is inserted through the nares into the posterior nasopharynx and allowed to remain there during a paroxysm. The swab, saturated with mucus, is then planted on Bordet-Gengou medium with added penicillin. The organism can rarely be cultured after the fourth week of the disease.
3. The fluorescent-antibody technique provides a rapid diagnosis of pertussis, and there are serologic tests (agglutinating and complement-fixing antibodies) which become positive during the third week. A positive skin test to the agglutinogen also develops about the same time. All these serologic tests are unreliable. Recently, an agar gel double diffusion test has been described which is probably the most consistent and reliable serologic test for pertussis.

Complications If the temperature rises above 101°F (38.3°C) a complication should be suspected. In the respiratory tract, bronchopneumonia, atelectasis, mediastinal emphysema, dissemination of a preexisting primary tuberculosis, and bronchiectasis are not uncommon. Digestive-tract complications are diarrhea, vomiting, ulceration of the frenulum of the tongue, prolapse of the rectum, and hernia. Hemorrhage, such as epistaxis, hemoptysis, subconjunctival, or cerebral, is usually mechanical in origin. Convulsions are not uncommon but may be due to hypoxia or intracranial hemorrhage as a result of the paroxysm or as a symptom of encephalitis which on occasion follows pertussis. The cause of the encephalitis is unknown. It may represent a hypersensitivity reaction to the organism itself or a toxic action on intracerebral vessels. The most common cause of death is pneumonia.

Treatment Infants must be observed continuously. They may require repeated suctioning and periodic oxygen administration. Erythromycin is the drug of choice. It shortens the period of infectivity (cultures become negative in 2 to 4 days) and, if administered during the incubation period or catarrhal phase, can abort the clinical course. If the paroxysmal stage has begun, antibiotics will not influence the course of the disease. Appropriate antibiotics should be given for bacterial complications, e.g., staphylococcal or *H. influenzae* pneumonia.

Hyperimmune globulin (PIG) is not effective after the disease has started. Diet should consist of small frequent feedings, and if vomiting occurs, feedings can be repeated in 15 to 20 minutes. Special nursing care is important in infancy to maintain a clear airway and prevent aspiration of vomitus and mucus. Sedation may be necessary to reduce coughing, lessen vomiting, and prevent convulsions. Careful attention must be paid to fluid and electrolyte balance and nutrition.

Public health aspects

1. Active immunization—see Chapter 4, "Preventive Pediatrics."
2. Care of exposed susceptibles—(*a*) Contacts under 6 years of age previously immunized against pertussis should be given a booster dose of pertussis vaccine and erythromycin. (*b*) Contacts not previously immunized against pertussis should be given erythromycin for a period of 10 days after the contact is broken or if it is impossible to break the contact for duration of cough in the infected contact. PIG may be of some use in prophylaxis, but erythromycin appears to be more effective.
3. Isolation of the patient—4 weeks from onset of disease or until the cough has stopped, or until the culture becomes negative if antibiotic therapy is given.

Prognosis The prognosis is good in older children but guarded in infants below 1 year, where the mortality is highest.

DIPHTHERIA

Etiology   Diphtheria is caused by *Corynebacterium diphtheriae* (Klebs-Loeffler bacillus).

Mode of transmission   Infection is spread by contact with active cases or carriers and fomites. Rarely, contaminated milk is a source of infection.

Incubation period   Incubation is from 2 to 6 days.

Pathogenesis   Diphtheria in its classical form is characterized by a local pseudomembranous lesion, usually located on the tonsils, pharynx, and adjacent tissues. A powerful toxin is produced, the absorption of which causes both local and constitutional symptoms. This toxin, shown to be a heat-coagulable protein in its chemically pure state, accounts for practically all the clinical manifestations of the disease. It is a potent tissue toxin, which, within a few hours after absorption, brings about characteristic cellular changes. For this reason, it is most important to administer antitoxin in adequate amounts without waiting for laboratory confirmation when dealing with a patient who presents the clinical signs and symptoms of diphtheria. Once the toxin has become fixed to the tissue cells, antitoxin will have no effect, for it neutralizes only the circulating toxin. The toxin also has special affinity for the cardiac, renal, liver, adrenal, and nervous tissues.

Faucial diphtheria

Local signs   The first day, there is congestion and slight swelling of the tonsillar and pharyngeal tissues, with minimal cervical lymphadenopathy; the second day, grayish small white spots appear on the surface of the tonsils and can be removed only with difficulty. The spots rapidly coalesce and spread to the pillars, uvula, soft palate, and posterior pharyngeal wall forming a pseudomembrane which, if forcibly removed, leaves a bleeding surface.

Constitutional symptoms   There is low-grade fever, tachycardia, malaise, toxicity, and weakness.

Laboratory findings   Leukocytosis and a positive throat culture are evident.

Clinical features of laryngotracheal diphtheria   The disease may be primary in the larynx or may be an extension from the pharyngeal fauces. There are edema and congestion of the tissues and a pseudomembrane in or over the laryngeal orifice which can be seen on laryngoscopy. The signs and symptoms of obstruction are restlessness, noisy breathing, brassy cough, hoarseness, retractions of the suprasternal and infrasternal notches on inspiration, "pulling" (use of accessory muscles of respiration), and cyanosis. If the obstruction is not relieved, death will result from hypoxia, cardiac failure, and exhaustion. Restlessness is an early danger sign that may appear well before the other obstructive signs.

Clinical features of nasal diphtheria Locally the obstructing membrane can be visualized with a nasal speculum. Serosanguineous discharge and excoriation of the upper lip are common. When the diphtheria is primary in the nose, there are mild constitutional symptoms because of poor absorption of toxin in this area. However, it may extend to the throat and larynx. A carrier state frequently develops in this type of diphtheria. When it is secondary to diphtheria in another location, the membrane is also found at the primary site and the constitutional symptoms are severe.

Other rare forms are vulvovaginal, skin, surgical, umbilical, and conjunctival diphtheria.

Complications

1. "Bull neck" is due to cervical adenitis, lymphangitis, and edema of the skin and subcutaneous tissue of the neck.
2. Respiratory complications are bronchopneumonia, atelectasis, and obstruction of the airway.
3. Circulatory complications: toxic myocarditis, with or without superimposed damage to the conduction system, is most common between the fifth and the twelfth days. It is characterized by fatigue, dyspnea, and tachycardia or bradycardia (heart block). The electrocardiogram often shows an increased P-R interval and elevation of the S-T segment. Cardiac failure may ensue.
4. Neural complications may appear at any time. They tend to be bilateral with motor rather than sensory involvement. There may be a toxic peripheral neuritis, which is painless and usually persists for several days or weeks. There may be palatal paralysis, strabismus, dilatation of the pupils, and ptosis of the eyelid in the third week or later. Phrenic-nerve paralysis is indicated by thoracic breathing, weak cough, dyspnea, apprehension, and cyanosis. Progressive general paralysis is extremely rare. If the patient survives, there is complete recovery from the various forms of diphtheritic paralysis, although recovery may not take place for several weeks or months.
5. Toxic nephritis.

Diagnosis The diagnosis of diphtheria is based on

1. Clinical manifestations.
2. History of immunization.

3. Positive Schick test.
4. Laboratory findings from smears taken from the nose and throat or suspected lesions and stained with methylene blue or by Gram's method. Cultures are made on special media including the rapid-culture method with horse serum. Identification of the organism by fluorescent-antibody technique is possible. A guinea pig virulence test may be done.

Differential diagnosis Faucial diphtheria may be confused with streptococcal acute follicular tonsillitis, posttonsillectomy membrane, infectious mononucleosis, Vincent's infection, agranulocytosis, leukemia, syphilis, candida infection, Coxsackie group A or adenovirus infections, plague, and tularemia.

Nasal diphtheria may be confused with syphilis, foreign body in the nose, common cold, and trauma to nasal mucosa.

Laryngeal diphtheria must be differentiated from acute nonspecific laryngotracheobronchitis, spasmodic croup, epiglottitis, aspiration of a foreign body, bronchopneumonia, tetany, asthma, peritonsillar abscess, and retropharyngeal abscess.

Treatment If the clinical diagnosis is suggestive of diphtheria, it is best to give antitoxin immediately. Do not wait for culture report. When giving antitoxin, a syringe containing epinephrine must be at hand.

1. Antitoxin—preferred route of administration is intravenous. The antitoxin is diluted with physiologic saline (1:20) and given at the rate of 15 drops per minute. Dosage is as follows: (*a*) 20,000 to 40,000 units in pharyngeal and laryngeal disease of 48-hours duration; (*b*) 40,000 to 60,000 units in nasopharyngeal lesions; (*c*) 80,000 to 120,000 units in extensive disease of 3 or more days duration or in any patient with brawny swelling of the neck. Before the antitoxin is administered, a test for sensitivity to horse serum must be done. This may be either a skin test (0.1 ml of 1:1,000 dilution of diphtheria antitoxin, DAT, in physiologic saline solution intracutaneously) or an eye test (1 drop of a 1:10 dilution of DAT in physiologic saline instilled inside the lower eyelid on one side and 1 drop of physiologic saline instilled in the other eye as a control). If the patient is sensitive to horse serum, he must be desensitized before treatment.
2. Antimicrobial therapy—erythromycin and penicillin are the drugs of choice. It must be strongly emphasized that antimicrobials in no way substitute for the antitoxin. They are adjunctive therapy to the antitoxin in rendering the patient noninfectious and in reducing the multiplication of other organisms in the upper respiratory tract, particularly beta-hemolytic streptococci. Therapy should be continued for about 7 to 10 days. Topical antimicrobials, e.g., bacitracin, may be used for skin diphtheria.

3. Nonspecific treatment
   a. Strict need for rest for at least 3 weeks.
   b. Electrocardiogram should be repeated twice weekly for 4 weeks.
   c. Observation for loss of the voice and gag reflex.
   d. In severe cases adrenal corticosteroids may be administered for approximately 2 weeks to lessen the incidence of myocarditis.
   e. A diet high in vitamin C and carbohydrates has been shown to be useful.
   f. Digitalization may be of value for myocarditis with cardiac enlargement.
   g. Respiratory obstruction (nasopharyngeal and laryngeal) may necessitate a tracheostomy. Cool moist oxygen as well as frequent suctioning and saline irrigations of the pharynx may be beneficial.

Public health aspects   Quarantined patients may be removed from isolation after three negative cultures, at least 24 hours apart, from both the nose and throat after all discontinuation of antimicrobial therapy. If cultures continue to be positive for 3 weeks, a virulence test should be done. Household contacts and contacts who are closely associated with children through their occupations, etc., should be quarantined until cultures from nose, throat, and skin lesions are negative.

Prevention (care of exposed susceptibles)   All contacts should be carefully examined for possible signs and symptoms of early diphtheria. If present, nose and throat cultures should be taken and the patient treated. If asymptomatic, those who have been previously inoculated with diphtheria toxoid should be given a booster, oral penicillin or erythromycin, and have daily surveillance. Asymptomatic persons not previously immunized against diphtheria should receive diphtheria toxoid and penicillin (preferably parenterally) for 5 to 7 days, and if not under daily surveillance, 10,000 units of DAT.

Congenital passive immunity (transplacental from an immune mother) is almost absolute for the first 3 months of life and partial until about the sixth month of life, if the mother has had experience with the disease or has been immunized recently. Passive immunity resulting from DAT affords protection for about 3 weeks. Active immunity may be acquired from diphtheria toxoid or from the disease if the patient received no antitoxin. Early administration of antitoxin interferes with production of active immunity, hence all patients should be actively immunized about one month after its use.

The Schick test formally used to determine the immune status of an individual is no longer in widespread use.

A carrier is defined as an asymptomatic individual who harbors virulent diphtheria bacteria in the nasopharynx. This condition is rare in the United States, but each carrier should be treated with procaine penicillin, 600,000 to 2,000,000 units intramuscularly, for 7 to 10 days or given a course of erythromycin orally. If antimicrobial treatment fails, tonsillectomy should be performed but not until 3 months after the acute illness.

TETANUS

Etiology   Tetanus is caused by *Clostridium tetani.*

Incubation period   Incubation ranges from 3 days to 3 weeks but is usually 8 days.

Clinical features

1. There is a history of skin wound or mucous-membrane abrasion. (There may be no history of trauma.)
2. Neonatal tetanus results from contamination of the cord and usually occurs at birth.
3. Onset is gradual—there is progressively increasing stiffness of the voluntary muscles—those of the neck and jaw are usually the first to be involved, swallowing becomes difficult.
4. There are systemic symptoms—increased irritability, headache, chills, low-grade fever and generalized pain.
5. Risus sardonicus and trismus are marked. Opisthotonus develops. These latter three signs are prominent during the tonic convulsions (painful paroxysmal spasms) which occur with minimal stimuli, e.g., bright light, noise.

Prophylaxis   Active immunization, produced by the use of toxoids, has been discussed in Chapter 4, "Preventive Pediatrics." Proper care of wounds contaminated with soil, feces, etc., is essential. At the time of cleansing and debridement, prophylactic use of antitoxin and penicillin depends on history of previous immunization against tetanus. The following table is a guide to treatment.

History of tetanus immunization (doses)	Clean minor wound		All other wounds	
	Td*	TIG†	Td	TIG
Uncertain, none or 1	Yes	No	Yes	Yes
2	Yes	No	Yes	No‡
3 or more	No§	No	No¶	No

* Td = tetanus diphtheria toxoid.
† TIG = tetanus immune globulin.
‡ Unless wound is more than 24 hr old.
§ Unless it has been more than 10 years since last dose.
¶ Unless it has been more than 5 years since last dose.

Tetanus antitoxin can neutralize only circulating toxin. Tetanus human immune globulin (TIG) is the preferred product and is used in the dose of 250 units for wounds of average severity. (A dose as high as 500 units may be given if necessary.) TIG lasts longer than animal antitoxin and is free from undesirable side effects. If TIG is not available, animal antitoxin (1,500 to 6,000 units) may be used after sensitivity tests have been made. Active immunization with tetanus toxoid should always accompany antitoxic prophylaxis using separate syringes and separate sites.

Treatment

1. The efficacy of antitoxin for patients with symptoms of tetanus is doubtful except in neonatal tetanus. Here TIG (500 units) or equine antitoxin (10,000 units) may be lifesaving.
2. Antibiotics—penicillin or oxytetracycline.
3. Sedatives and muscle relaxants, e.g., chlorpromazine, diazepam, methocarbamol.
4. The patient should be kept in a dark quiet room.
5. Fluid and electrolyte balance, caloric intake, a patent airway (tracheostomy may be necessary) and proper gaseous exchange must be maintained.
6. Intratracheal positive pressure respiration and curarization are effective.

Prognosis   The prognosis is poor. Mortality rate is 35 to 60 percent. If the patient recovers, his cure is complete; there are no residua.

SALMONELLOSES

Etiology   Over 1,200 serotypes have been identified. Most are primarily animal pathogens; a few, such as *Salmonella typhosa* (*S. typhi*) and the paratyphoid group (A, B, and C), are found only in man. Traditionally, the salmonelloses and typhoid fever are discussed separately. In recent years, the incidence of salmonellosis (non–*S. typhi*) has been increasing at an alarming rate in the United States and is presently an even larger public health problem than typhoid fever in some areas of the world. Furthermore, typhoid fever in children is a less severe disease than in adults and simulates other salmonelloses. For these two reasons typhoid fever will be discussed as one of the salmonelloses, rather than as a separate entity.

Mode of transmission   The organisms enter via the oral route and are spread through fecal contamination of food and drink or by direct or indirect contact with an infected person or animal (pets). The following sources are important:

1. Water contaminated with feces

2. Milk and other dairy products having inadequate pasteurization, improper handling, or contaminated with feces
3. Shellfish from contaminated water
4. Dried or frozen eggs from infected fowl or contamination during processing
5. Dried coconut
6. Meats and meat products either from infected animals (poultry) or by contamination with feces of rodents or man
7. Animal dyes used in drugs, foods, or cosmetics
8. Household pets such as turtles, dogs, and cats
9. Powdered milk and candies

The origin of contamination is more likely to be the feces of subclinical cases or carriers than of the frank, clinical cases, who are promptly isolated. This is especially dangerous if food handlers are shedding the organism. Many fowl, animals, cattle, and rodents are naturally infected with salmonelloses and have the bacteria in their meat, eggs, and excreta—hence there are immeasurable ways for food supply to be easily contaminated with this group of organisms.

Clinical manifestations

There are four types of clinical syndrome of salmonella infection. Table 14-5 compares the main clinical manifestations.

1. Acute gastroenteritis (food poisoning). This is by far the most common and accounts for about 65 percent of the salmonella infections—commonly due to *S. typhimurium, S. enteritidis, S. newport,* and many others.
2. Enteric fever (salmonella fever), usually caused by *S. typhi* and the paratyphoid group—*S. paratyphi* (A), *S. schottmülleri* (para B), *S. hirschfeldii* (para C).
3. Septicemia with or without focal lesions, often caused by *S. choleraesuis*—found with many of the other animal types of salmonellosis in the pediatric age group, particularly infants. As a general rule, the younger the child the more likely he is to develop the septicemia-focal lesion form.
4. Inapparent infection and carrier state.

Carrier state Persons with inapparent infections are becoming an increasing problem as salmonellosis becomes more prevalent and the bacteria more resistant to antibiotics. About 30 percent of those with manifest disease become convalescent carriers. Approximately 0.2 percent of the population is considered to be the permanent carrier rate for salmonellae in general, whereas 3 percent of survivors with typhoid fever become permanent carriers. The organisms are harbored mainly in the gastrointestinal tract. They are also harbored in the gallbladder, biliary ducts, and urine in typhoid and paratyphoid carriers. Anti-

Table 14-5. A comparison of clinical syndromes induced by salmonellae

	Gastroenteritis (food poisoning)	Enteric fever	Septicemia with focal infections
Incubation period	6–72 hr (usually 12 hr)	7–20 days—typhoid fever 1–10 days—paratyphoid fever	Variable—probably 1–7 days
Onset	Abrupt	Insidious—older children; abrupt—children under 2 years	Abrupt
Fever	Usually low—may be high, especially infants	Gradual rise in steplike manner over 2–7 day period—then high plateau for 3–4 weeks—older children; sudden high fever—younger children	Rapid rise then spiking septic temperature
Duration of disease	2–5 days, occasionally 1 week or longer	Several weeks—older children; 2 weeks—children under 2 years	Variable—several weeks—may be a cause of "fever of undetermined origin"
Gastro-intestinal symptoms	Abdominal pain, nausea, vomiting and diarrhea at onset; blood-streaked stools, especially infants; stools contain mucus and pus	Constipation early, later bloody diarrhea; younger children, marked diarrhea	Often none
Other signs and symptoms	Weakness, chills, headache occasionally, prostration, signs of dehydration, shock	Headache, malaise, rose spots early, splenomegaly, slow pulse in relation to fever, lethargy, stupor; young children: vomiting, no rose spots, no slow pulse, spleen is enlarged, often have convulsions and meningeal signs, intestinal ulceration and hemorrhage	Headache, malaise, may manifest itself as meningitis, pneumonia, osteomyelitis, endocarditis, pyarthrosis, abscesses, and pyelonephritis
Blood culture	Negative	Positive 1st and 2d week of disease	Positive during high fever

Stool culture	Positive soon after onset	Positive from 2d week on, urine also	Infrequently positive
Serologic tests	None	Positive agglutination test (Widal), rising titer of both O and H agglutinins, positive after 1st week—Group specific	Positive agglutination test—rise of both O and H agglutinins, after 1st week. Group-specific
WBC	Slight polynucleosis 10,000 to 15,000	Leukopenia—older children; leukocytosis (20,000–25,000) with polymorphonuclears 60–70% in younger children	Mild leukocytosis—polymorphonuclear
Treatment	Symptomatic—isolation, restoration of fluids and electrolyte balance—specific therapy usually not necessary. Chloramphenicol or ampicillin if very severe, particularly in a young infant or if patient has a hemoglobinopathy, hematopoietic disorder or underlying gastrointestinal disease (these all predispose to systemic invasion)	Isolation, symptomatic, chloramphenicol or ampicillin, depending on susceptibility of organism, for no longer than 14 days.	Isolation—symptomatic, chloramphenicol or ampicillin, depending on severity, localization of infection, and susceptibility of the organism

biotic treatment of children with gastroenteritis is of questionable value and tends to increase the long-term carrier rate. This is particularly true of infants less than a year of age.

Control measures for carriers are directed primarly toward food handlers, who must have three negative stool cultures before resuming their occupation. Antibiotic treatment is disappointing and contraindicated except for *S. typhi* intestinal or urine carriers, who may respond to a 3 to 6 week course of ampicillin. Gallbladder–infected carriers require cholecystectomy in addition to ampicillin.

Prevention and control   Immunization is successful only against typhoid fever (70 to 90 percent effective in children). Indications include (1) exposure to carrier or case in a household; (2) outbreak of typhoid in a community; (3) travel to an area where typhoid fever is endemic. See Chapter 4, "Preventive Pediatrics."

Public health measures

1. Sanitation measures must be taken to prevent contamination of food and water by rodents and other animals which excrete salmonellae.
2. The food industry must be compelled to monitor their products for contamination and be required to market only safe, uncontaminated food.
3. Public education is necessary as to the proper cooking of meats, poultry, etc., and proper personal hygiene is a must.

SHIGELLOSIS (Bacillary Dysentery)

Etiology   There are four main groups of shigella, each group comprising a number of types that differ serologically: Group A—*Shigella dysenteriae;* Group B—*S. flexneri* (common); Group C—*S. goydii;* Group D—*S. sonnei.*

Incubation period   Incubation is 1 to 7 days, usually 3 to 4 days.

Mode of transmission   Hand-to-mouth transfer of contaminated material ("food, fingers, feces and flies from man to man") spreads the infection.

Clinical features

1. The onset is usually sudden, with some fever, abdominal pain, cramps, vomiting, and occasionally meningeal signs, delirium, and convulsions.
2. Diarrhea with mucus, pus, and blood is typical and tenesmus is common. Most cases, however, have simple watery diarrhea or loose stools for a few days, with mild or absent constitutional symptoms.

3. The colon is principally involved, and sigmoidoscopy reveals markedly inflamed mucosa which bleeds easily, a pseudomembrane, and ulcerations.

Laboratory findings

1. Leukocytosis with marked shift to the left
2. Finding of the organism in stool cultures (direct rectal swab is preferable)
3. Rise in agglutination titers after the first week

Treatment

1. Isolation technique should be practiced.
2. Fluid and electrolyte balance should be maintained.
3. No antimicrobial therapy is needed in cases that respond to symptomatic therapy. Ampicillin is the drug of choice in severe cases. If there is no response in 72 hours, chloramphenicol, the tetracyclines, or furazolidone may be tried. All these drugs are bacteriostatic for shigella, and although they often suppress the acute attack, they fail to eradicate the organism. Hence, resistant shigella infections are widespread, and the carrier state is increasing at a rapid rate.

Public health aspects

1. Isolate the patient. Observe enteric precautions (proper disposal and disinfection of fecal material), personal hygiene, and frequent hand washing.
2. Community measures include sanitary control of water, food, and milk, and sewage disposal and fly control.
3. Subclinical cases should be detected, particularly in food handlers, and such people should be excluded from that occupation.

GONORRHEA

This disease has reached epidemic proportions in the United States and is now one of the most common infectious diseases reported. It is very prevalent among adolescents and has been diagnosed with increasing frequency in the young. Gonorrhea ophthalmia, however, is still quite rare—see Chapter 12, "Diseases of the Newborn."

Etiology   Gonorrhea is caused by *Neisseria gonorrhea* (pathogenic for man only).

Mode of transmission   Spread of infection is by contact with exudate from infected mucous membranes. It usually requires intimate contact such as sexual or parturient, but also is spread indirectly through intermediary objects, e.g., hands, bed clothes. The latter causes are being reported with increasing frequency in young children. The period of infectivity lasts as long as the patient harbors the organism.

Incubation period   Incubation averages 3 to 5 days (range 1 to 14 days).

Clinical features

1. Ophthalmia: (*a*) neonatorum (see Chapter 12); (*b*) older infants and young children—there is usually unilateral inflammation of the orbit with occasional spread to the infraorbital area of the face, severe edema and erythema of the conjunctivae with a thick greenish-yellow mucoid exudate. Keratoconjunctivitis may also be present, and occasional scarring of the cornea may result, particularly if untreated.
2. Urethritis and vaginitis: any discharge in infants or children may be gonococcal in origin. The symptoms are usually (*a*) presence of yellowish-green, thick, copious discharge, (*b*) burning on urination, frequency, and dysuria, (*c*) in females there is excoriation of the labia and inner aspects of the thighs and tenderness of the vulva with marked erythema of the hymen, vagina, and urethral meatus.
3. Constitutional symptoms are rare.
4. Complications, more frequent in the adolescent, include salpingitis and pelvic inflammatory disease, occasionally septicemia with resultant arthritis, meningitis, pericarditis, or endocarditis.

Laboratory findings

1. A smear and culture of the discharge should be done. The best culture medium is the Thayer-Martin VCN medium. Any discharge from the urethra or vagina in an infant, child, or adolescent should be cultured for gonococcus.
2. Many authorities believe that any sexually active adolescent girl from the age of 15 years and up should be routinely cultured from the urethra, cervix (if not possible, deep vagina), pharynx, and rectum, since 80 percent of infected females are asymptomatic.

Treatment

1. Nonspecific treatment should be directed toward removal of the exudate, e.g., frequent irrigations and good hygiene.
2. Penicillin is the drug of choice, although the organism is becoming increasingly resistant. There are no standardized regimens for the treatment of infants and young children, but in general, high doses over a period of 3 to 5 days should be used. For adolescent males and females the following regimen should be used in uncomplicated gonorrhea: aqueous procaine penicillin G, 4.8 million units, divided into two doses and injected into different intramuscular

sites together with probenecid, 1 Gm, orally given at least 30 minutes prior to the penicillin.

An alternate regimen consists of ampicillin, 3.5 Gm, orally with 1 Gm probenecid given simultaneously. For those allergic to the penicillins, spectinomycin may be used.

3. Accurate reporting and follow-up of all cases is essential.

There is no immunity to urethral, genital, and occular gonorrhea, hence the patient may become infected repeatedly.

PRIMARY TUBERCULOSIS

Primary, or childhood, tuberculosis means the first infection of an individual with tubercle bacilli. Primary tuberculosis may not occur until adulthood.

Etiology   The causative agent is *Mycobacterium tuberculosis*, var. *hominis*, occasionally *bovis*.

Mode of transmission   Infection is almost always by droplet infection from an adult. Contaminated fomites are not considered to be a common source of infection. Bovine tuberculosis (infection through milk) is practically nonexistent in this country. Rarely, tuberculosis may be acquired through the placenta.

Incubation period   Average incubation is 5 to 6 weeks; from the time of infection before development of allergy to tuberculin may be as long as 3 months.

Pathogenesis   The lung is involved in over 90 percent of cases:

1. The primary focus (Ghon tubercle) is the initial tissue lesion.
2. Transmission of tubercle bacilli is through the lymphatic vessels to the regional lymph nodes. A primary pulmonary complex would consist of primary focus in the lung, lymphangitis, and hilar lymphadenopathy.

Diagnosis   A diagnosis of primary tuberculosis is based on

1. History or evidence of contact with an open case of tuberculosis.
2. Positive tuberculin test.
3. Roentgenograms suggestive of tuberculosis.
4. Recovery of tubercle bacilli from gastric lavage, sputum, or other material, e.g., spinal fluid, stool, or urine, by direct smear, culture, or following injection into a guinea pig.
5. The clinical picture is most variable. The child may be entirely

symptom-free or may show any or all the following: elevated temperature (especially in the late afternoon or evening), persistent cough, anorexia, fatigue, loss of weight, night sweats (in older children), upper respiratory tract infection signs, croupy cough and stridor, and elevated sedimentation rate. Erythema nodosum and phlyctenular conjunctivitis may appear with the development of allergy.

Tuberculin tests   Intradermal (Mantoux) Test: Purified protein derivative (PPD)—screening (intermediate) dose is 0.0001 mg or 0.0002 mg (5 or 10 tuberculin units—TU); with old tuberculin (OT)—0.1 mg (10 TU). If positive, there is induration of 10 mm or more after 48 hours. Induration of between 5 and 9 mm is doubtful, and the test should be repeated in 6 weeks. A reaction of less than 5 mm is negative.

If tuberculosis is suspected, a dose of 1 TU (first strength PPD) is used. PPD second strength (250 TU) is used only to confirm a negative intermediate PPD.

PPD tablets must be used immediately (within 30 minutes) after reconstitution with diluent. Rapid deterioration of the solution may give rise to false-negative reactions. Recently, a new fluid PPD "stabilized solution" which has been guaranteed for 1 year under proper storage conditions has been made available.

Heaf test   This is a multiple puncture test using a special gun and disposable cartridge. Fluid concentrated PPD (about 100 TU) is applied either to the skin of the patient or the cartridge. Six punctures are made through the layer of PPD. The reaction is read 3 to 7 days later. Four or more papules are considered a positive test. Many false-positive tests and adverse reactions occur with this method. A positive test should be confirmed with a PPD (5 TU) Mantoux test.

Tine test (Rosenthal)   The unit consists of four stainless steel points, each 2 mm long, attached to a plastic handle. The teeth of the tines are precoated with OT, 5 TU. The points are pressed to the skin of the forearm. Tests are read at 48 to 72 hours. Induration of 5 mm or more is positive. Induration of 2 to 4 mm is a doubtful test and must be confirmed (see Heaf test). Induration of less than 2 mm is negative.

The significance of the tuberculin test in different age groups   A positive tuberculin test indicates that the person is or has been infected at some time with the tubercle bacillus and has become sensitized to the tuberculoprotein. (Previous vaccination with BCG gives positive tuberculin test.)

1.   In children under 1 year of age, it means active tuberculosis, with usually a guarded prognosis, even if there are no clinical or roentgenographic findings, since miliary tuberculosis and tubercular meningitis are common complications at this age.

2. In ages from 1 to 3 years, it probably means active tuberculosis with a good prognosis, if the child can be removed from the source of infection and treated.
3. Over 3 years of age, it indicates evidence of a past infection, which may or may not be active. Prognosis in this group is excellent.

The tuberculin test may be negative in infected persons under the following circumstances:

1. It may be negative for 2 to 8 months following the initial infection until an allergy is established to the tuberculoprotein, although this usually takes only 6 weeks.
2. A positive reactor may become negative during measles (or following active immunization), infectious mononucleosis, other virus diseases, scarlet fever, and pertussis.
3. In the course of miliary tuberculosis or tubercular meningitis, especially if the patient is in extremis, the tuberculin test may become negative.
4. During ACTH, hydrocortisone, or other immunosuppressive therapy.
5. Subcutaneous rather than intradermal injection of tuberculin may account for a false-negative reaction.
6. Patients under isoniazed therapy, particularly with a mild infection, may occasionally lose their reactivity to tuberculin.

The tuberculin test is markedly positive in

1. Tubercular infection of the bones or joints.
2. Tuberculosis in a diabetic child
3. Tubercular pleurisy
4. Erythema nodosum
5. Phlyctenular conjunctivitis

Roentgenograms of the chest

1. May show nothing or very little, since the primary tuberculosis may heal by resorption, fibrosis, or calcification (calcified nodules near periphery of the lung)
2. May show an exudative process about the primary focus (pneumonic or parenchymatous type)
3. May show a typical picture of enlarged hilar glands (hilar type)
4. May show a combination of the above (hilar and parenchymatous)
5. May show pleural effusion (unilateral) atalectasis or emphysema

Complications Dissemination occurs in unfavorable cases when the tubercle bacilli are too numerous or too virulent, or when the patient's resistance is poor.

1. Hematogenous spread is due to erosion of a blood vessel, leading to tuberculosis of any other organ of the body. Miliary tuberculosis and tubercular meningitis are discussed later. (Tuberculosis of the kidneys is rare in children except as part of a generalized miliary tuberculosis.)
2. Lymphogenous spread results in cervical or other node involvement.
3. Aspiration of the child's own sputum may result in spread to other areas of the lung (caseous pneumonia).
4. Caseous bronchopneumonia may result when material from a tubercular focus in the parenchyma or from a lymph node gets discharged into a bronchus in a state of liquefaction and is then spread to another part of the lung.
5. Endobronchial tuberculosis results from erosion through the bronchial wall from a contiguous process (usually an infected lymph node) with the production of large amounts of intraluminal polypoid material resulting in either emphysema (partial obstruction) or atelectasis (complete obstruction).
6. Ingestion of positive sputum leads to enteritis, mesenteric glandular tuberculosis, and tuberculous peritonitis.

"Reinfection tuberculosis" is a term used for a second infection with tubercle bacilli after the primary infection has been brought under control, whether the new infection is endogenous or exogenous.

Prognosis   The prognosis depends on

1. Age: It is worse in infants below 1 year and improves directly with increase in age.
2. Individual resistance to tuberculosis and the number and virulence of the tubercle bacilli.
3. Good nutrition and hygienic environment.
4. Adequate chemotherapy, the single most important factor.

Prophylaxis

1. Exposure to persons with known positive cases should be avoided.
2. Continued search for infected children (in schools, day-care centers, clinics, doctors' offices, and hospitals) by periodic tuberculin testing and periodic roentgenograms of all members of the community.
3. Chemoprophylaxis—if a tuberculin-positive child is identified, all his child associates and all child associates of the presumptive adult source case should be tuberculin-tested and if positive, x-rayed, cultured, and placed in treatment. The tuberculin-negative newborn infant, older infant, or child in contact with or recently exposed to an infectious case of tuberculosis should receive chemoprophylaxis throughout the period of exposure and for 6 months after the contact has been broken. Isoniazid (INH) is used in both of these situations.

4. BCG—vaccination with bacillus Calmette-Guérin is still a controversial subject in this country. One important objection to its use is interference with the interpretation of the tuberculin test; other objections are inability to judge its true effectiveness and an occasional dissemination of the bacillus with disastrous results. Children who have skin infections, positive tuberculin tests, burns, recent smallpox vaccinations, or who have immunoglobulin defects should not be given BCG. The major indications are

a. Children exposed to tuberculosis but who cannot be observed serially.

b. Children in households with adults under treatment or recently off treatment.

c. Children who live in or expect to travel to areas where tuberculosis is prevalent.

Children who are less than 2 months of age need not be tuberculin-tested prior to vaccination with BCG. Ten weeks after vaccination, a tuberculin test (250 TU) should be made. It is usually positive; if negative, revaccinate. BCG should not be given with INH because the latter inhibits the former.

Treatment

1. General measures
   a. Treat child at home unless seriously ill, persistently communicable, or home conditions are poor.
   b. Bed rest during toxic and febrile phase.
   c. Nutritious diet and supplementary vitamins.
   d. Protection from intercurrent infections.
2. Specific chemotheraphy
   a. Major drugs
      Isoniazid (INH)
      Ethambutol
      Streptomycin
      Rifampin
      Para-aminosalicylic acid (PAS)
   b. Secondary drugs
      Pyrizinamide
      Ethionamide
      Cycloserine
      Viomycin
      Kanamycin
      Capreomycin
   Dosage and side effects
   a. INH—5 to 30 mg per kg per day, orally or intramuscularly, one or two doses per day; the lower dosage is used for prophylaxis (newborn, 5 mg per kg per day; older infants and children, 10 mg per kg per day) and long-term therapy (usu-

ally after 12 to 18 months). The higher dosage is used for severe involvement. Side effects are vertigo, syncope, drowsiness or restlessness, hyperreflexia, neuritis, occasionally liver damage, diarrhea, or constipation. Adults show signs of pyridoxine deficiency, but this has not been reported in children; however, pyridoxine may be given if desired. All side effects are rare in children, and the drug is exceedingly well-tolerated.

b. Ethambutol—15 to 25 mg per kg per day orally can be given in one dose. Optic neuritis is an uncommon side effect.

c. Streptomycin—20 to 50 mg per kg per day, intramuscularly usually 1 Gm per day. Severe 8th nerve damage may occur.

d. PAS—0.2 to 0.5 Gm per kg per day (up to 12 Gm), orally, divided into three to four doses. Side effects include frequent nausea, vomiting, and diarrhea; it is difficult for children to take.

e. Rifampin—10 to 20 mg per kg per day, one to two doses daily. Causes occasional transitory elevation of the transaminases and impairs hepatic clearance of bilirubin; rarely, hearing loss occurs.

3. Surgery—Extirpation of infected portion of the lung and lymph node, joint, and bone surgery.

Principal indications for treatment

1. INH is recommended for 1 year for the following groups at high risk:
   a. All patients with active or possibly active disease—may be treated with INH alone or with INH plus PAS or ethambutol.
   b. Infants and preschool children with a positive tuberculin test.
   c. Adolescents with a positive tuberculin test not previously treated and adolescents, particularly girls, who had serious tuberculosis in childhood.
   d. Recent tuberculin reactors at any age.
   e. All children with a positive Mantoux test regardless of time of conversion in the presence of demonstrable disease.
2. Known tuberculin reactors with diabetes, leukemia, and malnutrition should probably be treated with INH continuously or in the case of malnutrition, until it is corrected.
3. Known tuberculin reactors with measles, measles immunization, pertussis, and those undergoing surgery should be given INH for 3 months.
4. Tuberculin reactors who are being treated with steroids, alkylating agents, or antimetabolites should receive INH during the period of therapy with these drugs and for 3 months afterward.
5. All children with more than just a simple primary infection should be treated with at least two drugs and if very seriously ill (e.g., miliary, meningitis, endobronchial, renal cavitation), with three

drugs. The usual combination of two is INH with ethambutol or PAS; and with three it is INH, streptomycin, and rifampin. The secondary drugs are used in various combinations with the major drugs in cases of antimicrobial resistance.

MILIARY TUBERCULOSIS

Miliary tuberculosis is the result of dissemination of the tubercle bacilli into the general circulation, usually from a primary caseous tracheobronchial lymph node that ulcerates into a large vein or into the thoracic duct. It is seen most frequently in infants and young children and is often difficult to recognize in the early stages. The clinical features are irregular fever, irritability, anorexia, loss of weight, mild respiratory distress, palpable spleen and liver, and leukocytosis. As the disease progresses, fine rales can be heard and the respiratory rate increases. Later, emaciation and pronounced debility occur. Roentgenograms reveal a characteristic "snowflake" appearance.

TUBERCULAR MENINGITIS

Clinical features

1. The onset is gradual, and this stage lasts from 1 to 2 weeks. The first abnormalities noted are changes in personality, with irritability, anorexia, drowsiness, and vomiting.
2. Then meningeal signs (second stage) appear (see The Meningitides, below). Ocular palsies and other eye signs are common during this stage.
3. As the meningeal involvement increases, the cerebral symptoms become more severe, with convulsions and localized muscular twitchings; then stupor and coma (third stage) with decerebrate rigidity, opisthotonus, hyperpyrexia, irregular pulse and respirations, and death.
4. Roentgenograms of the chest may reveal a primary complex or miliary tuberculosis.
5. The spinal fluid examination is most important. It reveals increased pressure; clear or ground-glass appearance; 50 to 500 cells, with lymphocytes predominate; glucose decreased, ranging usually from 18 to 36 mg per 100 ml; total protein increased; and tubercle bacilli in smear and culture. (Pellicle formation in cerebrospinal fluid is a particularly good source for bacteria.)

Treatment of tubercular meningitis and miliary tuberculosis

1. Drugs: see above.
2. Fluids and electrolytes to maintain balance during period of hypotonicity.

3. Adrenal corticosteroids (prednisone, 1 mg per kg per day, for 6 to 8 weeks) have been tried in association with the antitubercular agents and appear to be beneficial.

ATYPICAL MYCOBACTERIA

These are mostly saprophytes which have increasingly been implicated in human disease but are not communicable from person to person.

The following table is a classification of disorders produced by these atypical mycobacteria.

Type	Group (Runyon)	Organism	Disease produced
Photochromogens (yellow-orange colonies on exposure to light)	I	*M. kansasii*	Pulmonary infection indistinguishable from tuberculosis, disseminated lesions, lymphadenitis, and skin granulomas.
Scotochromogens (yellow-orange colonies in either light or dark)	II	*M. balnei* (*marinum*) "scrofula type"	"Swimming pool" granuloma—skin, lymph gland, and bone lesions.
Nonphotochromogens (buff or light-tan colonies)	III	Battey-avion-swine group (mainly in Southeast U.S.)	Pulmonary and occasional disseminated lesion, lymphadenitis, bone lesions.
"Rapid growing" (nonpigmented)	IV	*M. fortuitum,* etc., *M. ulcerans*	Rare cause of pulmonary and disseminated disease, lymphadenitis, deep skin ulcers.

Diagnosis

1. By skin tests: Many atypical mycobacteria give weakly positive (less than 10 mm) reactions to the tuberculin skin test. Comparative tuberculin tests using PPD-S (tuberculin) with PPD–atypical myobacteria may be of use. If the reaction to the PPD–atypical mycobacteria is larger than the reaction to the PPD-S, infection with atypical mycobacteria is probable, and tuberculous infection is highly unlikely. The PPD–atypical mycobacteria may also be used alone and may be positive in tuberculin-negative persons. In those in whom there is a dermal reaction to one or more strains of these bacteria, the largest reaction is likely to be produced by the antigen of the offending organism. These antigens are generally available from state or local health departments.
2. By culture of material from gastric washings, lymph nodes, skin scrapings, etc.

Treatment

1. Many atypical mycobacteria are relatively resistant to INH and streptomycin. Most are susceptible to rifampin.
2. Combinations of drugs including rifampin should be used and changed in accordance with sensitivity studies.

THE PURULENT MENINGITIDES

All the purulent meningitides may present any or many of the following clinical features: fever, headache, vomiting, nuchal rigidity, tense fontanel, intracranial bruit, opisthotonos, increased muscle tone, hyperreflexia, positive Kernig's and Brudzinski's signs, occasionally twitchings, convulsions, or somnolence. (Kernig's sign—the leg cannot be extended passively at the knee when the thigh is flexed to a right angle at the hip; Brudzinski's sign—an involuntary flexion of the thighs and knees when the neck is flexed.) Newborn infants may have a paucity of signs and symptoms—see Chapter 12, "Diseases of the Newborn." Infants beyond the newborn period often present with just fever and marked inconsolable irritability. They may also have a tense anterior fontanel and some of the other aforementioned signs.

The differential diagnosis of the meningitides may be aided by certain symptoms and signs but is confirmed only by the spinal fluid examination.

Lumbar punctures are a necessity for diagnosis and to ascertain the results of therapy. Table 14-6 shows the characteristic spinal fluid findings in the various meningitides and other conditions.

In addition to spinal fluid smear and culture, the use of fluorescent-antibody techniques may be of great value in the identification of specific organisms. When the organism causing the meningitis is not known, ampicillin is the drug of choice. It should be given in doses of 200 to 400 mg per kg per day, intravenously, every 4 hours. When the specific causative agent is identified by culture, other indicated drugs may be used instead, or if the patient is improving, it may be continued. Supportive therapy, e.g., fluids and electrolytes, is important.

MENINGISMUS

Meningismus is characterized by the signs and symptoms of meningeal irritation with normal spinal fluid. Meningismus in infants and children may be found with any acute infection. It is not uncommon in pneumonia (especially of the upper lobe), diarrhea, roseola infantum, otitis media, tonsillitis, pyelonephritis, and cervical adenitis.

The spinal fluid is increased in amount and pressure, but the cytologic and chemical findings are normal.

The treatment should be directed toward the primary disease. Lumbar punctures to relieve increased pressure are unnecessary.

Table 14-6. Spinal fluid findings

Disease	Cytology, cells/cu mm	Protein, mg/100 ml	Sugar, mg/100 ml	Bacteriology	Miscellaneous
Meningismus	Normal; 5–10 lymphocytes	Normal; 20–40	Normal; 50–80	Negative, by smear and culture	Increased pressure—over 200 mm H_2O
Aseptic meningitis (usually viral)	Increased; usually 50–500, predominantly lymphocytes	Normal or increased; 45–80	Normal (at least ½ blood sugar)	Negative, by smear and culture	Increased pressure—over 200 mm H_2O; mumps may reveal low sugar; enteric viruses, LCM virus may reveal polymorphonuclear, early
Purulent meningitis, e.g., pneumococcus, streptococcus, meningococcus, *H. influenza*	Increased; 500–3,000 or more, predominantly polymorphonuclear	Increased; 60–100 or higher	Decreased; 0–45 (less than ½ blood sugar)	Infecting organism by smear and culture. Type with specific antisera	Increased pressure—over 200 mm H_2O
Tuberculous meningitis	Increased; 50–500, usually lymphocytes, early polymorphonuclear	Increased; 45–120 or higher	Decreased; 0–45 (less than ½ blood sugar)	Tubercle bacilli by smear, culture, and guinea-pig inoculation	Increased pressure—over 200 mm H_2O. Chlorides often reduced below 600 mg per 100 ml; pellicle formation
Partially treated bacterial meningitis	Increased; 50–300	40–80	Normal or slight decrease	May be negative by smear and culture	Increased pressure—over 200 mm H_2O
Postinfectious or postvaccinal encephalitis	Increased; 20–500, usually lymphocytes	May be increased	Normal	Negative for bacteria by smear and culture	Increased pressure—over 200 mm H_2O. Usually follows primary disease, e.g., measles, rubella, chickenpox, or smallpox, rabies, or pertussis vaccination

318

Disease	Cells	Protein	Sugar	Bacteria	Remarks
Landry-Guillain-Barré syndrome (infectious neuronitis)	Slightly increased; usually 20–50, predominantly lymphocytes	Markedly increased; 80–200	Normal	Negative for bacteria by smear and culture	Increased pressure—over 200 mm H_2O. There is albuminocytologic dissociation
Brain tumor	Increased; usually 20–100, usually lymphocytes	Normal or increased; 40–100 or higher	Normal or low	Negative by smear and culture	Increased pressure—over 200 mm H_2O. Medulloblastoma may reveal low sugar
Intracranial hemorrhage	May be increased red blood cells; if old blood, the cells are crenated	Increased; 40–60	Normal or slightly elevated	Negative by smear and culture	Increased pressure—over 200 mm H_2O. Supernatant fluid is xanthochromic, with positive benzidine test, and does not clot on standing
Traumatic puncture	Red blood cells are round and normal	Normal to increased	Normal to increased	Negative	Fluid clears as it flows; blood clots on standing. Supernatant fluid is clear, with negative benzidine test. Ratio of red to white blood cells is the same as in peripheral blood

MENINGOCOCCAL MENINGITIS AND MENINGOCOCCEMIA

Etiology   The diseases are caused by the meningococcus (types A, B, C, and D).

Mode of transmission   Infection is spread by droplet infection from active cases or carriers.

Pathogenesis   Pathogenesis is probably from nasopharynx to bloodstream to central nervous system.

Clinical features   The septicemic form has a sudden onset with hyperpyrexia, chills, vomiting, malaise, occasionally joint pains and tenderness. Purpuric lesions—petechiae or ecchymoses—most marked over the pressure areas are highly suggestive.

The meningitic form presents symptoms and signs of meningitis, plus those of septicemia.

Endotoxic shock with disseminated intravascular coagulation (DIC) leading to adrenal hemorrhage and circulatory collapse (Waterhouse-Friderichsen syndrome) occurs frequently with meningococcemia. The patient shows widespread purpura, cloudy sensorium leading to confusion and coma, rapid thready pulse, and hypotension. With DIC there will be thrombocytopenia and a diminution of coagulation factors I, II, V, and VIII and an increase in fibrin-split products.

Treatment for endotoxic shock and its consequences includes vigorous antimicrobial therapy against the meningococcus, maintenance of adequate blood volume, restoration of arterial circulation using such drugs as isoproterenol or pharmacologic doses of hydrocortisone (which also has other antiendotoxic effects), and correction of metabolic acidemia. The use of heparin in DIC is quite controversial. Exchange transfusion has been helpful in some cases. Meningococcal disease may be mimicked by enteric viruses—particularly ECHO 9, staphylococcal endocarditis, or streptococcal septicemia.

Laboratory findings

1. Spinal fluid reveals few to several thousand polymorphonuclear leukocytes, reduced sugar, elevated protein, and intracellular Gram-negative diplococci found in smears and cultures.
2. Blood culture may be positive. Nose and throat culture may reveal meningococci. Scraping or aspirating skin lesions by injecting 0.1 ml saline solution may reveal the organism by smear and culture.
3. Polynucleosis of 20,000 to 30,000 in the blood.
4. Where cultures are negative, the serum of the patient on recovery can be agglutinated against meningococci, and a retrospective diagnosis can be made.

Complications Deafness, blindness, hydrocephalus, pneumonia, arthritis, and endocarditis may complicate the infection.

Prognosis The prognosis is good, except in fulminating types.

Treatment

1. Penicillin (aqueous crystalline penicillin G) 400,000 units per kg per day, intravenously, in six divided doses until afebrile for 7 days.
2. Care of contacts and carriers:
   a. Contacts should be treated with surveillance and throat cultures. If throat culture is positive, rifampin may be given for approximately 4 days, and penicillin, although it cannot eradicate the organisms from the pharynx, may prevent bacteremia.
   b. Carrier state—rifampin and minocycline are effective, particularly in adults.

Prophylaxis A vaccine against meningococcus type C (the most prevalent type) has been developed and is in use in the U.S. Armed Forces. Present indications are that it is highly effective and may soon be used for civilian populations. A vaccine against type A organisms is under study.

PNEUMOCOCCAL MENINGITIS

Pneumococcal meningitis is more common among infants than among older children. It usually follows otitis media or sinusitis, rarely an upper respiratory infection, pneumonia, or skull fracture.

Etiology The agent is the pneumococcus.

Diagnosis

1. Clinical features of meningitis.
2. Spinal fluid findings are the same as in other purulent meningitides, with positive smear and culture (intra- and extracellular Gram-positive diplococci).
3. Nose and throat cultures and blood culture may also reveal pneumococci.

Complications Pneumococcal complications include: pneumonia, empyema, peritonitis, and pericarditis; central nervous system complications include: brain abscess, paralyses, mental retardation, nerve deafness, and seizure disorders.

Prognosis The prognosis is guarded.

Treatment Treatment consists of penicillin G (aqueous, crystalline), 5 to 20 million units per day, intravenously, divided in six doses depending on age and severity of the infection for 1 to 2 weeks followed by 2 million units per day, intramuscularly for 1 week.

INFLUENZAL MENINGITIS

Etiology   The causative agent is *Hemophilus influenza,* almost invariably type B.

Clinical features   All those listed under the other purulent meningitides are true of influenzal meningitis with the following important differences: influenzal meningitis is the most frequent cause of bacterial meningitis. It occurs most often between 4 and 36 months of age with a peak incidence between 6 and 18 months; it is often preceded or accompanied by an upper respiratory infection and otitis media; purpura is uncommon.

Incubation period   Incubation is 3 to 5 days usually but may be variable.

Laboratory findings

1. Spinal fluid: cytologic and chemical findings as in other purulent meningitides; smear and culture on chocolate agar reveal a Gram-negative pleomorphic coccobacillus.
2. Nose and throat cultures and blood culture may reveal the organism.

Complications

1. As in other purulent meningitides.
2. Subdural collections of fluid may be associated with meningitis, particularly *H. influenza* meningitis. This complication should be suspected if focal neurologic signs or fever persist and the spinal fluid does not become sterile following adequate treatment. Subdural taps should be made, and if fluid is found, it should be removed by repeated aspirations.
3. Persistence or recurrence of fever may be caused by (2) above, brain abscess, or other foci of infection. Rarely, it may be due to phlebitis (following intravenous therapy), drug fever, or intercurrent infection.

Treatment

1. Supportive therapy—maintain fluid and electrolyte balance, maintain adequate airway.
2. Ampicillin—200 to 400 mg per kg per day, intravenously in six divided doses for 8 days after child is afebrile. If lower dose is given early, it should be increased after 2 to 3 days when meningeal

inflammation is diminished and blood-brain barrier is less permeable.

3. Chloramphenicol—100 mg per kg per day, intravenously, in four divided doses if the organism is resistant to ampicillin.

Prognosis   The prognosis is good if the disease is treated promptly.

STREPTOCOCCAL AND STAPHYLOCOCCAL MENINGITIS

Rarely staphylococcal meningitis may occur in the newborn period, postoperatively, or as a complication of endocarditis. Streptococcal meningitis usually due to group B beta-hemolytic type may also occur in the newborn. Streptococcal meningitis may occur as a complication of endocarditis (alpha streptococci) or as a result of a lesion of the skin, scalp, or throat.

For a discussion of bacterial meningitis of the newborn, see Chapter 12, "Diseases of the Newborn."

PARTIALLY TREATED BACTERIAL MENINGITIS

Partially treated bacterial meningitis is becoming a particularly difficult problem because of widespread and often indiscriminate antimicrobial use. Many children with early meningitis have been treated with enough antimicrobial therapy to distort the cerebrospinal fluid and peripheral blood findings so that in many instances the organism cannot be grown in culture and the typical polynucleosis and hypoglycorrachia may be absent. This then mimics an aseptic meningitis and causes a dilemma for the clinician. A test involving the ability of the white cells to reduce a specific dye, nitroblue tetrazolium (NBT) may be helpful in making the differential between an aseptic meningitis and a bacterial meningitis. A positive test is based on the ratio of NBT-positive neutrophils to the absolute number of neutrophils.

TULAREMIA

Etiology   Tularemia is caused by *Pasteurella tularensis* (*Francisella tularensis*).

Mode of transmission   Ingestion of improperly cooked rabbits, handling of squirrels and rabbits, tick bites, and bites of species of deer fly, and rarely, contaminated water can all cause tularemia.

Incubation period   Incubation is 1 to 10 days, averaging 3 days.

Clinical features   Symptoms depend on the mode and site of infection. Several types are known:

1. Ulceroglandular and glandular: primary cutaneous lesions which progress from papule to pustule to necrosis and finally to ulceration with scar formation associated with regional lymphadenopathy.
2. Oropharyngeal (pharyngotonsillar): The lesions in the mucous membrane of the oropharynx resemble those of the skin. There may be a follicular tonsillitis with a shaggy necrotic exudate and marked cervical lymphadenopathy. Vomiting, abdominal pain, and diarrhea may be present.
3. Typhoid-like (gastrointestinal): fever, toxemia, drowsiness, and prostration.
4. Oculoglandular: lacrimation, pruritus, and pain are followed by the appearance of yellow nodules on the conjunctiva. These nodules progress through the same stages as the skin lesions. There is regional adenopathy.
5. Pleuropulmonary: cough and frequently pleuritic pain.

Laboratory findings

1. Skin test (Foshay's test).
2. Agglutination test—none specific; cross-agglutination to brucella and proteus organisms may occur as well as heterophile antibody.
3. Culture of lesion or of blood.
4. Roentgenograms, which reveal infiltration in the pleuropulmonary type.

Treatment Tetracycline is the drug of choice; chloramphenicol is also effective and may be used as an adjuvant.

Prognosis Prognosis is good when treatment is instituted early.

BRUCELLOSIS

Brucellosis is an infectious disease caused by *Brucella abortus, Br. suis,* or *Br. melitensis,* which have their reservoir usually in the cow, hog, or goat, respectively. In children the infection is usually caused by *Br. abortus* and is acquired by drinking raw milk or other dairy products. The severity of the disease and symptoms depends on the etiologic strain. *Abortus* is the mildest, and *melitensis* is the most virulent.

Incubation period Incubation is 5 to 30 days.

Clinical features

1. The onset may be very insidious, with intermittent fever, malaise, weakness, and sweats, then subsidence for varied periods followed by acute flare-ups. Fever characteristically rises in the afternoon. Patients often present with "fever of undetermined origin."

2. Generalized lymphadenopathy and splenomegaly are more common in acute than in chronic cases. Hepatitis and jaundice may occur.
3. Arthritis; various skin lesions, e.g., erythema and purpura; ulceration of the mucous membranes; paralysis of extraocular muscles; pulmonary infiltrations; osteomyelitis; encephalitis; and meningitis have all been described.
4. Chronic form—low-grade fever, easy fatigability, pallor, irritability, and failure to gain weight—may persist for months or years.

Laboratory findings

1. Leukocyte counts are normal or low, with a lymphocytic predominance.
2. Isolation and culture of brucella from the blood, bone marrow, lymph node, or urine.
3. Serology: (a) agglutination test is helpful but false-positive and false-negative reactions occur. If negative in the face of strong clinical evidence of brucellosis, blocking antibodies may be present. (b) Blocking antibodies appear during the subacute phase and persist for years. (c) Precipitin test is a good indicator of active infection (after the acute phase).
4. Intradermal test: positive reaction indicates past contact but not necessarily active infection.

Treatment   Brucellosis should be treated with tetracyclines; in severe cases streptomycin may be added.

RAT–BITE FEVER

There are two types of rat-bite fever:

1. Sodoku, caused by *Spirillum minus* (*Spirillum morsus muris*), lasting usually more than 7 days with an incubation period of 1 to 3 weeks
2. Rat-bite fever (erythema arthriticum epidemicum), caused by *Streptobacillus moniliformis* (*Streptothrix muris rattis*), with an incubation period of 3 to 10 days, rarely longer

Sodoku is characterized by ulceration at the site of the bite and regional lymphadenitis, 3 to 4 days of elevated temperature, and a macular rash on the face and trunk; then, after an interval of 3 to 5 days, the febrile episode with rash is repeated.

Rat-bite fever, due to *S. moniliformis*, is characterized by irregular fever, a macular rash (the macules are smaller than those seen in sodoku), and polyarthritis involving both large and small joints. The local lesion may or may not ulcerate, and the febrile paroxysms have no regularity of recurrence. Haverhill fever is an *S. moniliformis* infection when the organism is ingested in milk.

Laboratory findings   A smear from the primary lesion or animal inoculation of blood and infected material will usually demonstrate the spirillum or streptobacillus. Agglutination test may be positive for streptobacillus.

Treatment   Penicillin is effective in both types of rat-bite fever.

LEPTOSPIROSIS

Leptospirosis (Weil's disease) is caused by many species of the genus *Leptospira*, most commonly *L. pomona*, *L. canicola*, and *L. icterohaemorrhagiae*. It is usually contracted while swimming in water or by eating food contaminated by the urine of infected wild rodents. Some domestic animals, for example, dogs and cattle, may also be infected. Incubation period is about 6 to 15 days. Leptospirosis is characterized in the early stages by septicemia and aseptic meningitis; later there are jaundice and hemorrhage into the skin and mucous membranes. Conjunctival injection occurs often as well as muscle pain and renal involvement resulting in albuminuria and azotemia. The clinical manifestations are very varied and will depend on the type of leptospira causing the infection. *L. icterohaemorrhagiae* and *L. canicola* cause severe disease. *L. pomona* causes most cases in the United States and only rarely causes jaundice. Diagnosis is based early in the course on finding the organism in the blood by dark-field preparation, by culturing whole blood, by inoculating animals with fresh plasma or urine, and by serum antibodies (agglutinating), complement-fixing, and lytic. Treatment is administration of tetracycline drugs and penicillin.

SYPHILIS

Congenital syphilis is not uncommon, and the incidence is increasing. It can only be eradicated through constant surveillance, an awareness that it exists, and through the pediatrician's insistence that public health authorities provide proper education and adequate treatment facilities.

Acquired syphilis is very rare in children but it is an increasing problem in adolescents. The symptoms and signs are similar to those in the adult.

EARLY CONGENITAL SYPHILIS

Etiology   The causative organism in syphilis is *Treponema pallidum*.

Source Maternal infection is the source.

Mode of transmission Congenital syphilis is passed in utero through the placenta about the fifth month of pregnancy. Infection prior to the fourth month is uncommon.

Clinical and laboratory features Any of the following may be found, or there may be practically no findings.

1. Rhinitis ("snuffles") is usually protracted and is characterized by a mucopurulent discharge, occasionally bloody, with upper-lip excoriation.
2. Skin and mucous membrane lesions: skin lesions are usually maculopapular, circular, elevated, and nonitching and involve the extremities; at first they are bright red, later becoming brown, and upon clearing there is a residual staining. The palms and soles may show redness and desquamation. There may be fissures around the corners of the mouth which become rhagades (radiating fissured scars). Condylomata lata are flat raised plaques that occur in the anogenital area. Mucous patches are flattened grayish-white lesions that appear on the buccal mucosa. All the above lesions are infectious.
3. Osseous lesions—the patient often presents with pseudoparalysis (Parrot's paralysis). Radiographically there is a multifocal, osteochondritis at the metaphyses of the elbows, wrists, knees, and ankles; symmetrical periostitis; and osteomyelitis of the long bones and occasionally of the skull. These bone lesions are often present at birth; if not, they appear within 2 months. The humeri and tibiae are often involved. The bilateral moth-eaten appearance of the medial aspects of the proximal tibiae (Wimberger's sign) is a highly characteristic finding of early congenital lues. There may also be widened and serrated epiphyseal lines and sometimes actual separation of the epiphyses. The lesions of osteochondritis and myelitis are present early. They are the most constant finding in early congenital lues and heal spontaneously without scarring within a few months. The periostitis, however, may continue actively for about 2 years, leaving a thickened cortex which results in the deformities of saber shin and frontal bossing. Later in infancy there may be recurrence of bone lesions frequently asymmetrical and frequently involving the hands and feet.
4. Hepatosplenomegaly is usually moderate and is accompanied by some degree of jaundice.
5. Central nervous system: meningitis signs and symptoms are rare, but there may be convulsions and hydrocephalus. One-third of all cases of congenital syphilis, with or without meningeal symptoms, show spinal fluid changes.
6. There are usually malnutrition, anemia, lymphadenopathy (par-

ticularly epitrochlear), chorioretinitis, pneumonia (alba), and renal involvement. Early congenital lues must be differentiated from congenital rubella, herpes, toxoplasmosis, and cytomegalovirus infection.

LATE CONGENITAL SYPHILIS

Late congenital syphilis may show any of the following:

1. Interstitial keratitis usually is found from 6 to 12 years of age and may be bilateral; it is resistant to treatment.
2. Meningovascular involvement with mental retardation and hemiplegia may be found.
3. Periostitis is shown by a saber shin.
4. Hutchinson's triad consists of deafness, which is now rarely found; central incisor notching and pegging, which is of moderate frequency; and keratitis, which occurs more often.
5. Paroxysmal hemoglobinuria (after exposure to cold), saddle nose, rhagades, bossing of head, and typical facies are infrequent.
6. Mulberry molars, Clutton's joints (synovial effusion), and subcutaneous gumma also occur.

Diagnosis   Diagnosis depends on the following:

1. Careful history and physical examination.
2. Roentgenograms of the bones: periostitis and osteochondritis (changes are usually present after the neonatal period).
3. Laboratory tests
   a. Dark-field examinations—material from skin or mucous membrane lesions or sentinel lymph node draining area of primary lesion—identification of typical motile spirochetes.
   b. Immunofluorescence
   c. Serologic test for syphilis (STS)
      (1) Tests for reagin (nonspecific antibodies): flocculation tests—VDRL, Kahn, and others; complement-fixation tests—Wassermann, Kolman. These tests sometimes give rise to biologic false-positive (BFP) reactions. In the absence of negative clinical features, other serologic tests should be made and a family history taken.
      (2) Tests for antitreponema antibodies—these are specific and hence more diagnostic. TPI (treponema pallidum immobilization) tests—demonstration of specific antibodies in the patient's serum—not readily available. FTA-ABS (fluorescent treponemal antibody test)—the most sensitive serologic test for syphilis; the first to become positive in early syphilis. False-positive tests have been reported in patients with immunoglobulin abnormalities. The IgM FTA-ABS test is especially helpful in the diag-

nosis of congenital syphilis particularly in infants whose mother's treatment failed to eradicate the infection in the fetus. *T. pallidum* complement-fixation test is too difficult to perform for routine use. Cerebrospinal fluid tests—both reagin and FTA-ABS tests can be performed.

4. Reagin tests are good screening tests. In questionable cases a series (every 3 to 4 weeks) of quantitative titrations is helpful for diagnosis. A rising titer indicates infection; a falling titer indicates absence of infection (of material antibody). With a falling titer the test will probably become negative by 3 to 4 months of age. When there is doubt, particularly in an asymptomatic baby, the FTA-ABS and IgM-FTA-ABS tests should be done to clarify the situation.

Treatment

1. Congenital syphilis
   a. Prenatal treatment—comprises early diagnosis and adequate treatment of the syphilitic pregnant mother.
2. Postnatal treatment—treat all infants and children with a definite diagnosis of congenital syphilis, also infants of untreated syphilitic mothers born with a reactive STS or with any clinical or x-ray manifestations compatible with syphilis or under certain conditions even with no serologic, clinical, or x-ray evidence of lues. If in doubt, treat! The drug of choice is penicillin.

Treatment of congenital syphilis

	Benzathine penicillin G	or	Aqueous procaine penicillin
Under 2 years of age	50,000 units/kg intramuscularly in one injection		100,000 units/kg intramuscularly daily for 10 days
Over 2 years of age but under 70 lb	50,000 units/kg intramuscularly in one injection		100,000 units/kg intramuscularly daily for 10 days

3. Acquired syphilis
   a. Benzathine penicillin G 2.4 million units intramuscularly, once (1.2 million units in each buttock)
   b. With patients who are allergic to penicillin, tetracycline or erythromycin may be used.
4. In adequately treated patients, serologic tests should show a definite fall in titer—80 percent of patients treated during the primary stage become seronegative after 6 months of treatment, 90 percent are seronegative after 12 months, and almost all after 2 years.

Treatment given at the latter stages of the disease may result in reactive serologic tests in low titer for life. The adolescent who has syphilis should be screened for other venereal diseases, particularly gonorrhea.

MYCOTIC INFECTIONS

ACTINOMYCOSIS

Etiology   This infection is caused by *Actinomyces israelii*.

Source   The source is endogenous, found in the oral cavity of asymptomatic individuals.

Clinical course   The course is characterized by chronic granulomatous lesions in various parts of the body which begin as red, relatively nontender swellings which usually develop slowly. In over half the cases, the initial lesion is cervicofacial involving the tissues of the neck, face, tongue, and often the mandible. The lungs and abdominal organs may also be the primary site. These lesions tend to break down and form multiple draining sinuses. The discharge typically contains "sulfur granules," which consist of a mass of filamentous mycelia of the organism.

Diagnosis   Demonstration of "sulfur granules" in the pus and identification of the organism on smear and culture.

Treatment   Penicillin, tetracycline, chloramphenicol, or sulfonamides are effective. Penicillin is preferred because high doses are needed for a long period of time. Surgical drainage and extirpation are recommended.

HISTOPLASMOSIS

Etiology and transmission   Endemic in the Eastern and Central United States and many other areas of the world, histoplasmosis is caused by the fungus *Histoplasma capsulatum*. The organism may be found in soil or dust in chicken coops, barnyards, caves, or other locations contaminated by bird, bat, chicken, and other animal droppings, and is probably transmitted through inhalation of airborne spores.

Incubation period   Incubation is 5 to 18 days, averaging 10 days.

Clinical features   The disease is generally benign and may be suggested by the following:

1. A positive skin test for histoplasmosis without any signs, symptoms, or history of infection.
2. A positive skin test with symptomless pulmonary calcification, either mediastinal nodes or in a miliary distribution. (Tuberculosis should be excluded, e.g., results of the Mantoux test should be negative.)
3. Pulmonary infiltrations with or without cavitation which persist in spite of the usual treatment for such lesions.
4. Disseminated infection with intermittent fever, weight loss, lymphadenopathy (not marked in children), hepatosplenomegaly, ulcerations of the nose, mouth, tongue, and colon, joint and muscle pain, purpura and meningitis (the severe form which may be fatal).

Laboratory findings

1. Anemia (hypochromic)
2. Leukopenia with a relative lymphocytosis
3. Smears of blood, bone marrow, sputum, or ulcerations and biopsy from lymph nodes, spleen, or liver may reveal the organism
4. The above-mentioned material may be cultured
5. Positive skin test with histoplasmin (May be negative in severe disseminated disease)
6. Serology—latex agglutination; complement-fixation, and precipitin tests become positive within a few weeks after infection.

Treatment   There is usually no treatment. Amphotericin B is given for disseminated, progressive disease, especially in infants. It should be given intravenously, over a period of several hours, for 7 to 30 days in the dose of 1 mg per kg per day. It is extremely nephrotoxic, especially in older children. The blood urea nitrogen should be monitored (hydrocortisone may lessen reactions).

COCCIDIOIDOMYCOSIS (San Joaquin Valley Fever, Desert Arthritis)

Etiology   *Coccidioides immitis;* it is endemic in Southwestern United States, Mexico, and Argentina.

Mode of transmission   Transmission is by inhalation of spore-laden dust.

Incubation period   Incubation is 7 to 21 days.

Clinical features

1. The primary infection is usually asymptomatic (60 percent); in others, influenza-like illness with anorexia, fever, chills, malaise, night sweats, persistent dry cough, headache, backache, and chest

pain, also erythema nodosum with or without erythema multiforme. Arthritis and phlyctenular conjunctivitis may occur. Cavities may develop in the lung. Complete recovery occurs spontaneously in almost all cases.

2. Disseminated granulomatous infection occurs in fewer than 1 percent of infected persons and apparently denotes a defect in the individual's ability to localize and control the infection. It is ten times more frequent in blacks and Orientals and more common in males. It resembles progressive primary tuberculosis, disseminating to viscera, bone, and central nervous system, and it is usually fatal. The skin test may be negative.

Diagnosis

1. The skin test becomes positive 4 to 6 weeks after infection.
2. A smear of gastric washings, sputum, and lesions reveal the organism.
3. Mice injected intraperitoneally with infected material develop the disease.
4. Serology.
   a. Precipitating IgM antibodies develop early then diminish.
   b. Complement-fixing IgG antibodies are present in high titer only in disseminated disease.

Treatment

1. Amphotericin B as in histoplasmosis (see above)
2. Surgery for pulmonary cavities

CRYPTOCOCCOSIS (Torulosis)

The causative organism is *Cryptococcus neoformans*. It is spread through inhalation of pigeon excreta and contaminated soil particles containing *C. neoformans* yeasts. Pulmonary or skin infections apparently take place primarily and then spread to the viscera, bones, and particularly, the central nervous system. It causes a severe meningitis resembling tuberculous meningitis, brain abscess, brain tumor, or a degenerative disease of the central nervous system. Wet india ink preparations of sputum, pus, or spinal fluid sediment demonstrate the encapsulated yeasts. The organism can be cultured on Sabouraud's media. Amphotericin B or 5-fluorocytosine is used for treatment.

PROTOZOAN INFECTIONS

MALARIA

Etiology *Plasmodium vivax, P. falciparum, P. malariae,* or *P. knowlesi* are causative agents.

Mode of transmission Transmission is by several species of Anopheles mosquito; occasionally it is passed by blood transfusion.

Incubation period Incubation with *P. vivax* is 8 to 31 days; with *P. falciparum,* 6 to 25 days; with *P. malariae,* 28 to 37 days; and with *P. ovale,* 11 to 16 days.

Clinical features Symptoms vary depending on whether (*a*) infection is a primary one in a child with no immunity or (*b*) in a child who has been repeatedly exposed since birth and has partial immunity. Malaria can be transmitted through the placenta.

Primary disease This is a severe illness with behavioral changes, headache, anorexia, unusual crying, drowsiness, and disturbance of sleep. Fever may vary from gradual increase and short paroxysmal elevations to sudden onset of high fever (105 to 107°F) with continuous elevation (falciparum) or remittent fever with either gradual or sudden onset. Chills and sweats may or may not be present. Convulsions are common. Generalized aches and pains (particularly the back and abdomen), enlarged, tender spleen (vivax). The liver may become enlarged and tender, and jaundice may evolve into hepatic failure. Cerebral complications are manifest mainly by continued convulsions and coma with a paucity of neurologic signs and normal cerebrospinal fluid. Anemia (normocytic) is severe and kidney function may be impaired. The child may develop Blackwater fever (hemoglobinuria falciparum). Death may result from central nervous system involvement, ruptured spleen or kidney, or hepatic failure.

Chronic disease Chronic disease is present in children in endemic areas. These children may have no acute episode but often show chronic malaise, "failure to thrive," with splenomegaly and frequent intercurrent infections. *P. malaria* may cause nephrotic syndrome.

Diagnosis Diagnosis may be made by demonstration of plasmodium parasites in blood smears—thick and thin.

Prevention Prevention includes destruction of mosquitoes and their breeding places and use of mosquito netting, repellants, etc. Chemoprophylaxis includes chloroquine or amodiaquine (see table).

Treatment
1. Acute attack—chloroquine diphosphate, orally; if vomiting or comatose, intramuscularly.
2. *P. falciparum* may not respond to or may become resistant to chloroquine. Quinine, 15 mg per kg, three times per day, for 10 days should be given along with pyrimethamine and sulfadiazine.
3. For prevention of relapse and eradication of exoerythrocytic forms of *P. malariae, vivax,* and *ovale*—Primaquine, 7.5 mg (base) daily,

Malarial chemotherapy with chloroquine

Dose* (mg)	Age (years)				
	0–1	1–3	3–6	6–12	12 and over
Initial	150	200	300	450	600
6 hr	75	100	150	225	300
24 hr	75	100	150	225	300
48 hr‡	75	100	150	225	300

* Dosage of base.
‡ Patient is usually afebrile after 48 to 72 hr.

for older children, for 14 days. Children less than 4 years of age rarely need to be treated for exoerythrocytic forms. (Children with a deficiency of glucose-6-phosphate dehydrogenase must be observed for signs of drug toxicity.)

Chemosuppression for malaria

Age (in years)	Chloroquine (base) or amodiaquine (in mg) (as a single weekly dose)
0–1	37.5
1–3	100
4–6	133
7–10	200
11–16	300
Over 16	400

These dosages should be given throughout the period of exposure and for 4 weeks after leaving the endemic area.

TOXOPLASMOSIS

Toxoplasmosis is caused by the protozoan *Toxoplasma gondii* and may be congenital (see p. 228) or acquired. The domestic cat is the main source of *T. gondii* infection. Most acquired primary infections are probably subclinical and may be found in any age group. However, several clinical patterns have emerged.

1. An infectious mononucleosis–like syndrome with fever, malaise, generalized lymphadenopathy, and splenomegaly but without heterophile antibody.
2. A typhus-like illness with fever, rash, and pneumonitis

3. Encephalitis
4. Chorioretinitis
5. Myocarditis and myositis

Spontaneous recovery usually occurs; some deaths from encephalitis and typhus-like syndrome have occurred.

Diagnosis

1. Identification of the organism on smears and tissue sections is suggestive.
2. Inoculation of susceptible animals, e.g., mice-definitive.
3. Serology
    a. The Sabin-Feldman Dye Test is a reliable test—antibodies rise in 2–3 weeks and remain high for years.
    b. Complement-fixation antibody is positive after 4 weeks but falls rapidly.

Treatment   Combined therapy of pyrimethamine and trisulfapyrimidines for 30 days is not highly effective.

REVIEW QUESTIONS

1. The following statements concerning measles (rubeola) are true except for one: (*a*) leukopenia with lymphocytic predominance; (*b*) bronchitis is an integral part of the disease; (*c*) there is a diminished reaction to the tuberculin test; (*d*) the prodromal stage lasts 7 to 10 days.
2. The following statements concerning cat-scratch disease are true except for one: (*a*) cultures from involved lymph nodes are sterile; (*b*) constitutional symptoms are mild or absent; (*c*) biopsy of a lesion reveals a granulomatous process; (*d*) treatment of choice is erythromycin.

    The following questions are of the matching type. In the blank next to the item in column I, put the letter of the item in column II with which it is most closely associated. (A letter may be used more than once.)

I		II	
3.	Herpangina _____	(*a*)	Coxsackie group A virus
4.	Hand-foot-mouth disease _____	(*b*)	Coxsackie group B virus
5.	Epidemic myalgia (pleurodynia) _____		
6.	Neonatal myocarditis _____		

7. A patient with pertussis is considered noninfectious (*a*) 2 weeks; (*b*) 4 weeks; (*c*) 6 weeks; (*d*) 8 weeks after onset of symptoms.
8. The drug of choice for pertussis is (*a*) erythromycin; (*b*) penicillin; (*c*) sulfisoxazole (Gantrisin); (*d*) ampicillin.
9. The following statements are true concerning gonorrhea except for one: (*a*) average incubation period is 14 to 21 days; (*b*) this disease has reached epi-

demic proportions in the United States; (*c*) it is very prevalent among adolescents; (*d*) penicillin is the drug of choice.

10. The tuberculin test may be negative in infected persons under the following circumstances except for one: (*a*) for 6 weeks to 8 months following an initial infection; (*b*) during immunosuppressive therapy; (*c*) in tuberculosis of bone; (*d*) in miliary tuberculosis.

11. "Swimming pool" granuloma with skin, lymph gland, and bone lesions is caused by the following type of atypical mycobacteria: (*a*) scotochromogens; (*b*) photochromogens; (*c*) nonphotochromogens; (*d*) "rapid growing" (nonpigmented).

12. In treating a patient who has meningitis in which the causative organism is not known, the drug of choice is (*a*) chloramphenicol; (*b*) erythromycin; (*c*) ampicillin; (*d*) Gantrisin.

13. The highest incidence of *H. influenzae* meningitis occurs in (*a*) adults; (*b*) children over 5 years of age; (*c*) infants 6 to 36 months of age; (*d*) infants below 3 months of age.

14. One of the following is not a feature of congenital toxoplasmosis: (*a*) jaundice; (*b*) hepatosplenomegaly; (*c*) caused by a fungus; (*d*) hydrocephalus; (*e*) chorioretinitis.

The following questions are the matching type. In each blank in column I, insert the letter corresponding to the word or phrase which is associated most appropriately.

I		II	
15.	Meningoencephalitis may occur as the only finding or may precede characteristic manifestations _____	(*a*)	Rubella
		(*b*)	Pertussis
		(*c*)	Mumps
16.	Koplik's spots _____	(*d*)	Scarlet fever
17.	Hemolytic streptococci _____	(*e*)	Rubeola
18.	Prominent postauricular lymphadenopathy _____	(*f*)	Cat-scratch disease
19.	Leukemoid blood picture _____		

20. The following are true concerning immunization for typhoid and paratyphoid fever except (*a*) immunization against paratyphoid fever is not effective; (*b*) children should be immunized against typhoid fever prior to entering school; (*c*) a child immunized against typhoid fever may contract the disease; (*d*) children traveling to an endemic area should be immunized against typhoid prior to age 5.

21. The following children should receive INH for a year except (*a*) preschool children with a positive tuberculin skin test; (*b*) adolescent female who had miliary tuberculosis at age 5 and is now cured; (*c*) recent tuberculin reactor; (*d*) sib of a child with a positive tuberculin skin test.

22. The following statements about congenital syphilis are true except (*a*) transplacental infection occurs during the first trimester; (*b*) a mother having negative serologic tests for syphilis at 5-months gestation can have a baby with congenital syphilis; (*c*) a nurse can contract syphilis from an infant with congenital syphilis; (*d*) bone lesions may be present at birth.

23. Measles encephalitis may occur at the following times: (*a*) only after the exanthem; (*b*) without the exanthem ever occurring; (*c*) before, during, or after the exanthem; (*d*) only during or after the exanthem.

15 RESPIRATORY DISEASES

UPPER RESPIRATORY TRACT INFECTIONS
(URI, Common Cold)

The URI is the most frequent of all pediatric illnesses. For clarity, it is perhaps easier to limit the meaning of "URI" to an acute viral infection of the nasopharynx and sinuses, associated with mild, if any, constitutional symptoms.

Etiology A large number of viruses are implicated: myxoviruses, adenoviruses, rhinoviruses (more than 90 types), enteroviruses, and reoviruses. Mycoplasmataceae are also implicated. (See Table 15-3, page 358, which deals with all viral etiologic agents for both upper and lower respiratory tract infections.)

Incubation period   Incubation is short, probably 12 to 72 hours; usually 24 hours.

Period and mode of transmission   Transmission is probably in the first 2 days, by droplet infection.

Predisposing factors   Individual variations of susceptibility and resistance, respiratory allergy, poor nutrition, and teething are probably important as predisposing factors. The frequency with which URI occurs in children is directly proportional to the number of exposures. Thus, an infant who lives in poor, overcrowded housing conditions frequently has colds before 6 months of age and is likely to have more colds during a season than an infant living in healthful surroundings. In the latter group, the occurrence of colds under 6 months of age is relatively rare. Dampness and exposure to cold probably do not increase susceptibility to the virus.

Immunity   Immunity is transient, probably lasting no more than a few weeks, and related to secretory IgA rather than humoral antibodies.

Clinical and laboratory features   These consist mainly of local manifestations. A mild constitutional reaction may precede the local symptoms by several hours. In general, the younger the child, the more prevalent are the constitutional manifestations. The older the child, the more the local findings tend to predominate. There is usually either a leukopenia or an absence of leukocytosis unless there is a complication.

Constitutional   The fever, if any, is slight. There may be restlessness or somnolence, malaise, anorexia, and occasionally vomiting and diarrhea.

Local   Early there may be a sore or "scratchy" throat with fever. The young child who cannot verbalize a sore throat usually becomes somewhat irritable and refuses to eat. Then there are sneezing and a nasal discharge which is watery at first and later becomes thicker, mucopurulent, and green and yellow in color. The nasal mucosa and the pharynx are hyperemic. The nasal passages are blocked, and mouth breathing is common. The nares are often excoriated; the eyes water; there is usually a hacking, nonproductive cough which later becomes productive. (Children do not actually expectorate sputum until about the age of 7 years, but cough it up out of the respiratory tract and swallow it.) The lymphoid tissue on the posterior pharyngeal wall becomes enlarged, as do the cervical lymph nodes.

Course   URI usually lasts 5 to 10 days provided no complications occur.

Differential diagnosis

1. The various viral agents of URI can only be distinguished by viral studies.
2. Other viral disease entities may begin with the above picture, e.g., measles, pertussis, poliomyelitis. In others, it is an integral part of the disease, e.g., influenza.
3. Allergic rhinitis is characterized by recurrent episodes of rhinorrhea, pale, boggy nasal mucous membranes, many eosinophils in the nasal discharge, and response to specific antiallergic therapy.
4. When there is a serosanguineous discharge, diphtheria, foreign body (unilateral discharge), and congenital syphilis must be considered.
5. Streptococcosis in infants under 6 months of age is characterized by nasopharyngitis associated with a thin mucopurulent discharge and irregular fever.

Complications   Complications are frequent and largely due to the secondary bacterial invaders.

1. Otitis media is more frequent in infants and younger children because their eustachian tubes are shorter, straighter, and wider.
2. Cervical adenitis is common.
3. Laryngitis, bronchitis, and pneumonia are more often encountered in infancy and may represent extension of the viral infection rather than secondary infection.
4. Sinusitis, particularly in older children.
5. Tonsillitis and adenoiditis occurs most often from 2 to 7 years of age.

Prophylaxis   There are no satisfactory prophylactic measures.

Treatment

1. General measures have been discussed in Chapter 6, "Drugs and Treatment."
2. Symptomatic: analgesics and antipyretics may be used when necessary, e.g., aspirin, acetaminophen, to reduce restlessness and discomfort.
3. Nasal decongestants sometimes are helpful. These are particularly indicated when there are nasal occlusion, difficulty in sucking due to obstructed breathing, and a postnasal drip with a cough. Solutions commonly used are ephedrine $\frac{1}{2}\%$ in older children and phenylephrine $\frac{1}{8}$ to $\frac{1}{4}\%$ in infants older than 3 months of age. In administration of nose drops, the child is kept in a head-low position; the drops are usually given 15 minutes before a feeding. Topical nasal applications may also be used in older children. Nose drops probably should not be continued for more than 3 or 4 days, since prolonged use is injurious to the mucous membrane and

causes a "rebound" phenomenon. Physiologic saline nose drops are often helpful when the nasal discharge is either very thick or inspissated. Oral decongestants are not particularly useful in young children, and may only serve to excite them. There is no advantage to combining decongestants with expectorants.

4. A highly humidified environment obtained with a vaporizer or cool humidifier may be quite beneficial.
5. Antihistamines are of no value.
6. Antimicrobials are not indicated unless there are complications from secondary bacterial invaders.

ACUTE PHARYNGITIS

"Acute pharyngitis" refers to all acute infectious conditions of the pharynx including tonsillitis and pharyngotonsillitis. Although pharyngeal involvement is part of most URI and found in many generalized infections, when used as above, it refers to conditions where the primary involvement is in the throat.

Etiology   Generally caused by viruses (see URI and Table 15-3). There are only two bacteria which are definitely known to cause acute pharyngitis. *C. diphtheriae* and the group A beta-hemolytic streptococcus. The only reliable method for differentiating viral from bacterial pharyngitis is by means of a culture.

Clinical and laboratory features

1. Pharyngitis is more common beyond infancy and reaches its peak between the fourth and seventh years.
2. A viral pharyngitis is usually of gradual onset, with fever, malaise, and anorexia. A painful throat is variable (soreness of the throat is very difficult to determine in a young child). Hoarseness, cough, and rhinitis may be present. Inflammation of the throat varies from mild to severe. There may be small ulcers on the palate and posterior pharyngeal wall and exudate on the lymphoid follicles of the posterior pharynx and tonsils. The cervical nodes are often moderately enlarged and somewhat tender. Conjunctivitis may also be present. Leukocytes range from 6,000 to over 30,000 often with an early predominance of polymorphonuclear cells. The course of illness is usually 1 to 5 days.
3. Bacterial—diphtheria pharyngitis is discussed in Chapter 14. Group A beta-hemolytic streptococcal pharyngitis is most often seen in children over 2 years of age, but may be encountered in those 16 to 18 months and older. It begins suddenly with headache, abdominal pain, vomiting, and fever of 103 to 105°F. Hours later the throat becomes sore in approximately one-third of the patients. There is enlargement of the tonsils, which appear beefy red with

exudate on them. The exudate may vary from a few yellowish-white discrete follicles to larger patches to a complete pseudomembrane. There is hyperemia of the pharynx, and the pain varies from slight to severe enough to make swallowing difficult. The other two-thirds of patients have only mild hyperemia with no particular tonsillar enlargement or exudate. Anterior cervical adenopathy occurs frequently with streptococcal pharyngitis, and the nodes are quite tender. Fever usually continues from 1 to 4 days but may last as long as 2 weeks. Hoarseness, rhinitis, cough, and conjunctivitis are noticeably absent. The white blood count is generally high with a persistent polynucleosis. Treatment is specific, namely, penicillin (erythromycin in patients who are allergic to penicillin), and the response is dramatic. Usually within 24 hours (sometimes as long as 36 to 48 hours) the child is afebrile and feeling well. (For dosage schedule see Scarlet Fever in Chapter 14.) Acute complications include otitis media, mastoiditis, cervical adenitis, sinusitis, peritonsillar abscess, and retropharyngeal abscess. In those children treated promptly mastoiditis and the latter two conditions are very rare. Late complications include acute rheumatic fever and acute glomerulonephritis.
4.   Mesenteric adenitis giving rise to abdominal pain and vomiting often simulates acute appendicitis. This may occur with both viral and streptococcal pharyngitis.

SPECIFIC TYPES OF PHARYNGOTONSILLITIS

1.   The herpangina syndrome is caused mainly by Coxsackie group A, a few Coxsackie B viruses, and sometimes by ECHO virus. Characterized by fever of 101 to 105°F and vesiculoulcerative lesions on the anterior pillars, fauces, and soft palate, common between the ages of 1 and 7 years. (See Chapter 14.)
2.   Acute lymphonodular pharnygitis is caused by Coxsackie A. Characterized by small white or yellowish nodular lesions of the uvula, anterior pillars, and posterior pharynx which do not vesiculate or ulcerate.
3.   Pharyngoconjunctival fever is caused by adenovirus type 3 and occasionally types 7 or 14. Characterized by fever (to 104°F lasting 1 to 10 days); mild sore throat; conjunctivitis (follicular and often monocular); often headaches and listlessness; and submaxillary, submandibular and posterior cervical adenopathy. The lymph follicles on the posterior pharyngeal wall are prominent, and there may or may not be an exudative tonsillitis. (Patches of grayish white exudate, which may be coalescent, may also be present on the posterior pharyngeal wall.) Pharyngoconjunctival fever occurs in outbreaks, mostly in the summer in school-age children who live and swim together, but may also occur sporadically at any time.
4.   Acute febrile pharyngitis is caused by adenovirus, particularly

types 1, 2, and 5. It occurs mainly in infants and young children. This is usually a mild disease consisting of low-grade fever and sore throat with or without conjunctivitis or rhinitis.

5. Acute exudative (membranous) pharyngotonsillitis is caused by both viruses and bacteria and may be found as part of other disease entities such as viral infections—infectious mononucleosis (discussed in Chapter 14), adenovirus infections, herpangina, herpetic gingivostomatitis, and ECHO 9 infections; bacterial infections—diphtheria, group A beta-hemolytic streptococcus, and *Mycoplasma hominis;* other diseases—monilia, agranulocytosis, and leukemia.

TONSILS AND ADENOIDS

The tonsils and adenoids are present at birth and increase in size through the preschool period. After this time, in the absence of infection, there follows a gradual decrease in their size. Two chief functions have been ascribed to them:

1. The whole of Waldeyer's lymphoid ring, of which the tonsils and adenoids are an integral part, probably acts as a defense mechanism for the respiratory tract; a system which filters and protects against invasion by pathogenic microorganisms. The problem arises when its defense mechanism is overwhelmed and the tissue itself becomes infected.
2. These lymphoid tissues play a role in the formation of immunoglobulins.

It is significant that the tonsils and adenoids have their major growth up to the age of 5, and it is during these early years that the susceptibility to respiratory infection usually is greatest. As the child's immunity increases, the protective function of the tonsils and adenoids appears to be of less importance. Thus when considering tonsillectomy, surgery should be delayed, if possible, until about 4 to 5 years of age. By that time the problem most likely has resolved itself.

Indications for tonsillectomy   This is a tremendously controversial subject mainly because of the lack of good controlled studies. However, there is general agreement on the following three recommendations:

1. Hypertrophy sufficient to produce symptoms of obstruction, i.e., inability to swallow in the absence of acute infection, respiratory distress, or cor pulmonale
2. Tumor of the tonsil
3. Diphtheria carrier who does not respond to antimicrobial therapy

Chronic or repeated infection of the tonsils with chronic infection of the cervical lymph nodes, middle ear and sinuses, peritonsillar abscess, and tuberculosis of the tonsils, were at one time considered indications for tonsillectomy, but with adequate and vigorous antimicrobial therapy, tonsillectomy should not be necessary.

Indications for adenoidectomy During infancy and early childhood adenoidectomy alone may be done; later in childhood, combined tonsillectomy and adenoidectomy are usually performed.

1. Persistent nasal obstruction with mouth breathing
2. Recurrent or chronic otitis media
3. Impaired hearing due to infection or hypertrophy of adenoids with eustachian tube obstruction, particularly if serous otitis media occurs and it is unresponsive to other measures
4. Interference with swallowing (requires tonsillectomy and adenoidectomy)

Allergy frequently plays a role in many of the above conditions. Surgery alone is frequently of less benefit than anticipated. Control of the allergic symptoms often lessens the need for surgery.

Rheumatic fever, glomerulonephritis, and systemic infections are not indications for tonsillectomy and adenoidectomy. Each child should be evaluated, keeping in mind the indications enumerated above.

Tonsillectomy and adenoidectomy should be postponed until the child has completely recovered from any acute infection. The presence of an epidemic of poliomyelitis in the community is an absolute contraindication to tonsillectomy or adenoidectomy. If poliomyelitis occurs in a child with a recent tonsillectomy, it is more apt to be of the bulbar type.

ACUTE OTITIS MEDIA

This is a common complication of upper respiratory diseases in young children. With increasing age the incidence decreases because of the changes which occur in the anatomy of the eustachian tube—it becomes longer and narrower.

Etiology The most common cause of acute otitis media is viral (as part of a URI). The pneumococcus is the most common bacterial pathogen and the most common cause of exudative otitis media. *H. influenza* is the second most common bacterial pathogen and is particularly prevalent before 4 years of age. Other bacterial causes are beta-hemolytic streptococci, neisseria, and many enteric organisms. In the young infant (less than 6 weeks) *E. coli,* staphylococcus, and *Klebsiella pneumoniae* are the most common bacterial agents.

Clinical features An acute catarrhal otitis media usually accompanies an upper respiratory infection. Routine examination of the eardrum in these cases will frequently reveal mild injection at the periphery which disappears as the upper respiratory infection subsides. If bacterial infection occurs, the otitis progresses. There is a sudden rise in temperature accompanied by pain in the ear. In infants who are unable to complain of pain, there may be pulling or rubbing of the affected ear. At this time otoscopic examination reveals a diffuse injection, perhaps with some bulging or fullness of the tympanic membrane. The normal landmarks—cone of light, umbo, and short process of the malleus—are still observed. If proper treatment is instituted, the otitis will not progress beyond this stage but will regress, leaving a normal membrane.

When the condition is untreated, or if the causative organism is not susceptible to the particular antibiotic used, there is an increased bulging, owing to the collection of purulent material in the middle ear, and loss or marked distortion of landmarks (acute purulent otitis media). If the tympanic membrane does not rupture spontaneously at this time, it should be incised (myringotomy), permitting free drainage. Adequate drainage with medical treatment usually results in a return to normal if the organism is susceptible. When drainage continues for more than 2 to 3 weeks, in spite of treatment, the condition is considered chronic. Diagnosis must be made from middle ear aspirate because cultures made from nasopharyngeal secretions are unreliable.

Acute otitis media should be differentiated from otitis externa (see Chapter 26, "Skin Disorders") and from acute bullous myringitis with or without hemorrhage and probably due to mycoplasma infection. Fever may or may not be present, and examination of the drum shows tense vesicles filled either with fluid or with blood.

Complications Complications are unusual since the advent of antimicrobials. Those which may occur are chronic otitis media, mastoiditis, labyrinthitis, petrositis, venous sinus thrombosis, meningitis, and brain abscess.

Treatment

1. Antimicrobial therapy for children under 4 years of age—penicillin and sulfisoxazole or ampicillin (advocated by many, although best reserved for severe or life-threatening infections; for children over 4 years of age—penicillin. All regimens are given for at least 10 days and until the tympanic membrane and discharge (if present) clears.
2. Nasal decongestants.
3. In the catarrhal stage, local heat or warm ear drops (antipyrine 5% in glycerine) may be used to relieve pain.
4. Myringotomy is indicated if the drum is bulging and there is

severe pain, or when the constitutional manifestations are severe and do not disappear in response to therapy. Once drainage is instituted, the only local treatment should be dry wipes.

Following an acute otitis media, the child's hearing should be evaluated. This may be accomplished by testing it with the whispered voice or a watch. If any deficiency is suspected, more definite audiometric tests should be made.

RECURRENT OR CHRONIC OTITIS MEDIA

Features and treatment

Recurrent type

1. Recurrent otitis occurs frequently (especially in infants) and may recur shortly after antimicrobial therapy has been discontinued.
2. Organisms commonly involved include *S. aureus, H. influenza,* and other Gram-negative rods. The organism should be obtained from middle ear aspirate.
3. The tympanic membrane is thickened but intact. No discharge is present.
4. The eustachian tube is blocked due to allergy, infection, or both.
5. Treatment includes myringotomy, antimicrobials in accordance with antibiogram and as indicated tympanostomy tube insertion (placement of plastic tube into middle ear cavity for continuous drainage), adenoidectomy, and treatment of allergy. Test hearing.

Chronic type

1. Hallmark—painless persistent drainage from middle ear and loss of hearing.
2. Discharge reveals mixed bacterial flora including staphylococci and Gram-negative organisms (particularly pseudomonas and proteus).
3. Cholesteatoma formation and destruction of the ossicles.
4. Mastoiditis is almost always present. X-rays should be made.
5. Treatment: (*a*) local therapy to cleanse the canal; (*b*) tympanoplasty (remove cholesteatoma and granulation tissue and reconstruct ossicles); (*c*) mastoidectomy if indicated; (*d*) appropriate antimicrobial therapy; (*e*) test hearing.

SEROUS OTITIS MEDIA (Secretory Otitis, Chronic Otitis with Effusion, Glue Ear)

Etiology The cause of the condition is unknown, but bacterial otitis media inadequately treated with antimicrobials, viral infections, and allergy have been implicated.

Clinical and laboratory features

1. Probably due to blockage of eustachian tube and negative pressure within the middle ear.
2. Impaired hearing (conduction type), sense of fullness in the ear, popping or clicking sensation on swallowing, and an absence of constitutional signs are characteristic.
3. Thin, serous, mucoid or gelatinous, sterile fluid is present in the middle ear.
4. Tympanic membrane appears dull. It may be retracted or bulging depending on amount of fluid present.

Treatment

1. Nasopharyngeal decongestants and antihistamines may be helpful.
2. Desensitization for the child with allergy.
3. Instillation of urea in the middle is efficacious in some cases.
4. Myringotomy and aspiration of fluid.
5. Tympanostomy and tube insertion.
6. Adenoidectomy.

CERVICAL ADENITIS

This is a common accompaniment of upper respiratory infection in children and usually subsides as the URI does. It may also be a complication of a URI or acute pharyngitis, in which case, it may be bilateral. It is most often unilateral, and the involved lymph node is usually enlarged, very tender, and warm. The child may have high fever. Group A streptococcus is the major offender but staphylococcus and pneumococcus have also been responsible. Proper antimicrobial therapy (high-dose penicillin is the drug of choice) usually causes recession of the node in 1 to 2, or at the most, 3 weeks. If fluctuation occurs, an incision and drainage should be done. Infectious cervical adenitis must be differentiated from the following:

1. Specific infection: tuberculosis, infectious mononucleosis, brucellosis, syphilis, Boeck's sarcoid, cat-scratch disease, tularemia, toxoplasmosis, cytomegalic virus disease
2. Neoplastic disease: leukemia, Hodgkin's disease, lymphosarcoma
3. Reticuloendothelioses: Gaucher's disease, Niemann-Pick disease, Hand-Schüller-Christian disease
4. Congenital anomalies: cystic hygroma, branchial-cleft cyst
5. Infected skin lesions of the head and neck: pyoderma, pediculosis, tinea with secondary lymphadenitis, external otitis
6. Collagen diseases

(The above diseases are discussed individually in various sections of this book.)

SINUSITIS

The paranasal sinuses may be involved in any upper respiratory infection (they are lined by mucous membrane continuous with that of the nasal cavity). Occasionally, the sinusitis persists after the upper respiratory infection subsides, usually because of secondary bacterial invasion, and produces the following syndrome:

Clinical features

1. Persistent purulent nasal discharge, often unilateral; fever (low-grade or high); localized pain and tenderness or a sense of fullness, headache, and edema over the affected sinus; nasal quality to the voice.
2. Acute ethmoiditis is not uncommon in infants and young children and presents as periorbital cellulitis with edema of the subcutaneous tissues and erythema of the skin.
3. Roentgenograms may reveal clouding of the involved sinus. Edema alone, however, may also cause clouding. A fluid level is sometimes observed.
4. Transillumination may be of diagnostic value in older children.

Treatment

1. Antimicrobial therapy—primarily penicillin since group A beta-hemolytic streptococci is the main organism involved.
2. Nasal decongestants.
3. Occasionally in older children aspiration of the sinus may be necessary or desirable.

In cases of chronic sinusitis some underlying pathologic condition, for example, allergy, nasal deformities, or chronically infected adenoids, is often present and requires correction. Rarely, surgical drainage may be necessary. Chronic infection of the sinuses or contiguous tissues will retard the normal development of the paranasal sinuses.

RETROPHARYNGEAL ABSCESS AND PERITONSILLAR ABSCESS

Both of these entities have become rare since the introduction of antimicrobials. The former is more common in infants, and the latter after 5 years of age. Retropharyngeal abscess may result from extension of pharyngitis (streptococcal) to the lymph nodes in the retropharyngeal space with consequent swelling and suppuration through the posterior pharyngeal wall. Peritonsillar abscess results as a direct extension of a tonsillar infection. In peritonsillar abscess, there is trismus and displacement of the uvula to the opposite side. Treatment for both consists of vigorous antimicrobial therapy and incision and drainage of the abscess at the proper time.

CROUP

Croup is a symptom complex consisting of (1) hoarseness or change in the voice; (2) noisy inspiration; (3) barklike cough; and (4) difficult respiration (inspiration), tachypnea, and retractions of the chest wall (due to use of accessory muscles of respiration), particularly substernal, suprasternal, and supraclavicular. (Aspiration of a foreign body and angioneurotic edema can cause all the signs of croup. Infantile hypocalcemic tetany—rare in the croup age group—and tumors or trauma of the larynx must be differentiated from croup.)

There are two major categories of croup:

A.   Spasmodic croup (midnight croup, allergic croup)
B.   Infectious croup
    1.   Viral—may cause laryngitis, laryngotracheitis or laryngo-tracheobronchitis (descending croup).
    2.   Bacterial
        a.   Diphtheric croup (true croup) (See Chapter 14)
        b.   Acute epiglottitis

The croup diathesis is seen most commonly in "the chubby boy" from an allergic family.

Table 15-1.   Comparison of viral and bacterial (nondiphtheritic) croup

	Viral	Bacterial
Etiology	1. Parainfluenza viruses—types 1, 2, 3, particularly 1 and 2 (the "croup viruses") 2. RS virus 3. Adenoviruses 4. Influenza 5. Measles 6. ECHO (many types)	1. *H. influenzae* type B (vast majority) 2. Group A streptococcus 3. Pneumococcus
Onset	Slow—usually 1–3 days of URI symptoms before signs of croup develop, any time of day or night	Sudden, rapid, progressive, any time of day or night
Signs and symptoms (see above)	Fever 101–104°F, acutely ill, usually alert, signs of croup, hoarseness, may also have expiratory difficulty, wheezes,	Prostration, toxicity, high fever 103–105°F, anxious infant lies with hyperextension of neck; older child sits up, leaning forward,

	Viral	Bacterial
	and rhonchi which may change from time to time. Pharnyx usually inflamed; epiglottis not visualized or slightly hyperemic but retains normal shape. Restlessness and increasing respiratory difficulty leading to cyanosis.	eyes bulge, sternocleidomastoid muscles taut. In addition to other croup signs, voice is muffled ("mouth full of mush" sound). Throat shows typical enlargement of epiglottis, which appears as a round, red cherry at base of tongue. Poor breath sounds in lungs.
Pathology	Subglottic edema, edema of vocal cords, and exudate on tracheal wall and throughout the respiratory tract—if bronchioles and bronchi involved—patchy atelectasis and obstructive emphysema.	Epiglottis inflamed and edematous, supraglottic edema.
Radiography	Chest—often shows patchy pneumonia, usually unilateral. Neck—may show subglottic narrowing of trachea.	Neck—distension of hypopharynx by a large swelling in the region of the epiglottis.
Laboratory findings	White blood count—normal or slightly elevated. Blood culture—negative. Pharyngeal culture—positive for specific virus.	Leukocytosis—15–25,000 predominantly polymorphonuclear. Blood culture may be positive, throat cultures—positive for specific bacteria (usually *H. influenza* type B).
Treatment	1. Tracheostomy or intubation may be necessary (not often). 2. Cool humidity. 3. Intermittent positive-pressure breathing (IPPB) with racemic epinephrine. 4. Pharmacologic doses of corticosteroids may be helpful. 5. Adequate fluids and electrolytes.	1. Probably $\frac{1}{3}$–$\frac{1}{2}$ need tracheostomy. 2. Antimicrobial therapy—ampicillin 100–150 mg/kg/day. 3. Cool humidity. 4. Pharmacologic doses of corticosteroids may be helpful. 5. Adequate fluids and electrolytes.
Prognosis	Good.	High fatality rate if untreated. If treated vigorously, rapid recovery.

SPASMODIC CROUP

Spasmodic croup usually occurs between 2 and 4 years of age. The cause has not been determined, but it is generally believed to be of infectious or allergic origin. Certain children seem predisposed to develop this severe laryngospasm with little or no apparent cause. It is often associated with a mild URI.

Clinical features   (in addition to those listed above for all types of croup)

1. The onset is late at night usually between 11:00 P.M. and 2:00 A.M.
2. Anxiety and restlessness may become marked.
3. No matter how ill these patients look, they rarely become cyanotic and never become so obstructed that dramatic measures need to be taken.
4. After a few hours, the severity decreases, the cough loosens, and the child seems well during the following daytime except for a mild URI.
5. There is no more than a low-grade fever, if any.
6. These attacks may recur two or three nights in succession.
7. They tend to recur each winter during early childhood.

Treatment

1. Relief of this spasm is accomplished by subemetic doses of syrup of ipecac, ½ to 1 tsp. If no relief occurs in 15 to 20 minutes, emesis may be induced.
2. Humidification is helpful; cool humidity is preferred over warm.
3. Phenobarbital or an antihistamine for sedation and humidity should be given after emesis and on successive nights before retiring to prevent further attacks.

INFECTIOUS CROUP (See Table 15-1)

The patient with croup must be watched very carefully. The essence of good care, besides recognition of epiglottitis and vigorous antibiotic treatment, is recognizing the proper time to perform a tracheostomy if it is needed. Waiting until the patient is cyanotic is too late! Increasing restlessness (the first sign of air hunger) with increasing respiratory rate and worsening of retractions are indications for a tracheostomy. Good nursing care is fundamental in the care of the patient with croup before and after tracheostomy. An x-ray should always be made following insertion of a tracheotomy tube to be certain that it is not occluding a major bronchus and causing atelectasis.

CONGENITAL LARYNGEAL STRIDOR (Laryngomalacia)

Congenital laryngeal stridor is usually due to relaxed vocal cords or a flabby epiglottis which causes more than the usual amount of collapse on inspiration. There are stridulous, crowing inspirations in the new-born infant and sometimes marked dyspnea. A laryngoscopic examination is necessary to confirm the diagnosis and rule out other conditions, e.g., papilloma of the vocal cords, stenosis, cysts, or congenital membrane. There is no specific treatment. The prognosis is good, since the condition disappears in 6 to 24 months.

BRONCHITIS

Bronchitis should be termed more accurately acute tracheobronchitis. It is most often viral in origin and usually preceded by a URI. Pain in the chest and a dry, hacking unproductive cough with low-grade or no fever are characteristic. The cough becomes productive in 2 to 3 days, and the entire syndrome subsides within 7 to 10 days.

ACUTE BRONCHIOLITIS

This is a very common entity found in infants and young children from about the age of 4 to 18 months. The basic pathology is obstructive emphysema due to the presence of edema, thick secretions, and exudate in the terminal bronchioles creating a ball-valve effect and small scattered areas of atelectasis.

Etiology   Viral: most cases are due to the respiratory syncytial (RS) virus, some to the parainfluenza group, adenoviruses, rhinoviruses, influenza, and measles and occasionally to mycoplasma.

Clinical and laboratory features

1. Coryza, sneezing, and cough for 1 to 3 days.
2. Wheezing and respiratory distress varies from mild to severe.
3. Cough is staccato in character and may be almost constant.
4. Fever may be absent, low-grade, or high depending on the causative agent.
5. Respiratory distress is largely expiratory with prolongation of this phase. Subcostal and intercostal retractions (usually shallow) peak in 48 to 72 hours then gradually lessen. Cyanosis may develop.
6. Respiratory rate varies from 60 to 100 per minute.
7. Percussion and auscultation of the chest reveal hyperresonance and a "noisy" chest, i.e., coarse rales, rhonchi, wheezes, and coarse breath sounds. Crepitant rales may be present. If obstruction is nearly complete, breath sounds may be barely audible.
8. The liver and spleen may be palpable considerably below the costal margins because of emphysema which depresses the diaphragm.
9. Radiographic findings reveal hyperaeration, increase in anterior-posterior diameter of the chest as seen in the lateral view, and

depression of the diaphragmatic leaflets. There may be some scattered areas of increased density probably due to atelectasis.

Treatment

1. Humidified oxygen
2. Maintain fluid and electrolyte balance (large amounts of water are lost via the lungs)
3. Monitor blood gases (acidosis, both respiratory and metabolic, is apt to occur)

PNEUMONIA

The pneumonias are a group of diseases caused by various agents, e.g., fungi, bacteria, mycoplasma, viruses, foreign bodies, which have characteristic pathologic findings in common.

Anatomic classification Lobar pneumonia—consolidation of all or part of a lobe; disseminated lobular pneumonia—an involvement of scattered lobules in both lung fields; interstitial pneumonia—a diffuse bronchiolitis and peribronchiolitis in both lung fields; bronchopneumonia—a loose term usually covering the latter two, namely, disseminated lobular and interstitial pneumonias.

Etiologic classification This is preferable to anatomic classification because it aids in selecting the proper therapeutic agent and suggests the prognosis.
   Pneumonia may be caused by viruses, e.g., respiratory syncytial, adenovirus (types 3, 4, and 7), parainfluenza; chlamydiae, e.g., psittacosis; rickettsia, e.g., Q fever; bacteria, e.g., mycoplasma, pneumococcus, *H. influenza,* staphylococcus, Klebsiella, *E. coli*; mycotic infections, e.g., *Candida albicans, Histoplasma capsulatum;* protozoa, e.g., toxoplasmosis; parasites, e.g., ascariasis; chemicals, e.g., following aspiration of oils or volatile hydrocarbons; allergy, e.g., Loeffler's syndrome.

VIRAL PNEUMONIA

Viral pneumonia is characterized by bronchiolitis, peribronchiolitis, and interstitial pneumonia. It is the most common pneumonia in all age groups except the newborn.

Etiology Causes are similar to those discussed under bronchiolitis: RS virus; adenoviruses 3, 4, 7, and 7*a;* parainfluenza and influenza viruses; measles; and enteroviruses.

Mode of transmission Pneumonia is transmitted by droplet infection from upper or lower respiratory infections caused by the above viruses.

Table 15-2. Comparative importance of the respiratory viruses and mycoplasma in various respiratory entities in children

Group	URI (Upper Respiratory Infection)	Croup	Bronchitis	Bronchiolitis	Pneumonia
Myxovirus					
1. Influenza	++	+	+	+	+
2. Parainfluenza	+++	++++	+++	+++	++
3. Respiratory synctial (RS)	+++	++	+++	++++	++++
Adenovirus	+++	+	+++	++	+++
Picornovirus					
1. Rhinovirus	++		+		
2. Enterovirus					
(Echo,	+				
Coxsackie,	++				
poliomyelitis)	+				
Diplornovirus					
1. Reovirus	+		+		
Coronavirus	+		++		
Mycoplasma	+		++	+	++

Incubation period   Incubation is 3 days to 3 weeks.

Clinical features

1. There is usually an insidious onset and a variable course, lasting anywhere from 1 week to several weeks.
2. The temperatures may vary from 100 to 104°F (37.2 to 40°C) and may be fluctuant in type.
3. A dry, tight cough is prominent, but there is usually only slight if any dyspnea and little to moderate malaise.
4. Headache is frequent and severe, and an injected pharynx is common.
5. In the early stages there may be no physical findings. In the later stages, scattered rales and dullness may appear. Characteristically, the auscultatory findings change within a short time, rales may appear and disappear or shift from one area to another. On physical examination there may be much heard but little seen on x-ray, or vice versa.

Laboratory findings

1. The total and differential white cell counts are not diagnostic— they may be slightly elevated or depressed. There may be a lymphocytosis or polymorphonucleosis.
2. The sedimentation rate is elevated or normal.
3. Roentgenographic findings are out of proportion to the clinical signs and change rapidly. There is usually an infiltration which

extends from the hilar regions and branches out as it approaches the periphery; there may be diffuse nodular shadows or a patchy infiltrate.

4. See Table 14-4.

Differential diagnosis   Other types of pneumonia should be ruled out.

Treatment   The care is supportive. Secondary bacterial infection is usually due to contamination by equpiment, e.g., croupettes, oxygen tents.

PNEUMOCOCCAL PNEUMONIA

Pneumococcal pneumonia may present either a lobar or a bronchopneumonia picture. Bronchopneumonia is seen more often in infants, while lobar pneumonia is found in infants and children.

Clinical and laboratory features

1. Usually begins with coryza, cough, low-grade or no fever; then in 48 to 72 hours, respiratory difficulty occurs.
2. The baby is in marked respiratory distress with wheezing, rapid respiratory rate (60 to 100 per minute), subcostal and intercostal retractions—expiration is difficult and prolonged. Cough becomes severe—hacking or staccato.
3. Hyperresonance and a very noisy chest are characteristic. The breath sounds are loud and harsh with wheezes; rhonchi and rales are scattered throughout. At times there are numerous fine crepitant rales, and if the process is severe, breath sounds are diminished.
4. The respiratory distress reaches its peak in 36 to 72 hours, following which there is a gradual recovery.
5. Radiographs of the chest show hyperaeration, increased bronchovascular markings, depression of the diaphragm and widening of the intercostal spaces, and patchy areas of atelectasis.
6. Bacterial complications are rare.

Clinical features of lobar pneumonia

1. It may be preceded by an upper respiratory infection but often comes on suddenly.
2. Frequently chills usher in the onset in older children; in infancy convulsions may occur.
3. There is a rapid rise in temperature to 103 to 105°F (39.4 to 40.6°C); usually the fever is of the continuous type but occasionally may be remittent.
4. Prostration, pain in the chest with splinting of the affected side, and hacking cough are more common in older children. Abdominal pain occurs particularly in the right lower quadrant.
5. The tachypnea is out of proportion to the tachycardia; there is

flaring of the alae nasi, grunting respirations, and intercostal retractions. There may be cyanosis.

6. Over the involved lobe, the physical findings are dullness or percussion, crepitant rales at the onset and subcrepitant rales at resolution, suppressed breath sounds or bronchial breathing with increased voice transmission; occasionally a friction rub may be heard early.
7. Meningismus is found with upper-lobe involvement particularly.
8. The untreated case terminates in crisis, usually in 5 to 9 days.

Laboratory findings

1. High white cell count (20,000 to 30,000) with increased polymorphonuclear cells and a shift to young forms.
2. The invading organism can be identified in cultures of the sputum, or tracheal or lung aspirate.
3. Roentgenograms reveal the lobar involvement.
4. Blood cultures are positive in about 30 percent of the cases.

Clinical features of bronchopneumonia

1. Bronchopneumonia usually follows an upper respiratory infection.
2. There is a spiking temperature of 102 to 104°F (38.9 to 40°C) or more, with marked prostration, toxicity, restlessness, and occasionally convulsions.
3. Associated gastrointestinal findings, e.g., vomiting and diarrhea, are common. Paralytic ileus is rather frequent.
4. The respirations are rapid and shallow, with flaring of the alae nasi, an expiratory grunt, intercostal retractions, and usually cyanosis.
5. The physical findings are scattered—bilateral rales, small areas of impaired percussion, and suppressed breath sounds. If the smaller patches become confluent, the typical signs of consolidation found in the lobar form are noted.
6. Early in the course it should be remembered that the involved areas may be minute and undetectable by physical signs or even by roentgenogram.
7. The untreated course is usually 2 to 3 weeks, with gradual recovery by lysis.
8. Meningismus is common.

Laboratory findings

1. White cell count is 12,000 to 15,000, with a polymorphonuclear leukocyte predominance.
2. Tracheal aspirate and lung aspirate cultures will help in identification of the organism.
3. Roentgenogram usually shows the patchy consolidation in both lung fields.

It may be difficult to differentiate between pneumococcal broncho-pneumonia and lobar pneumonia; the treatment, however, is the same for both.

Treatment   Penicillin is the drug of choice, and the response is dramatic. The patient is afebrile and feels well within 24 hours. Resolution begins at about the same time. Continue therapy for 7 to 10 days. Supportive measures, e.g., oxygen, fluids and electrolytes, may be indicated during the acute phase.

Complications

1.   Otitis media is common.
2.   Other complications such as empyema, lung abscesses, septicemia, and meningitis are rather rare.

Prognosis   The prognosis is good, with proper antimicrobial therapy.

STAPHYLOCOCCAL PNEUMONIA

Staphylococcal pneumonia is principally seen in infancy. It is probably second in prevalence to pneumococcal pneumonias. Most staphylococcal pneumonias are due to penicillin-resistant coagulase-positive strains of staphylococcus. Staphylococcal pneumonia often complicates measles, varicella, influenza, or cystic fibrosis, but primary infection also occurs. Very early it is indistinguishable from other pneumonias. Characteristically, though, it progresses rapidly from a simple infiltration to consolidation, multiple abscesses, and the formation of fluid. Empyema, pyopneumothorax, and the formation of pneumatoceles (air cysts) are typical of staphylococcal pneumonia. The disease spreads rapidly from one lobe to the other and is almost always bilateral. The empyema may be loculated.

Clinical and laboratory features

1.   Early—cough, nasal obstruction, high fever, anorexia, and toxicity.
2.   Moderate to severe respiratory distress develops rapidly.
3.   Respiratory distress increases. Abdominal distension, pallor, cyanosis, and prostration occur. Signs of lobar pneumonia and pleural effusion are present.
4.   There is usually a marked leukocytosis with the presence of immature cell types. White blood cell count may be normal in very young infants.
5.   Recovery is usually complete. Scoliosis may occur due to pleural thickening and adhesions (may require decortication of lung). Pneumatoceles usually disappear spontaneously in 2 to 4 months.

Diagnosis is based on history of prior infection, e.g., skin, umbilical cord; typical clinical course; typical radiographic findings; and positive culture from pleural fluid or blood culture.

Treatment

1. Vigorous antimicrobial therapy—methicillin or oxacillin is the drug of choice, 250 to 300 mg per kg per day; cephalothin may be used as second choice. Chloramphenicol, bacitracin (parenterally), and kanamycin are also effective. Antimocrobial therapy is continued for at least 6 weeks.
2. Supportive—humidity, oxygen, and fluids and electrolytes. High-protein diet during recovery phase.
3. Empyema and pyopneumothorax—early establishment of closed suction drainage which may be removed when drainage ceases.

Prognosis   Mortality rate is high, 5 to 40 percent.

STREPTOCOCCAL PNEUMONIA

Streptococcal pneumonia is also usually due to a secondary invasion, particularly as a complication of a contagious disease. There are tracheitis, bronchiolitis, and interstitial pneumonia. The clinical picture is the same as described for bronchopneumonia. Specific antimicrobial therapy should be used in treatment.

INFLUENZAL PNEUMONIA

Hemophilus influenzae pneumonia is principally caused by type B influenza (the same organism which frequently causes acute epiglottitis). It is seen mainly in infants and young children but is distinctly uncommon. Being lobar in type, it mimics pneumococcal pneumonia but has an insidious onset and a more prolonged course. Bacteremia and empyema are frequent, thus making it possible to establish a diagnosis. It sometimes complicates measles, varicella, pertussis, or influenza. Ampicillin is the drug of choice.

FRIEDLANDER'S BACILLUS PNEUMONIA

Klebsiella pneumonia is rather rare, and it usually produces a severe lobar pneumonia, especially in debilitated children or newborn infants. Abscess and empyema may complicate the pneumonia. The diagnosis is based on finding the encapsulated organism in tracheal secretions, lung aspirates, pleural fluid, or blood. The characteristic x-ray of pulmonary abscesses and cavitation along with bulging interlobar fissures and lobar involvement help to make the diagnosis.

PRIMARY ATYPICAL PNEUMONIA

This condition is caused by *Mycoplasma pneumoniae*. It occurs rarely in infants but is common in adolescents. In some instances, cold

Table 15-3. Viruses and mycoplasmataceae important in respiratory diseases of children

Virus	Group	Incubation period (days)	Mode of transmission	Infectivity (including duration)	Epidemiology
I. Respiratory syncytial (RS)	Paramyxovirus	3–7	Droplet or direct contact	High. Duration unknown; virus recovered up to 1 week	Fall and winter, endemic
II. Parainfluenza types 1, 2, 3 (4)	Paramyxovirus	2–6	Droplet or direct contact	High. Duration unknown; virus recovered after 1 week	Fall and winter, endemic
III. Influenza types A, B, C	Orthomyxovirus	1–3	Droplet, contaminated articles, direct contact	High. Duration from just prior to onset to 1 week after	A and B—recurrent epidemics every 3–5 years, winter. C—local outbreaks, winter
IV. Adenoviruses types 1, 2, 5, 3, 7, 7a, 8, 9, 14, 21	Adenovirus	5–7	Direct contact with secretions from respiratory and gastrointestinal tracts, eye	High. Duration 1–4 days or longer; virus latent in adenoids and tonsils	(1) endemic (2) summer (3) military camp outbreaks (4)–(8) endemic, winter
V. Rhinoviruses	Picornavirus	Unknown, probably several days	Droplet or direct contact	Probably high. Duration unknown; virus recovered after 2–3 weeks	Mainly fall-winter, endemic
VI. Coxsackie viruses	Picornavirus	3–5 (2–14)	Direct contact—fecal-oral and pharyngeal-oral contact	Moderately high. Duration 2 days prior to onset to several days after	Summer and early fall

VII. ECHO viruses	Picornavirus	3–5 average	Same as above	Moderately high. Duration from a few days prior to onset to a few days after	Summer and early fall
VIII. *Mycoplasma pneumoniae*	Mycoplasmataceae	7–14	Probably droplet or direct contact	Unknown. Organism persists for several weeks after asymptomatic	Any time of year, endemic
IX. *Mycoplasma hominis*	Mycoplasmataceae	Unknown	As above	Unknown	As above

Table 15-3. Continued

Clinical syndrome and virus types	Signs and symptoms
I.*(1) Bronchiolitis	(1) Most common agent causing bronchiolitis, striking lack of fever or low (less than 101°F), asthma-like picture, wheezing respiratory distress (expiratory), tachypnea
(2) Pneumonia	(2) Cough, respiratory distress
(3) Croup	(3) Croup symptoms
(4) URI	(4) Coryza, cough
II. (1) Croup—1, 3, 2	(1) Most common agents causing croup. Fever 101–104°F, barking cough, stridor, substernal retractions, hoarseness.
(2) Bronchiolitis—3	(2) Second to RS virus as cause of bronchiolitis, fever—101–104°F, signs as above
(3) URI—1, 2, 3	(3) Fever, coryza, cough
(4) Pneumonia—3	(4) High fever, hacking cough
III. Influenza	
(1) "The Flu," A, B, C	(1) and (2) Fever (102–105°F), chills, headaches, malaise, chest pain, myalgia—lasts 3–7 days—may have secondary bacterial pneumonia. Infants and young children less ill—URI, rarely pneumonia.
(2) "Asian Flu," A₂	
IV. (1) Acute febrile pharyngitis—1, 2, 5	(1) Low-grade fever, sore throat, mild disease
(2) Pharyngo-conjunctival fever—7, 14	(2) Fever, conjunctivitis, sore throat, headache, tonsillar exudate, adenopathy
(3) Acute respiratory disease (ARD)—4, 7, 21	(3) Flulike, headache, fever, malaise, myalgia, cough, adenopathy, tonsillar exudate
(4) Pneumonia—3, 7, 7a	(4) Fever, cough, respiratory distress (severe, perhaps respiratory failure and death)
(5) Acute follicular conjunctivitis—3, 6, 7, 9	(5) Erythema, follicles on palpebral and bulbar conjunctivae
(6) Epidemic kerato conjunctivitis (EKC)—8	(6) Marked involvement of conjunctivae with edema pseudomembrane and subconjunctival hemorrhages
(7) Pertussis syndrome—2	(7) Paroxysmal cough, low-grade fever, three clinical stages
(8) Bronchiolitis—2	(8) Fever, noisy breathing, wheezing, marked cough, expiratory distress
V. "Common Cold" (URI)—all types	Cough, coryza, sore throat, sneezing, low-grade fever, "stuffy nose"
VI. Herpangina mostly A, some B	Fever 103–105°F, vesicles and ulcers on fauces, soft palate, and tonsillar pillars
VII. (1) Herpangina—3, 6, 16	(1) As above
(2) URI—Diarrhea—20	(2) Cough, coryza, sore throat, numerous loose mucoid stools
(3) Exudative tonsillitis—9	(3) Fever, sore throat, exudate (yellowish-white) on tonsils, maculopapular rash, signs of meningitis
VIII. (1) Primary atypical pneumonia	(1) Fever, cough, malaise, chest pain, hemoptysis, mild respiratory distress
(2) URI	(2) Fever, coryza, sore throat
(3) Myringitis	(3) Hemorrhagic or serous bullae on tympanic membranes
IX. Exudative tonsillitis	Afebrile, sore throat, tonsillar exudate

* Refer to corresponding roman numerals in first section of table, pp. 358–359.

agglutinins or agglutinins against streptococcus MG may be found in the blood of these patients. The diagnosis can be made by culturing the organism from the throat and sputum. Immunofluorescent staining of mononuclear cells from the throat may reveal the organism. Specific serologic tests (complement fixation, immunofluorescence, passive

Age predominance	Diagnosis (see Table 14-4)	Treatment	Prophylaxis
I. (1) Infants and young children; 3 months–18 months (2) Infants and young children (3) 6 months–3 years (4) Older children	(1) Typical x-ray of bronchiolitis, culture and serology	Symptomatic	Live attenuated vaccine, experimental
II. (1)–(4) Infants and young children	(1) X-ray of neck—edema of subglottid area and vocal cords (4) X-ray of lungs—infiltrate	Symptomatic	Live attenuated vaccine, experimental
III. (1) and (2) Older children and adults Infants and young children	Epidemic in area, culture	Symptomatic	Amantadine against A₂ (not effective as therapy), polyvalent vaccine for high-risk groups
IV. (1) Infants and young children (2) Any age (3) Young adults and teen-agers (4) Infants, young children, and occasionally adults (5) Adults and older children (6) Adults and older children (7) Infants (8) Infants	Culture and serology (3) WBC may be up to 30,000—predominantly polymorphonuclears (6) WBC normal or low (7) WBC up to 35,000 or more—predominantly lymphocytes, adenoviruses cause from 5–10 % of respiratory disease in children.	Symptomatic No specific	Live attenuated vaccine against types 4, 7—in trial
V. Adults and older children	Isolation of virus difficult	Symptomatic	None
VI. Young children	WBC elevated—polymorphonuclear early, culture and serology	Symptomatic	None
VII. (1) Young children (2) Infants (3) School-age children	(1) As above (2) As above (3) As above plus rash and aseptic meningitis	Symptomatic	None
VIII. (1) Older children and young adults (2) Older children (3) Younger and school-age children.	X-ray of chest demonstrates more pathology than found on physical examination, culture and serology	Tetracycline or erythromycin	None
IX. Older children	Culture	As above	None

hemagglutination, and growth inhibition) are available. The clinical course is similar to that of the viral pneumonias. The tetracyclines and erythromycin are effective.

Psittacosis (Ornithosis)   A disease of birds, spread directly to man, resembles influenza or atypical pneumonia, or sometimes, typhoid fever. Responds well to tetracyclines.

ASPIRATION PNEUMONIA

Debilitated or newborn or premature infants may aspirate formula or food or regurgitate and then aspirate the regurgitated contents. This is particularly easy to do in the supine position—pneumonitis may result, particularly in the right upper lobe and may be a lipoid pneumonia if the aspirated food contained milk or some other fat-containing substance. Lipoid pneumonia may also result from aspiration of either oily nose drops or vitamin preparations. Depending upon the type of oil aspirated or the amount of food aspirated, infants will have variable symptoms and signs. Nothing specific is seen on the x-ray, although often widening hilar densities are present. Secondary infection is common and should be treated with antibacterial drugs. Adrenal corticosteroids may be of value when used early.

FOREIGN BODY IN THE RESPIRATORY TRACT

The clinical findings will depend on the location of the foreign body, the degree of obstruction produced, and whether there is an inflammatory reaction or secondary infection. A careful history will usually reveal a spasm of coughing, choking, difficult respiration, or gagging at the time when the object could have been aspirated, usually followed by a "silent" period of no symptoms, lasting for several hours, days, or even weeks. Then the clinical manifestations appear. Roentgenograms will reveal radiopaque objects.

FOREIGN BODY IN THE LARYNX

A croupy cough, hoarseness, and inspiratory dyspnea, which may go on to cyanosis, characterize this condition. Hemoptysis is rare. Direct laryngoscopic examination is diagnostic.

FOREIGN BODY IN THE TRACHEA

The condition is characterized by a croupy cough, hoarseness, and inspiratory dyspnea, which may go on to cyanosis, plus a typical "audible slap and palpable thud" over the trachea with each respiration. Bronchoscopy is usually necessary to confirm the diagnosis.

FOREIGN BODY IN THE BRONCHI

If there is no obstruction, there may be no clinical findings for a long time. Slight obstruction, with free ingress and egress of air, produces a wheezing type of respiration. Obstruction that permits ingress but interferes with egress (check valve) produces emphysema. An obstruction that does not permit ingress or egress of air (stop valve) produces atelectasis.

The peanut is the foreign body most commonly encountered. In addition to the possible obstructive findings described above, there is a generalized necrotizing inflammation (vegetal bronchitis), which is characterized by septic temperature, dyspnea, and toxicity. The diagnosis depends on history, physical findings, roentgenograms, and bronchoscopic examination.

Prognosis   The prognosis is excellent if foreign bodies are removed but very poor when they are not removed, since chronic suppuration usually supervenes.

Prevention   This is most important since aspiration of a foreign body is usually due to adult carelessness.

Treatment   Requires removal of the foreign body by bronchoscopy if necessary, plus antibiotics if secondary infection occurs.

ATELECTASIS OF THE LUNG

Etiology   Any factor that does not permit ingress of air (stop valve) may produce atelectasis.

1. Extrinsic pressure on a bronchus or the parenchyma, e.g., from hilar lymph nodes or tumors
2. Obstruction within the lumen or in the bronchial wall, e.g., mucous plugs (allergy), foreign body, edema of mucosa, tumor, abscess, or endobronchial tuberculosis

Clinical features

1. There may be dyspnea, cyanosis, and asymmetric respiratory excursions.
2. On percussion, dullness is noted, and breath sounds are absent or diminished over the atelectatic area.
3. The trachea and cardiac apex beat tend to be displaced toward the involved side.
4. Roentgenogram reveals an area of density, the mediastinum displaced toward the affected side, and narrowed intercostal spaces.
5. If the atelectasis is untreated or prolonged, bronchiectasis usually results.

Treatment

1. The cause should be removed, if possible, by bronchoscopic aspiration.
2. The child should be placed on the normal side and may be given breathing exercises; in infants, crying or coughing is stimulated.
3. Inhalation of oxygen 95% and carbon dioxide 5% may be helpful.
4. Postural drainage is helpful in eliminating secretions.
5. If atelectasis does not clear within 8 weeks after adequate medical therapy, bronchoscopy must be performed.

EMPHYSEMA OF THE LUNG

Emphysema may be compensatory in unaffected lung tissue when another part of the lung is not functioning; it is obstructive when there is anything that acts as a check valve, allowing air in but not out.

Etiology   The cause is the same as for atelectasis (see above).

Clinical features

1. There may be shallow, rapid breathing with small excursions.
2. The breath sounds are decreased, with hyperresonance on percussion over the affected area.
3. Roentgenogram and fluoroscopic examination show a shift of the mediastinum toward the normal side on forced expiration, widened intercostal spaces, decreased density, diminished lung markings, and depressed diaphragm.

Treatment   The cause should be removed wherever possible. Postural drainage and breathing exercises should be instituted. Bronchoscopy is indicated if the condition does not clear in 8 weeks.

BRONCHIECTASIS

Bronchiectasis is a localized or generalized dilatation of the bronchi. It consists of inflammatory destruction of bronchial and peribronchial tissue which permits accumulation of exudative material in dependent bronchi, and hence distension in some instances.

Etiology and pathogenesis

1. Prolonged bronchial obstruction from any cause (see Atelectasis above) is the most important factor. Mucoviscidosis is the single most common underlying condition.
2. There is also a superimposed secondary infection. (Sinusitis is frequently found as a concomitant condition.)
3. Patients with an immunoglobulin abnormality may have repeated attacks of bacterial pneumonia and bronchitis leading to bronchiectasis.
4. "Right-middle-lobe syndrome" is not unusual in pediatrics. It is generally caused by extensive compression by hilar nodes, mucous plugs (in asthmatic children), or a congenital anomaly of the bronchus, and consists of chronic pneumonitis, bronchial obstruction, atelectasis, and destruction of the lobe.
5. "Reversible bronchiectasis" occurs frequently after pertussis and lobar and interstitial pneumonias. Shortly after these illnesses the bronchi appear cylindrically dilated on bronchography. Some months later these changes usually disappear.
6. Situs inversus (Kartagener's syndrome) may be the cause.

Clinical features

1. Cough—always present—productive of copious mucopurulent sputum. Change in position or physical activity commonly initiates a bout of coughing.
2. Recurrent and persistent infections of the lower respiratory tract are common.
3. May be afebrile, or fever may be the only symptom.
4. Hemoptysis—occurs late and usually during acute exacerbations.
5. Follows a remitting and relapsing course.
6. Rales present especially during exacerbations.
7. Finally develops persistent dyspnea and retardation of development.

Diagnosis

1. Roentgenogram is suggestive of atelectasis, mediastineal lymph nodes, demonstration of a foreign body, or increased bronchovascular markings near the hilus of the lung.
2. Ventilatory and diffusion studies may reveal widespread and severe pulmonary involvement.
3. Presence of pulmonary osteoarthropathy—late.
4. Bronchography—diagnostic.

Differential diagnosis When a cough persists for more than a month, pertussis, tuberculosis, asthma, sinusitis, foreign body, and bronchiectasis should be considered.

Treatment Prophylactic: Diagnosis and treatment of the bronchial obstruction before it becomes secondarily infected and goes on to irreversible changes. Medical: (1) Elimination of all foci of infection in the respiratory tract; (2) intensive postural draining with cupped-hand percussion; (3) systemic antimicrobial therapy during acute exacerbations in short courses of 5 to 7 days, followed by antibiograms of bronchial aspirates; (4) aerosol inhalation of antibiotics following postural drainage; (5) good nutrition; (6) bronchoscopic aspiration helps to secure drainage if all the above fail; (7) surgery is indicated—segmental or lobar resection or removal of extrinsic obstruction of the bronchus, e.g., node or tumor.

LUNG ABSCESS

Lung abscess is most commonly secondary to pneumonia or bronchiectasis or to aspiration of blood or vomitus following oropharyngeal operation, e.g., tonsillectomy and adenoidectomy. Mixed infections are common. They may be aerobic or anaerobic organisms.

Clinical features

1. At the onset, cough and slight or moderate remittent fever are the only findings.
2. A careful history may reveal the causative factor, for example, tonsillectomy 10 days before, or tooth extraction.
3. If the abscess communicates with a bronchus, the cough will become productive. The sputum is putrid.
4. Hemoptysis is rare but may be seen along with clubbing of the fingers.
5. If the abscess cavity is close to the chest wall, dullness and high-pitched breath sounds may be found.

Laboratory findings

1. Leukocytosis.
2. Roentgenograms (anteroposterior and lateral views should be taken) will usually reveal the abscess cavity in the lung.
3. In chronic lung disease of unknown causation, lung puncture with culture may be indicated; if no fluid or tissue juice is obtained, sterile saline solution is injected and withdrawn; it is smeared and cultured.

Treatment

1. Prophylaxis—adequate treatment of primary condition, e.g., pneumonia.
2. Intensive antimicrobial therapy.
3. Postural drainage is important in those cases where the abscess communicates with a bronchus.
4. Good nutrition—high protein diet.
5. Bronchoscopy—removal of foreign body if present, and aspiration of purulent material.
6. If cavity is not eliminated in 1 month, surgical removal is necessary.

PLEURISY AND EMPYEMA

In the former there is serofibrinous fluid, in the latter, purulent fluid, in the pleural cavity. These conditions are always secondary to a primary disease, e.g., pulmonary infection, chest trauma, extension from surrounding tissues, or septicemia. Serofibrinous pleurisy is more often tuberculous or rheumatic in origin; empyema usually follows pneumonia.

Clinical features

1. The signs and symptoms are those of the primary disease plus those due to the pleural effusion.
2. The extent of dyspnea depends on the degree of mediastinal dis-

placement (which embarrasses cardiac action) and lung compression by the fluid.

3. Physical examination of the chest reveals flatness to percussion; decreased tactile fremitus, breath and voice sounds; and displacement of the cardiac apex away from the effusion. (Interlobar effusion may give no discernible physical signs except in area of dullness.)

Diagnosis is established by roentgenograms and aspiration. Roentgenograms reveal the presence of fluid in the chest and possibly a shift of the mediastinum away from the side of the pathologic condition. Thoracentesis confirms the diagnosis; the fluid should be examined and cultured.

Treatment

1. Repeated aspirations for pleurisy or closed drainage for empyema.
2. Appropriate antimicrobial therapy should be given.

Prognosis With proper antimicrobial therapy the disease has become infrequent; when it does occur, the prognosis is markedly improved.

ACUTE PULMONARY INTERSTITIAL AND MEDIASTINAL EMPHYSEMA (Air Block) AND PNEUMOTHORAX

This condition is characterized by extraneous collections of air in the interstitial tissues of the lungs, the mediastinum, and their fascial extensions, which interfere with the normal circulatory and respiratory functions.

Etiology and pathogenesis Operative or accidental trauma, over-inflation of the lungs with alveolar rupture during resuscitation, acute or chronic infection, atelectasis, or congenital anomalies may lead to rupture of the alveoli, with release of air into the perivascular sheaths. The air then diffuses along artificial channels, with the formation of mediastinal emphysema. With further increase of pressure, air is forced into the pleural space, causing pneumothorax, and it may even extend into the subcutaneous tissues.

Clinical features The onset is usually acute, with pain, cyanosis, and dyspnea as the outstanding features. Even in severe cases there may be few other physical findings. Roentgenograms establish the diagnosis; both anteroposterior and lateral views should be taken.

Prophylaxis Prophylaxis is very important. Since most cases occur in the newborn infant, every effort should be made to avoid injury during birth and during resuscitation.

Treatment In mild cases, oxygen is needed for relief of dyspnea. If cyanosis and dyspnea are progressive in spite of this treatment, it may be necessary to aspirate the mediastinum. If infection is present, it should be treated with antibiotics.

REVIEW QUESTIONS

1. Children do not expectorate sputum until the age of (a) 3 years; (b) 5 years; (c) 7 years; (d) 10 years.
2. Contraindications to tonsillectomy or adenoidectomy include two of the following: (a) summer; (b) acute infection in the patient; (c) presence of an epidemic of poliomyelitis in the community; (d) chronic glomerulonephritis.
3. The most common cause of acute otitis media is (a) pneumococcus; (b) viral; (c) H. influenza; (d) beta-hemolytic streptococcus.
4. Diagnosis of the causative organism in the case of bacterial infection of the middle ear is best made from (a) nasopharyngeal secretion; (b) middle ear aspirate; (c) blood culture; (d) none of the above is of value.
5. Following an acute attack of otitis media, the child should be managed as follows: (a) he should be taught to "blow" his nose properly; (b) he should have cerumen removed from auditory canal regularly; (c) his hearing should be tested; (d) he should wear a hat with earmuffs.
6. Peritonsillar abscess occurs most commonly (a) in infancy; (b) after 5 years of age; (c) with equal frequency at all ages; (d) in females.
7. The following characterize spasmodic croup except for one: (a) it usually occurs between 2 and 4 years of age; (b) the onset is late at night; (c) fever is greater than 102°F; (d) it tends to recur.
8. The following characterize congenital laryngeal stridor except (a) onset in the newborn infant; (b) crowing on inspiration; (c) necessity for surgical treatment; (d) visualization of a flabby epiglottis on laryngoscopic examination; (e) possible presence of dyspnea.
9. The following statements concerning acute bronchiolitis are true except for one: (a) usually occurs in infants and yound children; (b) basic pathology is obstructive emphysema; (c) most cases are due to bacterial etiology; (d) acidosis is prone to occur.
10. The following clinical features characterize bronchopneumonia except for one: (a) meningismus is common; (b) paralytic ileus is seen frequently; (c) leukocytosis of 20,000 to 30,000; (d) identification of organism is made by tracheal or lung aspirate.

The following questions are of the matching type. In the space next to the respiratory disease in column I, insert the letter of the phrase in column II which characterizes the epidemiology of the disease:

I	II
11. Respiratory syncytial virus (RS) _____	(a) Summer and early fall
12. Coxsackie virus _____	(b) Recurrent epidemics every 3 to 5 years during winter
13. Influenza types A and B _____	(c) Endemic during fall season

14. The single most common underlying condition in bronchiectasis is (*a*) ascariasis; (*b*) IgM abnormality; (*c*) mucoviscidosis; (*d*) aspiration of a foreign body.

15. The most common viruses causing upper respiratory infections are (*a*) myxoviruses and adenoviruses; (*b*) rhinoviruses and adenoviruses; (*c*) enteroviruses and rhinoviruses; (*d*) reoviruses and myxoviruses.

16. The following statements except one are true for upper respiratory infection: (*a*) it is uncommon in infants less than 6 months of age raised in healthful surroundings; (*b*) the younger the child, the milder the constitutional symptoms; (*c*) the cervical lymph nodes may become enlarged; (*d*) it may simulate rubeola.

17. Group A beta-hemolytic streptococcal pharyngitis is (*a*) common in the neonate; (*b*) uncommon before age 2 years; (*c*) uncommon before age 6; (*d*) not age-related.

16
HEART DISEASES

Diseases of the heart in children may be classified into two categories —congenital and acquired. Rheumatic fever is by far the most common cause of acquired heart disease in children. Myocarditis occurs as a complication of the common contagious diseases, infectious mononucleosis, and the acute respiratory and enteric viral infections (probably with greater frequency in the latter instance than is realized). Degenerative diseases of the heart and those due to metabolic disturbances occur in children infrequently.

CONGENITAL MALFORMATIONS OF THE HEART

Etiology In Chapter 12, "Diseases of the Newborn," the major causative factors in congenital malformations have been mentioned.

It is estimated that 6 infants of every 1,000 born have congenital heart disease. The incidence of individual congenital cardiac malformations is unknown, and many of these children have multiple lesions. It has been suggested that the order of frequency of 13 noncyanotic types is as follows: ventricular septal defect, patent ductus arteriosus, atrial septal defect, coarctation of the aorta, isolated pulmonary stenosis, aortic and subaortic stenosis, primary endocardial fibroelastosis, idiopathic dilatation of the pulmonary artery, vascular rings, anomalous left coronary artery, aortic pulmonary window, ruptured sinus of Valsalva, and glycogen-storage disease. The order of frequency of eight cyanotic types is the following: tetralogy of Fallot, complete transposition of the great vessels, pulmonary stenosis with atrial and ventricular septal defects, Eisenmenger's complex, tricuspid atresia, persistent truncus arteriosus, levocardia, and anomalous drainage of all pulmonary veins.

Abnormal physiology of congenital heart diseases   The signs, symptoms, and sequelae of the morbid anatomy of congenital cardiac malformations are in most cases due to one of the following disturbances of cardiac hemodynamics:

The heart may be considered to consist of paired structures—right-sided (low pressure–low oxygen content) and left-sided (high pressure–high oxygen content). The paired structures are the vena cava and pulmonary veins, right and left atrium, right and left ventricle, pulmonary artery and aorta. The pressure (P) within a chamber or vessel is the resultant of volume of flow (F) and the resistance (R) against forward flow $(P = F \times R)$.

The two sides of the heart have no communication in postnatal life after closure of the ductus arteriosus and the foramen ovale. Venous blood from the low-pressure right side enters the high-pressure left side through the pulmonary capillary bed. Arterial or oxygenated blood from the left side enters the right side via the systemic capillary bed. The presence of an abnormal connection between paired structures of the left and right usually causes blood to flow from the left to the right, e.g., from the pulmonary vein to the vena cava, from the left to right atrium or ventricle, from the aorta to the pulmonary artery, because of the higher pressures on the left side. However, this applies only when the communication is small (approximately less than one-half the diameter of the aortic valve orifice, as in ventricular septal defects). When the defect is larger, then the two compartments or chambers have the same pressure and the direction of blood flow— left to right or right to left—is a function of resistance (pulmonary versus systemic). This increased volume of blood entering the lungs is characterized radiologically by increased vascular markings, but the oxygen content of the blood passing into the peripheral circulation is normal, and therefore cyanosis is not present.

Blood passes from the right to the left side if in addition to an abnormal communication the pressure is higher on the right than on the left side of the heart. The increased right-sided pressure is due to an obstruction to the blood flow lying distal to the abnormal communication. The obstruction may be congenital, e.g., stenosis or atresia of the tricuspid or pulmonary valve, or acquired, e.g., progressive pulmonary arteriolar sclerosis. Initial left-to-right shunts may change to right-to-left shunts as the resistance rises on the right side to exceed that of the left, as in atrial or ventricular septal defects complicated by progressive pulmonary arteriolar sclerosis. The blood flow through the pulmonary arterial circulation will gradually decrease, because of the arteriolar sclerosis, and ultimately cyanosis will appear. This phenomenon is almost invariably associated with large defects with pressures equal on both sides of the defect so that the direction of flow is determined by the resistance difference between the left and right side. The pressure remains equal on both sides even as shunting changes from left to right to right to left.

Visible cyanosis is present when the magnitude of the right-(venous) to-left (arterial) shunt is sufficient to cause a concentration of 5 Gm reduced hemoglobin per 100 ml blood in the systemic capillary blood or when arterial oxygen saturation is below 80 percent.

Classification of congenital heart disease

1. Left-to-right shunt: cyanosis is absent; the pulmonary vascular markings are increased on roentgenogram, depending on the volume of the shunt and the related increase in pulmonary blood flow.
    a. Atrial septal defect
    b. Ventricular septal defect
    c. Patent ductus arteriosus
    d. Aortic-pulmonary window
    e. Anomalous pulmonary venous return
2. Right-to-left shunt: cyanosis is present—the time of onset depends on the volume of the shunt bypassing the pulmonary capillary bed and thus decreasing the oxygen content in the systemic arterial circulation.
    a. Tetralogy of Fallot
    b. Tricuspid atresia
    c. Transposition of the great vessels
    d. Eisenmenger's complex
    e. Pulmonary valve stenosis with an atrial septal defect
    f. Ebstein's anomaly of the tricuspid valve
    g. Truncus arteriosus
3. Absence of shunt: associated with cardiac disability due to either increased pressure or an intrinsic derangement of normal cardiac function.
    a. Aortic stenosis or isolated pulmonary stenosis
    b. Coarctation of the aorta
    c. Vascular ring (double aortic arch)
    d. Subendocardial fibroelastosis

    e. Anomalous origin of the left coronary artery
    f. Myocarditis of infancy
    g. Glycogen-storage disease

Diagnostic techniques in congenital heart disease Whenever possible the diagnosis should be made on the basis of careful history, clinical findings, x-ray, and other routine laboratory studies. The various precise methods of cardiac catheterization, angiography, etc., have been developed for more accurate anatomic diagnosis, determination of size of flows and shunts, and evaluation of important hemodynamic factors—cardiac output, pressure changes in venous chambers, oxygen saturation, pulmonary function. These help to diagnose the exact nature of the malformation and its immediate and remote effect on the physiology of the cardiovascular system. Cardiac catheterization makes possible the following measurements:

1. Oxygen saturation:
    a. All right-sided chambers, vena cava, and pulmonary artery—about 70 percent. (The inferior vena cava usually is 3 to 5 percent higher than the superior vena cava.)
    b. All left-sided chambers, pulmonary veins and aorta—about 95 to 97 percent.
2. Pressures (mmHg):
    a. Right atrium—3 to 5
    b. Right ventricle—20 to 30/0
    c. Pulmonary artery—20 to 30/10–15
    d. Left atrium—5 to 7
    e. Left ventricle—80 to 110/5
    f. Aorta—80 to 110/50–80

LEFT–TO–RIGHT SHUNT (Noncyanotic)

ATRIAL SEPTAL DEFECT

This defect is a deficiency in the septum dividing the two atria. There are three types, each derived from a different arrest of development of the heart.

Foramen secundum defect This defect occurs in the midpart of the septum (in the area of the fossa ovalis) and is surrounded by remnants of the septum.

Clinical features
1. The defect of average size is consistent with a relatively normal lifespan. Retardation of growth is less frequent than in other defects. Symptoms of cardiac disability, if they occur, usually appear after 50 years of age except in the larger defects, which cause disability in infancy and childhood.

2. Physical examination discloses a soft, ejection, systolic murmur in the 2d and 3d intercostal spaces to the left of the sternum. The pulmonary second sound is prominent with a wide, fixed split. A thrill is not palpable, but a right ventricular heave is present. The pulmonary artery pulsation may be palpable in the slim child. The heart is mildly enlarged. With large defects, cardiac enlargement is more marked, and a short early diastolic murmur may be audible over the lower precordium.

Laboratory features
1. Electrocardiogram shows right axis deviation and right ventricular hypertrophy with an incomplete right bundle branch block, best seen in the V_1 lead.
2. Roentgenographic and fluoroscopic examination reveal enlargement of the right atrium and the right ventricle. The main pulmonary artery is dilated and pulsates. The pulmonary vascular markings are increased and show a pulsating hilar movement (hilar dance).
3. Cardiac catheterization reveals an oxygen-saturation increase in the blood of the right atrium. Pulmonary artery pressure usually does not exceed 50 mmHg in children.
4. Angiocardiography following injection of radiopaque material into the left atrium may give added detail of the anatomy of the defect.

Treatment   Open-heart surgery to close the defect is indicated only if cardiac enlargement is present.

Ostium primum defect   This occurs in the lower part of the septum where it adjoins the atrioventricular valves; usually it is associated with a cleft in the mitral and/or tricuspid valves, making them incompetent.

Clinical features
1. Variable, depending on the size of the defect and the extent of valvular involvement.
2. The physical findings resemble a ventricular septal defect more than a simple atrial septal defect. Examination discloses a harsh, blowing, systolic murmur in the 4th and 5th interspaces to the left of the sternum. A mid-diastolic rumble is usually heard to the left of the systolic murmur area. A slight thrill is frequent in the 4th and 5th left interspaces. The second pulmonary sound is accentuated and split. If the mitral value is cleft, an apical systolic murmur, which is transmitted to the axilla, is also heard.

Laboratory features
1. Electrocardiogram is very helpful: evidence of right ventricular hypertrophy and incomplete right bundle branch block is present. The limb leads show a superior axis with a progressive dominance of S waves from leads 1 to 3. The vectorcardiogram describes a

counterclockwise rotation above the base line in the frontal plane.
2. The roentgenographic and fluoroscopic pictures resemble those of the larger secundum defect.
3. Cardiac catheterization results are similar to those of a secundum defect, with a tendency toward more marked pulmonary hypertension.
4. Angiocardiographic examination may demonstrate mitral incompetence if dye can be injected into the left ventricle.

Treatment   This has a worse prognosis than the secundum defect because of the left ventricular burden produced by the cleft mitral valve. Open-heart surgery should be performed to correct these defects, preferably at 5 to 8 years of age.

Common atrioventricular canal   This is essentially an ostium primum defect with cleft tricuspid and mitral valves, and it is continuous with a defect in the ventricular septum. Thus all four cardiac chambers are in communication.

Clinical features   Physical examination reveals findings similar to those of an ostium primum defect. The systolic thrill is usually more marked in the atrioventricular canal defect. Because of pulmonary hypertension and increasing pulmonary vascular resistance, mild cyanosis is common with increasing age. (The shunt, though predominantly left-to-right, becomes increasingly bidirectional.) Cardiac failure and repeated respiratory infections are more common in the two previous types of atrial defect.

Laboratory features
1. Electrocardiogram resembles that of the ostium primum defect.
2. Cardiac catheterization results resemble those of the ostium primum defect except that the right ventricular and pulmonary artery pressures approach the systemic pressure because of the large size of the ventricular septal defect, and arterial oxygen saturations are usually below 90 percent.

Treatment   Open-heart surgery should be attempted despite a relatively higher risk than in the correction of simple atrial or ventricular septal defects.

Lutembacher's syndrome   This defect consists of an atrial septal defect accompanied by mitral stenosis, usually acquired. This lesion is rare.

VENTRICULAR SEPTAL DEFECT

This defect commonly occurs at the base of the heart in the membranous part of the septum, rather than in the muscular section. Classically it lies close by the aortic valve behind the septal leaflet of the tricuspid valve. (This proximity to the aortic valve probably explains the rare complication of a prolapsed aortic valve cusp and resulting aortic insufficiency.)

Clinical features
1. The heart is enlarged, the degree of enlargement depending on the size of the defect and its position in the septum. Severe pulmonary hypertension associated with the larger defects complicates the clinical picture.
2. A thrill, usually marked, is palpable along the left sternal border from the 3d to the 6th intercostal spaces. A loud, harsh, systolic murmur is heard in this area, radiating toward, but not beyond the apex. The enlargement of the heart and displacement of the apex are downward and to the left. The apical impulse is usually diffuse. The second heart sound is often accentuated but is rarely split as in atrial defects. Infants with a large defect and severe pulmonary hypertension may have a blowing murmur and no thrill. The second sound in these infants is very loud. (Transmission of the thrill and murmur to the left base of the heart is usually associated with acquired hypertrophy of the outflow tract of the right ventricle, or occasionally with an associated congenital infundibular obstruction.)

Laboratory features
1. The electrocardiagram varies with the extent or predominance of the burden imposed on either the right or left ventricles. In the smaller defects, the axis is balanced or left and there is evidence of hypertrophy of the left ventricle or of both ventricles. The cardiogram may appear normal in the latter case except for wide excursions of the R and S components of the QRS complex. In the larger defects, especially those complicated by pulmonary hypertension of severe degree (above 60 mmHg), right axis deviation and predominant right ventricular hypertrophy are usually seen.
2. Roentgenograms and fluoroscopic examination show variable degrees of cardiac enlargement and increased pulmonary markings. The apex is displaced downward and to the left; the pulmonary artery is prominent; and the left atrium is mildly dilated. The right ventricle is enlarged as well as the left, although this is difficult to determine radiologically. A hilar dance may be present.
3. Cardiac catheterization reveals an increased oxygen content of blood in the right ventricle. Pressure levels in the right ventricle and pulmonary artery may vary from normal to those equal to systemic pressure. Pressure gradients across the outflow tract of the right ventricle are found frequently and are due to a large flow of blood across the pulmonary valve or to hypertrophy of the outflow tract of the right ventricle accounts for a higher pressure in the right ventricle than in the pulmonary artery.
4. Angiocardiography: injections from the left ventricle are neces-

sary to delineate the anatomy of the defect. The presence of aortic insufficiency is best demonstrated by an aortogram. A right ventricular angiocardiogram will demonstrate any associated infundibular or valvular obstruction.

Treatment
1. Cardiac failure if it occurs will appear between 3 weeks and 4 months of age. If it is uncontrolled by medical therapy, banding of the pulmonary artery can be performed to decrease the volume flow across the septal defect.
2. Elective closure of the defects are performed at age 5 to 6 years, except in those larger defects associated with systolic pulmonary artery pressure greater than 75 mmHg, where surgery is recommended between 15 and 18 months.

PATENT DUCTUS ARTERIOSUS

This is an abnormal persistence of the fetal connection between the aorta and the pulmonary artery. The structure normally ceases to function at birth or several days later, but is usually not anatomically closed until the age of 3 or 4 weeks. A ventricular septal defect is often associated with a patent ductus arteriosus.

Clinical features   The degree of cardiac disability varies with the diameter of the ductus. Frequently if the ductus is large, cardiac failure and death may occur in infancy. The physical findings in such cases resemble those of a ventricular septal defect, and the continuous or machinery murmur at the left base, characteristic of a patent ductus, is absent. The pulses are full and bounding, with a pulse pressure of over 40 mmHg.

Laboratory features

1. In the smaller or asymptomatic lesions the electrocardiogram is normal or reveals left ventricular hypertrophy. In patients with a large ductus, the electrocardiogram reveals combined right and left ventricular hypertrophy or predominant right ventricular hypertrophy if sufficient pulmonary hypertension is present.
2. Roentgenograms and fluoroscopic examination may reveal normal cardiac size or enlargement of the left ventricle and left atrium. In the more severe defects the right ventricle is also enlarged. The main pulmonary artery is dilated, and the lung fields reveal increased vascular markings.
3. Cardiac catheterization in patients with a small ductus demonstrates a rise in blood oxygen content in the pulmonary artery with mild elevation of pulmonary artery pressure. In the presence of a larger ductus, especially if it is associated with moderate or severe pulmonary hypertension, the first rise of oxygen content appears in the blood of the outflow tract of the right ventricle, as

is seen with a high ventricular septal defect. A retrograde aortogram revealing the passage of dye from the aorta to the pulmonary arteries differentiates the ductus from the septal defect.

Treatment   If cardiac failure occurs at any age, cardiac catheterization should be performed and an aortogram made. If the diagnosis is corroborated, prompt surgical closure of the ductus is advised.

Every patent ductus, even if asymptomatic, should be closed soon after the child is 1 year of age.

AORTIC–PULMONARY WINDOW

This defect occurs in the septum dividing the aorta and the pulmonary artery at the base of the heart; it is very rare when compared with the occurrence of patent ductus arteriosus.

In infancy, this lesion presents the same problem as the patent ductus in that it resembles a ventricular septal defect. It is best diagnosed by retrograde aortography, which delineates the site of entry of radiopaque material from the aorta to the pulmonary artery. In older children the physical findings are similar to those of a patent ductus. Some patients have a continuous machinery murmur at the left base; others have a harsh, systolic murmur with a blowing diastolic murmur transmitted inferiorly along the left sternal border.

Treatment   Closure by cardiac pump bypass surgery is indicated after the child is 3 years of age.

ANOMALOUS PULMONARY VENOUS RETURN

Several anatomic variations occur, but in all of them there is an abnormal return of some or all of the pulmonary veins, either to the venae cavae or to the right atrium. The site of entrance of the pulmonary veins may present an obstruction to the flow of blood or, more commonly, it may cause no obstruction. The following descriptions apply to the unobstructive type.

Clinical features

1.   The degree of disability and cardiac insufficiency is related to the number of aberrant veins (one to four). One or two anomalous veins usually do not distress the heart. If three or four veins are involved, cardiac failure occurs during infancy or early childhood.
2.   The physical findings are variable and are related to the number of veins involved and to their location. If the pulmonary veins enter the superior vena cava, there is a systolic or a continuous murmur at the base of the heart. If these veins enter the right atrium, there may be no murmur, or there is a soft systolic or a continuous murmur over the lower precordium. Mild cyanosis may be present.

Laboratory features

1. Roentgenogram: in the severe type, there is right-sided cardiac enlargement with marked increase of pulmonary vascular markings. If the veins enter the superior vena cava, there is a classical rounded density of the right and left bases of the heart, because of dilatation of the superior vena cava and innominate veins.
2. The electrocardiogram reveals marked right axis deviation and right ventricular hypertrophy.
3. Cardiac catheterization shows a marked increase in amount of oxygen in the blood samples taken from the site where the veins enter the vena cava. In the case of total anomalous drainage, the oxygen content in the pulmonary artery equals or exceeds that of the aorta.
4. The angiocardiogram shows earlier visualization of the aorta than normal. A dye-dilution curve is also helpful in demonstrating a right-to-left shunt at the auricular level, if none of the veins enters the left atrium.

Treatment   Surgical correction should be attempted in infancy if cardiac failure occurs. If possible, surgical correction is delayed until after 3 years of age.

RIGHT–TO–LEFT SHUNT (Cyanotic)

TETRALOGY OF FALLOT

This malformation is a combination of:

1. Pulmonary stenosis: due to infundibular stenosis (crista superventricularis) and/or hypoplasia or stenosis of the pulmonary valves. The main pulmonary arteries are also hypoplastic.
2. Ventricular septal defect: in the membranous portion of the septum proximal to the crista supraventricularis.
3. Aortic involvement: the aortic valve is in immediate proximity to the large ventricular septal defect so that in spite of the normally arising aortic root and valve, right ventricular blood easily enters the aorta.
4. Hypertrophy of the right ventricle.

Clinical features

1. Cyanosis is usually noted at 3 to 6 months of age. It may be seen at birth if severe pulmonary stenosis or atresia is present, or it may not appear until later childhood if only a mild degree of obstruction to pulmonary flow is present. The cyanosis deepens with activity (e.g., crying, exercise), dyspnea occurs, and fainting may ensue because of cerebral hypoxia if the fall in oxygen saturation of the blood is rapid and marked. After exertion these children

characteristically assume a squatting position. Clubbing of the fingers and toes, and polycythemia are also found. Physical growth is mildly retarded.

2. The heart is not enlarged. The heart sounds are loud and clear. The second sound at the left base is loud and pure even with pulmonary valvular stenosis, in which case the pure, loud second sound is probably due to closure of the aortic valve. A systolic murmur is heard along the left sternal border in the 3d and 4th intercostal spaces. It is soft and blowing with severe stenosis and louder and harsher with mild stenosis. A murmur is not heard with pulmonary atresia. A mild right ventricular heave is noted in young and thin children. A mild systolic thrill may be present.

Laboratory features

1. Roentgenograms reveal a normal-sized, boot-shaped heart with variable degrees of hypoplasia of the pulmonary arteries and a decrease in pulmonary markings directly related to the severity of the pulmonary stenosis. The aortic knob is large; when it is not easily visible, a right aortic arch should be suspected. (This is present in 20 to 25 percent of the cases.)
2. Electrocardiogram: right axis deviation and pure right ventricular hypertrophy.
3. Cardiac catheterization: pressure in the right ventricle is equal to the systemic arterial pressure, and the pulmonary artery pressure is low or normal. Arterial oxygen saturation is decreased.
4. Angiocardiogram: injection of radiopaque material into the right ventricle can demonstrate the anatomic details of its outflow tract, the diameter of the pulmonary valve orifice, and the size of the pulmonary arteries, in addition to the simultaneous opacification of the aorta and the pulmonary artery.

Complications

1. Brain abscess
2. Cerebral thrombosis

Medical treatment

1. Close observation of the hemogram to keep hemoglobin and red cell count in balance (color index, at least 0.9). Routine use of iron may increase polycythemia to unduly high levels and increase the incidence of spontaneous thrombosis. However, anemia (color index below 0.9) should be treated with iron.
2. Prompt treatment of illness and prevention of dehydration, particularly during warm weather.

Surgical treatment

1. Blalock or Pott's procedure is indicated if syncope occurs before the age of 4 years or if polycythemia is severe enough to raise the

hematocrit level above 75 percent, hemoglobin above 20 Gm per 100 ml, and red cell count above 7.5 million per cu mm. A Blalock procedure (subclavian artery–pulmonary artery anastomosis) is preferable to a Pott's procedure (aorta–pulmonary artery anastomosis) because it is easier to undo when definitive open-heart surgical repair is performed at a later date.

2. Open-heart surgical repair of the septal defect and resection of the pulmonary stenosis is performed after the age of 4 years.

TRICUSPID ATRESIA

Atresia of the tricuspid valve causes blood to flow from the right atrium to the left atrium (via a patent foramen ovale or septal defect). The right ventricle is hypoplastic and receives blood only from the left ventricle (via a small septal defect). The pulmonary artery is usually hypoplastic with a small deformed valve. Occasionally the great vessels are transposed or both arise from one ventricle.

Clinical features

1. Cyanosis is severe and present at birth unless the pulmonary artery arises from the left ventricle. In this circumstance, cyanosis is mild or absent because of increased pulmonary blood flow until pulmonary resistance rises, after which cyanosis increases progressively.
2. Physical examination may reveal no murmur, or there may be a soft systolic murmur along the left sternal border. The second sound is pure.

Laboratory features

1. Roentgenogram: The heart is not enlarged except when the great vessels are transposed. The shape of the heart has the appearance of a square in the posterior-anterior view and has a straight instead of a mildly convex anterior border in the left anterior oblique view. The pulmonary vascular markings are decreased except when the pulmonary artery is transposed, in which case the markings are increased.
2. Electrocardiogram: There is left axis deviation and left ventricular preponderance. P waves are usually peaked.
3. Cardiac catheterization has limited value. Angiocardiography may help to delineate the hypoplastic right ventricle and the origin of the great vessels.

Treatment   Surgical intervention is indicated; superior vena cava–pulmonary artery anastomosis is the procedure of choice. However surgery is usually necessary before 1 year of age, in which case a subclavian artery–pulmonary artery anastomosis is used.

TRANSPOSITION OF THE GREAT VESSELS

In this defect the aorta originates from the right ventricle and the pulmonary artery from the left ventricle. The systemic and pulmonary veins drain normally into their respective atria.

The continuation of life beyond a few days is possible only if co-existing communications, e.g., patent ductus arteriosus or septal defects, permit passage of oxygenated blood from the left side to the right or if pulmonic valve stenosis is present. Other variations occur in which one or both major vessels arise from both chambers astride a ventricular septal defect.

Clinical features

1. Cyanosis and dyspnea are intense and are observed within the first week of life.
2. Auscultation of the heart is not helpful—murmurs may or may not be present. When heard, they indicate the presence of associated anomalies.
3. Cardiac failure usually occurs shortly after birth, except when pulmonary stenosis is present.

Laboratory features

1. Electrocardiogram: right axis deviation and right ventricular hypertrophy.
2. Roentgenogram: shows rapid and progressive cardiac enlargement and increased pulmonary vascular markings. When pulmonary stenosis is present the heart size is normal and the shape resembles that in tetralogy of Fallot.
3. Angiocardiogram: delineates the position of the vessels and shows whether the transposition is partial or complete.
4. Cardiac catheterization reveals characteristic findings:
   a. Pressure in the systemic artery is normal. Pressure in the pulmonary artery is usually equal to the systemic pressure if a ventricular septal defect is present.
   b. Catheter passes directly into the aorta from the right ventricle, where the pressure is systemic in level.
   c. Oxygen content in the pulmonary artery is higher than in the aorta.

Prognosis   Death occurs in the first days or weeks of life. The life-span may be prolonged months or years if there are associated defects, especially pulmonary stenosis or partial overriding of the pulmonary artery.

Treatment

1. Digitalis for the management of cardiac failure.
2. At the time of cardiac catheterization if no atrial septal defect is

present, the atrial septum is ruptured by an inflated balloon pulled from the left to the right atrium. If this fails, the atrial septum can be partially removed surgically (Blalock-Hanlon) at this time. If successful, the surgical procedure may be done at a later date.

3. If a large ventricular septal defect is present, the pulmonary artery must be banded by 3 months of age to prevent the development of obstructive pulmonary vascular disease.

4. After the age of 3 years an open-heart procedure is performed to change the direction of venous flow—pulmonary to the right and systemic to the left (Mustard).

EISENMENGER'S COMPLEX

Anatomically this lesion is characterized by a large, high or membranous ventricular septal defect and pulmonary arteriolar sclerosis.

Clinical features

1. In infancy and early childhood cyanosis is usually absent. It appears and increases progressively after the age of 4 years. The onset of cyanosis coincides with the change of direction of the flow of blood through the shunt from left to right to right to left, because the increasing pulmonary artery resistance ultimately exceeds the systemic vascular resistance.

2. In the cyanotic phase a soft, blowing systolic murmur is audible. A pulmonary diastolic murmur due to pulmonary valve regurgitation may be present. The second pulmonary sound is single and cracking.

3. Physical capacity progressively decreases with increasing age, and death usually occurs from massive pulmonary hemorrhage.

Laboratory features

1. Electrocardiogram: right axis deviation and right ventricular hypertrophy.

2. Roentgenogram: mild cardiac enlargement involving the right ventricle, and a convex main pulmonary artery silhouette. The pulmonary vascular markings are increased in the central hilar area and may be decreased in the peripheral lung fields. Fluoroscopic examination: a central hilar dance is visible.

3. Cardiac catheterization is diagnostic, revealing equal pulmonary artery and right ventricular pressures. This pressure equals the systemic arterial pressure. The arterial blood is mildly desaturated of oxygen.

4. Angiocardiogram: large pulmonary arteries and peripheral blockade; the aorta opacifies as radiopaque material enters it from the right ventricle.

Prognosis   No treatment is available. Death occurs in late childhood or early adult life.

PULMONARY VALVE STENOSIS

In about one-third of the cases there is an associated atrial septal defect.

Clinical features

1. Cyanosis and decreased exercise capacity occur only in the more severe degrees of valvular obstruction. The right atrial pressure rises, and a right-to-left shunt develops via either the atrial septal defect, if present, on the foramen ovale.
2. The heart is enlarged relative to the degree of pulmonary stenosis. A rasping systolic murmur is heard at the left base and a thrill is palpable in this region. The second pulmonary sound is normal or decreased.

Laboratory features

1. Electrocardiogram: variable degree of right axis deviation and right ventricular hypertrophy, depending on the severity of the stenosis. The P waves are usually tall and peaked in the severe lesions.
2. Roentgenogram: enlarged right atrium and ventricle. The main pulmonary artery is very much dilated (poststenotic) after the first 2 years of life. The peripheral pulmonary vascular markings are normal or decreased. Fluoroscopic examination: the main pulmonary artery pulsates while the peripheral pulmonary arteries are quiet.
3. Cardiac catheterization reveals a high right ventricular pressure, reaching levels up to 300 mmHg. The pulmonary artery pressure is normal or decreased.
4. Angiocardiogram reveals the thickened, domed pulmonary valve and the dilated pulmonary artery.

Prognosis The prognosis varies from a normal lifespan for patients with mild lesions to acute failure of the right side of the heart occurring in infants with severe lesions.

Treatment Surgery offers complete relief of the obstruction and can be performed at any age.

EBSTEIN'S ANOMALY OF THE TRICUSPID VALVE

This defect consists of a large tricuspid valve which prolapses into the right ventricle. Part of the valve is adherent to the wall of the right ventricle. The outflow tract of the right ventricle is normal. If blood flow is obstructed across the valve, blood may shunt to the left atrium through a foramen ovale, and cyanosis will be present. There may be no murmur, a soft systolic murmur, or to-and-fro systolic and diastolic murmurs.

The electrocardiogram shows arrhythmia, prolonged P-R interval due to tall, widened P waves, and right ventricular conduction disturbances with widened, notched, and often low-voltage QRS complexes. The roentgenogram usually shows an enlarged heart; the pulmonary vascular markings are decreased. On fluoroscopic examination, the heart presents diminished pulsatile activity of the right ventricle. Making an angiocardiogram is dangerous, but it shows slow ejection of the radiopaque material from the right atrium and in the posteroanterior view a large right atrial chamber with an indentation in the region of the tricuspid valve ring on the undersurface of the heart. An atrialized pressure curve distal to the tricuspid valve ring is found.

The prognosis varies with the degree of obstruction to blood flow; death occurs either in infancy or in early adult life. No corrective surgical procedure is possible. A superior vena cava–right pulmonary artery anastomosis is of help in decreasing blood flow to the right atrium and increasing flow to the right lung.

TRUNCUS ARTERIOSUS

A single vessel, the truncus arteriosus, arises from both ventricles astride a large ventricular septal defect. The vessel is large and guarded by an abnormal valve. The single vessel or several vessels going to the lungs may originate from the aorta anywhere from its base to the descending aorta.

Initially, the amount of blood going to the lungs is increased, normal, or decreased, depending on the size of the vessels. Secondarily, if the lungs receive blood under systemic pressure, pulmonary hypertensive changes develop which decrease pulmonary blood flow, with consequent lowering of the systemic arterial blood oxygen saturation.

Cyanosis will usually appear in late infancy or early childhood unless there are inadequate or absent pulmonary arteries, in which case cyanosis will be present at birth.

The heart is slightly enlarged. A right ventricular heave is present, and the apex is in the 4th or 5th intercostal space but lateral to the nipple line. Early in infancy a systolic murmur may be heard; later, a continuous blowing murmur is heard to the left and right at the base of the heart. This continuous murmur can be heard best over the lateral or posterior aspect of the chest. Prior to 2 years of age a roentgenogram reveals transverse enlargement of the heart and a markedly upturned apex. The electrocardiogram varies, demonstrating right or combined right-and-left ventricular hypertrophy. The angiocardiogram demonstrates the truncus and subsequently the nature of the blood flow to the lungs.

Treatment   In those cases with large pulmonary flow and no cyanosis, banding of the pulmonary artery or arteries will delay the development of pulmonary arteriosclerotic changes. Surgical correction of the defect (separating the pulmonary arteries from the aorta, connecting these arteries to the right ventricle, and closing the septal defect) can be performed.

ABSENCE OF SHUNT

AORTIC STENOSIS

Obstruction of the outlet of the left ventricle occurs at one of four sites.

1. Aortic valve stenosis (most common type): due to fusion of two or three cusps of the valve and usually accompanied by marked distortion and irregularity of cusp size. This distortion is responsible for a high incidence of regurgitation phenomenon due to prolapse of a cusp not only before but also after surgical correction.
2. Subaortic stenosis: due to a diaphragm about 1 cm proximal to the valve or a fibrous band encircling the outlet of the left ventricle.
3. Congenital progressive hypertrophy of the muscular wall of the left ventricle producing stenosis of the outlet (obstruction is most marked during systole).
4. Supravalvular stenosis: due to a fibrous band or diaphragm on the inner surface of the aorta immediately distal to the origin of the coronary arteries. Some patients may show associated peripheral pulmonary artery stenosis, an elflike facies, mental retardation, and hypercalcemia in infancy.

Clinical features of aortic valve stenosis and subaortic stenosis

1. In infancy and early childhood, a harsh systolic murmur is heard at the lower sternal border to the right of the apex. A thrill is present in this area. (A ventricular septal defect is often suspected initially.) Later the localization of the murmur and the thrill change to the upper sternum and they are transmitted to the suprasternal notch and along the vessels of the neck. The second aortic sound may be diminished, but its usefulness in differentiating aortic valve from subaortic stenosis is limited as the second sound may be present or diminished in either lesion. A diastolic murmur at the aortic area or at Erb's point usually appears in late childhood (more often in subaortic than in aortic stenosis). The heart is normal or enlarged, depending on the degree of stenosis. The peripheral pulses are weak, and a narrow pulse pressure is present in the severe lesions.
2. Easy fatigability, lightheadedness, and syncope may occur. A change in play habits to a more sedentary type, often producing an increase in weight gain, should be interpreted as an indication for surgical intervention.

Laboratory features

1. Electrocardiogram: in early childhood the milder lesions are associated with normal right-sided preponderance, but evidence of left ventricular hypertrophy and strain occur in cases with more severe stenosis. The presence of S-T or T-wave depression and inversion is a sign of myocardial hypoxia and is an indication for surgery.
2. Roentgenogram: variable degrees, usually mild, of left ventricular enlargement are noted in childhood, even in the presence of severe lesions. The proximal aorta is often dilated and pulsates.
3. An angiocardiogram following injection of radiopaque material into the left ventricle is the only useful diagnostic tool to delineate the anatomy of the defect.
4. Catheterization of the left ventricle and aorta demonstrates the pressure gradient across the valve. A systolic gradient of 60 mmHg or greater is an indication for surgery.

Prognosis   Progressive cardiac failure and death usually occur in the young adult, but sudden death may occur earlier, probably due to ventricular fibrillation.

Treatment   Surgical repair of the lesion is indicated when the pressure gradient across the obstruction exceeds 60 mmHg. About 20 to 25 percent of the cases will have an aortic regurgitation after surgery, but this causes less strain on the heart than stenosis and may be repaired later by a valve prosthesis.

COARCTATION OF THE AORTA

This lesion occurs in two forms.

Postductal (adult) type   There is a narrowing of the aorta at, or distal to, the ductus arteriosus. Although marked hypertension (over 200 mmHg pressure in the upper extremities) may occur early in life, this type of coarctation infrequently causes cardiac difficulty in infancy. A concomitant widely patent ductus proximal to the narrowing of the aorta produces a large blood flow from the aorta to the lungs via the ductus under high pressure and causes early cardiac failure.

Clinical features
1. Physical examination discloses weak or absent femoral pulses and strong radial pulses. Occasionally the right arm pulse is stronger and the pressure higher than in the left. The blood pressure is higher in the upper than in the lower extremities. The heart is usually not enlarged except in the infrequent cases developing cardiac failure.
2. In infancy and early childhood murmurs are usually absent, or a soft systolic murmur may be heard. In the occasional patient with

a patent ductus there is a continuous machinery murmur. With increasing age, a systolic murmur becomes more evident, especially at the base of the heart, and it is loudest at the posterior chest between the scapulae. Later a continuous blowing murmur is heard posteriorly with palpable pulsations reflecting the passage of blood through large collateral vessels. (Frequently there is an associated bicuspid aortic valve which will produce a loud systolic murmur over the aortic valve, especially in later childhood.)

Laboratory features
1. Roentgenogram: Children having mild hypertension usually will have normal-sized hearts. In the more severe cases, especially those with a large patent ductus arteriosus, the heart will be enlarged and increased pulmonary vascular markings due to the functioning patent ductus will be seen. Notching of the ribs is present after the age of 4 years.
2. Electrocardiogram: usually right-sided preponderance of infancy is present. In later childhood evidence of left ventricular hypertrophy becomes apparent.
3. A retrograde aortogram via the left brachial artery is the most valuable procedure to demonstrate this lesion.

Treatment   In the asymptomatic child, the lesion is repaired surgically after 6 years of age.

In the rare case developing cardiac failure in the newborn period, failure to respond to medical treatment is an indication for prompt surgical treatment.

Preductal (infantile) type   There is a narrowing of the aorta proximal to the ductus arteriosus. Most often the ductus distal to the coarctation is widely patent, and blood flows in a reversed direction from the pulmonary artery to the descending aorta. Since this is venous blood, that portion of the body (below the pelvic brim) which it supplies may be mildly cyanotic. A commonly associated ventricular septal defect will prevent the appearance of differential cyanosis. The presence of severe pulmonary hypertension, plus the commonly associated aortic and mitral valve lesions, produces a high incidence of early cardiac failure and death.

The femoral arterial pulses may be weakly palpable in this type of coarctation after the first 2 or 3 days of life. The infant with preductal coarctation usually develops cardiac failure between the second and sixth weeks of life. Medical treatment usually fails, consequently surgery is indicated. The coarctated segment is usually long, in which case it should not be resected or anastomosed. The patent ductus should be ligated and if pulmonary artery pressure remains above 80 mmHg because of the presence of a large ventricular septal defect, the pulmonary artery is banded. If the coarcted segment is short, it is resected. Whether the pulmonary artery is banded again depends upon the presence of a ventricular septal defect and the presence of pulmonary hypertension.

The combination of a long hypoplastic aortic segment, underdevelopment of the left side of the heart and aortic atresia produces a characteristic clinical picture—hypoplastic left heart syndrome. The infant, apparently normal at birth, develops intractable cardiac failure after the second day of life. There are absent pulses in all four extremities, frequently a gallop rhythm, mild-to-moderate cardiac enlargement, mild cyanosis, and an electrocardiogram showing right-sided preponderance. This syndrome probably accounts for one-half of all deaths from cardiac disease occurring in the first week of life. Surgical correction is not possible.

VASCULAR RING (Double Aortic Arch)

This anomaly is subject to wide anatomic variation. The most common type is due to a persistence of both the right and left 4th aortic arches, which encircle the esophagus and trachea and join the descending thoracic aorta.

The infant has a coarse stridor, predominantly expiratory, and a high-pitched brassy or tracheal cough. The stridor becomes worse on ventral flexion of the head and decreases on dorsiflexion.

An esophagram will reveal a double indentation, anteriorly and posteriorly, where the vascular ring impinges upon it.

Surgical correction of the ring is indicated; the mortality rate from pneumonia and aspiration in untreated patients is about 50 percent during the first year of life.

SUBENDOCARDIAL FIBROELASTOSIS

A marked increase in elastic tissue occurs immediately beneath the endocardium of the heart. The left-sided chambers, especially the ventricle, show the most marked change, but the right side may also be involved.

The clinical features, which usually are apparent at 3 to 6 months of age, include cardiomegaly, cardiac failure, tachycardia with a gallop rhythm, and no significant murmurs.

The electrocardiogram shows a balanced or left axis deviation and a pattern of left ventricular hypertrophy with inverted T waves in the left precordial leads. Cardiac catheterization demonstrates a normal or high end diastolic pressure in the left and right ventricles. An angiocardiogram reveals a large, globular left ventricle with very slow ejection of opaque dye from the chamber.

Cardiac failure and death occur in early infancy when the aortic and mitral valves are distorted and stenosed by the disease. Occasionally, children may be asymptomatic until later childhood.

The essential hemodynamic change is a restriction in the ability of the heart to contract and relax properly. Digitalization is indicated;

often it is effective for a long period of time. A few cases have become normal after a period of years.

ANOMALOUS ORIGIN OF THE LEFT CORONARY ARTERY

The left coronary artery originates from the pulmonary artery, causing progressive cardiac enlargement and cardiac failure at about 3 to 4 months of age. These findings occur because coronary flow originates from a vessel whose pressure is lower than that of the aorta, not because the left ventricle is being supplied with venous blood. There is evidence to indicate that because of the low pressure, coronary blood flows from the right coronary artery through collateral vessels to the left coronary artery and then into the pulmonary artery. If this collateral supply is well developed, cardiac symptoms may be delayed until childhood or early adult life.

An aortogram demonstrating the flow from the right to the left coronary artery and then into the pulmonary artery proves the adequacy of the collateral channels. Cardiac catheterization may demonstrate increased oxygen saturation in the pulmonary artery. In this type of defect, surgical ligation of the left coronary artery is beneficial.

The electrocardiogram reveals left ventricular hypertrophy and flat or inverted T waves over the left precordium. In addition, a pattern of anterior myocardial infarction is often seen. Unfortunately, this infarction pattern may be present in fibroelastosis and severe viral myocarditis in infancy, which makes it an inadequate criterion for differential diagnosis.

The presence of collateral channels produces a systolic or soft continuous murmur heard over the apex of the heart. No murmur is present in the absence of collateral vessels between the right and left coronary arteries, in which case failure occurs in infancy.

RHEUMATIC FEVER

Etiology and pathogenesis These are still not fully understood, but there is convincing evidence that rheumatic fever is a type of tissue hypersensitivity to a streptococcal (group A beta-hemolytic) infection occurring in a susceptible host. The mesodermal tissue throughout the body may be affected by exudative and proliferative reactions. Histologically the characteristic lesion is the Aschoff body, which may be found in the involved tissue.

Predisposing factors Socioeconomic status of the family is the most important predisposing factor. Rheumatic fever is found most commonly in crowded environments, often in those characterized by poverty, poor hygiene, and malnutrition. There is a seasonal rise in incidence, but the season varies in different locations, for example, along the Eastern seaboard, spring; on the West Coast, winter. The incidence is high in a climate characterized by cold, dampness, and sudden variability of temperature, such as that of the Temperate Zone. In short, it usually follows the epidemiology of the streptococcal infection, and there is a 3 percent chance of developing rheumatic fever after the infection. In children, the onset usually occurs at from 4 to 12 years of age.

Clinical features   The picture varies greatly in intensity, from a mild, unsuspected case to one of high toxicity producing severe symptoms. The acute or active form subsides in its natural course to the inactive stage. The child may show no sign of rheumatic activity for months or even years, and then the symptoms of acute rheumatic fever may recur, usually following another clinical or subclinical attack of streptococcal infection. During the acute stage any of the following may occur:

1. Upper respiratory infection, e.g., sore throat and tonsillitis, precedes or accompanies the attack in about 50 percent of the acute cases.
2. Slight to high fever, pallor, malaise, and easy fatigability.
3. Carditis is manifested by tachycardia, or less commonly by sinus bradycardia, heart enlargement, cardiac murmurs, or change of the character of the already present murmur; heart sounds of poor quality; gallop rhythm; embryocardia (tic-tac rhythm); occasionally increased venous pressure, edema, dyspnea, and decreased vital capacity occur as signs of decompensation. Pericarditis may be present, and for variable periods a friction rub is audible.
4. Migratory polyarthritis may be mild or severe with varying degrees of redness and swelling. The large joints are primarily involved, e.g., ankle, knee, and wrist. Pain is more severe than the degree of visible joint involvement (redness and swelling) would indicate. Muscle and tendon pain are common in children and are located in the anterior thigh, calf, and posterior aspect of the knee.

    These muscle and tendon pains must be differentiated from so-called "growing pains," which are nonrheumatic, occur more often at night or at the end of the day, and do not occur in the morning. There is no pain on motion and the child is vague in pointing out the site of the pain. They may be due to poor sleeping posture, strenuous exercise, strain, etc. These growing pains are often relieved by such nonspecific therapy as hot or cold compresses and alcohol rubs. When there is doubt as to the origin of the pains, prolonged critical observation and careful evaluation including laboratory tests are necessary to rule out rheumatic fever.
5. Chorea occurs more often in girls than in boys and may be the only manifestation of rheumatic fever. It may occur during the acute stage as well as in the inactive stage. (Chorea is discussed in detail at the end of this section.)
6. Subcutaneous nodules vary in size from 3 to 10 mm and are located

along the prominences of the bones and tendon. They are often indicative of a severe attack, and when present they are strongly suggestive of acute rheumatic fever. Occasionally they are found in rheumatoid arthritis and disseminated lupus erythematosus.

7. Erythema marginatum (annulare), erythema nodosum, erythema multiforme, and purpuric manifestations are occasionally seen.
8. Abdominal pains, shifting or sometimes constant, are not uncommon. They may be difficult to distinguish from an acute surgical condition of the abdomen. The salicylate test may be helpful in the differential diagnosis; rheumatic abdominal pain responds promptly to adequate doses of salicylate intravenously or orally.
9. Epistaxis should be differentiated from nosebleeds due to "picking," e.g., during upper respiratory tract infection.

Laboratory findings

1. Acute-phase reaction tests: e.g., sedimentation rate. Levels of C-reactive protein, mucopolysaccharide, and mucoprotein are usually elevated during the acute phase. They may be normal in certain cases with chorea or erythema marginatum. The sedimentation rate may decrease to normal in the presence of congestive heart failure and become elevated when the congestive heart failure improves.
2. Electrocardiogram may show various changes, which may be only transient. Serial electrocardiograms may be helpful. The most common findings are sinus tachycardia, prolongation of the P-R interval, S-T and T-wave changes, prolongation of the corrected Q-T interval (Q-Tc). Atrial fibrillation, bradycardia, bundle branch block, and arrhythmias (paroxysmal tachycardia) are infrequent.
3. There may be leukocytosis, with a predominance of polymorphonuclear neutrophils, and anemia may also be present during the acute phase.
4. A rising streptococcal antibody titer is present in 70 percent of the cases, e.g., antistreptolysin O (over 500 Todd units) and antistreptokinase.
5. Roentgenogram and fluoroscopic examination may reveal cardiac enlargement, especially of the left atrium and ventricle.

Diagnosis   Rheumatic manifestations may be divided into major and minor.

Major   Carditis, polyarthritis, chorea, subcutaneous nodules, and erythema marginatum (annulare).

Minor   Fever, polyarthralgia, positive acute-phase reaction tests, prolonged P-R interval, preceding streptococcal infection, and history of previous rheumatic fever.

Diagnostic criteria of rheumatic fever are generally fulfilled if either one major and two or more minor or two or more major manifestations are present.

Differential diagnosis Diagnosis may be difficult because of the number of diseases simulating rheumatic fever. Some of these are rheumatoid arthritis and other collagen diseases, septic arthritis, osteomyelitis, poliomyelitis, sickle-cell anemia, leukemia, salmonella infection, febrile disease with an associated functional murmur, bacterial endocarditis, tuberculous allergic arthritis with fever and elevated sedimentation rate (Poncet's disease), lymphomas. The problem is more acute at present because corticosteroids frequently given to rheumatic fever patients would be generally contraindicated in bacterial and viral infections, for example, in osteomyelitis, poliomyelitis, subacute bacterial endocarditis.

Course and prognosis Rarely an acute attack may be rapidly fatal; more commonly there is a prolonged course with eventual subsidence. The amount of heart damage is the final determinant of prognosis. Death may result from carditis and heart failure. Rheumatic fever has been declining in its severity and recurrence rate, perhaps because of improved general hygiene, better nutrition, good public health measures to prevent the spreading of the streptococcal infection, and the advent of the antibiotics. If the patient has been put on continuous antibiotic prophylaxis and observes it strictly, the recurrence rate of rheumatic fever is minimal (less than 3 percent).

INACTIVE RHEUMATIC HEART DISEASE

Inactive rheumatic heart disease is characterized by a past history of rheumatic fever and signs of heart disease—a murmur and an enlarged heart if the residual valvular lesion constitutes a significant mechanical burden to the heart. The common lesions are mitral insufficiency, mitral stenosis, and aortic insufficiency. Tricuspid lesions and aortic stenosis occasionally occur; they may occur together with the others as combined valvular disease.

Mitral insufficiency There is a long (at least half of the systolic phase) blowing systolic murmur, best heard over the mitral area and transmitted to the axilla. An enlarged left ventricle is demonstrated by fluoroscopic examination and roentgenograms. The left auricle may also be enlarged in severe cases. The electrocardiogram shows left ventricular hypertrophy occasionally with "P mitrale" (see Mitral Stenosis, below). This murmur must be differentiated from the frequently heard functional murmurs which may be due to anemia (hemic murmur), a febrile disease, or an unknown cause. The functional murmur is unassociated with any organic cardiac defect. It is estimated that 60 percent of children have a functional murmur between the age of 2 years and adolescence, at which time these murmurs tend to disappear.

There are two types of functional murmur:

1. A soft, blowing murmur, present usually at the left base of the heart and the upper left sternal border, less frequently to the right of the apex. This murmur is more common in adolescents.
2. A low-pitched, musical murmur, heard best to the right of the apex and transmitted to the left sternal border. This murmur is more common in young children.

Functional murmurs are always short in duration and midsystolic in time, and never diastolic. Characteristically, the intensity of these murmurs increases after expiration (often a groaning or squeaking quality of the murmur is heard). The loudness of the murmur varies with positional changes of the body or after exercise. In some children these murmurs may only be heard during febrile illnesses. The roentgenogram and electrocardiogram are normal.

A venous hum is heard most frequently in the supraclavicular areas but may be at the base of the heart. It is continuous in timing and therefore simulates a patent ductus arteriosus or even a truncus arteriosus. The venous hum has a diastolic accentuation and is altered markedly by changing the position of the head either by rotation or by flexion. It is usually heard best in the upright position. The murmur associated with a patent ductus arteriosus is best heard in the supine position and though continuous has a systolic accentuation. The electrocardiogram and roentgenogram are normal.

Cardiorespiratory murmurs also require differentiation (decrease in intensity with deep inspiration) and disappear when the breath is held.

Mitral stenosis There is a low-pitched, rumbling, diastolic murmur, usually late, best heard at the apex, accentuated second pulmonary and apical first sounds, and occasionally palpable presystolic thrill over the apex. The left atrium is enlarged on fluoroscopy and roentgenograms. The electrocardiogram shows right axis deviation, vertical heart, right ventricular hypertrophy, and a widened, notched P wave in leads I and II (P mitrale) related to the severity of pulmonary hypertension.

Aortic insufficiency This problem usually occurs with an associated mitral insufficiency. There is a high-pitched decrescendo diastolic murmur, best heard in the 3d intercostal space to the left of the sternum, transmitted down the sternal border toward the apex. Radiologically, the left ventricle is enlarged. The electrocardiogram reveals left ventricular hypertrophy or mild strain with S-T and T changes in the severe lesions. When there are hemodynamic changes of significant aortic regurgitation, a wide pulse pressure and a low diastolic pressure are present.

DIFFERENTIAL DIAGNOSIS: RHEUMATIC VERSUS CONGENITAL HEART DISEASE

History

1. Age: Murmurs or other abnormal cardiac findings in the first year of life are suggestive of congenital heart disease. Rheumatic heart disease is rare before 3 years of age.
2. A history of any of the major manifestations of rheumatic fever discussed above is strong evidence for rheumatic heart disease. In congenital heart disease, there may be a maternal history of infections early in pregnancy, or other anomalies may be present, e.g., cataracts or mongolism.
3. Infrequently in children there may be the characteristic presystolic or mid-diastolic murmur (mitral stenosis) or the aortic diastolic murmur of insufficiency which is also characteristic of rheumatic heart disease. The criteria for diagnosis of these rheumatic murmurs have been discussed in the previous paragraphs.

Laboratory findings

Active rheumatic heart disease   Polymorphonucleosis, anemia, elevated sedimentation rate, elevated serum antistreptococcal titers are noted.

Inactive heart disease   Findings may be normal with the above-mentioned tests.

Congenital heart disease   Laboratory findings are normal, or in cyanotic-type congenital heart disease there may be polycythemia and reduced oxygen saturation.

Roentgenographic and electrocardiographic findings   Rheumatic heart disease in children causes either mitral insufficiency and/or aortic insufficiency, so that the left ventricle and left atrium are the chambers enlarged, if any. The pulmonary vascular markings are normal.

In congenital heart disease, enlargement of the left-sided chambers is usually associated with left-to-right shunts. Therefore, the pulmonary markings are increased. Since obstructive valvular lesions of the left side in children are rarely acquired, they should be considered congenital. Such lesions would produce left-sided enlargement with normal vascular markings.

Right-sided enlargement in children with or without a change from normal pulmonary vascular markings should be considered nonrheumatic and usually congenital.

The electrocardiogram in inactive rheumatic heart disease with residual valvular lesions is usually normal except when left ventricular or left atrial hypertrophy with severe aortic or mitral insufficiency is present.

An electrocardiogram demonstrating evidence of right or combined hypertrophy can be considered to be due to a congenital cardiac defect.

Treatment of the active or acute phase   Therapy is symptomatic and suppressive. The carditis may be influenced favorably if the suppressing therapy is instituted early, the dosage is adequate, and the duration is long enough.

1. General measures include bed rest, which is necessary during the acute phase (see Chapter 6, "Drugs and Treatment"), and proper nutrition, e.g., dietary and vitamin intake should be adequate during this long illness. Psychologic care is also important. Occupational therapy and schooling should be carried on in bed as soon as the child is ready.
2. Eradication of group A streptococci, which may persist after obvious infection has subsided and may be the source of hypersensitive reaction or recurrence. The use of penicillin which persists in the serum for 10 days can eradicate the streptococci, e.g., benzathine penicillin G (Bicillin), 600,000 to 1,200,000 units intramuscularly once, or procaine penicillin, 300,000 units daily intramuscularly for 10 days.
3. Suppressive therapy
    a. For rheumatic fever without carditis: salicylates, 100 to 120 mg per kg per day for 6 weeks. For maximal suppression of inflammation, a blood-salicylate level of 25 to 30 mg per 100 ml is necessary, although *arthritis* is usually relieved at lower levels.
    b. For carditis: Adrenal corticosteroid therapy is advised (most effective if started within 2 to 3 weeks of the onset of symptoms). The dosage of prednisone is 1 mg per lb per day. The adrenal corticosteroids are continued for 6 to 8 weeks; then, with disappearance of evidence of carditis, they are gradually discontinued over a 2-week period. If there is an exacerbation within 2 weeks after discontinuance of adrenal corticosteroids, therapeutic dosages of salicylate, as outlined above, are used. (It has been suggested that salicylates be given initially in conjunction with adrenal corticosteroids.) A low-sodium diet with added potassium and vitamin C is advised during the period of adrenal corticosteroid therapy.

    Withdrawal rebound: Reappearance of rheumatic activity, e.g., fever, tachycardia, elevated C-reactive protein, or sedimentation rate, may follow the sudden cessation or the end of the suppressive treatment. Most of these findings are mild and transitory and require no treatment, but if a symptom is severe and persistent, corticosteroid therapy may be reinstituted with a small dosage and for a short time. Withdrawal rebound usually occurs within 2 weeks after cessation of treatment.

   c. Chorea (discussed in detail at the end of this chapter).
4. Prophylactic treatment: Prevention of streptococcal infections is the most effective measure against the recurrence of rheumatic fever. Benzathine penicillin, 1.2 million units intramuscularly once monthly, or oral penicillin, 250,000 to 300,000 units twice daily, is effective. If there is an allergy to penicillin, erythromycin or sulfonamides may be used. Prophylaxis should begin following therapy for the eradication of the streptococcal infection and should be continued indefinitely.

Criteria for discontinuation of rest: Children should be kept at rest during the acute phase. If the acute-phase reaction tests, e.g., C-reactive protein, sedimentation rate, are negative for two consecutive weeks, if the child appears clinically well, and if the cardiac status is stable, gradual resumption of activity may be attempted, with the child under close observation. During this convalescent period, close watch should be kept for signs and symptoms of rebound phenomena due to withdrawal of suppressive therapy.

TREATMENT OF ACTIVE CARDITIS WITH CONGESTIVE HEART FAILURE

In addition to treatment of the active or acute phase to suppress the acute carditis, the following are used for congestive heart failure:

1. Oxygen
2. Digitalization
3. Diuretics
4. Sedation: morphine, phenobarbital
5. Low-salt diet (high-potassium diet if renal function is normal)

Digitalis   The total oral digitalizing dosage of digoxin is

Premature infants: 0.45 mg per kg
Birth to 2 years: 0.06 mg per kg
2 to 6 years: 0.04 to 0.05 mg per kg
More than 6 years: 0.03 to 0.04 mg per kg
(Intramuscularly: 80 percent of the above dosage)

It is given, orally or intramuscularly, over a 12- to 36-hour period. One-half of the total dosage is given at the start, and this is followed by two doses, each one-fourth of the total dosage. Following this, a daily maintenance dosage, usually of one-quarter the digitalization dosage, is given. A rapidly acting intravenous glycoside, lanatoside C

(Cedilanid), may be used; its total digitalizing dosage is 0.01 to 0.02 mg per lb of body weight, and two-thirds of this dosage is given at the start, followed by one-third after 1 hour. Six hours later, oral digoxin is started—one-fourth of the digitalizing dosage, every 6 hours for four doses followed by the usual maintenance dosage.

In premature infants the dosage of digoxin may be lower—0.045 mg per kg usually does not cause toxicity, but a dose as low as 0.03 mg per kg may be sufficient. The use of electrocardiographic follow-up is essential to prevent digitalis intoxication in premature infants.

This regimen is a general guide to digitalization. Each patient must be observed closely and the dosage adjusted according to individual needs. The pulse and the clinical response are guides to proper dosage; a normal pulse rate for the age is indicative of a digitalization response. Reduction of edema, of the size of the liver, and of body weight as well as clinical improvement, signify a good response. Vomiting and nausea are the common and first clinical manifestations of digitalis toxicity. Congestive heart failure itself, however, sometimes produces vomiting and nausea. Neurologic complaints, e.g., yellow vision, headache, are rare signs of toxicity in the pediatric age group. If there is evidence of digitalis toxicity, the dosage of digitalis should be reduced by skipping one or two doses and decreasing the total daily dosage. When there is a change in the character of the pulse, e.g., irregular pulse, bigeminal pulse, electrocardiographic study is indicated to help differentiate digitalis effect from digitalis toxicity. The change of ST-T configuration, P-R interval prolongation, and ventricular slowing are the signs of digitalis effect. Digitalis should be continued in these cases. Atrial fibrillation, atrial tachycardia with irregular ventricular response, nodal tachycardia with atrioventricular dissociation, partial and complete atrioventricular block are signs due to excessive amount of digitalis; the dosage of digitalis should be reduced. Ventricular premature systoles, ventricular paroxysmal tachycardia, and ventricular fibrillation are the electrocardiographic signs of severe digitalis toxicity. Digitalis treatment should be discontinued when these occur.

Diuretics, e.g., Mercuhydrin, 0.1 to 1.0 ml, intramuscularly; ethacrynic acid, 1 mg per kg, intravenously or orally in a dose of 25 to 50 mg daily; or furosamide, 1 mg per kg, intravenously may be given.

CLASSIFICATION OF HEART DISEASE

The following functional and therapeutic classification of heart disease (by the New York Heart Association) is helpful when prescribing activity for the patient.

Functional classification (according to degree of cardiac disability):
Class I. Ordinary physical activity does not cause discomfort or other cardiac complaint.
Class II. Ordinary physical activity causes slight discomfort or other cardiac complaint.

Class III. Ordinary physical activity causes marked discomfort or other cardiac complaint.

Class IV. Discomfort or other cardiac complaint even when at rest.

Therapeutic classification (according to recommendation for physical activity):

Class A. Physical activity need not be restricted.

Class B. Ordinary physical activity need not be restricted, but child should be advised against unusually strenuous or competitive efforts.

Class C. Ordinary physical activity should be moderately restricted and more strenuous efforts should be discontinued.

Class D. Ordinary physical activity should be markedly restricted.

Class E. Should be at complete bed rest, confined to bed or chair.

No heart disease: Predisposing etiologic factors (no limitation of activity).

No heart disease: Undiagnosed manifestations (no limitation of activity).

CHOREA

Chorea is a disorder of the central nervous system, probably resulting from rheumatic fever and characterized by emotional instability, incoordinated movements, and muscular weakness. It occurs more often in females (2:1) and usually from 5 to 15 years of age. A large number of children with rheumatic fever present this manifestation at some time, while 75 percent of children with chorea have other rheumatic fever manifestations.

Clinical features

1. Emotional instability: change in disposition, child becoming irritable, moody, restless, unhappy, and easily provoked to tears or laughter. Occasionally a child may become almost maniacal (chorea insaniens).
2. Purposeless, incoordinated movements, e.g., writing becomes illegible, dressing and other simple tasks are carried out in a clumsy fashion. There may be facial grimaces and sudden contraction of the tongue, drawing it to the floor of the mouth and causing "choreic cluck." Speech may be indistinct; in counting, the enunciation is clear at first and then becomes thick, indistinct, and hesitant; finally, there is a complete block. The movements of the upper extremities are usually more marked on one side. When the patient is asked to shake hands, there is momentary hesitation, and then the movement is executed quickly for fear that the goal may not be reached. The gait is unsteady. The breathing may be irregular when the respiratory muscles are involved.
3. Muscular weakness is demonstrated by a feeble hand clasp.
4. "Hung-up" reflex: in the knee jerk, the knee rises promptly but returns to the original position more slowly and hesitantly than is normal. Czerny's sign: when the patient takes a deep breath, the diaphragm does not descend on inspiration, but instead is drawn up and results in an indrawing of the abdomen.

5. Laboratory data: the acute-phase reaction test, e.g., C-reactive protein, sedimentation rate, mucoprotein can be elevated or normal (isolated chorea).

Differential diagnosis Tic, postencephalitis neurologic complication, hyperthyroidism, athetoid movements, emotionally disturbed children with hypermotility are all possible diagnoses.

Prognosis In uncomplicated cases the prognosis is good although the course is variable. There is usually subsidence in 1 to 3 months; rarely it may last for many months. Recurrence is frequent, particularly during emotional strain. In about half the patients there are associated heart lesions.

Treatment Physical and mental rest are desirable. Occupational therapy, depending on the severity of the case, is helpful to achieve rest. Sedative and psychotherapeutic drugs, e.g., phenobarbital, Thorazine, antihistamines (see Chapter 6, "Drugs and Treatment"), are often of aid in securing rest and quiet. Adrenal corticosteroids may be effective in some severe cases. If there are complicating psychogenic factors, psychotherapy is indicated in the treatment and in the prevention of recurrences.

RHEUMATIC PNEUMONIA

Rheumatic pneumonia is characterized by pulmonary infiltration and is not related to congestive heart failure. It is rare and when present is associated with a severe carditis. The exact pathogenesis is unknown. This consolidation is probably due to rheumatic infiltration in the lung through increased vascular transudate. The pathologic findings are similar to those found in other rheumatic lesions. The treatment is directed to the acute rheumatic fever.

NONRHEUMATIC HEART DISEASE

BACTERIAL ENDOCARDITIS

SUBACUTE BACTERIAL ENDOCARDITIS

Subacute bacterial endocarditis is an infectious disease caused in the majority of cases by *Streptococcus viridans* or resistant staphylococcus and involves abnormal heart tissue, e.g., old rheumatic lesions or congenital anomalies of the cardiovascular system. An ulcerative-vegetative process spreading over the endocardium, beyond the initial seat of infection, is the characteristic finding. Vegetations are friable and break off, causing emboli, which are a prominent feature of the disease.

Clinical features

1. Often a history of a preceding infection, frequently of the upper respiratory tract, or of preceding oral surgery.
2. Onset is insidious, with fever, irritability, and weakness.
3. Spleen is usually enlarged and tender.
4. There may be petechiae, embolic phenomena, or pathognomonic erythematous painful nodules in the finger tips (Osler's nodes), palms, and toes.
5. Murmurs are heard that change in character; heart action is forceful and rapid, and a gallop rhythm may be present.
6. Hemiplegia may occur.

Laboratory findings

1. Leukocytosis, anemia, albuminuria, and, occasionally, hematuria.
2. Positive blood cultures (many cultures, including bone-marrow cultures, may have to be done before a positive one is obtained; negative cultures should not cause treatment to be delayed if bacterial endocarditis is suspected).
3. Electrocardiogram may show prolongation of the P-R interval or changes of the T wave.
4. Roentgenogram may show cardiac enlargement.

Treatment

1. Antibiotics in large dosages for prolonged periods. Choice of drug will depend upon the organism.
2. If congenital anomalies, e.g., patent ductus arteriosus or arteriovenous fistula, are present, corrective surgery should be performed when the infection has been controlled.
3. Patients must be observed for at least 4 months after completion of therapy. Blood culture should be done at each follow-up examination.

Prophylaxis

1. Operable cardiovascular abnormalities should be corrected as early as feasible.
2. Penicillin should be given to children with cardiovascular disease undergoing dental or surgical procedures and during an acute respiratory disease.

Prognosis The prognosis has improved with antibiotic therapy but is still grave. It depends upon the duration of the disease before diagnosis.

ACUTE BACTERIAL ENDOCARDITIS

This is a rare disease and is usually secondary to a septic focus elsewhere in the body caused by any organism. Heart action is tumultuous, and murmurs change rapidly because of rapid valvular destruction. The course is usually rapidly fatal.

Treatment   Indicated antibiotics in large dosages is the usual treatment.

MYOCARDITIS

Primary myocarditis in infancy and childhood is usually of viral etiology (Coxsackie, ECHO). Myocarditis may also occur secondary to other infections, e.g., measles, poliomyelitis, diphtheria, typhoid fever.

Tachycardia, poor heart sounds, and cardiomegaly occur. The electrocardiogram usually shows the rapid rate and very mild T-wave changes, if any. Low-voltage waves in the heart leads are described but may be difficult to evaluate in infancy. In infancy, especially during the neonatal period, there may be marked electrocardiographic changes suggestive of severe coronary and myocardial insufficiency (Q and ST-T changes). The severity of illness is usually not reflected by changes in the electrocardiogram. Treatment is supportive and the prognosis is guarded.

PERICARDITIS

Pericarditis is an inflammation of the parietal and visceral surfaces of the pericardium. There may be a serofibrinous, hemorrhagic, or purulent exudate, which may be absorbed completely or may lead to variable pericardial thickening or to obliteration of the sac with or without chronic constriction of the heart. Pericarditis may occur in rheumatic fever, rheumatoid arthritis, in bacterial infections from extracardiac foci, or by direct extension from neighboring infections, e.g., pneumonia, mediastinal tuberculosis. A viral form (Coxsackie B), usually benign, has also been recognized. The causation is usually determined by identification of the underlying disease, for example, rheumatic carditis.

Clinically there may be dull, aching, or stabbing chest pain localized to the left side of the chest, the shoulder, or the neck and exaggerated on lying down in bed. On examination a friction rub can be heard; this is the earliest sign of pericarditis but is often missed because it is transient. Later, when fluid is present and the rub has disappeared, symptoms and signs may arise from compression of the heart and the surrounding structures. If intrapericardial pressure is great enough to interfere with diastolic filling and venous return, both systolic and pulse pressures decrease, the neck veins distend, the liver enlarges, and respiratory distress becomes manifest. Roentgenograms and fluoroscopic examination reveal diminished cardiac pulsations in a rapidly enlarging cardiac shadow which changes in contour with change of body position. The electrocardiogram is of value only when changes are present—elevation of the S-T segment, followed later by T-wave inversion and low voltage of the ventricular deflections. Treatment consists of caring for the primary disease and the cardiac failure. Anti-inflammatory agents, e.g., aspirin and steroids, are useful.

In cases of rapid or massive effusions with progressive symptoms and signs of heart tamponade, it is necessary to perform pericardial paracentesis. Prognosis is guarded because the disease may vary unpredictably. It may be present as a fleeting complication without cardiac consequence, it may progress to the chronic constrictive form, or it may be rapidly fatal.

HYPERTENSION

The normal blood pressure in the various age groups has been described in Chapter 1, "Growth and Development." Hypertension may be brought about in children by the following:

1. Renal disease: glomerulonephritis, nephritis secondary to anaphylactoid purpura, polycystic kidney disease, anomalies (ectopic), chronic pyelonephritis, hydronephrosis, Wilms's tumor, neuroblastoma, polyarteritis, hypoplastic kidney, unilateral vascular conditions causing ischemia.
2. Endocrine and metabolic disease: pheochromocytoma, adrenocortical hyperplasia or tumor, hyperthyroidism, idiopathic hypercalcemia, during adrenal corticosteroid therapy, porphyria.
3. Central nervous system lesions with increased intracranial pressure: brain tumor, Riley-Day syndrome, encephalitis.
4. Congenital vascular anomalies: coarctation of the aorta, renal vascular anomalies (see above).
5. Acquired cardiovascular disease: rheumatic aortic insufficiency, collagen diseases.
6. Reflex hypertension: for example, from fright, excitement, or after exercise. (This rise is not sustained, and the blood pressure shortly returns to normal.)
7. Drugs, e.g., epinephrine, and poisons, e.g., mercury (acrodynia), lead, thallium, vitamin D, carbon monoxide.
8. Familial hypercholesterolemic xanthomatosis.

9. Essential hypertension. (Diagnosis is made only after all other possible conditions have been ruled out.) Uncommon in children.
10. Malignant hypertension (arteriolar sclerosis) is extremely rare in infancy and childhood.

If hypertension persists for long periods of time without treatment, hypertensive heart disease develops, with left ventricular hypertrophy, cardiac failure, and occasionally cerebral hemorrhage.

Treatment

1. Discovery and treatment of the underlying cause
2. Antihypertensive drugs: reserpine, hydralazine, hexamethonium, chlorthiazide, etc.

PULMONARY HEART DISEASE (Cor Pulmonale)

Pulmonary heart disease occurs secondary to pathologic changes in the pulmonary parenchyma or in the pulmonary vessels, resulting in right ventricular enlargement and failure. It is relatively uncommon in children. Acute cor pulmonale may be caused by thromboembolic phenomena, e.g., subacute bacterial endocarditis. The subacute type may be secondary to hyaline membrane disease and atelectasis of the newborn. The chronic type is seen in chronic pulmonary disease, e.g., chronic bronchitis, bronchiectasis, tuberculosis, chronic asthma, etc.; fibrocystic disease of the pancreas; and primary pulmonary hypertension.

CARDIAC TUMORS

Cardiac tumors are rare in children. Primary tumors include myxoma, rhabdomyoma, fibroma, and sarcoma. Metastatic tumors include bronchiogenic carcinoma, sarcoma, etc.

In metastatic tumors the clinical picture is dominated by the primary lesion. In primary tumors, the symptoms depend upon the location of the tumor. When the valves are involved, murmurs are prominent. If the tumor invades intramurally, arrhythmias and conductive disturbances may occur. Progressive cardiac enlargement and cardiac failure become evident later. Diagnosis is made by exclusion and by electrocardiographic and angiographic studies.

Treatment In primary tumor, exploratory thoracotomy may be indicated.

HEART DISEASE ASSOCIATED WITH
MISCELLANEOUS DISEASES

In this group are included diseases that may have cardiac manifestations in their clinical picture. The clinical manifestations are those of heart failure in addition to the symptoms of the primary disease.

HEART DISEASE IN ANEMIA

When the hemoglobin drops below 7 Gm, cardiac output increases. When the hemoglobin falls to 3.5 Gm or below, cardiac dilatation or hypertrophy occurs, and there is beginning congestive failure.

HEART DISEASE IN DISEASE OF THE THYROID

Hyperthyroidism Tachycardia, high systolic and pulse pressure, cardiac enlargement, atrial fibrillation, and congestive heart failure may be prominent clinical findings.

Hypothyroidism Bradycardia, low blood pressure, weak pulse, pericardial effusion, and cardiac enlargement are the usual clinical manifestations. Electrocardiogram shows low voltage.

HEART DISEASE IN DIPHTHERIA (See p. 297)

HEART DISEASE IN PROGRESSIVE MUSCULAR DYSTROPHY (See p. 531)

The characteristic findings are myocardial cellular atrophy with fibrous and fatty infiltration.

HEART DIEASE IN GARGOYLISM (See p. 540)

The characteristic findings are endocardial thickening, valvular lesions, coronary insufficiency, cardiac hypertrophy, and congestive failure. The particular structures are involved due to deposits of mucopolysaccharides.

GLYCOGEN–STORAGE DISEASE OF THE HEART

This disease (see p. 167) may cause cardiac failure in the 3- to 6-month age group.

The electrocardiogram is helpful in confirming the diagnosis because of the marked S-T depression and inversion of T waves in the precordial leads. In no other lesion is there such a degree of inversion (3 to 10 mm). The prognosis is poor.

HEART DISEASE IN FRIEDREICH'S ATAXIA (See p. 517)

The clinical picture may show coronary disease and myocardial fibrosis and abnormal electrocardiographic findings.

HEART DISEASE IN MARFAN'S SYNDROME (See p. 539)

The characteristic findings are aortic dilatation with regurgitation and aneurysm of the ascending portion. This is probably due to a defect of the elastic fibers resulting in a weakness of the media.

ARRHYTHMIAS

Arrhythmia is any disturbance of the regular automaticity of the cardiac impulses or of the pattern of cardiac conduction. An electrocardiogram is important in defining the diagnosis.

ATRIOVENTRICULAR BLOCK

This condition may be congenital or acquired. There are three degrees of severity:

1. P-R interval longer than normal for the age of the child (frequently seen in rheumatic carditis).
2. Atrial impulse occasionally not transmitted to the ventricle (rare in children).
3. Complete atrioventricular block—auricle and ventricle beat independently.

The first- and second-degree atrioventricular blocks do not produce symptoms per se. Complete heart block is usually congenital and may produce fatigue, fainting spells, and decompensation. These symptoms usually occur when there are associated cardiac defects, which is not the usual situation. Acquired heart block may occur as a sequela of contagious diseases, e.g., varicella, rubella.

PAROXYSMAL TACHYCARDIA

Paroxysmal tachycardia may occur in utero, during the neonatal period, or any time thereafter. It may be congenital or acquired, for example, in rheumatic fever, digitalis toxicity, congestive heart failure, or during cardiac catheterization. Paroxysmal tachycardia is most common during early infancy, with recurrences during the first year and rarely thereafter. Infrequently Wolff-Parkinson-White (WPW) syndrome is the cause. It is usually supraventricular in origin, and the heart rate exceeds 220 per minute. The attacks may be accompanied by dyspnea, pallor, syncope, and palpitation, and may last from a few minutes to several days. Those of longer duration may result in cardiac dilatation and failure (this happens more rapidly in children under 2 years of age) and may lead to death if not recognized and treated early.

Wolff-Parkinson-White syndrome is characterized by recurrent paroxysmal tachycardia with typical electrocardiogram—short P-R interval, widening of the QRS complex, and marked notching of the ascending limb of the R wave (delta wave). There is a rare form of tachycardia which consists of continuously recurring short runs of premature beats (*tachycardie en salves*); it is diagnosed only by electrocardiogram and is usually asymptomatic.

Treatment   Simple procedures, e.g., pressure on the eyeballs or carotid sinus, which stimulate the vagus, may halt an attack promptly (however, this is usually unsuccessful in infancy and during early childhood). Such measures are more effective in the supraventricular type. Digitalis is usually effective. Quinidine sulfate, 6 mg per kg every 3 hours, has also been recommended. Prostigmine (1:4,000, intramuscularly) is useful when digitalis alone does not decrease the tachycardia. Lidocaine, 1 mg per kg, can be tried if other therapy fails.

In children under 2 years of age digitalis should be continued for 6 months to a year because of the high rate of recurrences.

ATRIAL FIBRILLATION

Atrial fibrillation may occur in rheumatic heart disease, congestive heart failure, digitalis toxicity, or other heart disease. It indicates marked cardiac damage. There are complete irregularity in rhythm and intensity of heart beats and pulse, pulse deficit, and fractional blood pressure; the electrocardiogram reveals absence of P waves and irregularity of rhythm. Digitalization is the treatment of choice. Quinidine, procaine amide (Pronestyl), or a combination of these may occasionally be indicated.

CONGESTIVE HEART FAILURE

Congestive heart failure develops when the cardiac output and cardiac reserve are unable to deliver the nutritional components, including oxygen, for cellular or systemic metabolism. The inability to empty the heart completely results in a high venous filling pressure and decreased effective cardiac muscle work. Increased load leads to cardiac hypertrophy.

Although it is often classified into two types, left-sided and right-sided, congestive heart failure is usually a combination of both. The left-sided failure is manifested clinically by dyspnea, orthopnea, cardiac asthma, pulmonary rales, gallop rhythm, and pulsus alternans. The right-sided failure is manifested by increased venous pressure (distended neck veins), enlargement of the liver, and edema of the lower extremities.

Laboratory findings include increased venous pressure and prolongation of circulation time. Roentgenograms of the chest reveal cardiac enlargement, congested lung fields, and pulmonary edema. The electrocardiogram may show prominent P waves, arrhythmia, or ventricular hypertrophy.

Treatment for right-sided and mixed heart failure is as described earlier in this chapter under Rheumatic Heart Disease; for severe left-sided failure, rapidly acting diuretics, sedation, e.g., morphine, and oxygen are indicated.

REVIEW QUESTIONS

1. The incidence of congenital heart disease per 1,000 live-born infants is (a) 2; (b) 6; (c) 20; (d) 30.
2. Of the following noncyanotic congenital cardiac malformations select the one that occurs most frequently: (a) patent ductus arteriosus; (b) atrial septal defect; (c) ventricular septal defect; (d) coarctation of the aorta.
3. All the following types of congenital heart disease represent a left-to-right shunt except for one: (a) ventricular septal defect; (b) tetralogy of Fallot; (c) patent ductus arteriosus; (d) anomalous pulmonary venous return.
4. The normal oxygen saturation of blood of right-sided chambers of the heart is about (a) 35 percent; (b) 50 percent; (c) 70 percent; (d) 95 percent.
5. The normal oxygen saturation of blood of left-sided chambers of the heart is about (a) 35 percent; (b) 50 percent; (c) 70 percent; (d) 95 percent.
6. Ventricular septal defect is associated with the following except (a) a palpable thrill and systolic murmur along the lower left sternal border; (b) ECG may show left, right, or combined hypertrophy; (c) pulmonary artery is prominent on x-rays; (d) it is one of the common defects causing cyanosis in infancy; (e) the level of pulmonary artery pressure is a primary factor in determining the age for surgical repair.
7. An asymptomatic patent ductus arteriosus should be closed soon after (a) birth; (b) 1 year; (c) 2 years; (d) not at all.
8. Right-sided cardiac enlargement with marked increase of pulmonary vascular markings, ECG reveals right-axis deviation and earlier visualization of the aorta than normal on angiocardiography are suggestive of (a) anomalous pulmonary venous return; (b) patent ductus arteriosus; (c) tetralogy of Fallot.
9. The following statements concerning tetralogy of Fallot are true except for one: (a) cyanosis is severe and usually noted at birth; (b) x-ray reveals a normal-sized boot-shaped heart; (c) ECG shows right-axis deviation and pure right ventricular hypertrophy; (d) a frequent complication is brain abscess.
10. The following statements concerning transposition of the great vessels are true except for one: (a) murmurs may or may not be present; (b) no treatment is available; (c) on cardiac catheterization the catheter passes directly into the aorta from the right ventricle; (d) after 3 years of age an open-heart procedure is performed.
11. The following are consistent with Eisenmenger's complex except (a) right ventricular hypertrophy; (b) pulmonary artery pressure and right ventricular pressure are equal on cardiac catheterization; (c) cyanosis present at birth; (d) systolic murmur heard best at the lower half of the sternum.
12. An elflike facies, mental retardation, and hypercalcemia in infancy are likely to be associated with (a) tetralogy of Fallot; (b) Eisenmenger's complex; (c) supravalvular aortic stenosis.
13. The infant with preductal (infantile) coarctation of the aorta usually develops cardiac failure at (a) birth to 2 weeks of age; (b) 2 to 6 weeks; (c) 7 to 10 weeks; (d) after 3 months of age.

14. An infant with a coarse expiratory stridor and a high-pitched brassy cough which becomes worse on ventral flexion of the head may be suspected to have (a) subendocardial fibroelastosis; (b) coarctation of the aorta; (c) vascular ring; (d) anomalous origin of the left coronary artery.

15. The following statements concerning rheumatic fever are true except for one: (a) socioeconomic status is an important predisposing factor; (b) there is a 3 percent chance of developing rheumatic fever after any streptococcal infection; (c) abdominal pains are not uncommon; (d) prolonged P-R interval on ECG is included as one of the major manifestations of rheumatic fever.

16. It is estimated that at some time (a) 20 percent; (b) 40 percent; (c) 60 percent; (d) 75 percent of children between the age of 2 years and adolescence have a functional murmur.

17. The following statements concerning functional murmurs are true except for one: (a) they are always short in duration; (b) they are diastolic; (c) the intensity of the murmur increases after expiration; (d) the loudness of the murmur varies with positional changes or after exercise.

18. Enlargement of the chambers of the heart in rheumatic fever as opposed to congenital heart disease can be categorized as follows: (a) enlargement of the right side of the heart is more likely to be associated with rheumatic fever than congenital heart disease; (b) enlargement of the right side of the heart is more likely to be associated with congenital heart disease than rheumatic fever; (c) there is no specific frequency with which enlargement of either side of the heart occurs in these two conditions.

19. Maximal suppression of inflammation in rheumatic fever by salicylates is usually achieved at a blood level of (a) 10 to 25 mg per 100 ml; (b) 25 to 30 mg per 100 ml; (c) 50 to 60 mg per 100 ml; (d) 100 mg per 100 ml.

20. Chorea occurs more frequently in (a) males; (b) females; (c) there is no difference in frequency of occurrence in the two sexes.

21. The following statements concerning subacute bacterial endocarditis are true except for one: (a) *Streptococcus viridans* is involved in the majority of cases; (b) gallop rhythm may be present; (c) ECG may show prolongation of the P-R interval; (d) leukopenia is a common laboratory finding.

22. When the hemoglobin drops, congestive heart failure ensues. A critical level is about (a) 3.5 Gm per 100 ml; (b) 7 Gm per 100 ml; (c) 9.5 Gm per 100 ml.

17 GASTRO-INTESTINAL DISEASES

COLIC OF EARLY INFANCY

Colic is characterized by recurrent paroxysmal attacks of severe abdominal pain and crying, occurring during the first 3 or 6 months of life. It has a striking periodicity, usually occurring in the late afternoon or evening, starts suddenly, and ends just as suddenly. During an attack the face is congested, the abdominal wall is tense, and the legs and thighs are held in a flexed position. Colic is found mainly in the so-called "hypertonic" type of infant, i.e., one who responds excessively to the environment, is tense, and is easily alarmed by noises or movements.

EDITORS' NOTE: The section on Intestinal Parasites was prepared by Eileen Halsey Pike, Ph. D.

Etiology   The cause of colic is unknown. There is probably no single cause; rather, colic may be due to any or several of the following:

1. Parental or environmental tension
2. Excessive peristaltic contractions from hunger or distension from air swallowing
3. Indigestion from overfeeding quantitatively or qualitatively, e.g., feeding of excess carbohydrate
4. Gastrointestinal allergy
5. Imbalance of the autonomic nervous system
6. Inguinal hernia

Treatment

1. Palliative: the body position may be changed to favor elimination of gas—holding the infant up over the shoulder as for "bubbling" or placing him face down over mother's lap. Applying heat to the abdomen with a hot-water bottle may be helpful. Antispasmodics and sedatives, particularly phenobarbital, are used frequently but usually with little success. Occasionally an antihistamine, e.g., Benadryl, or rarely a psychotherapeutic agent—tranquilizers (see Chapter 6, "Drugs and Treatment")—may be effective when sedatives fail. Carminatives, e.g., catnip and fennel, are of questionable value.
2. Corrective: if there is an underlying demonstrable cause, it should be removed; e.g., the diet should be made adequate and a qualitatively proper formula provided. When allergy to cow's milk exists, utilizing substitutes such as soybean or meat base may provide relief.
3. A quiet, restful environment for the infant and reassurance for the family to give them confidence are important.
4. Inguinal hernia should be repaired as soon as it is discovered.

Prognosis   The prognosis is excellent, since colic usually subsides by 3 to 6 months of age.

VOMITING IN INFANCY

Etiology

1. Febrile diseases: vomiting is usually marked only at the onset but occasionally may persist as long as the fever is high. (In pyelonephritis gastrointestinal symptoms, i.e., vomiting, abdominal pain, or diarrhea, are second in frequency to fever.)
2. Gastroenteritis or ingestion of poisons or of foreign bodies.
3. Overdistension of the stomach from air swallowing or excessive food.

4. Indigestion: for example, as a result of an improperly constructed formula.
5. Environmental causes: excessive handling after feedings.
6. Gastrointestinal allergy.
7. Intestinal obstruction: early in life, such congenital anomalies of the gastrointestinal tract as esophageal atresia, pyloric stenosis, duodenal atresia, or congenital bands; later in life, mechanical causes producing extrinsic pressure, e.g., neoplasm, bands, or adhesions, or obstruction from within, such as intussusception, foreign bodies, tumor, or parasites.
8. Diseases of the liver, e.g., infectious hepatitis, or of the pancreas.
9. Increased intracranial pressure: subdural hematoma, brain tumor.
10. Psychogenic or emotional factors: these rarely may be associated with a characteristic form of regurgitation called "rumination," in which the food is rechewed and reswallowed.
11. Riley-Day syndrome (familial dysautonomia).

Diagnosis   Diagnosis depends on a careful history, complete physical examination, and indicated laboratory tests, e.g., roentgenograms.

Treatment   Removal of the cause and correction of the dehydration and acidosis or alkalosis that may be present is the indicated treatment.

CYCLIC VOMITING
(Recurrent Vomiting or Acetonemic Vomiting)

This condition is characterized by recurrent episodes of vomiting and ketosis and usually occurs in a child from 3 to 7 years of age. The cause is unknown, but allergy, psychogenic factors, abdominal epilepsy, and infection may initiate an episode. The acute phase is treated by sedation and restoration of fluid and electrolyte balance. Psychotherapeutic agents (tranquilizers), see Chapter 6, "Drugs and Treatment," are often helpful. The prognosis is good, and attacks usually become less frequent and of shorter duration as the child grows older, usually subsiding by puberty.

CONSTIPATION

Constipation is characterized by infrequent defecation, hard, dry stools, and difficulty in evacuation as compared with the individual child's usual stool habits. Paradoxic diarrhea can occur with oozing of stool and soiling.

Etiology

1. Diet: e.g., high-protein content, deficiency of carbohydrates, insufficient fluid, and low residue, as well as insufficient total intake.

2. Psychogenic causes or poor training: undue stress placed upon toileting may frighten the child, and several months may be required to allay his fears and to reeducate the parents.
3. Anal fissure very frequently results in constipation because of the pain and spasm associated with defecation. Constipation in turn may cause anal fissuring, and this cycle frequently results in the formation of skin tags.
4. Prolonged use of enemas, suppositories, and cathartics is a frequent cause of constipation.
5. Decreased muscle tone in abdomen or intestines: may be due to lack of exercise, malnutrition, chronic illness, rickets, or hypothyroidism.
6. Allergy: especially to milk. Constipation frequently dates back to introduction of whole milk.
7. Anatomic abnormalities such as anal stenosis or congenital megacolon (Hirschsprung's disease).

Treatment

1. Any of the causes mentioned above that contribute to the constipation should be removed or corrected.
2. A proper diet should be constructed with sufficient residue and enough fluids. Prune juice (1 to 3 oz), coarse cereals, vegetables, and raw fruits may be helpful.
3. Mineral oil, 1 to 3 tbsp, or milk of magnesia, 1 to 3 tsp, may be given temporarily for rapid results, then gradually discontinued as improvement takes place. It is unwise to use cathartics, enemas, or suppositories for any prolonged period.
4. Surface-active agent, dioctyl sodium sulfosuccinate, e.g., Colace, orally, under 3 years of age—10 to 40 mg daily; 3 to 6 years of age—20 to 60 mg; 6 to 12 years of age—40 to 120 mg; older children—50 to 200 mg. The higher doses are used for initial treatment and then may be reduced.

CONGENITAL MEGACOLON (Aganglionic)

Congenital megacolon (Hirschsprung's disease) is to be distinguished from dilatation of the colon due to other causes, e.g., psychogenic constipation, anorectal stenosis, tumors, thiamine deficiency. In this condition, distal to the dilatation there is a congenital defect of the parasympathetic ganglion cells in Auerbach's plexus in the constricted rectum and rectosigmoid, and sometimes even more proximally, resulting in an absence of peristalsis and propulsive movement. There is a familial incidence with about 90 percent of cases occurring in males and involving the rectum and rectosigmoid. A longer segment or possibly the entire intestine may be affected, and these infants may have signs and symptoms of intestinal obstruction at birth. In mild cases there is usually only a short aganglionic segment.

Clinical features

1. There is a history of constipation frequently beginning at birth or shortly thereafter, becoming progressively worse with enlargement of the abdomen. Abdominal pain is usually not present.
2. In the newborn infant there may be no meconium passed or it may be passed sparingly. A meconium plug may occur, and perforation of the cecum, appendix, or colon have been reported. Less frequently a profuse watery diarrhea is found, or the condition may simulate ileal obstruction (vomiting, distension, hyperactive peristalsis, and scanty stools).
3. Infants are prone to develop severe enterocolitis.
4. Stools are pelletlike or ribbonlike.
5. Examination reveals an empty rectum. (In psychogenic megacolon the rectum is packed with feces.)
6. Rectal biopsy reveals absence of ganglion cells.
7. Fluoroscopy and roentgenograms following insertion of a small amount of a thin mixture of barium just beyond the rectal sphincter reveal dilatation of that portion of the colon proximal to the narrowed rectosigmoid and absence of haustral markings.
8. In long-standing cases there are retardation of growth, malnutrition, and anemia.

Treatment

1. Surgery: the Swenson operation (resection of the contracted portion of the rectosigmoid and rectum distal to the dilatation with a pull-through anastomosis) has been successful.
2. Enemas: the use of solutions other than normal saline should be avoided. Water and magnesium intoxication resulting in death have been reported.
3. Pyschotherapy is important, as in any chronic disease.

DIARRHEA

Diarrhea is characterized by an increase in the frequency and fluidity of stools. It may be a serious condition in young infants.

Etiology

1. Enteral infections: virus; bacteria, e.g., salmonella, Shiga bacillus, staphylococcus; protozoa; and amebic dysentery.
2. Parenteral infections: otitis media, pneumonia, pyelitis.
3. Dietary: overfeeding, quantitatively or qualitatively, for example, too much carbohydrate or fat.
4. Oral antibiotics may induce diarrhea by direct action on the gastrointestinal tract or by inhibiting the normal bacterial flora and permitting overgrowth of pathogens.

5. Enzyme deficiencies, either primary (see Chapter 8), or secondary to diarrhea from any other cause.
6. Enteritis or colitis.
7. Gastrointestinal allergy.
8. Endocrine: hypoadrenalism and hyperthyroidism.
9. Psychogenic: emotional upset or excitement.
10. Vitamin deficiency: pellagra.
11. Chemical poisoning: arsenic, sodium fluoride, cadmium, zinc.
12. Food poisoning: some types of mushroom, new sprouted potatoes.

Classification according to severity

1. Mild diarrhea: an increase in stools to about five to eight daily, with no dehydration and no acidosis. There may be vomiting and slight fever but no toxicity.
2. Moderate diarrhea: frequent fluid stools with mild to moderate dehydration but no clinical acidosis. There may be moderate fever and slight toxicity.
3. Severe diarrhea: usually 15 or more fluid stools daily. There are marked dehydration (see p. 131), acidosis (see pp. 129–137), and prostration, and often the infant is semicomatose.

Usually the number of stools reflects the severity of the dehydration; however, severe inflammatory reaction may result in marked edema of the intestines with severe dehydration following the passage of only a few stools.

General rules for therapy in diarrhea

1. The etiologic factors are eradicated if possible.
2. The gastrointestinal tract is rested.
3. Dehydration, electrolyte imbalance, and shock are combated.
4. Adjuvant therapy may be helpful (see below).

Treatment of mild diarrhea

1. Ordinarily no food is offered for several hours; clear fluids, e.g., weak sweetened tea, ginger ale, or water with added electrolytes and carbohydrate (1 qt water + ½ tsp salt + ½ tsp sodium bicarbonate + 10 tsp sugar) is given by mouth during this time.
2. Then a weakened formula may be started.
3. When the stools have improved, there can be a gradual return to full-strength formula and regular diet.

Treatment of moderate diarrhea

1. All food may be withheld for 12 to 24 hours, during which time water with added electrolytes and carbohydrates is given (see above).

2. Enough total fluid and electrolytes by oral and parenteral routes should be supplied to prevent progression of dehydration and development of acidosis.
3. Diluted milk may be used for interim feeding for 24 to 48 hours until the stools are improved.
4. Finally there is a gradual return to the regular feedings.

Treatment of severe diarrhea This condition is considered a medical emergency.

1. An intravenous infusion should be started immediately (cutting down on a vein if necessary). In addition to the tests suggested earlier, a blood culture and a stool culture should be made.
2. Oral feedings may be started on the second day with the water, electrolyte, and carbohydrate solution suggested above.
3. If oral fluids are tolerated, diluted milk may be given, followed by a gradual return to normal feedings.
4. It should be emphasized that as soon as an etiologic factor, for example, acute purulent otitis media or shigella in the stool, has been ascertained, it should be treated promptly.

Adjuvants Antibiotics and chemotherapy are used according to the known or presumptive etiologic organisms. Adsorbents, e.g., kaolin, and antispasmodics, e.g., Lomotil, are of limited value. Water-soluble vitamins (C—500 mg, B_1—5 mg, B_2—5 mg, and niacin—20 mg) should be added to the infusions to prevent deficiency; as the infant improves, rarely tetany may occur and calcium can be used prophylactically.

CHRONIC NONSPECIFIC DIARRHEA

Chronic nonspecific diarrhea is an ill-defined syndrome characterized by the appearance at 6 to 36 months of age of persistent, loose, foul-smelling stools containing mucus. Growth and weight gain are little affected by the chronic gastrointestinal disturbance that is frequently associated with an intercurrent infection. Partial response to diet and antibiotics may occur, but the administration of diiodohydroxyquin (Diodoquin), 0.32 to 0.65 Gm, daily in two or three divided doses is efficacious. Although the condition may last several months, the prognosis is very good.

CELIAC SYNDROME

Celiac syndrome (malabsorption) is a chronic nutritional disturbance of infancy and childhood in which the fundamental defect appears to be faulty absorption and assimilation of complex sugars and fats. Familial incidence is common.

Etiologic classification of celiac syndrome

1. Idiopathic celiac disease (chronic idiopathic steatorrhea, Gee-Herter disease): The metabolic defect is unknown but there is basically a disturbance of fat absorption from the intestine. Symptoms usually appear between 6 and 18 months of age.
2. Gluten-induced enteropathy: The clinical picture is identical with that of idiopathic celiac disease but is caused by an intolerance to the gluten (the amino acid glutamine, found in the gliadin fraction, is probably the offending substance) present in wheat, rye, and oats. There is probably an unknown basic defect in enzymatic activity or metabolism or a biochemical dysfunction of mucosal cells.
3. Exudative enteropathy (idiopathic hypoproteinemia): The defect is an excessive loss of serum proteins through the gastrointestinal tract. There is apparently impaired function of the intestinal lymphatic vessels with abnormal permeability to serum proteins, which are lost in the stool.
4. Congenital pancreatic insufficiencies (cystic fibrosis of the pancreas) will be discussed separately.
5. Other conditions causing celiac syndrome: chronic incomplete obstruction of the small intestine or intestinal lymphatic vessels; extensive surgical resection of the small bowel; chronic parenteral infection, e.g., genitourinary; chronic intestinal infection, e.g., *Giardia lamblia;* hypo- or agamma globulinemia; oral antibiotics, e.g., neomycin; gastrointestinal allergy; colitis; deficiency of sugar-splitting enzymes (see p. 162), e.g., lactase, sucrase; exclusion of bile from the intestines, e.g., atresia of the bile ducts, biliary cirrhosis; and acanthocytosis. Acanthocytosis (abetalipoproteinemia) occurs mostly in Jewish children. It is probably transmitted as a recessive gene, being characterized by ataxia (diarrhea begins at an age characteristic for celiac syndrome, but central nervous system symptoms begin after 2 years of age), retinopathy with progressive loss of vision, and thornlike projections on the red blood cells.

Clinical features Although the etiology of the several diseases causing a celiac syndrome varies, the clinical features are similar.

1. Diarrhea and steatorrhea: Passage of bulky, frothy, frequent, foul stools, often exacerbated by respiratory infections.
2. Malnutrition (appetite is usually poor but may be excessive): weak, wasting muscles, especially of the buttocks and extremities, while the face tends to be spared (eyelashes are long).
3. Stunted growth: height and weight frequently below average.
4. Irritability, vomiting, and abdominal pain are common.
5. Hydrolability leading to crises of dehydration and electrolyte disturbances.

6. Findings of deficiency diseases of various minerals and vitamins, such as osteoporosis, rickets, tetany, and anemia. Subclinical deficiencies of vitamin C and vitamin B complex are rather common. Hemorrhagic diathesis (vitamin K deficiency) is uncommon.

Laboratory findings

1. Feces: Dried stool of a celiac patient on a normal diet contains 30 to 60 percent fat (mostly split), while normal stool fat content does not usually exceed 10 percent of the dietary fat; increased excretion of fat may be detected by microscopic examination of fecal smears, and there may be an excess of extracellular starch granules.
2. Glucose-tolerance test: There is a flat curve when glucose is given orally but a normal curve after intravenous administration.
3. Roentgenograms of the bones frequently show osteoporosis and rarely rickets; in the gastrointestinal x-ray series, the jejunum is most frequently involved revealing mucosal pattern abnormalities, dilatation and segmentation (puddling of barium).
4. Blood picture: The anemia is usually microcytic and hypochromic, but rarely is it macrocytic; total cholesterol level—100 to 140 mg per 100 ml—is low; serum carotene level is low.
5. Special tests: Vitamin A–tolerance test may reveal a flat curve (rise of less than 50 micrograms per 100 ml), and xylose absorption may be reduced (less than 20 percent being excreted in the urine during a 5-hour period following test dose).

In addition, the following specific tests aid in differentiating causes of malabsorption:

6. Serum protein: Albumin may be low in the idiopathic and gluten-induced forms and is an indication of severe disease but it is markedly diminished in exudative enteropathy. Serum-globulin level is usually normal in all types except in the exudative enteropathy and those cases associated with hypo- or agammaglobulinemia in which it is low.
7. Oral gluten leads to marked increase in content of fecal fat in gluten-induced celiac disease. Antibodies against gluten can be demonstrated in serum, small-bowel secretions, and stool.
8. Radioactive iodine (^{131}I) tagging of albumin reveals rapid disappearance from the serum. Polyvinylpyrrolidone (PVP) test also demonstrates loss of serum protein via the intestinal tract and is useful in cases of exudative enteropathy.
9. Disaccharidase deficiencies result in the excess production of short-chain acids and a lowered pH of the stool which cause excoriation of the skin of the buttocks.
10. Absorption tests for lactase, amylase, maltase, and sucrase ac-

tivity: after a loading dose of lactose, starch, maltose, and sucrose, respectively, an appropriate rise in blood glucose is expected if normal enzyme activity is present.

11. Peroral tube biopsy of the intestinal mucosa may demonstrate dilation of the lymphatic vessels with exudative enteropathy. Gluten-induced enteropathy is characterized by a mucosa which is atrophic with blunting, fusion, or absence of the villi, diminution of the surface goblet cells and increase in plasma cells and eosinophilic and polymorphonuclear leukocytes in the lamina propria. Similar findings may be seen in other forms of celiac syndrome, e.g., neomycin toxicity. Sugar-splitting enzyme deficiencies can be demonstrated chemically on small intestinal biopsy material.

Treatment

1. Dietary management: The diet should be high in calories, high in protein, and low in fat. Fat is best given as medium-chain triglycerides rather than longer-chain ones which are the common forms found in the average diet. Absorption of medium-chain triglycerides is not affected by absence of bile and affected only to a limited degree by absence of pancreatic lipase. It should contain no starch. Sugars should be simple (mono- and disaccharides), and in indicated cases specific sugars should be eliminated. The following is a suggested program for adding food to the diet: milk (Pregestimil—contains glucose, medium-chain triglycerides, and protein hydrolysate) and banana powder; then scraped beef and tomato juice; then ripe bananas, two to ten daily; then pot cheese and gelatin; puréed squash, peas, and celery; other meats and egg; scraped apple and other fruits and vegetables; cereal (other than wheat and rye) and potatoes; whole milk and butter would be added last.

2. Vitamin and mineral supplements: ascorbic acid, 100 mg daily; nonoily vitamins A and D, in amounts two to three times the prophylactic dosages; vitamin B complex in large dosages; iron for the anemia.

3. Additional parenteral therapy may be necessary early in treatment, for example, crude liver extract, starting with two units three times a week and increasing to ten units three times a week; vitamin B complex two times a week.

4. Prompt treatment of secondary infections is necessary.

5. When in crisis, immediate and vigorous treatment of the severe diarrhea and resulting acidosis and dehydration is essential. Adrenal corticosteroids are helpful.

Prognosis The prognosis is usually good, but the regular diet may have to be modified for some years. There may be recurrences during adulthood, especially during pregnancy. Anemia is common during adulthood.

CYSTIC FIBROSIS OF THE PANCREAS (Mucoviscidosis)

Cystic fibrosis of the pancreas is a congenital and familial (autosomal recessive trait) disease involving the exocrine glands; it presents the clinical findings of the celiac syndrome plus chronic pulmonary disease. There is a characteristic disturbance in the exocrine glands of the entire body, resulting in the secretion of abnormally viscid mucus (mucoviscidosis). In the pancreas the inspissated secretion produces the obstruction of the pancreatic ducts and acini which leads to the pathologic changes of cystic fibrosis, with an absence or gross deficiency of the secretion of pancreatic enzymes. Diabetes mellitus due to this disease occurs, but only infrequently. In the lungs, the tracheobronchial mucous glands are also affected, leading to the chronic pulmonary disease. In the liver, cirrhosis is not uncommon and frequently leads to portal hypertension. There is also consistent involvement of the sweat and salivary glands. The disease is uncommon among blacks.

Clinical features

1. Neonatal: There may be intestinal obstruction from a meconium ileus, because the meconium has not been liquefied in the fetal intestinal tract by the pancreatic juices. Meconium peritonitis and congenital peritoneal adhesions may occur as a result of perforation in utero. (See Chapter 18, "Surgical Conditions of the Abdomen.")
2. Neonatal to 6 months of age: failure to gain weight on a good dietary intake; large foul stools; and chronic respiratory infection, e.g., bronchitis, bronchopneumonia, and bronchiectasis.
3. From 6 months on: the gradual appearance of the celiac syndrome and the respiratory tract infections; these may be slight at first but become progressively worse. Lobar atelectasis, hemoptysis, spontaneous pneumothorax, clubbing of fingers and toes, and cor pulmonale are common complications in chronically ill patients.
4. Excessive loss of sodium and chloride in the sweat; acute disturbances of fluid and electrolyte balance (especially in hot weather).
5. Involvement of the paranasal sinuses with polyp formation is common.
6. Rectal prolapse occurs often during infancy or childhood.
7. Intestinal obstruction may occur at any age due to inspissated fecal masses.
8. Delayed sexual maturity occurs, and sterility is common in males.

9. Mild or incomplete forms of the disease may occur which usually are not diagnosed early in life.
10. Exudative retinopathy (dilation of vessels and papilledema) is prone to occur in patients with marked pulmonary involvement.

Laboratory findings

1. Sweat-electrolyte levels are elevated—sodium and chloride are about three times the normal value (chloride levels above 60 meq per liter are significant). These are best measured following pilocarpine iontophoresed into the skin.
2. Hypoalbuminemia may occur due to improper absorption and utilization of protein (especially if soybean milk is used); there is also impairment of liver function and hemodilution secondary to chronic pulmonary disease. Gamma globulin levels may be elevated in response to repeated pulmonary infection.
3. Examination of duodenal juice usually reveals no trypsin and increased viscosity.
4. Gelatin film test with stool shows failure of digestion because of lack of trypsin in stool. (This test has now been modified to rule out possible proteolytic action of intestinal bacteria. Care should be taken in collecting the specimen, as urine has a proteolytic action.)
5. Progressively abnormal glucose-tolerance curves appear in some patients with increasing age. Ketonuria, acidosis, and vascular changes as seen in true diabetes mellitus are uncommon.
6. Microscopic examination of the stool shows excessive fat droplets.
7. Vitamin A absorption is poor (except in alcoholic form), and the serum-carotene level is always low. The blood-cholesterol level is low, secondary to the poor fat absorption.
8. Roentgenograms of the chest usually show pulmonary lesions. Gastrointestinal series reveals puddling in small intestines, as in celiac disease.
9. The xylose-tolerance test, tests for protein loss via the gastrointestinal tract, and histologic examination of intestinal mucosa are normal (see Celiac Disease, p. 419).

Treatment

1. Dietary therapy: diet high in calories, 180 Cal per kg; high in protein, 10 to 12 Gm per kg (preferably in the amino acid state). Vitamin supplement: 20,000 to 40,000 units of vitamin A and 10,000 units of vitamin D (both water-soluble preparations); vitamin K parenterally; ascorbic acid, 200 to 300 mg daily; vitamin B complex orally and parenterally. Fat is best given as medium-chain triglycerides (see p. 420).
2. Pancreatin should be given (5 to 10 Gm daily). Dosage depends

upon the patient's clinical response. Anorexia and constipation are symptoms of overdosage. Viokase, 0.3 to 0.6 Gm, or Cotazyme, 0.3 to 0.6 mg with each feeding, may be used.
3. The respiratory infections should be treated in the incipient stages and prevented, if possible, by the administration of antibiotics for prolonged periods. They are usually *Staphylococcus aureus* infections, but occasionally other resistant organisms, e.g., *Pseudomonas aeruginosa, Monilia albicans,* may develop. Single and, if necessary, combined antibiotics (see Chapter 6, "Drugs and Treatment") should be employed for both treatment and prophylaxis of infections. Penicillin, methicillin, oxacillin, streptomycin, polymyxin B, bacitracin, cephalothin, oxytetracycline, and neomycin may also be given as aerosols. Postural drainage, breathing exercises, and chest clapping are important adjuvants in the treatment of pulmonary involvement.
4. Aerosol therapy (propylene glycol 10% in saline) with ultrasonic nebulizers may be used at home during sleep, prior to postural drainage, and for short periods repeated several times during the day.
5. During hot weather, adequate amounts of salt (2 Gm or more per day) and water should be offered.
6. Hospitalization should be avoided whenever possible to prevent infection with resistant organisms.
7. Every effort to treat the child as normally as possible should be made. Cystic fibrosis has a severe effect upon the social, emotional, and economic aspects of both the patient and his family. A multidisciplinary approach to the many problems encountered is needed.

Prognosis The prognosis is poor, but as the child grows older dietary restrictions appear to be less necessary.

REGIONAL ENTERITIS

Regional enteritis is a chronic granulomatous condition of unknown cause, involving part of the small intestines, usually the terminal ileum. The colon may be involved (granulomatous colitis). Clinical features are usually abdominal discomfort, nausea, vomiting, diarrhea or constipation, and low-grade fever; there may be acute exacerbations simulating acute appendicitis. The condition may clear spontaneously or be slowly progressive. Diagnosis can be made by roentgenograms showing extreme narrowing of the terminal ileum and by laparotomy. Early surgery is recommended by some, while others prefer to use adrenal corticosteroids or Azulfidine (see p. 424) and wait since occasionally there is a spontaneous cure. Surgery must be performed for complications, e.g., obstruction, fistula, and abscess formation.

CHRONIC ULCERATIVE COLITIS

This is a chronic inflammatory disease of unknown etiology. Various causes, e.g., infection, allergy, and psychosomatic factors, have been implicated. The mucous membrane becomes hyperemic and friable, ulcerates, and tends to form pseudopolyps which are subject to malignant degeneration.

Clinical features

1. The onset is usually insidious but may occur suddenly. Diarrhea is the most common presenting symptom.
2. Frequent small stools containing mucus, pus, and blood occur.
3. Pain and tenesmus may or may not be present.
4. Low-grade fever may occur occasionally and precede other symptoms.
5. Anorexia, loss of weight, and increased irritability are present.
6. Arthralgia, skin lesions, iritis, liver damage, and hemorrhagic manifestations may occur.

Laboratory findings

1. Anemia and leukocytosis are present.
2. Sedimentation rate may be increased.
3. Serum albumin–globulin ratio may be reversed.
4. Roentgenograms of the colon following barium enema reveal spasm and on postevacuation films, thickened mucosal marking; later they reveal lack of haustrations and marginal irregularities; with progression there is a "lead pipe" appearance due to thickening, shortening, and loss of haustrations.
5. Sigmoidoscopic examination early reveals a hyperemic, friable mucosa and later the ulcerations.

Treatment

1. Diet should be bland and should contain little residue during periods of exacerbation.
2. Psychotherapy is important; tranquilizing drugs, e.g., meprobamate, may be helpful.
3. Antibacterial therapy, e.g., sulfonamides (Azulfidine—150 mg per kg per day), may be helpful during periods of exacerbation.
4. Supplementary vitamins B and C should be given, along with iron for anemia.
5. ACTH and cortisone have been employed to induce remissions and lessen the severity of relapses.
6. In progressive cases, surgery may be indicated.

Prognosis   Recurrences are common, and there is a high incidence of malignant changes in cases that persist into adulthood.

LIVER–FUNCTION TESTS

Many tests have been devised for the numerous functions of the liver. No test is specific, and it is better to do several well-selected tests serially than to rely on a single one. These tests may be divided into several groups.

1. Biliary function: Normally, after the red blood cells are broken down by the reticuloendothelial system, part of the released hemoglobin is transformed to bilirubin. This is further acted upon, and a bilirubin-protein compound is formed which is called bilirubin type I (this type is insoluble in water and gives an indirect van den Bergh reaction). By enzymatic action, the liver then conjugates this to a bilirubin glucuronide (water-soluble) or type II, which is excreted in the bile. (Type II gives a direct van den Bergh reaction and represents the 1-minute fraction.) In the intestines, bilirubin type II is converted by bacterial action to urobilinogen, most of which is excreted in the feces as stercobilinogen. The portion that is reabsorbed is excreted, in part by the kidneys and in part by the liver.

   Tests associated with the formation and excretion of bile pigments are: icterus index (normal 3 to 5 units), determination of serum bilirubin (normal, 1-minute fraction—0.1 to 0.2 mg per 100 ml; normal, indirect—0.1 to 1.0 mg per 100 ml), quantitative determination of urinary bilirubin (normal, 0 to 0.25 mg per 100 ml) and urobilinogen (normal, 1.0 Ehrlich unit), and stool examination for stercobilinogen (normal, 100 to 200 mg per day).

2. Enzyme levels: Enzymes and substrates involved in metabolism and stored in high concentration in the liver are often released when there is acute cell damage, with a subsequent rise in blood levels. They are also present in other tissue so that interpretation of elevated levels requires knowledge to rule out other causes of such rises. Serum glutamic oxaloacetic transaminase (SGOT) is also present in the heart, skeletal muscle, and kidney. Serum glutamic pyruvic transaminase (SGPT) is present to a greater extent in liver than cardiac or skeletal muscle. It is therefore a more specific index of hepatocellular injury. Normal levels of SGOT and SGPT in the neonate are much higher than in infants and children (see p. 13). Lactase dehydrogenase (LD) is found in many tissues including red blood cells. LD found in the liver can be separated by starch gel electrophoresis from other isoenzymes.

   Cephalin flocculation and thymol turbidity tests are also employed to demonstrate liver cell damage. Abnormalities of the former are related to changes in gamma globulin; in the latter case they are due to a relative increase in gamma globulin and beta lipoproteins.

   Alkaline phosphatase is elevated (normal, 3 to 13 Bodansky units) in biliary tract obstruction but normal or slightly elevated in hepatitis (slight elevation is probably due to swelling of liver cells causing pressure on finer biliary passages). In bone disease, the clinical features, roentgenograms, and electrophoretic demonstration of elevated alkaline phosphatase in the beta globulin (bone) rather than in the alpha globulin (liver) usually permit differentiation.

3. Dye excretion: Following the injection of a dye, e.g., Bromsulphalein, that is excreted by the liver, the amount remaining in the blood is measured after a given period of time (normal after 5 minutes—20 to 50 percent, after 45 minutes—none); retention indicates liver disease. (This test is of no value in the presence of jaundice.) Radioiodinated (^{131}I) rose bengal is valuable to demonstrate biliary obstruction in the presence of hyperbilirubinemia. This is particularly true in the newborn infant with suspected biliary atresia.

4. Carbohydrate metabolism: In the presence of liver damage there is faulty metabolism of one or more of the saccharides (glucose, galactose, levulose), resulting in elevated and prolonged blood-sugar curves following their administration (tolerance test).

5. Fat metabolism: e.g., serum-cholesterol level and percentage of esterification (normal, 120 to 250 mg per 100 ml with 50 percent or more esterification). An increase in total cholesterol indicates obstructive jaundice; a decrease, hepatocellular disease.

6. Protein metabolism: for example, serum-albumin levels (normal, 4.5 to 5.5 mg per 100 ml) and serum globulin (normal, 1.8 to 2.7 mg per 100 ml), cephalin flocculation (normal, 0 to 1+), thymol turbidity (0 to 3 units), prothrombin time (normal, 12 to 15 seconds, Quick method).

7. Ammonia fixation: Blood ammonia fasting arterial levels (normal, 20 to 50 mg per ml) may be elevated in severe liver disease due to failure of fixation. Normal individuals or those with mild liver disease have no rise in blood ammonia after a test meal of protein or a dose of ammonium chloride.

8. Detoxification: e.g., conversion of orally administered sodium benzoate to hippuric acid, which is then excreted (normal, 90 percent excretion in 4 hours; if decreased, indicates liver damage).

9. Biopsy: Biopsy of the liver may be of value in making a diagnosis if the disease is generalized, for example, in glycogen-storage disease or Wilson's disease; or for following patients with chronic liver disease, e.g., hemosiderosis.

Jaundice usually becomes manifest when the plasma-bilirubin level is about 2.0 mg per 100 ml, though in the newborn infant, higher levels are necessary.

The elevation of bilirubin occurs when (1) excessive amounts of hemoglobin are destroyed, or (2) there is interference with the process of excretion.

Jaundice may be classified as obstructive (regurgitation) or hemolytic (retention). The obstructive types of jaundice include those due to true obstruction of the bile ducts and those due to parenchymal damage to the polygonal cells of the liver by infectious or toxic agents. The hemolytic group occurs when excessive amounts of bilirubin are produced and the liver is unable to remove them from the circulating blood.

The primary laboratory differences are as shown in Table 17-1.

INFECTIOUS HEPATITIS

Two clinically, epidemiologically, and immunologically distinct types of hepatitis have been described, the short-incubation type (IH or HA) and the long-incubation type (SH or HB). The SH infection is consistently associated with Australian antigen (HB_{ag}). Infectious mononucleosis and other viruses, e.g., Coxsackie, herpes virus, have been implicated in some cases of hepatitis.

Mode of transmission IH is highly contagious and transmitted by fecal contamination. It occurs most commonly in young adults. SH has a low rate of contact transmission and is more often transmitted by contaminated blood, blood products, or instruments, e.g., needles. It occurs in all age groups.

Clinical features

1. Incubation period: IH—about 1 month; SH—about 1 to 3 months.
2. The onset is usually characterized by malaise, anorexia, abdominal discomfort, vomiting. IH usually has a more abrupt onset and may be associated with fever.
3. Several days later jaundice usually appears, and occasionally

Table 17-1.   Two types of jaundice

Test	Obstructive	Hemolytic
Urine:		
Bilirubin	Present	Absent
Urobilin	Not increased	Markedly increased
Stools:		
Bilirubin	Absent	Increased
Urobilin	Decreased	Increased
Blood:		
Alkaline phosphatase	Elevated (with true* obstructive type)	Normal
Van den Bergh	Direct—biphasic	Indirect

Parenchymal jaundice usually has more positive cephalin flocculation but less elevation of alkaline phosphatase than the true obstructive type.

pruritus may be present. This is often preceded by the presence of increased amounts of urobilinogen in the urine.
4.   The stools may become clay-colored.
5.   The liver is enlarged and tender.

Laboratory findings

1.   Serum enzyme levels, e.g., SGOT, SGPT, are increased.
2.   Van den Bergh's reaction is at first direct and later biphasic.
3.   The icterus index, serum-bilirubin, and urinary urobilin levels are increased. Later in the course, little bilirubin is excreted; consequently urobilin levels fall. With recovery there is a second rise in the level.
4.   The serum alkaline phosphatase level is raised.
5.   Stercobilinogen is reduced resulting in clay-colored stools.
6.   There is leukopenia in the preicteric stage, leukocytosis later.
7.   Virus can be detected in the stools during the incubation period and early in the disease in IH infection.

Prophylaxis   The role of gamma globulin (0.02 to 0.06 ml per kg) in IH disease is not clearly understood. It may not prevent the hepatitis but only suppress the jaundice and modify the disease, so that it occurs in a subclinical form and the patient develops active immunity.

Treatment   There is no specific therapy. Ad lib diet with fat as tolerated and confinement to home with no restriction of activity is recommended. In severe or chronic cases adrenal corticosteroids appear to be of benefit.

Prognosis   The prognosis is good. A small percentage of patients, however, may develop acute yellow atrophy. The role of infectious hepatitis as a cause of cirrhosis has not been evaluated.

REYE'S SYNDROME

Reye's syndrome consists of encephalopathy associated with fatty infiltration of the liver, pancreas, and kidneys. The etiology is unknown, but there is almost always an associated viral infection, not infrequently varicella. Protracted vomiting, lethargy, and stupor rapidly progress to death in a few days. Abnormal laboratory findings include hypoglycemia, elevated serum transaminase, elevated blood ammonia, and altered blood-clotting factors produced in the liver. Treatment consists of 10 percent glucose intravenously, cleansing enemas, and neomycin. Exchange transfusion with fresh blood is recommended for progressively deepening coma. This may have to be repeated. The prognosis is grave. Improvement occurs rapidly in survivors, and recovery is usually complete, but neurologic sequelae may occur.

CIRRHOSIS OF THE LIVER

Cirrhosis is a chronic diffuse fibrosis of the liver. It may be due to congenital anomalies, e.g., atresia of bile ducts; hereditary disorders, e.g., hepatolenticular degeneration, glycogen or other storage diseases; infection, either congenital, e.g., neonatal hepatitis, or acquired; hemolytic anemia; nutritional deficiency; drug toxicity; poisonings; autoimmune disease, e.g., plasma cell hepatitis, as well as a number of other miscellaneous disorders, e.g., amyloidosis. Two main varieties exist:

1. Portal cirrhosis (Laennec's), in which the fibrosis extends from the portal venules
2. Biliary cirrhosis, in which there is obstruction of the bile ducts and the fibrosis extends from these ducts

In children the pure forms of cirrhosis are rarely seen; a combination of both is the more usual picture. The clinical features depend upon which type predominates. In biliary cirrhosis, jaundice, acholic stools, and enlarged liver are found. In portal cirrhosis, vague abdominal pains, loss of weight, hematemesis, and spider nevi are often found; later in the course of the disease, ascites develops. In both forms of the disease, one or more of the liver-function tests give abnormal results. There is no specific therapy unless a definite primary disease such as syphilis is found. A high-vitamin (especially vitamin B), high-protein diet is recommended. Choline and methionine (3 Gm of each per day) may be of value. Paracentesis may be necessary to relieve respiratory distress caused by ascites. Adrenal corticosteroids may also be of value.

CONGESTIVE SPLENOMEGALY

Congestive splenomegaly (portal hypertension, Banti's disease) is due to interference, from any cause, with the return flow of blood through the portal vein or the spleen. Omphalitis in the neonatal period, cannulation of the umbilical vein and anomalies of the portal vascular system, and rarely cirrhosis of the liver may cause congestive splenomegaly. However, not infrequently massive hematemesis is the first evidence of the disease. It is characterized by enlargement of the spleen and development of collateral circulation. The increased collateral circulation may result in esophageal varicosities with hematemesis and dilatation of superficial abdominal veins. Eventually, if death does not supervene, hepatomegaly and frequently ascites develop. There are usually an anemia and leukopenia. Diagnosis of operable portal hypertension is aided by percutaneous and transplenic vasography, which indicate the size and positioning of splenic and portal veins. Portal venous pressure (normal—about 7 mmHg) and presinusoidal pressure in the spleen (normal—slightly above portal vein pressure) can be measured diagnostically and to evaluate the effectiveness or shunting procedures. For treatment see p. 469.

DIAGNOSIS AND TREATMENT OF INTESTINAL PARASITES

The prevalence of parasitic infections is generally either global, e.g., enterobiasis, giardiasis, or geographically more restricted, i.e., schistosomiasis, taeniasis, and many others. A broader distribution of these previously less-cosmopolitan infections can now be expected as man travels with ever increasing ease and frequency. The presence of intestinal parasitic infections, either single or multiple, should therefore be considered, particularly in those children presenting with gastrointestinal complaints.

Occurrence and extent of clinical manifestations depend upon the magnitude of the parasite burden, host response or immune status, and adequacy of the host's diet. Light infections, generally asymptomatic, may be accidentally discovered when adult worms responding to a stimulus, e.g., pyrexia, migrate into ectopic sites and are vomited or otherwise passed.

Definitive diagnosis of patent gastrointestinal parasitism may be established by the finding in the child's feces, of either the egg, larval, segmental (proglottid), adult, trophozoite, or cyst stage of the causative parasite. During the prepatent period, and in certain infections, e.g., trichinosis, the use of special tests is indicated, as outlined below.

ASCARIASIS

Etiology *Ascaris lumbricoides,* large roundworm of man, is the etiologic agent.

Mode of acquisition Ingestion of fertilized embryonated eggs is the mode of acquisition.

Clinical features Symptoms may occur during two phases of worm's life cycle in the child. (From ingestion of eggs to development of mature worms requires from 8 to 12 weeks.)

1. Larval phase: During part of their development the larvae transverse the lungs, forcing their way through the capillary and alveolar walls. Fever, hemoptysis, dyspnea, and eosinophilia may develop. Radiologically, lungs exhibit mottling. Only rarely are larvae

demonstrable in the sputum. Clinical resolution of this phase gradually follows in 7 to 10 days. Host sensitization resulting in allergic asthmatic manifestations may occur in heavy or repeated infections.

2. Adult phase: Adult male and female ascaris, 6 to 8 and 7 to 10 in. long respectively, live in the lumen of the jejunum. If they are few in number (5 to 10), the host may be asymptomatic. A moderate-to-heavy worm burden may cause colicky pain, diarrhea or constipation, anorexia, and abdominal distension and place a nutritional burden upon the child. During fever, anesthesia, and administration of certain oral medications worms may wander. They may ball up causing intestinal obstruction, perforate into the peritoneal cavity, enter the biliary and pancreatic ducts, or penetrate the appendix. Their normal lifespan is from 1 to 1½ years. Worms may be passed via the nose, vomited, or coughed up.

Diagnosis

1. Established by finding eggs of ascaris in the feces
2. Established by the presence of adult worms in stools and vomitus
3. Established radiologically following barium meal as barium may be visualized in the worm's intestinal tract
4. Suggested by the presence of eosinophilia during the larval phase, with low or normal levels during adult phase of life cycle

Treatment

1. If polyparasitism is present, it is advisable to first treat for ascaris. This will reduce the chance of ectopic wandering by adult worms as may occur if partially ascaricidal drugs are used, i.e., tetrachlorethylene for hookworm.
2. Pyrantel pamoate: One oral dose, 11 mg (base) per kg (not to exceed 1 Gm) or 1 ml per 10 lb. No laxatives or starvation are necessary. Side effects include abdominal cramping, nausea, vomiting, headache, and transient elevation of SGOT.
3. Piperazine: salts of the drug are available as tablets and wafers, each containing 250 or 500 mg; or as syrup and suspensions containing 100 mg per ml, calculated as the hexahydrate. No laxatives or starvation are necessary before giving the following daily doses:

Up to 30 lb	1.0 Gm	
30–50 lb	2.0 Gm	once daily for two consecutive days.
50–100 lb	3.0 Gm	
Over 100 lb	3.5 Gm	

Rarely urticaria, dizziness, headache, and blurred vision may be experienced, but disappear when drug is discontinued. Efficacy of

treatment should be evaluated by follow-up stool examination 1 week later.
4.   Thiabendazole: See Strongyloidiasis, below.

VISCERAL LARVA MIGRANS

Etiology   Larvae of dog and cat ascarids, *Toxocara canis, T. cati,* and of other nonhuman nematodes, are etiologic agents.

Mode of acquisition   Larvae are acquired by ingestion of fertilized eggs.

Clinical features   Larvae, in the strange host, wander in the child's liver, lungs, brain, eye, and other regions. Granulomata may be formed. Leukocytosis and persistent eosinophilia of 30 to 90 percent occurs. Child may be asymptomatic or have low-grade fever, cough, nervous symptoms, hepatomegaly, pulmonary infiltration, and hyperglobulinemia. General ill health may persist for many months.

Diagnosis   Demonstration of larvae in biopsy specimens confirms the diagnosis. Hemagglutination and flocculation tests may be helpful.

Treatment and prognosis   Specific treatment is lacking. Thiabendazole and diethylcarbamazine may be helpful. Prognosis is good with eventual complete recovery.

ENTEROBIASIS (Pinworm or Seatworm Infection)

Etiology   *Enterobius vermicularis* is the etiologic agent.

Mode of acquisition   Eggs are acquired through anus-to-mouth transmission via ova on hands, either from scratching the perianal region or handling contaminated night clothes, bedding, towels and fomites, inhalation of ova-laden dust, and retrofection via the anus.

Clinical features   Three to six weeks after egg ingestion gravid female worms migrate out of the cecum into the perianal folds to deposit their ova. The pruritis, which results in scratching, may be moderate or severe, especially at night. The ova mature and are infective in a few hours. Insomnia, restlessness, irritability, and psychologic disorders characterize this infection. Vaginitis, frequency of micturition, appendiceal inflammation, and gastrointestinal disorders may occasionally occur in heavy infections due to the presence of worms and ova in the genital tract, appendix, and large intestine, respectively.

Diagnosis

1. Adult worms in anal region or on surface of stool.
2. Ova in the perianal region via cellophane-tape swab (eggs are seldom present in stool). Before the child's early morning toiletry a strip of sticky cellophane tape is applied to the perianal region, removed, and spread on a glass slide for microscopic examination. The gravid female worms migrate irregularly, therefore repeated examinations on consecutive days may be necessary.

Treatment, control, and prognosis

1. Piperazine (see ascariasis above) is given orally for 7 consecutive days as follows:

   Up to 15 lb: 250 mg daily
   15 to 30 lb: 250 mg twice daily
   30 to 60 lb: 500 mg twice daily
   Over 60 lb: 1 Gm twice daily

   If necessary the course may be repeated after 1 week.
2. Pyrvinium pamoate is given as a single oral dose of 5 mg per kg, and the dose may be repeated in 1 week. A suspension containing 10 mg per ml and tablets of 50 mg are available. The latter should not be chewed. The drug occasionally causes vomiting. (It colors the stool and vomitis red.)
3. Pyrantel pamoate is also effective (see p. 431).
4. Thiabendazole (see strongyloidiasis below) should be given in doses of 10 mg per lb orally twice daily for 1 day. This procedure should be repeated in 1 week unless poorly tolerated.
5. Adjuvant hygienic precautions:
   a. The entire household and close contacts should be studied and all treated if more than one person is found infected.
   b. Hands should be washed with a brush frequently and especially before eating; trim fingernails close.
   c. Infected children should wear close-fitting underpants during the night and day, changing them on arising and retiring. The underpants should be boiled for 10 minutes before laundering.
   d. The toilet seat should be cleaned frequently.
   e. The floors of the sleeping quarters should be scrubbed with strong soap at least at the end of each period of therapy.
6. Prognosis: Good, but there is no immunity to reinfection.

HOOKWORM DISEASE (Necatoriasis, Ancylostomiasis)

Etiology   The etiologic agents are *Necator americanus* and *Ancylostoma duodenale.*

Mode of acquisition   The infection results from penetration of skin by filariform larvae present in contaminated soil. (Additionally, infection with ancylostoma may become established following ingestion of larvae on leafy vegetables.) Following skin penetration, the larvae migrate through the lungs, going finally to the small intestine where they develop into sexually mature worms. This requires approximately 6 weeks.

Clinical features   The "ground itch" syndrome, or penetration dermatitis, is characterized by itching and burning at the site of larval penetration followed by erythema, edema, and papular vasicular rash lasting about 2 weeks. Similar symptomatology is evidenced in creeping eruption and strongyloidiasis (see below).

The pulmonary signs resultant from the larval migration resemble those observed in ascariasis (see above) but generally are more mild.

As they reach maturity the worms attach to the intestinal mucosa causing ulceration and blood leakage. The latter recur frequently during the lifespan of the worms as they move about the mucosa. Additionally their blood-sucking habits add to the daily blood loss. The early phase of attachment may be marked by epigastric discomfort, fatigue, anorexia, weight loss, and eosinophilic leukocytosis.

The degree to which anemia develops depends upon the magnitude and duration of the infection, the iron content of the diet, and the state of the child's iron reserves. Hookworm infection should be differentiated from hookworm disease. Worm burdens of 50 to 100 may be symptomless. In children with heavy infections, in addition to the symptomatology commensurate with the marked anemia (rapid pulse, cardiac enlargement, hemic murmur, edema), there may be physical, mental, and sexual retardation. Hookworms have a lifespan of from 2 to 5 or more years.

Diagnosis   Finding the characteristic hookworm eggs in the feces establishes the diagnosis. Fecal egg counts aid in assessment of the worm burden.

Treatment

1. Tetrachlorethylene is the drug of choice for treating necator uncomplicated by ascaris (see Ascariasis above). Specific antihookworm treatment is indicated when there are 2,000 or more eggs per gram of feces. If there is marked anemia or nutritional deficiency, tetrachlorethylene administration should be delayed until the anemia is corrected with iron therapy and an adequate diet instituted.

    Tetrachlorethylene, as an emulsion in skimmed milk or in gelatin capsules, is given on an empty stomach in a single dose, 0.06 ml per lb body weight. A fat-free liquid diet should be given the day before. Food should be withheld for 4 hours, although water

may be taken, fatty foods should be avoided for the rest of the day. This will aid nonabsorption of the drug. Treatment may be repeated after 1 week if indicated by a continuing high egg count in the feces. A 90 percent worm-removal value can be anticipated for *N. americanus,* less for *A. duodenale.*
2. Bephenium hydroxynaphthoate (Alcopara) is the drug of choice for *A. duodenale.* A single dose will remove 90 percent of the worms. (Multiple dosing is required for *N. americanus.*) It has the advantage of low toxicity, is an effective ascaricide, and can be used in anemic children. It is distributed in packets of 5 Gm (2.5 Gm bephenium base). Because of its bitter taste, it is best administered by suspending the granules in sweetened milk or fruit juice and given 1 hour before food. For children weighing 50 lb or less, a single dose of 1.25 Gm base is used against ancylostoma, 1.25 Gm base on 3 successive days against necator.
3. Thiabendazole (Mintezol) is also effective against hookworm (see Strongyloidiasis below).

TRICHURIASIS (Whipworm Infection)

Etiology   *Trichuris (Trichocephalus) trichiura* is the agent.

Mode of acquisition   Acquisition is by ingestion of fertilized embryonated eggs. Adult worms develop in from 30 to 60 days.

Clinical features   The threadlike worms normally live with the slender anterior portion threaded in the cecal mucosa. In heavy infections the worms may also be found in the colon, rectum, appendix, and lower ileum. The worms may live for 14 years or longer.

Children with chronic heavy infections (200 or more worms) are anemic and experience abdominal discomfort, nausea, vomiting, headache, mild fever, and frequent blood-tinged diarrheic stools. There may be mild eosinophilia and rectal prolapse.

Many light infections are discovered upon routine stool examination.

Diagnosis   Finding the typical brownish lemon-shaped eggs in the feces establishes the diagnosis. Charcot-Leyden crystals and eosinophils are frequently present in diarrheic stools. Worms may be observed at sigmoidoscopy, attached to the prolapsed rectum, and occasionally in the feces.

Treatment

1. Hexylresorcinol 0.2% solution, 500 ml as a 1-hour retention enema (buttocks and thighs are covered with a protective coating of petroleum jelly to prevent burns).

2. Thiabendazole, 10 mg per lb per dose, twice daily for 2 days (maximum daily dose 3.0 Gm). This may yield a cure in about one-third of those treated. For side effects, see Strongyloidiasis below.
3. Dichlorvos is a good trichuricide but is presently not approved by the FDA.

STRONGYLOIDIASIS (Threadworm Infection)

Etiology   The etiologic agent is *Strongyloides stercoralis*.

Mode of acquisition   Acquisition is by skin penetration by filariform larvae present in contaminated soil. Autoinfection causes the infection to be self-perpetuating. Strongyloidiasis may thus be present long after the child has left an endemic zone. From skin penetration to the production of eggs and rhabditiform larvae requires approximately 4 weeks.

Clinical features   The larval stage, as with hookworm, is accompanied by itching and dermatitis, with the severity dependent upon the degree of prior sensitization. Serpiginous tracts form in the path of the larvae not unlike those observed in man with cutaneous larva migrans. This "creeping eruption" subsides as the larvae migrate to the lungs and eventually to the small intestine. During this phase there may be fever, anorexia, cough, and urticaria.

In moderate-to-heavy infections the intestinal phase is marked by midepigastric tenderness, nausea, vomiting, dyspepsia, weight loss, and diarrhea alternating with constipation. In chronic infections, malabsorption, steatorrhea, and anemia may develop. There is a persistent eosinophilia.

Diagnosis

1. Finding typical rhabditiform larvae in fresh stool specimens.
2. Rhabditiform, filariform (infective), and free-living adults in 48-hour stool cultures.
3. By duodenal intubation to obtain adults, larvae, or ova.
4. Eosinophil counts of 15 percent are suggestive.

Treatment   Other concomitant infestations should be treated first, e.g., ascaris, hookworm. Thiabendazole is the drug of choice. It is administered orally in a dose of 10 mg per lb twice daily for 2 days, maximum daily dose 3.0 Gm. Nausea, vomiting, drowsiness, headache, anorexia, and weakness are the major side effects. They are dose-related and not uncommon.

Prognosis is good except in cases of chronic autoinfection and altered immunity. The migrating larvae may initiate a generalized septicemia.

TRICHINOSIS (Trichiniasis)

Etiology   The etiologic agent is *Trichinella spiralis*.

Mode of acquisition   Organisms are acquired by ingestion of insufficiently cooked pork, bear, or walrus meat containing trichina larvae in the muscle, when eaten plain or in ground meat or sausage mixtures.

Clinical features

1. Gastrointestinal phase. Following ingestion of the trichinous pork the larvae excyst and during the next 24 to 48 hours grow into adult worms in the intestinal mucosa. Following fertilization the female worms begin to deposit larvae on or about the fifth day. These larvae are carried via the bloodstream to various parts of the body, eventually to encyst in striated muscle. Symptomatology during this early phase reflects the number of worms present, the immune status, and the age of the child. Often trichinosis resembles a mild intestinal upset and is otherwise clinically silent. In acute and severe cases there may be headache, nausea, vomiting, fever, abdominal pain, and diarrhea.
2. Larval migration, muscle invasion, and encystation. These may be accompanied by myalgia frequently causing difficulty in breathing, swallowing, masticating or locomotion, subungual hemorrhages, orbital edema, persistent fever, cough, and rapidly rising eosinophilia. Mild cases generally begin to recover after the fourth week; however, death may occur during weeks 3 to 6 as a result of exhaustion, pneumonia, cardiac failure, toxemia, and cerebral involvement.
3. Repair and calcification. Within 6 months the muscle pain subsides, the eosinophil count gradually decreases. Most of the larvae begin to calcify in from 12 to 18 months.

Diagnosis

1. Suggested by symptoms and associated epidemiology.
2. Steadily rising eosinophilia beginning at the end of the first week, peaking (range 20 to 80 percent) between weeks 3 and 4, followed after a variable time by a return to normal.
3. Bachman intradermal skin test, evident beginning in weeks 2 to 4. May remain positive for several years.
4. Diagnosis is established by finding living larvae in a muscle biopsy, e.g., deltoid or gastrocnemius.
5. Complement-fixation and precipitin tests generally become positive during the fourth week and remain positive for from 9 months to 2 years. Other tests include the bentonite-flocculation test and the indirect fluorescent-antibody test.

Treatment   Trichinosis may be mild, requiring only symptomatic treatment, or acute. In the latter instance ACTH or corticosteroids may be required to relieve the intense inflammatory response. Supportive treatment is indicated as is monitoring of cardiac function. Although all the larvae may not be killed, the use of thiabendazole, a larvicidal drug, is recommended. A dose of 10 mg per lb twice daily for 2 to 4 successive days is advocated. For side effects, see Strongyloidiasis above. If trichinosis is suspected following the early gastrointestinal phase the administration of sodium sulfate may help to eliminate some of the adult worms thereby reducing the number of larvae that would be produced to later invade the muscles.

CAPILLARIASIS

Etiology   The etiologic agent is *Capillaria philippinensis*.

Description   Intestinal capillariasis is a newly recognized disease of man first recorded in the Philippines. The etiologic agent is related to trichuris and trichinella. The tiny worms live in the jejunal mucosa and are responsible for marked changes in intestinal function, e.g., altered absorption, loss of fluid, electrolytes, and plasma proteins. The fatality rate may exceed 10 percent. The clinical features include intractable diarrhea, weakness, weight loss, anasarca, and emaciation. Eggs, larvae, and adults have been found at autopsy and in stool samples; autoinfection therefore cannot be ruled out. The mode of acquisition is ill-defined, although larval stages are known to occur in certain fish. Treatment is with thiabendazole.

CESTODIASIS (Tapeworm Infection)

General   Tapeworms may parasitize man in their adult and/or larval stage.

ADULT TAPEWORMS

Etiology   Man is the definitive host of *Taenia saginata*, the beef, and *T. solium*, the pork tapeworm. *Diphyllobothrium latum*, the fish tapeworm, occurs in numerous vertebrates including man. *Hymenolepis nana* and *H. diminuta* are tapeworms of rodents which also infect man. *Dipylidium caninum*, the common tapeworm of dogs and cats, occasionally parasitizes man, particularly children.

Mode of acquisition

1.   *Taenia saginata:* consumption of insufficiently cooked beef containing the cysts (*Cysticercus bovis*).

2. *T. solium:* consumption of insufficiently cooked pork containing the cysts (*Cysticercus cellulosae*). Swallowing of eggs causes visceral taeniasis, see below under Larval Tapeworms.
3. *D. latum:* consumption of insufficiently cooked fish harboring the larval plerocercoid stage.
4. *H. nana,* human strain: ingestion of eggs, anus-to-mouth transmission, particularly in children. Rodent strain: accidental swallowing of fleas or grain beetles harboring the larval stage.
5. *H. diminuta:* accidental swallowing of flour beetles or other arthropods harboring the larval stage.
6. *D. caninum:* accidental swallowing of dog fleas or lice harboring the larval stage, as when children hug and kiss an infected pet.

From ingestion of infected meat, fish, or arthropods, or via autoinfection, to development of mature tapeworms requires for *T. saginata* and *T. solium* 2 to 3 months, for each of the others from 3 to 5 weeks.

Clinical features Adult tapeworms live in the small intestine. The majority of infections are asymptomatic whether the child harbors one worm, as is generally the case in infections with the beef, pork, fish, or dog tapeworm, or many worms, as commonly occurs in hymenolepiasis. Abdominal discomfort, increase or loss of appetite, indigestion, weight loss, allergic and neurologic manifestations, diarrhea, mild eosinophilia, anemia (*D. latum*), and enteritis (*H. nana*) have been linked to tapeworm infections. The worms all have substantial carbohydrate requirements and, in the case of *D. latum,* vitamin B_{12} and other vitamins. These needs, their longevity, 10 to 20 or more years, mechanical factors, 5- to 10-meter length of beef, pork, and fish tapeworms, and their metabolic excretions, may all play a role.

Diagnosis

1. *T. saginata, T. solium:* Gravid segments may be found in the feces. Rarely eggs may be present in the feces or observed in cellophane-tape preparations (see Pinworm above).
2. *D. latum:* The operculate eggs are found in the feces. Gravid segments with central rosette uterine configuration also may be observed.
3. *H. nana, H. diminuta:* Characteristic eggs are found in the feces.
4. *D. caninum:* Presence in the feces of pumpkin-seed shaped segments containing egg capsules or released capsules each containing 15 to 25 eggs establishes diagnosis.

Treatment

1. Niclosamide (Yomesan) is the drug of choice for the elimination of all adult tapeworms. Its use should be cautioned in *T. solium,* see item 3 below. Omit breakfast. The tablets are crushed or

chewed and washed down with water. Children under 2 years of age: 2 doses of 250 mg 1 hour apart; children over 8 years of age: 2 doses of 1 Gm each 1 hour apart. In *H. nana* infections drug should be taken for 5 successive days to eliminate worms emerged from the larval state. Patient may eat 2 hours after the last dose. The drug disintegrates the worms, therefore recovering of the worm's scolex, necessary for complete cure, is not possible. Stools should thus be examined monthly for 4 months. If no eggs or segments are found, cure has been affected.

2. Dichlorophen (Antiphen): a single oral dose of 0.5 Gm per lb body weight. In treating children the dose should not be below 4.5 Gm, or failure to eliminate the worm may occur. Dose should be repeated in 3 weeks for *H. nana*. The drug has a laxative action and may cause slight colic. The drug also disintegrates the worm. Its use is contraindicated in liver disease.

3. Quinacrine hydrochloride (Atabrine) is effective against all tapeworms. The worm is eliminated without distintegration of segments thus preventing the release of eggs. The child should be hospitalized and given a liquid diet for 24 hours prior to treatment. A purge or enema is given the evening before treatment. The next morning a sedative is given to prevent vomiting. If segments of *T. solium* are regurgitated, eggs released by their digestion may lead to cysticercosis. A duodenal tube is inserted and through it the atabrine, suspended in water, is administered, for children weighing 100 lb or more 1 Gm, those weighing 40 to 75 lb 0.5 Gm. Wash down with additional water. If given orally divide the dose and give the tablets at 10-minute intervals not to exceed 30 minutes. Two hours later give a saline purge. Withhold food until bowels move then resume normal diet. During the subsequent 48 to 72 hours all stools should be saved and examined for the scolex. Ultimate proof of cure is lack of eggs or segments in the stool 4 to 6 months after treatment.

EXTRAINTESTINAL LARVAL TAPEWORMS

Although not intestinal, the diseases caused by larval tapeworms are included here for continuity of subject.

CYSTICERCOSIS

Etiology   *Cysticercus cellulosae*, larval stage of *T. solium*, is the agent.

Mode of acquisition   The cysticercus stage of *T. solium*, normally confined to the pig, may develop in man following ingestion of eggs. The source may be extraneous or if the child harbors an adult *T. solium* either via the anus-to-mouth route or by retroperistalsis of gravid segments.

Clinical features The cysticerci, frequently numerous, mature in from 7 to 10 weeks, when they vary in size from 4 to 20 mm. They remain viable for up to 6 years. The bladder worms have a propensity for voluntary muscles, connective tissues, and the central nervous system, although any tissue or organ may be involved. A fibrous capsule forms around the cysts except in the racemosus type. Symptomatology is related to the number, site, and age of the cysts. Often there are no symptoms during the early phases although muscle pain, headache, epileptic seizures, and other disturbances related to the central nervous system may occur. The central nervous system symptoms frequently follow the death and degeneration of the cysts. Palpable subcutaneous cysts or nodules occur.

Diagnosis

1. Palpation of a nodule, its removal, and microscopic examination for the typical single scolex.
2. X-ray of the musculature. The cysts are not visible prior to calcification.
3. Suspicion of cysticercosis in an older child who suffers epileptic attacks and is from an endemic area.
4. Encephalography and studies of visual functions.

Treatment There is no specific treatment. Anticonvulsant therapy in cases of cerebral cysticercosis is beneficial.

ECHINOCOCCOSIS, HYDATID DISEASE

Etiology The hydatid cyst stage of *Echinococcus granulosus* is the etiologic agent.

Mode of acquisition Dogs and other canines are the definitive hosts of this worm, which they acquire through ingestion of cyst-containing viscera of sheep and other herbivores, the normal intermediate hosts. Eggs are passed in the feces of the definitive host. Children become infected by accidentally swallowing eggs either while fondling an infected dog or from a contaminated source.

Clinical features Hydatid cysts may develop in any tissue or organ but are primarily found in the liver, secondarily in the lungs. The symptoms depend upon the age, size, and location of the cyst. The cysts are of three types: (1) unilocular, the most common; (2) osseous; (3) alveolar or multilocular of *E. multilocularis* origin involving wild carnivores and rodents. The latter type of cyst is not confined and behaves like a neoplasm. The unilocular cyst, consisting of two membranes, brood capsules, scolices, and hydatid fluid, becomes surrounded by compressed host adventitia. The cyst grows slowly, reaching a diameter of 1 cm in 5 months. Its future enlargement depends upon its location. Liver, lung, and abdominal cysts are frequently latent, being discovered only upon routine examination for other conditions. Cysts present in areas of confinement, brain, orbit, and spinal cord become manifest at a much earlier stage. Such cysts seldom occur singly; hepatic and/or pulmonary cysts are usually also present. Trauma to a cyst results in rupture with spillage of scolices (hydatid sand) and proteinaceous fluid. Allergic manifestations follow, their severity depending upon the site, speed, and extent of the leakage. Fatal anaphylactic shock may ensue, also dissemination via the released scolices.

Diagnosis

1. History of being in a sheep-raising endemic area and contact with infected dog.
2. Casoni intradermal test is positive in 85 to 90 percent of cases.
3. Complement-fixation test is useful in detection of living cysts.
4. Hemagglutination, Bentonite-flocculation, and Latex slide agglutination tests are also sensitive tests, useful in the differential diagnosis.
5. Radiologic examination, photoscan of the liver.
6. Definitive diagnosis is made by finding scolices, hooklets, and membrane fragments from a surgically removed cyst or one that has been infiltrated with hypertonic saline. Diagnostic aspiration should not be done because of anaphylaxis and seeding probabilities. Sputum and urine may contain hydated materials from a ruptured cyst.
7. Eosinophil count may be elevated or normal.

Treatment   Treatment consists of surgical removal of the intact cyst after a portion of the wall has been frozen and the cyst infiltrated with hydrogen peroxide, Lugol's iodine, or hypertonic saline.

Sparganosis and coenurus disease are additional, rarely found, larval cestode diseases of man.

SCHISTOSOMIASIS (BILHARZIASIS)

Etiology   *Schistosoma mansoni,* the blood fluke, is the agent.

Mode of acquisition   Acquisition is by penetration of intact skin or oral mucous membranes by free-swimming cercariae. The cercarial larvae are then carried via the bloodstream to the heart and lungs thence via the systemic circulation to the portal system where they mature, finally settling in the radicles of the inferior mesenteric veins. Cycle requires from 4 to 6 weeks.

Clinical features   There are three clinical phases in intestinal schistosomiasis; each reflects the host's immunologic response to the developmental stages of the blood fluke.

1. Cercarial dermatitis. As the cercariae penetrate the skin there is a pricking sensation; pruritic papules develop and persist for 2 to 3 days, longer in previously sensitized individuals.
2. Larval development, toxic and allergic phase, occurs during the subsequent 3 to 6 weeks. Antibodies formed in response to worm antigens, and subsequently to egg antigens, complex, exciting diverse host responses. These include urticaria, abdominal pain, fever, enlarged tender liver, splenomegaly, leukocytosis, and eosinophilia of 15 to 30 percent. With the maturation of the worms and their migration into the tributaries of the inferior mesenteric veins, egg production begins and continues for the life of the worms, up to 20 years. It is the eggs that are responsible for most of the ensuing pathology. Some of the eggs escape in the feces, many others become trapped in the intestinal mucosa and its lymph glands, the liver, and other tissues. Granulomata form around the eggs; ulceration, thrombosis of small blood vessels, and thickening and fibrosis of surrounding tissue follows.
3. Late manifestations. These begin within 1 year in heavy, later in light infections. During this period hepatic fibrosis, portal hypertension, Banti's syndrome, esophageal varices, nervous disorders, cor pulmonale, and hemoptysis may develop. The number of worms, sites of egg localization, host response, and magnitude and duration of the infection all govern the extent to which the above syndromes develop.

Diagnosis

1. Finding of lateral spined eggs in the feces, either by direct microscopic examination or following water sedimentation or other concentration techniques, or in saline squash preparations of a rectal biopsy establishes diagnosis. In chronic cases or in light infections it is often necessary to examine repeated stool specimens.
2. Physical findings and history of being in an endemic area.
3. Serologic tests are helpful aids but because of cross-reactions with other parasites are of limited diagnostic value.
4. Sigmoidoscopy, barium enema, splenoportography, and esophagoscopy aid in evaluating the extent of the disease and in the differential diagnosis.

Treatment

1. Lucanthone (Nilodin, miracil D) orally, 15 mg per kg per day in three divided doses (maximum dosage, 1 Gm per day) for 7 days. Vomiting, abdominal pain, or disturbance of cerebral function requires reduction of dosage or suspension of therapy. Yellow discoloration of the skin may occur, but it will disappear 3 to 4 weeks after therapy is discontinued. This is the drug of choice for children, but it should not be given to those more than 16 years of age because of the frequent occurrence of severe central nervous

symptoms in this age group. Following successful treatment, eggs may be found in stools for a period of 2 months and in tissue from rectal biopsy for 3 to 6 months.

2. Niridazole (Ambilhar) orally, 25 mg per kg daily in two divided doses, at meal times, for 7 days. During therapy the urine may be dark brown. Caution should be exercised in giving the drug to children with marked liver involvement or history of epilepsy and psychosis. Side effects include headache, dizziness, vomiting, mental confusion, and electrocardiographic changes.

3. Stibophen (Fuadin) intramuscularly, 1 ml per 9 kg three times a week for 20 doses. (The initial dose is divided and given on two successive days, one-third the first day and two-thirds the second day as a test for idiosyncrasy.) Increasing albuminuria, recurrent vomiting, symmetric skin eruption, cardiac abnormality, purpura, or severe intercurrent infection precludes further therapy.

4. Sodium antimony dimercaptosuccinate (Astiban) intramuscularly, 10 mg per kg dose on alternate days for a total of five doses. The drug is cardiotoxic and is therefore better administered when the child is resting in a hospital. In addition to tachycardia there may be nausea, vomiting, headache, urticaria, and generalized muscle pain. Although both stibophen and sodium antimony dimercapto-succinate are effective schistosomaticides, the serious side effects which they may produce and their painful intramuscular injection make their usage less advantageous in the treatment of children than does that of either lucanthone or niridazole.

5. Surgery and specific chemotherapy may be required in cases presenting with marked hepatic damage and other late manifestations of severe or chronic schistosomiasis.

6. Extracorporeal filtration of *S. mansoni* worms has been carried out in selected patients during local anesthesia. Worms are trapped as portal blood is filtered via umbilical vein catheterization.

7. Assessment of treatment should include periodic stool examinations over the subsequent 6 months to search for living eggs. If found, treatment may need to be reinstituted.

In addition to *S. mansoni*, other flukes such as *S. japonicum, Fasciolopsis buski, Heterophyes heterophyes, Metagonimus yokogawai,* and others may be responsible for intestinal trematodiasis.

AMEBIASIS

Etiology   *Entamoeba histolytica* is the etiologic agent.

Mode of acquisition   Ingestion of cysts via fecally contaminated water or food, fecal-oral transmission and in crowded institutions, via child-to-child contact are all modes of acquisition.

Clinical features The prepatent period varies from a few weeks to several months. It is influenced by the size of the infecting dose, invasiveness of the strain, the diet, stress factors, gut conditions, and the incidence of prior exposure of the child. *E. histolytica* initially parasitizes the colon. The ensuing symptomatology is extremely variable and is directly related to the ability of the amebas to colonize and invade the intestinal wall and to the host's defense reactions. The infection may be acute and chronic. Following ingestion and excystation of the cysts, the resultant motile trophozoites multiply. If unable to colonize, the trophozoites round up in the lumen, become cysts, and can be found in the feces. The infection may terminate, or the commensal carrier state becomes established. The child will continue to pass infective cysts which are of potential hazard to himself and others, but is otherwise asymptomatic. The preponderance of infections in temperate climates are of this type.

When colonic colonization is successful, microabscesses are formed. The amebas may lyse through from the mucosa to the submucosa and spread radically, creating the characteristic flask-shaped ulcers. Erosion of blood vessels initiates bleeding and the possibility of extraintestinal dissemination. Frequently the ulcers become secondarily infected, adding to the pain and discomfort of the dysentery. Fusion of the ulcers may result in severe necrosis and sloughing. The clinical expression reflects the extent and duration of the pathology and the sites involved.

In chronic amebic colitis there are episodes of diarrhea, with or without blood and mucus, alternating with constipation, mild abdominal discomfort (lower right quadrant), slight weight loss, and malaise. The liver is enlarged and tender, reflecting a toxic response to the colonic infection or to actual hepatic infection. Extraintestinal amebic abscesses, e.g., liver, are seldom encountered in children.

Acute dysenteric attacks may be precipitated by concurrent disease and other stressful situations. The onset is abrupt, with 15 or more explosive watery stools containing trophozoites, blood, mucus, flecks of fecal material, and minimal or no cellular exudate (the latter in contrast to bacillary dysentery). Abdominal cramping, chills, fever, dehydration, and prostration are common. The attack may end fatally particularly in infants. Intestinal hemorrhages, perforation, and peritonitis are rare complications. Less severe attacks generally last for several days or weeks and then spontaneously subside. If neglected, the attacks recur, and chronic ulcerative amebic colitis gradually develops over a period of years.

Diagnosis

1. Demonstration of either trophozoites in the acute dysenteric stool or cysts in the remission or formed stool establishes diagnosis. Unformed stools should be examined promptly as trophozoites quickly die and become distorted and difficult to identify. If this is not possible, specimen should be immediately placed in preserva-

tive. Differentiation must be made from other intestinal amebas, *E. hartmanni, E. coli, Iodamoeba, Endolimax,* and *Dientamoeba.*
2. Saline purgation may be useful for the detection of trophozoites in suspected cases in which cysts have not been revealed in formed stools.
3. Saline preparations of specimens obtained at sigmoidoscopy. Trophozoites must be differentiated from tissue cells.
4. Character of the dysenteric stool, acidic, scanty cellular exudate, blood and degenerate erythrocytes, Charcot-Leyden crystals and amebas.
5. In vitro culture of microscopically negative stools.
6. Immunologic tests, fluorescent-antibody, indirect hemagglutination, and gel-diffusion precipitin tests are useful aids both in intestinal and hepatic amebiasis.
7. Sigmoidoscopic examination for the presence of lesions.

Treatment   Therapy in amebiasis must be directed against amebas dwelling both in the tissue and in the lumen of the intestine, taking into consideration the severity of the disease and the child's general condition. More than one course of therapy using different drugs alone or in combination, amebicides and antibiotics, may be necessary to effect a cure.

1. Diidohydroxyquin (Diodoquin) for 20 days: for children weighing less than 20 kg, 0.32 Gm three times a day; to those weighing 20 to 40 kg, 0.65 Gm twice a day; to those weighing over 40 kg, 0.65 Gm three times a day. Contraindications, iodine sensitivity and liver damage. Cure rate is seldom 100 percent, therefore a second course of therapy with tetracycline is advisable.
2. Tetracycline, 25 to 50 mg per kg daily divided into 4 doses for 10 days; maximum daily dose, 2 Gm.

For severe colitis (dysentery) only:

1. Emetine hydrochloride: 1 mg per kg per day, subcutaneously (deep) in two divided doses (maximum dose 65 mg), until the frequency of stools is reduced to three or four per day, maximum duration 5 days. Bed rest, and because of cardiotoxicity, it is advisable to frequently monitor the pulse and blood pressure. If secondary infection causes persistent dysentery, tetracycline is used and followed by a course of Diodoquin.
3. Metronidazole (Flagyl), 750 mg three times a day for 10 days, is effective against hepatic and acute intestinal amebiasis, but side effects occur and include nausea, vomiting, rash, headache, weakness, vertigo, furry tongue, metallic taste, and not infrequently leukopenia.

Evaluation of cure   Three successive stools should be examined at the end of treatment, repeated 2 weeks later and, following clinical recovery, periodically repeated for a period of 1 year or whenever symptoms require. Sigmoidoscopy is additionally of value. If amebas are again found in the stool, check for sources of reinfection and reinstitute therapy.

Prognosis   In mild cases, 90 percent are cured by one course of therapy. (A cure is effected if the patient is asymptomatic for 1 year and has three negative stools after purging.) Even when a cure is not accomplished, symptomatic control is always possible with repeated therapy.

GIARDIASIS (Lambliasis)

Etiology   The agent is *Giardia lamblia*.

Mode of acquisition   The protozoan is acquired by ingestion of cysts in food and water contaminated with sewage, via food handlers or flies, and by hand to mouth.

Clinical features   The trophozoites live attached to the mucosa of the duodenum. Occasionally they may be present at lower levels of the small intestine, and in the gallbladder and bile ducts. Altered absorption of vitamin A and fats has been attributed to their presence. Children are more frequently infected than adults. It is not uncommon to encounter minor sporadic outbreaks among institutionalized children. Infections may be acute or chronic, asymptomatic or present with a celiac-like syndrome.

Celiac syndrome, colicky abdominal pain, abdominal distension, anorexia, nervousness, weight loss, and vomiting characterize heavy infections. Mild infections present with a history of intermittent watery diarrhea (with a moist sand appearance) and malaise.

Diagnosis   Diagnosis is established by finding cysts in formed stools and trophozoites and cysts in diarrheic specimens. Rarely it may be necessary to examine duodenal contents.

Treatment   Because of the possibility of household transmission and reinfection, all infected members of the family or household should be treated.

1.   Atabrine dihydrochloride, supplied in 0.5 and 0.1 Gm, plain, not sugar-coated tablets, is administered as follows: to children less than 4 years of age, 0.05 Gm twice daily for 5 days; to those be-

tween 4 and 8 years of age, 0.1 Gm twice daily; to those over 8 years of age, 0.1 Gm three times daily for 5 days.

2. Metronidazole (Flagyl) is administered as follows: to children less than 2 years of age, 125 mg daily for 5 days; to those between 2 and 4 years of age, 250 mg daily for 5 days; 4 to 8 years, 375 mg daily for 5 days; and over 9 years, 500 mg daily for 5 days. For side effects see under Amebiasis above.

Because of the relatively high incidence of relapse, as well as of reinfection, treatment may have to be repeated.

BALANTIDIASIS

Balantidium coli, the causative ciliated protozoan, parasitizes the large intestine in the same areas as *E. histolytica.* It is a common parasite of hogs and monkeys in warm climates. The disease in man is rarely encountered in temperate climates. It may simulate amebiasis, causing variable symptomatology. Tetracyclines are effective in treatment against this parasite.

REVIEW QUESTIONS

1. The following statements concerning colic are true except for one: (*a*) occurs most frequently in the first 3 to 6 months of life; (*b*) there is probably no single etiology; (*c*) antispasmodics and sedatives are usually helpful in eliminating the symptoms; (*d*) colic is found mainly in the hypertonic infant.
2. In the following question, column I lists symptoms involving the gastrointestinal tract and column II contains statements related to these symptoms. Match the two columns.

I	II
A. Vomiting in infancy _____	(*a*) 90 percent of cases occurs in males
B. Cyclic vomiting _____	(*b*) May be due to milk allergy
C. Constipation _____	(*c*) Usually occurs in children 3 to 7 years of age
D. Congenital aganglionic megacolon _____	(*d*) Riley-Day syndrome

3. The following are noted in Hirschsprung's disease except for (*a*) in the affected newborn there may be no meconium passed; (*b*) there is a familial incidence; (*c*) in some cases profuse watery diarrhea occurs; (*d*) abdominal pain usually is present; (*e*) the entire colon may be involved.
4. In celiac disease the typical curve following an intravenous glucose-tolerance test is (*a*) flat; (*b*) normal; (*c*) elevated; (*d*) biphasic.
5. The following statements about celiac syndrome are true except for one: (*a*) chronic intestinal infection with *Giardia lamblia;* (*b*) extensive surgical

resection of the small bowel; (c) an elevated serum-albumin level; (d) ingestion of gluten.

6. The following statements concerning celiac syndrome are true except for (a) abdominal pain and vomiting are common; (b) gastrointestinal mucosal pattern abnormalities found in the ileum; (c) total cholesterol level is usually low; (d) dried stool of a patient on a normal diet contains 30 to 60 percent fat.

7. Column I contains tests used in the diagnosis of celiac syndrome; column II contains some statements concerning these tests. Match the two:

I	II
A. Vitamin A–tolerance test _____	(a) Marked increase in fecal fat
B. Administration of oral gluten _____	(b) Rise of less than 50 micrograms per 100 ml
C. Loading dose of lactose, starch, maltose, and sucrose _____	(c) Rise in blood glucose
D. Small intestine biopsy _____	(d) Increase in plasma cells

8. The following statements regarding cystic fibrosis of the pancreas are true except for one: (a) vitamin A absorption is poor; (b) the xylose-tolerance test is normal; (c) intestinal obstruction may occur at any age; (d) sweat electrolyte levels are low.

9. The following statements concerning chronic ulcerative colitis are true except for one: (a) leukopenia is common; (b) barium enema shows "lead pipe" appearance; (c) serum albumin-globulin ratio may be reversed; (d) there is a high incidence of malignant changes in cases that persist into adulthood; (e) it may be associated with joint pains.

10. A specific index of hepatocellular injury can be best obtained by determining the level of: (a) SGOT; (b) SGPT; (c) both are of equal usefulness.

11. Column I lists several liver function tests; column II contains some statements concerning these tests in severe liver disease. Match the two:

I	II
A. Alkaline phosphatase _____	(a) Do not perform in the presence of jaundice
B. Bromsulphalein dye excretion _____	(b) Elevated curve
C. Ammonia fixation _____	(c) Normal or slightly elevated in hepatitis
D. Carbohydrate metabolism _____	(d) More than 50 mg per ml

12. Jaundice usually becomes manifest when the plasma bilirubin level is (a) 0.2 mg; (b) 0.8 mg; (c) 1 mg; (d) 2 mg per 100 ml.

13. Column I lists various tests used in jaundice; column II lists some statements regarding the results of these tests in obstructive jaundice. Match the two:

I	II
A. Urine bilirubin _____	(a) Decreased
B. Urine urobilin _____	(b) No change
C. Stool bilirubin _____	(c) Absent
D. Stool urobilin _____	(d) Elevated
E. Alkaline phosphatase _____	(e) Present

14. All the following statements concerning viral hepatitis of the HA form are true except: (*a*) incubation period is about 1 month; (*b*) occurs in all age groups; (*c*) virus can be detected in the stools during the incubation period and early in the disease; (*d*) there is a secondary rise in urobilin levels with recovery.

15. In cases of polyparasitism it is advisable to treat first for (*a*) ascaris; (*b*) hookworm; (*c*) trichuris; (*d*) strongyloides.

16. Pinworms may cause any of the following except (*a*) rectal itching; (*b*) vaginitis; (*c*) insomnia; (*d*) appendicitis; (*e*) vomiting.

17. Chronic amebic colitis is characterized by all the following except (*a*) bloody stools; (*b*) constipation; (*c*) hepatomegaly; (*d*) amebic abscess of the spleen.

18

SURGICAL CONDITIONS OF THE ABDOMEN

THE PERINATAL PERIOD

Abdominal surgery in the perinatal period is primarily focused on the correction of congenital anomalies. These disorders may exhibit a variety of symptoms and signs: respiratory distress, vomiting (especially if bile-stained), copious frothy sputum, jaundice, abdominal distension or masses, scaphoid abdomen, failure to pass meconium or urine, gastrointestinal bleeding, and umbilical abnormalities.

Early diagnosis is essential to success in the treatment of many of these congenital conditions. The clinician should be aware of certain telltale clues even before the birth of the infant.

Preoperative preparation

1. Intravenous catheter to administer blood and replace fluid and electrolytes.
2. Nasogastric tube to keep stomach empty.
3. Tracheal suction as needed.
4. Preoperative medication: only atropine or scopolamine is needed in newborn infants. From 6 months to 1 year, a barbiturate, e.g., pentobarbital, may be added, and over 1 year of age, morphine or Demerol has an excellent pacifying effect.
5. Temperature regulation: the proportionally greater surface area of an infant may produce rapid drops of body temperature, increased oxygen requirement, and more rapid fluid exchange. High fever should be reduced by cool sponging, an aspirin suppository, or the hypothermia blanket.

Intraoperative measures

1. Endotracheal intubation.
2. Frequent monitoring of vital signs—heart rate, blood pressure, and body temperature—is essential.
3. Blood in amounts to replace loss.
4. Assisted respiration as needed.

INTESTINAL OBSTRUCTIONS IN NEWBORN INFANTS

Meconium passage is rarely delayed beyond the twelfth hour of life. Such delay associated with a bout of vomiting should be investigated promptly. Even though other conditions such as brain damage, sepsis, and metabolic disturbances may cause vomiting, a mechanical or functional obstruction (paralytic ileus) of the gastrointestinal tract must be excluded. The physical signs will vary according to the level and completeness of the block. High obstructions are readily decompressed temporarily with early vomiting so that there is little abdominal distension, and, not infrequently, a delay in diagnosis. Obstructions below the midileum show generalized abdominal distension and a delay in vomiting. Stools are absent in complete obstructions and scanty in partial obstruction. The presence of normal meconium in the rectum does not exclude intestinal atresia since some atresias develop late in fetal life.

Air is the best and safest contrast medium to outline the level of obstruction by x-ray in a newborn. Normally gas reaches the rectum by about 12 hours of age. If the bowel is not outlined with gas, the stomach is aspirated and 50 ml of air is instilled. In 1 to 2 hours the air will progress down to the point of obstruction. Oral barium or other contrast media are usually unnecessary and only increase the difficulty in manipulating the fluid-laden intestine during surgery. When many loops of dilated bowel are generally distributed throughout the abdomen, it is usually impossible to distinguish small from large intestines. A contrast-medium enema is helpful in these instances to rule out the colon as the site of the trouble. A normal colon in a newborn infant with small-bowel obstruction appears as a narrow tube, the so-called "microcolon," because it has not yet been dilated with the passage of stool.

ESOPHAGEAL ATRESIA (See Chapter 12)

CONGENITAL DIAPHRAGMATIC HERNIA

Etiology   A variable number of abdominal organs gain access to the chest and may cause lethal respiratory distress with dramatic rapidity by compression of the lung and mediastinum. The defect is commonly located in the posterolateral part of the diaphragm where there is persistence of the pleuroperitoneal canal of Bochdalek. About 70 percent of hernias occur through the left diaphragm and 20 percent through the right, usually without a peritoneal sac. The remaining 10 percent occur either at the foramen of Morgagni (retrosternally) or through the esophageal hiatus. The latter types are not usually as severe or as dangerous as the Bochdalek variety.

Clinical features

1. Dyspnea.
2. Cyanosis.
3. Vomiting.
4. Absent breath sounds unilaterally with respiratory lag on one side.
5. The apex beat of the heart is shifted to the opposite side.
6. Bowel sounds are heard over the rib cage.
7. The abdomen is scaphoid.
8. Chest x-ray reveals intestinal loops outlined with gas situated in the thorax. The mediastinum is shifted to the opposite side.

Treatment   Reduction of the displaced abdominal organs, with repair of the diaphragmatic defect, is accomplished using the abdominal approach. Surgery is performed immediately after the diagnosis is established. No attempt is made to expand the compressed lung during the operation; it gradually returns to normal size.

The results are excellent except for those infants who have severe respiratory difficulty during the first 24 hours of life. For these infants the mortality rate is high, either because of hypoplasia of the lung or because of an inability to cope with the altered cardiorespiratory physiology.

CONGENITAL HYPERTROPHIC PYLORIC STENOSIS

The pyloric muscle fails to relax normally and hypertrophies, causing a progressive lengthening of the pyloric canal as seen on x-ray, and a partial obstruction.

Clinical features

1. More common in males (3.5:1) and in first-born infants. The symptoms usually begin in the second to third week, rarely as late as the second month. There is an increased familial incidence.
2. There is projectile vomiting directly after feeding, or often after several feedings have accumulated. The vomitus contains no bile. Hunger is constant in spite of the vomiting.
3. Constipation becomes progressively worse until there are no stools.
4. Gastric peristalsis is visible from left to right.
5. There is no weight gain but rather a loss.
6. There is an olive-sized, 2- to 3-cm, hard, smooth pyloric tumor in the region of the right costal margin and right rectus muscle, which is most palpable during a feeding or immediately after vomiting when the stomach is empty. When the stomach is distended, the mass is pushed toward the flank and toward the right lower quadrant of the abdomen.
7. Hypochloremic alkalosis may occur early because of loss of hydrochloric acid. Persistent vomiting, however, eventually leads to acidosis caused by the following factors—starvation and tissue destruction with increased production of acid metabolites; dehydration, hemoconcentration, and reduced kidney function with retention of acid metabolites; inflammatory reaction of the upper gastrointestinal tract with loss of all electrolytes (including fixed base) as a transudate.
8. Jaundice may be present.
9. If the above features are present, fluoroscopic and roentgenographic examinations are unnecessary to confirm the diagnosis. Contrast media ingestion reveals gastric retention, lengthened pyloric canal (string sign), and delayed pyloric opening time.
10. Gastric lavage will also reveal gastric retention, since ingested food can be recovered many hours after the last feeding.

Differential diagnosis

1. "Pylorospasm" may be difficult to differentiate. It occurs in hyperactive and hypertonic infants during the first week or two of life. Its cause is obscure, but it may be associated with an autonomic nerve imbalance. The vomiting is prominent, and there may be visible gastric peristalsis. None of the other criteria of pyloric stenosis is present. The infant with pylorospasm responds well

when given a quiet, placid environment and medical treatment as outlined below.

2. Achalasia (cardiospasm) is an uncommon condition causing an obstruction to the passage of food at the lower end of the esophagus probably due to an autonomic imbalance. The esophagus exhibits a characteristic abnormal muscle-contraction curve in balloon studies. Fluoroscopy following a barium meal demonstrates a dilated esophagus which funnels down to a narrowed area near the cardia. Repeated dilatations usually control the symptoms. More rarely, longitudinal surgical transection of the lower esophageal musculature may be required.

3. Cardioesophageal relaxation (chalasia) is another rare condition, caused by a temporary neuromuscular dysfunction, which produces repeated regurgitation (vomiting) in the newborn or young infant. Fluoroscopy following barium ingestion demonstrates reflux. Treatment consists in using a thickened formula and propping up the infant, especially after feedings.

4. Duodenal obstruction usually occurs below the ampulla of Vater, and the vomitus contains bile. If the obstruction is proximal to the ampulla, the clinical picture is similar to pyloric stenosis, except for the absence of a mass. The x-ray will reveal the characteristic "double-bubble" sign in which two dilated hollow viscera are seen in the upper abdomen, the stomach on the left and the dilated proximal duodenum on the right (see p. 456).

5. Intracranial lesions may cause projectile vomiting. (See Chapter 12, "Diseases of the Newborn.")

Medical treatment   A medical regimen may be tried if the diagnosis of pyloric stenosis is in doubt. Vomiting due to such causes as pylorospasm will usually respond.

1. The formula is thickened with cereal and fed through a nipple with the top cut off or by spoon.

2. Phenobarbital, ⅛ to ¼ gr (8 to 15 mg), 20 minutes before feedings is useful for sedation and also acts as an antispasmodic.

3. Gastric lavage with saline solution is performed one to several times a day before feedings.

4. Hydration and fluid balance can be maintained parenterally when necessary.

5. Atropine: a freshly prepared 1:1,000 solution can be started with one drop and increased drop by drop until signs of dry skin and mucous membranes, flushing, and dilation of pupils appear. This dosage or slightly less should relieve pylorospasm. (Atropine is not used too often because the margin of safety is small and the drug may be dangerously toxic in this age group.)

Surgical treatment When the diagnosis is definitely made, parenteral fluids and electrolytes are administered to correct any imbalance, and a Fredet-Ramstedt pyloromyotomy is performed. The hypertrophied pyloric muscle is split down to the mucosa so that the mucous membrane bulges to the level of the serosal surface. Inadvertent entrance into the duodenum is not a serious complication provided it is recognized at the time and closed.

Postoperatively a small glucose water feeding is begun after 4 to 6 hours, and the volume is increased as tolerated. Then half-strength formula is given and is gradually increased to full strength. Persistence of vomiting for several feedings may occur but has no significance. Where the duodenum was entered and closed, feeding is delayed and nasogastric suction is maintained for 24 hours.

DUODENAL OBSTRUCTIONS

The most common causes in newborn infants in order of frequency are

1. Malrotation with band formation
2. Duodenal atresia
3. Annular pancreas
4. Intrinsic webs

Malrotation Malrotation represents an arrest in rotation and absence of fixation of the mesentery to the posterior abdominal wall during early embryonic development. The entire small intestine hangs loosely from the superior mesenteric vessels, and the cecum is misplaced (lying at or near the right upper quadrant). Associated peritoneal bands which stretch from the cecum to the right lateral abdominal wall compress the duodenum, causing a complete or partial obstruction. Other adhesions may be present which attach the duodenojejunal junction in a kinked position. Volvulus of the small or large bowel may be present.

Duodenal atresia This denotes an intrinsic complete obliteration of the duodenal lumen. The dilated proximal bowel and the distal collapsed bowel may remain in continuity, lie entirely separated, or be connected by a fibrous cord. Several possible etiologies have been suggested but present evidence points to intrauterine gangrene and resorption of the developing bowel due to volvulus, intussusception or vascular accident.

Annular pancreas This is the result of the persistence of a portion of the ventral anlage of the pancreas which curves around the right side of the duodenum to fuse with the main body of the pancreas. It causes extrinsic, partial or complete obstruction at the descending duodenum.

Intrinsic webs   These webs are diaphragm-like partitions across the bowel lumen which have variable-sized central openings. A stenotic partial obstruction may become complete if the opening is blocked by edema or milk curds.

Clinical features of duodenal obstructions

1. The symptoms and signs are proportional to the completeness of the obstruction.
2. Vomiting is usually present early in life, within 24 hours in complete obstruction. The vomitus is bile-stained in over 90 percent of the cases.
3. Distension of the abdomen is absent. In fact, the abdomen is scaphoid in complete obstruction since no air or fluid has passed into the intestine. Sometimes gastric dilation may be noted in the left upper quadrant.
4. Dehydration and weight loss rapidly supervene.
5. Meconium passage is scant or absent. The stools are small, dry, and grayish white or green. In complete atresia, the meconium may contain squamous epithelial cells or lanugo hair (positive Farber test), which merely indicates that the bowel had a lumen at one time.
6. Jaundice may occur when the bile duct is constricted by an annular pancreas.
7. Bloody rectal discharge or hematemesis may forebode a volvulus associated with malrotation.
8. The "double-bubble" sign is demonstrated on an upright x-ray.
9. In most cases the intestinal obstruction becomes clinically apparent in the neonatal period. However, some infants go along for months or even years with only mild recurring pain, nausea, and vomiting, or a celiac syndrome-like picture.

Treatment   Obstructions due to malrotation are relieved by lysis of the peritoneal bands stretching across the duodenum. Adhesions around the duodenojejunal junction may require liberation. If present, an associated volvulus is untwisted. Nonviable bowel is resected, and bowel continuity is restored with an end-to-end anastomosis. (As much as 50 percent or more of the small intestine may be removed without permanent nutritional impairment.) The appendix is usually removed since acute appendicitis would present with left-upper-quadrant pain and may be misdiagnosed by another unsuspecting surgeon.

The blocked section of duodenum in atresia, internal web, and annular pancreas is left undisturbed, and intestinal continuity is restored by a side-to-side duodenoduodenostomy or duodenojejunostomy.

Other anomalies frequently accompany congenital duodenal obstructions (esophageal atresia and Down's syndrome). The patency of the remainder of the intestinal tract should be verified during the operation to avoid overlooking other areas of atresia.

Serious postoperative complications are: (1) leak in the anastomosis causing peritonitis, (2) recurring obstruction due to adhesions requiring a second operation, (3) wound infection which may cause dehiscence, (4) pulmonary lesions secondary to aspiration.

JEJUNAL OBSTRUCTIONS

Atresia, intrinsic webs, and congenital bands are the more common anomalies causing obstruction at this level.

Clinical features

1. Bile-stained vomiting occurs early in high jejunal obstruction.
2. Abdominal distension is confined to the upper abdomen and may not be apparent when the bowel is decompressed by vomiting.
3. Absence of stools; some abnormal meconium may be passed.
4. Roentgenograms taken with the infant in the upright position demonstrate one or two dilated intestinal loops in addition to the stomach. There is absence of gas beyond the dilated loops when obstruction is complete.

Treatment   Intestinal continuity is restored by an end-to-end anastomosis of the blind ends of the bowel on either side of the atresic area. Resection of a segment of the greatly ballooned proximal end is advisable because of its weakened peristaltic potential. An internal web may occasionally be removed by simple enterotomy, removal of the web, and closure of the enterotomy site. Usually it is best to resect the webbed segment of bowel and perform an anastomosis.

ILEAL OBSTRUCTIONS

Ileal atresia   While intestinal stenosis is most frequent in the duodenum, the ileum is the most common site of atresia.

Clinical features
1. Vomiting of green material usually occurs within 12 to 36 hours after birth.
2. Abdominal distension may be marked.
3. Passage of meconium is absent; a scant amount of whitish mucoid material may be passed.
4. Roentgenograms of the abdomen with the infant in the upright position reveal many distended loops of bowel with fluid levels. In doubtful cases, a barium enema will rule out a colonic lesion as the cause of the obstruction.

Treatment   End-to-end anastomosis of the proximal and distal bowel is performed. Many surgeons prefer to do a temporary double-barrel enterostomy of the loops on either side of the atresia. The anastomosis is then performed 10 to 14 days later. This has the advantage of accomplishing immediate decompression with a lesser operation; it is most useful in those babies who are poor surgical risks or who are otherwise frail.

Meconium ileus   This is the form of intestinal obstruction that occurs in newborn infants with cystic fibrosis of the pancreas (see Chapter 17, "Gastrointestinal Diseases"). Because of a deficiency of pancreatic enzyme, pebblelike hard masses of tenacious meconium block the terminal ileum; the bowel proximal to this area is greatly dilated and filled with pasty meconium. Volvulus and gangrene of the dilated loops may occur, sometimes with perforation (this may occur in utero). (See Meconium Peritonitis, p. 462). The clinical picture is similar to that of ileal atresia. Features which support the diagnosis are:

1. Family history of cystic fibrosis of the pancreas.
2. Abnormally elevated sweat electrolyte levels are characteristic, if sweat is obtained by chemical stimulation. Hair or nail clippings also can be analyzed for sodium and chloride content.
3. The abdomen feels doughy and intestinal loops may be felt.
4. X-ray of the abdomen may show a soap-bubble granularity of the bowel contents. There is variation in the caliber of the dilated intestinal loops; one unusually large prominent loop is frequently noted.

Treatment   Gastrografin enema with reflux into the terminal ileum occasionally may be successful. If not, enterotomy with irrigation of the loop with pancreatic enzyme or a very dilute solution of hydrogen peroxide is usually effective. With the latter substance, the anesthesiologist must be informed so that in the rare event of air embolism, proper measures can be taken. If this fails, the blocked terminal ileum together with the meconium-laden loop above it is resected. The remaining bowel may be either anastomosed or brought out as a double enterostomy. The latter has the advantage of immediate decompression and provides a route for the instillation of pancreatic enzyme to soften the residual meconium.

COLONIC OBSTRUCTIONS

Congenital megacolon   (See Chapter 17, "Gastrointestinal Disease") This is a congenital agenesis of the myenteric parasympathetic nerve ganglia in a segment of intestine extending proximally from the anus for a varying distance. The large majority of cases occur in males, and there is a 20 percent chance of occurrence in another male sib. The condition has an increased incidence in Down's syndrome.

Most infants with this disease have delayed passage of meconium. Rectal examination reveals an empty ampulla, and it is frequently followed by a rush of gas and meconium with relief of distension which may preclude radiologic demonstration of typical findings. This may be followed by an asymptomatic period which is deceptive. However, careful observation shows continued abnormality of bowel movements with constipation and at times paradoxical diarrhea. Barium studies do not show distended colon before 18 days to 5 weeks, but there is delayed emptying with even distribution of barium throughout the colon at 24 hours. Rectal biopsy showing no ganglion cells confirms the diagnosis.

Treatment   Daily gentle saline irrigations are used to keep the bowel decompressed. These must be done with a large (22 French) rubber rectal tube, very gently by an experienced physician, since colon perforation may occur. Definitive surgery to correct the defect may be carried out when the child is stable; however, this repair may be delayed until the child is 6 months to 1 year of age and pelvic structures are larger. In this event, temporary colostomy is performed at the most distal ganglionic area of the colon.

Atresia of the colon   This rare anomaly is diagnosed following a barium enema and fluoroscopic examination. The proximal dilated colon is brought out as a colostomy. Colonic continuity is restored at a later date.

MALFORMATION OF THE ANUS AND RECTUM

Diagnosis is usually apparent if rectal examination is routinely performed in all newborn infants. There are four types:

Type I   Stenosis of anus or rectum. The diagnosis is evident on digital examination. Symptoms appear soon after birth or not until months later, depending on the severity of the stricture. Distended abdomen, fecal impaction, and secondary megacolon may develop.

Treatment   Gentle daily dilatations usually establish normal function. Very narrow stenosis may require a plastic procedure.

Type II   Imperforate anus due to a membrane. The membrane may be discolored by the meconium which fills the rectum.

Treatment   The membrane is easily incised or excised. This is followed by anal dilatation until bowel function is normal. The prognosis is excellent.

Type III   Imperforate anus with the rectal pouch ending blindly a variable distance above the anus (80 percent or more are of this type). Most patients have associated fistulous tracts between the proximal rectum and the genitourinary system or the perineum. In the female, the fistula leads to the vagina (commonly at the fourchette) or the perineum. Since it is usually large enough to permit evacuation of stool, most females do not require immediate surgery. In the male, the fistula which enters the urethra, bladder, or perineum is usually small, and intestinal obstruction may develop rapidly.

Diagnosis Physical examination reveals absence of the anal opening. Presence of a fistula opening into the perineum or fourchette is evidence of a lesion below the levator sling. If meconium is passed from the vagina, a catheter should be inserted and Gastrografin injected under fluoroscopy to attempt to outline the fistula and locate the rectal pouch.

If no physical evidence of a fistula is found, a high lesion may be present. In the male, urinalysis will demonstrate the presence of meconium with rectourethral or rectovesical fistula. Catheterization and injection of Gastrografin is performed to give the surgeon as much information as possible concerning the location of the rectal pouch and fistula if present.

Finally, an x-ray is made with the infant upside down. If the air outlining the rectal pouch is below the pubococcygeal line, the rectum has penetrated the levator sling. If the rectal pouch appears above this level, a high imperforate anus may be present. If air does not reach the most distal rectum due to the presence of meconium, the x-ray may be incorrectly interpreted as demonstrating a high lesion. Thus, all above methods of diagnosis must be used to determine the level of the rectum before deciding upon colostomy or perineal proctoplasty. If in doubt, decompressing colostomy is preferred, since repeated surgery in the anal area destroys chances for anatomic reconstruction.

Treatment If the blind pouch ends below a line drawn from the tip of the coccyx to the symphysis pubis, it has theoretically penetrated the levator sling and can be repaired by anoproctoplasty from below.

If the pouch ends above the levator sling an abdominoperineal procedure is required. It is generally wise to perform immediate colostomy with definitive surgery deferred 6 months to 1 year at which time the infant is larger and stronger, especially in the presence of prematurity or other life-threatening anomalies. Later abdominoperineal proctoplasty is performed to provide normal anal function.

Type IV Atresia of the mid or upper rectum. A normal anus and rectal ampulla end blindly several centimeters above the perineum. Proximal to this lies the blind end of the rectosigmoid. This rare anomaly is discovered by a digital examination which reveals a complete block within reach of the little finger. An abdominoperineal approach is necessary for correction by anastomosis.

Meconium plug syndrome The distal colon is filled with inspissated meconium. There is lower intestinal obstruction with failure to pass meconium, abdominal distension, and vomiting. A rectal examination or enema may stimulate a bowel evacuation with total relief of the obstruction. There is no associated cystic fibrosis of the pancreas, although the altered character of the meconium suggests some pancreatic deficiency. Fluoroscopy following a barium enema reveals a distal ribbonlike unused colon. The characteristic distinguishing this condition from congenital megacolon is the return to normal intestinal function following the removal of the meconium plug.

MECONIUM PERITONITIS

This is a serious complication of intrauterine perforation of the gastrointestinal tract with leakage of sterile meconium into the peritoneal cavity. The perforation, which may be associated with meconium ileus, atresias, volvulus, etc., is often sealed off. Dense adhesions containing calcium deposits form between matted loops of bowel. The infant appears very ill with a weak cry, tachypnea, and tensely distended abdomen often with a somewhat red-violet discoloration of the skin. Roentgenograms of the abdomen reveal distended loops of bowel and calcific plaques in most cases.

Treatment   All entrapped bowel including the distended loop proximal to the obstruction is resected, and end-to-end anastomosis is performed. About one-third of the patients will survive.

OMPHALOCELE AND GASTROSCHISIS
(See Chapter 12, "Diseases of the Newborn")

Omphalocele is a variable-sized defect of the abdominal wall and umbilicus, covered by a thin sac consisting of amnion externally and peritoneum internally. This sac may rupture in utero or at any time during or after parturition. Most of these infants also have intestinal malrotation and about half have other serious congenital anomalies.

Gastroschisis is a defect in the abdominal wall lateral to the umbilicus, usually on the right. There is no covering membrane, and coexistence of other serious anomalies is uncommon. However, malrotation and poor bowel fixation due to abnormal mesentery is frequently found.

Treatment   If there is an intact sac covering the peritoneal cavity (unruptured omphalocele), treatment consists of application of local antiseptic solution and daily dressings. (In large defects, mercurochrome application carries the risk of mercury poisoning.) An eschar forms, and in about 8 to 10 weeks skin grows from the periphery to cover the defect. Growth of the child and contracture of the scar often results in a relatively small ventral hernia which may be repaired at about 1 year of age.

When the sac is ruptured, or if the abdominal contents have no covering, as in gastroschisis, the prognosis is poor, with death occurring in about 40 percent of cases. Dacron mesh coated with silastic to prevent adhesions (Silon) may be used to cover the defect, with gradual tightening and replacement of intestinal contents over a period of 14 to 16 days.

Another alternative, the Gross method, frees skin down to the flanks and provides immediate coverage with later repair of the ventral hernia. This procedure is limited by the amount of skin available to close the defect, and in the past infants have succumbed because of too tight a closure.

In both these conditions infection and intercurrent intestinal complications such as volvulus or duodenal obstruction may occur. These require medical treatment or surgical intervention. In the case of the unruptured omphalocele, the sac is removed and further treatment is by Silon mesh or skin closure as described above.

INTESTINAL OBSTRUCTIONS IN THE OLDER CHILD

CONGENITAL ANOMALIES

Intraabdominal anomalies, e.g., malrotation, annular pancreas, intestinal stenosis, internal hernia, congenital bands, present at birth will often be clinically inapparent for months or years. Others may exhibit signs and symptoms of a partial intestinal obstruction with intermittent bilious vomiting and recurrent crampy abdominal pain. The diagnosis is frequently delayed by assuming the vomiting to be due to allergy, gastritis, cyclic vomiting, emotional disturbances, etc. The obstruction may become complete as a result of plugging of a stenotic area, volvulus, or constriction of a congenital band.

The diagnosis of a partial obstruction is made by x-ray examination using contrast medium orally or by barium enema to disclose the site of the pathology.

ACQUIRED INTESTINAL OBSTRUCTIONS

Intussusception   Intussusception is an invagination of a length of bowel into an adjacent portion of bowel, telescope fashion. Eighty percent of the cases occur in the first year of life, most commonly from the fifth to the ninth month; it is more common in males.

Etiology   Diarrhea, constipation, cathartics, upper respiratory infections, gastrointestinal allergy, and increased mobility of the colon may play a role in the cause. Anatomic causes such as Meckel's diverticulum, intestinal polyp or tumor, and bowel duplication are the focal stimuli for intussusception in a small number of cases in infancy; they are responsible for the majority of the cases which occur after the age of 3 years.

Types of intussusception   The most common type, occurring in 95 percent or more of the cases, begins at or near the ileocecal valve (ileocecal or ileocecocolic). In a few cases intussusception occurs in the small bowel (enteroenteral); the least common variety is localized to the colon (colocolic).

Clinical features

1. Severe spasmodic pain, explosive in onset, frequently with vomiting, occurs in a previously sturdy infant. The infant looks startled, the thighs are often flexed, and as the pain recedes, the patient lies limp, pale, and sweaty.
2. Currant-jelly stools characteristically appear a number of hours after onset.
3. A tender, sausage-shaped mass can usually be felt in the region of the ascending or transverse colon. The remainder of the abdomen is usually soft and not tender; the right lower quadrant may feel empty.
4. Rectal examination: bloody mucus will often be seen on the gloved finger. Occasionally the intussusception descends low enough to be felt rectally.
5. Roentgenogram: plain films reveal dilated loops of bowel. A barium enema demonstrates the coiled-spring appearance of the barium between the walls of the intussusception.
6. Abdominal distension, rigidity, fever, and toxicity suggest strangulation with gangrene.
7. The condition may occur in more than one member of a family.

Treatment   An attempt is made to reduce the intussusception by a barium enema administered with fluoroscopic control. Safety in controlling hydrostatic pressure is increased by not raising the enema bag more than 3 feet above the child. This measure is frequently successful in early cases. Any difficulty or failure of reduction by barium requires immediate laporotomy and manual reduction. The bowel must be inspected for evidence of gangrene or perforation.

Prognosis   Spontaneous relief occasionally occurs without any definitive treatment. The condition may recur even after surgical reduction. Mortality and morbidity are related to the time which elapses between onset and reduction of the intussusception. The prognosis is excellent under 12 hours, good from 12 to 24 hours, and grave if strangulation has occurred.

Adhesions   Previous abdominal surgery or peritoneal infection may result in adhesions which cause mechanical intestinal obstruction. Abdominal cramps, distension, and vomiting, combined with the history, indicate the diagnosis. Auscultation of the abdomen reveals hyperperistaltic bowel sounds. The temperature and leukocyte count are usually normal. X-ray of the abdomen taken in an upright position shows distended loops of bowel with air-fluid levels.

Treatment Lysis of adhesions is necessary before strangulation occurs.

Paralytic ileus Paralytic ileus is a condition of the intestinal tract characterized by a failure of propulsion of intestinal contents. It is always present for hours to days following major surgery on the pleural, intraperitoneal, or retroperitoneal organs. Peritonitis from any cause, e.g., appendicitis, ruptured viscus, is usually associated with paralytic ileus. Intra- or retroperitoneal bleeding, e.g., following trauma, or systemic toxic or debilitating disease, e.g., pneumonia, and electrolyte imbalance, especially hypokalemia, may be causes.

Clinical features
1. Abdominal pain is not as severe and is usually more constant than in mechanical obstruction.
2. Fever and leukocytosis are often present.
3. The abdomen is quiet on auscultation.

Treatment
1. The underlying cause is treated and general supportive measures, e.g., correction of fluid and electrolyte imbalance, are instituted.
2. No oral feedings are given, and a nasogastric tube is used with or without intermittent suction for decompression.

INTRAABDOMINAL INFECTIONS

ACUTE APPENDICITIS

Acute appendicitis is rare before the age of 1 and occasional in the second year, after which time it is the most common condition requiring abdominal surgery in childhood. Contrasted with an adult, the pediatric patient presents a more rapid and virulent course as well as unique problems in diagnosis.

Clinical and laboratory features

1. There is a sudden onset, usually with generalized abdominal pain at first, which within several to 24 hours becomes localized in the right lower quadrant.
2. Soon after the onset, nausea and vomiting occur. Constipation is much more frequent than diarrhea.
3. Temperature is only moderately elevated, usually well under 102°F (38.8°C).
4. The child appears ill and does not wish to move. The right thigh may be held in a flexed position.
5. Persistent tenderness in the right lower quadrant is the single most important factor in establishing the diagnosis. There may be accompanying hyperesthesia and muscle spasm in this area.

6. Rectal examination discloses a right-sided tender induration in cases of pelvic appendicitis or abscess.
7. The white cell count is frequently elevated up to 15,000; polymorphonuclear leukocytes predominate, with a shift to the left. A count over 20,000 in unperforated cases is unusual. The sedimentation rate may be normal.
8. X-ray of the abdomen may reveal a fecolith in the appendix.

Differential diagnosis   In children, constipation, the most common cause of abdominal pain, may mimic appendicitis, especially if accompanied by vomiting. Mesenteric adenitis, pneumonia (especially of the right lower lobe), rheumatic fever, pyelitis, gastroenteritis, gastrointestinal allergy, and abdominal epilepsy usually must be ruled out.

Treatment   Appendectomy is performed as soon as feasible. An appendical abscess is evacuated, and an appendectomy is attempted provided the appendix is easily accessible without extensive dissection and manipulation. When perforation is present, intestinal decompression (usually by nasogastric tube) is essential in the postoperative period. Antibiotics are given when perforation and/or abscess is present. They should be started preoperatively if perforation or abscess is suspected.

Prognosis   The prognosis is excellent when surgery is performed before perforation. When the diagnosis is presumptive, operation is preferred to observation, in order to avoid rupture.

PRIMARY PERITONITIS

This is a rare condition in infancy and early childhood which is often associated with upper respiratory infection, septicemia, or other intraabdominal infections. Streptococci or pneumococci are the usual organisms encountered.

Clinical features

1. Vomiting and high fever.
2. Diffuse abdominal tenderness and distension.
3. Diarrhea often occurs early, followed by constipation.
4. Leukocytosis (20,000 to 40,000) is an important diagnostic sign.
5. Blood culture is frequently positive.
6. Positive smear and culture of peritoneal exudate (paracentesis).

Treatment   Antibiotics are the treatment of choice. Exploratory laparotomy may be necessary when the diagnosis is uncertain.

Prognosis   The prognosis is good.

MESENTERIC ADENITIS

Acute mesenteric adenitis is a frequent cause of abdominal pain in children. It is usually associated with an upper respiratory infection.

Clinical features

1. History of preceding upper respiratory infection or tonsillitis; temperature rise occurs prior to the onset of abdominal pain. Vomiting may precede the pain.
2. Abdominal pain which is colicky and frequently generalized.
3. Temperature is often over 102°F (38.8°C) ; the sedimentation rate is moderately increased ; and there may be leukocytosis.
4. Localized abdominal signs may simulate those of appendicitis.

Treatment   Treatment is directed toward the upper respiratory infection when it is present. Laparotomy is performed when the physical findings suggest possible appendicitis.

CHOLECYSTITIS AND CHOLELITHIASIS

Biliary infection and gallstones are uncommon during childhood. The diagnosis is often difficult to make because these conditions are not suspected. Roentgenographic studies are helpful.

Acute cholecystitis is associated with extraintestinal infections, e.g., streptococci, staphylococci, or it may be secondary to intestinal involvement, e.g., colon-typhoid group. There may be abdominal pain and tenderness in the right upper abdomen. Surgery is usually not required and is considered only if there is no response to antibiotics or if the signs point to empyema of the gallbladder with impending rupture.

Cholelithiasis in children is usually manifested as a collection of pigmented stones secondary to increased blood destruction (e.g., hemolytic and sickle-cell anemias). These stones are not radiopaque unless some calcium is deposited. Cholesterol stones are occasionally seen in the older child.

Treatment   Cholecystectomy is the treatment. Choledochotomy may be required in addition in cases of obstructive jaundice or to remove stones from the extrahepatic bile ducts.

SUBPHRENIC ABSCESS

This is usually secondary to appendiceal and other intraabdominal infections or to a perforated viscus. There may be upper abdominal or shoulder pain, tenderness, and muscle spasm. Tenderness to percussion over the lower rib cage on the involved side is a valuable sign. There is continued or increased septic temperature and rapid pulse rate.

Roentgenograms and fluoroscopy reveal decreased motion of the diaphragm on the affected side, which is displaced upward ; the liver is displaced downward. A subdiaphragmatic air-fluid level may be seen. Lateral views are taken to aid in the localization of the abscess.

Treatment   The abscess is drained either via an anterior subcostal incision or through the bed of the 11th or 12th rib, depending on the site of the infection. Antibiotics are selected according to the causative organism.

Prognosis   The prognosis is good if the diagnosis is not unduly delayed.

GASTROINTESTINAL BLEEDING

Bleeding from the gastrointestinal tract can be conveniently divided by location (upper versus lower) and age (newborn or older child). During the newborn period, care must be taken to distinguish true bleeding from swallowed maternal blood. The Apt test makes use of the fact that fetal hemoglobin, unlike the adult type, is resistant to alkaline denaturation. In all cases, care must be taken to rule out hemorrhagic diatheses, e.g., hemorrhagic disease of the newborn, leukemia in an older child.

In general, gross hematemesis or blood obtained on nasogastric aspiration point to a lesion above the ligament of Treitz. There may be occult blood, gross blood (hematochezia), or altered blood (melena) in the stool, depending on the rapidity of bleeding. Red or maroon blood in stool in the absence of gross blood from nasogastric aspiration signifies that the lesion is below the ligament of Treitz.

Causes of gastrointestinal bleeding

    I.   In the newborn
        A. Lower
            1. Fissure in ano
            2. Volvulus
        B. Upper acute
            1. Peptic ulcer usually secondary to stress, e.g., sepsis
   II.   In the infant
        A. Lower
            1. Fissure in ano
            2. Meckel's diverticulum
            3. Intussusception
        B. Upper
            1. Acute peptic ulcer usually secondary to stress, e.g., burns, pneumonia, increased intracranial pressure
 III.   Child
        A. Lower
            1. Polyps

   2. Meckel's diverticulum
   3. Duplications
   4. Ulcerative colitis
B. Upper
   1. Eosophageal varices
   2. Chronic peptic ulcer

ANAL FISSURE

This is not an uncommon condition in the newborn period, and it continues to occur in older children as well. Bleeding is usually minimal, occurs with constipated bowel movements, and is smeared on the outside of the stool. The most important factor in diagnosis is careful examination of the anus with gentle eversion of its edges to reveal the tiny crack in the mucosa. Treatment with stool softeners is usually successful.

PEPTIC ULCER

Massive upper GI bleeding in a newborn infant is generally due to acute peptic ulcer. The etiology is unknown, although often associated with stress, and there is no correlation with later-occurring chronic ulcer disease.

Therapy consists of vitamin K (to rule out hemorrhagic disease of the newborn) followed by cold saline lavage and blood transfusions. This is carried out in a warm incubator to avoid undue chilling of the infant.

Loss of more than 1.5 blood volumes with no sign of cessation of bleeding requires surgical exploration. Usually a major vessel, such as the gastroduodenal artery, is found to be the source of the bleeding, and simple suture ligature suffices to stop it. Pyloroplasty may be performed for better drainage of the stomach following closure of the duodenum, but vagotomy is not usually done. Prognosis is good and recurrence is rare.

Peptic ulcer in the older child appears to be the same disease as found in adults, and many adults have histories extending to late childhood. Medical management is used except for uncontrollable hemorrhage or obstruction. In the latter, vagotomy and a drainage procedure are most commonly employed, although occasionally for mechanical reasons a partial gastrectomy is preferred. Nutrition is relatively unimpaired in most cases.

ESOPHAGEAL VARICES

After age 2 years, massive upper bleeding is probably most frequently due to portal hypertension with esophageal varices. Unlike adults, cirrhosis is a rare cause, and most children have portal vein thrombosis. For clinical and laboratory features, see page 429.

Definitive therapy by splenorenal or mesentericocaval shunt is delayed until adolescence if possible because of the larger size of the vessels and diminished danger of shunt thrombosis. Prognosis is improved if liver function is unimpaired. Overtransfusion during acute bleeding episodes should be avoided, since this apparently prolongs and even worsens hemorrhage. Patients with hermatocrit levels of 9 or 10 percent are often alert with warm, dry extremities and no signs of shock.

RECTAL AND COLONIC POLYPS

These growths in children begin to appear at about age 2 years and may be conveniently divided histologically into the very common juvenile or inflammatory and the rare, but much more dangerous, adenomatous (the latter associated with familial polyposis).

Small amounts of blood completely mixed with stool or occult blood per rectum should prompt a search for polyps if other causes, e.g., fissure in ano, Meckel's diverticulum, intussusception, have not been found. The polyps may protrude from the anus, be noted by proctoscopy, or appear on x-rays following barium enema. If they are within reach of the proctoscope, they are removed and submitted for pathologic interpretation. If seen by barium study, in absence of rectal adenomatous polyps or family history of polyposis, they are not removed since most slough spontaneously causing no further damage. The polyp may cause intussusception.

Adenomatous polyps of the colon or rectum are usually associated with familial polyposis. Malignant degeneration occurs after adolescence but has never been reported before age 10 years. Parents must be informed of the nature of this disease and the fact that it is transmitted genetically. A total colectomy preserving the rectal segment is the treatment of choice. Follow-up is required for life, with recurring rectal polyps being destroyed from below.

After age 14, the chances of carcinoma occurring in the rectal stump increase with age. The safest procedure to avoid this is to perform a rectal resection with permanent ileostomy. It is certainly wise to defer this mutilating operation, however, since procedures for removing rectal mucosa and preserving sphincter function eventually may prove practical and safe.

The rare Peutz-Jeghers syndrome is a familial condition in which polyps of the small intestine (occasionally of the colon, too) are accompanied by melanin spots on the lips, buccal mucosa, and sometimes the fingers. Conservative management is preferable. Surgery may become necessary for intussusception or prolonged and serious bleeding. Radical resections are avoided, if possible. Malignant degeneration is thought not to occur.

DUPLICATIONS OF THE ALIMENTARY CANAL

Duplications of the esophagus appear as cystic masses adjacent to the esophagus. They may produce repeated attacks of pneumonitis due to pressure on the bronchi. Roentgenograms reveal a smooth mass projecting from the midline into the thoracic cavity; a barium meal may show deviation of the esophagus and occasionally may outline the duplication. The right side is more commonly involved (5:1). Perforation, ulceration, and hemorrhage are potential complications. Vertebral anomalies are sometimes noted. Rarely, extension below the diaphragm is manifested. Surgical removal is the best treatment, if feasible.

Beyond the esophagus, enterogenous cysts (which occur most frequently along the terminal ileum) may cause pain, fullness, and ulceration with bleeding, as well as intussusception and obstruction. A smooth, freely movable mass is often felt, and roentgenogram with barium may show pooling in the duplication if it communicates with the adjacent normal intestine.

Differential diagnosis   Mesenteric cyst, hydronephrosis, ovarian cysts, and teratoma.

Treatment   Segmental resection of the duplication together with the adjacent normal bowel is performed when both of these portions of bowel are intimately attached. If this is not possible because of extensive involvement or difficult location, windows are made between the normal and duplicated bowel for decompression of the duplication pouch.

MECKEL'S DIVERTICULUM

Meckel's diverticulum is the remnant of the omphalomesenteric duct which has a relationship to the terminal ileum. It is present in about 2 percent of the population and varies from a nipplelike outpouching to a complete fistula having egress at the umbilicus. Complications occur in 25 percent of the cases, most often in infancy, and about one-half within the first 2 years of life. The most common complications are

1. Peptic ulcer: arises from aberrant gastric mucosa lining the Meckel's diverticulum. Dark or bright-red rectal bleeding (often massive) may occur. Pain is usually absent, and if present, is generally not a prominent symptom. Positive roentgenographic signs are infrequent. Perforation of such an ulcer shows the usual signs and symptoms of a ruptured viscus, together with x-ray evidence of air under the diaphragm.
2. Intussusception of Meckel's diverticulum: presents the same findings as any other intussusception.
3. Meckel's diverticulitis: the clinical picture resembles acute appendicitis, and the true diagnosis may be disclosed only during the operation. The pain is often more colicky than in appendicitis and vomiting more persistent. Blood in the stools may be detected.
4. Umbilical fistula: discussed in Chapter 12, "Diseases of the Newborn."
5. Volvulus of Meckel's diverticulum: exhibits the features of in-

testinal obstruction. Obstruction may also occur by a twisting of the bowel around a bandlike remnant of the vitelline duct which may extend to the umbilicus.

Treatment   Except for umbilical fistula, the above complications require prompt surgery with removal of the diverticulum as soon as the diagnosis is suspected.

Prognosis   Good, provided the diagnosis is quickly made and the surgery is prompt. The mortality rate is highest when perforation and strangulating obstructions have occurred.

OTHER ABDOMINAL CONDITIONS

RUPTURE OF A VISCUS

Traumatic rupture of the liver, spleen, or kidney is accompanied by a variable amount of hemorrhage and shock. A diagnostic paracentesis is valuable if intraperitoneal hemorrhage is suspected. Local tenderness and muscle spasm are often present. Urinalysis may reveal hematuria.

Rupture of the stomach (which may be multiple) or intestine in the newborn infant usually occurs during the first week or two. It can be secondary to trauma, e.g., birth trauma, inflation of the stomach by tight-fitting oxygen masks, or accidental intubation of esophagus, acute peptic ulcer, and perforation by stiff plastic catheters. Many cases without clear evidence of trauma have a history of hypoxia during or after birth. The "diving reflex" causes spasm of blood vessels supplying the stomach and gastrointestinal tract resulting in weak points which will later rupture with minor trauma. A small number appear to be idiopathic. Perforation of the cecum in Hirschsprung's disease and of the colon in ulcerative colitis occasionally are seen in older children. Rapid abdominal distension and circulatory collapse ensue. Roentgenograms taken with the patient in the upright position reveal air under the diaphragm.

Treatment   Immediate surgery to repair a perforation is indicated. In the case of massive distension with air, as can occur with gastric or cecal rupture, needle aspiration may be used for immediate decompression. Subtotal colectomy, if feasible, is the preferred treatment when there is a perforation of the colon secondary to ulcerative colitis. Trauma to liver or spleen associated with intraperitoneal hemorrhage must be explored surgically. Intravenous pyelography is useful in revealing calyceal tears of the kidney. Characteristically dye remains trapped in the torn part after the remaining pelvis has drained. Such kidneys should be repaired to preserve function and to prevent later hypertension or delayed hemorrhage. Arteriography is usually done prior to surgery.

INGUINAL HERNIA

Inguinal hernia is more common in boys and is most frequently noted in the first year of life. It may be unilateral or bilateral and occurs as a result of a persistent processus vaginalis. The painless swelling in the inguinal canal, sometimes extending into the scrotum is usually reducible. After reduction, the bulge disappears, but a characteristic silky and sliding sensation when feeling the cord remains. (The presence of a hydrocele is presumptive evidence of a patent processus vaginalis.) In females, a fallopian tube or ovary which is irreducible is often found. Inguinal hernia must be differentiated from inguinal lymphadenopathy. Femoral hernia, which is found below and lateral to the pubic spine, occurs in less than 0.5 percent of groin hernias in children. It may be diagnosed preoperatively, but often is found on reexploration for "recurrent inguinal hernia."

UMBILICAL HERNIA
(See Chapter 12, "Diseases of the Newborn")

DIASTASIS RECTI

Separation is occasionally noted in the midline of the upper abdomen. There is no danger of incarceration. Usually no repair is required, although theoretically the linea alba could be reconstructed. Cosmetically, the scar is probably less desirable than the condition.

VOLVULUS

Acute small-bowel volvulus usually occurs in association with malrotation and poor fixation of the mesentery. The infant becomes distended, fails to pass stool or passes blood from his rectum, and vomits all feedings. Temperature may become subnormal. X-rays generally show a ground-glass appearance, since bowel loops are edematous and filled with fluid, although proximal small-bowel distension with air-fluid levels may be present due to the obstruction.

Immediate laparotomy is required. Delay will lead to gangrene, Gram-negative sepsis, and death. If reduced early, the bowel usually is not gangrenous. Nonviable bowel must be removed. In the event of doubt, where the entire midgut is involved and resection would lead to severe nutritional impairment, the abdomen may be closed after reduction of the volvulus and reoperated 8 hours later. Often apparently nonviable gut will appear better and a smaller resection might be possible.

REVIEW QUESTIONS

1. The onset of congenital hypertrophic pyloric stenosis usually occurs (*a*) at birth; (*b*) in the second to third week of life; (*c*) any time during the neonatal period; (*d*) in utero.

2. All the following statements concerning congenital hypertrophic pyloric stenosis are true except for (a) progressively worsening constipation; (b) hypochloremic alkalosis occurs early; (c) vomitus contains no bile; (d) gastric peristalsis is visible from right to left; (e) associated with an increased incidence of jaundice.

3. Column I lists some conditions which have to be considered in the differential diagnosis of hypertrophic pyloric stenosis; column II contains statements concerning these conditions. Match the two:

I	II
A. Pylorospasm _____	(a) Fluoroscopy with barium
B. Achalasia (cardiospasm) _____	(b) "Double-bubble" sign on x-ray
C. Cardioesophageal relaxation _____ (chalasia)	(c) May be associated with autonomic nerve imbalance
D. Distal duodenal obstruction _____	(d) Fluoroscopy shows marked narrowing at distal end of esophagus

4. The most common cause of duodenal obstruction in the newborn is (a) annular pancreas; (b) duodenal atresia; (c) malrotation of the intestine; (d) web formation.

5. An infant with a family history of cystic fibrosis of the pancreas is noted to have abdominal distension and vomits green material 20 hours after birth. Sweat electrolytes are elevated following chemical stimulation. The most likely diagnosis is (a) hypertrophic pyloric stenosis; (b) meconium ileus; (c) jejunal obstruction; (d) congenital diaphragmatic hernia; (e) hypertonic dehydration.

6. Barium studies in congenital megacolon do not show a distended colon before (a) 1 day; (b) 10 to 14 days; (c) 2 to 5 weeks; (d) 1 year.

7. Column I lists the three types of malformation of the anus and rectum in the newborn; column II contains statements concerning these malformations. Match the two:

I	II
A. Type I—stenosis of the anus and rectum _____	(a) Requires immediate surgical correction even in the female
B. Type II—imperforate anus due to a membrane _____	(b) 80% or more are of this type
C. Type III—imperforate anus with rectal pouch ending blindly _____	(c) May not be clinically evident for some months after birth

8. All the following statements concerning type III imperforate anus are true except for (a) most patients have associated fistulous tracts between the proximal rectum and the genitourinary system; (b) absence of a fistula usually means a high lesion; (c) to determine the level of the rectal pouch the infant must be in a supine position when the x-ray is made; (d) if definitive surgery cannot be performed immediately, then decompressing colostomy is the procedure of choice.

9. The most common kind of fistula seen in a male infant born with imperforate anus is (a) rectoperineal; (b) rectovesicle; (c) rectourethral; (d) abdominal.

10. In gastroschisis, the following statements are true except for (*a*) other serious anomalies are usually present; (*b*) there is a defect in the abdominal wall lateral to the umbilicus and usually on the right; (*c*) there is no covering membrane; (*d*) malrotation may be associated.

11. The most common type of intussusception is (*a*) ileocecal; (*b*) enteroenteral; (*c*) colocolic; (*d*) none of the above.

12. The following statements concerning intussusception are true except for (*a*) left lower quadrant may feel empty on palpation of the abdomen; (*b*) currant-jelly stools are characteristic; (*c*) dilated loops of bowel are seen on x-ray; (*d*) attempts may be made to reduce the intussusception by barium enema.

13. The most frequent cause of lower gastrointestinal bleeding in an infant is (*a*) fissure in ano; (*b*) Meckel's diverticulum; (*c*) intussusception; (*d*) polyps.

14. The most frequent cause of lower gastrointestinal bleeding in the older child is (*a*) fissure in ano; (*b*) Meckel's diverticulum; (*c*) intussusception; (*d*) polyps.

15. Peutz-Jeghers syndrome is related to all the following except for (*a*) familial condition; (*b*) melanin spots; (*c*) polyps; (*d*) surgery is the treatment of choice.

16. Inguinal hernia occurs (*a*) most frequently in males during the first year of life; (*b*) most frequently in males after the first year of life; (*c*) with equal frequency in both sexes; (*d*) most frequently in females during child-bearing age.

19

GENITO-URINARY DISEASES

ACUTE GLOMERULONEPHRITIS

Etiology Acute glomerulonephritis, or postinfectious hemorrhagic nephritis, is probably due to hypersensitivity to an extrarenal infection with certain types of beta-hemolytic streptococci, e.g., group A type 12.

Clinical features

1. From 1 to 3 weeks prior to the onset there may be a history of any of the following: upper respiratory infection, tonsillitis, otitis media, scarlet fever, impetigo or other coccal skin infection.
2. Moderate fever, malaise, and pallor usually occur.

EDITORS' NOTE: The section on Urologic Conditions was prepared by David T. Mininberg, M.D.

3. Hematuria, reported as smoky or "Coca-Cola"–colored urine, and mild proteinuria are frequent.
4. Edema, periorbital (especially apparent in the morning) or pretibial, is common; more widespread edema develops infrequently.
5. Hypertension: there is frequently an increased blood pressure, systolic and diastolic.
6. Cardiac failure with an enlarged tender liver or pulmonary edema may complicate the disease.
7. Hypertensive encephalopathy (headaches, vomiting, convulsions) occasionally is seen, and less frequently there is marked cerebral edema with neuroretinopathy (papilledema and capillary changes).

Laboratory findings

1. Transient macroscopic or microscopic hematuria is a characteristic finding. The urine may also contain an increased amount of protein, red cell, or granular casts and an increased number of white cells. There usually is oliguria (less than 300 ml per sq meter per day) and hypervolemia.
2. The urea nitrogen (BUN) and nonprotein nitrogen (NPN) levels are usually elevated, and inulin and urea clearance are frequently depressed during the acute phase.
3. Serum complement is diminished during the acute phase.
4. Increased sedimentation rate, moderate leukocytosis, and anemia are usually found. The anemia is primarily due to increased plasma volume rather than to blood loss in the urine.
5. The antistreptolysin O titer as well as levels of other antistreptococcal antibodies are usually elevated.

Treatment   All patients should receive penicillin therapy to eradicate the primary streptococcal infection. For purposes of further treatment, the BUN level and blood pressure may be used as criteria for dividing patients with acute glomerulonephritis into four groups:

Those patients showing normal or only slightly elevated BUN and blood pressure need receive no special treatment beyond the general measures previously described in Chapter 6, "Drugs and Treatment."

Those patients showing markedly increased BUN and decreased urinary output but normal or only slightly elevated blood pressure should receive the following:

1. General measures of treatment as in the first group.
2. During periods of oliguria, fluid should be restricted to an amount equal to insensible water loss plus an amount equal to the previous day's urinary output. Fluid balance is best evaluated by daily weighing.
3. Hyperkalemia is treated with Kayexalate (1 Gm per kg will reduce potassium level approximately 1 meq per liter).

Those patients showing markedly increased blood pressure but normal or slightly elevated BUN should receive:

1. Salt-intake restriction (less than 1 Gm per day) and sedation (barbiturates) may be all that is necessary because hypertension is mostly of short duration.
2. Combined use of reserpine, 0.07 mg per kg, and hydralazine, 0.10 mg per kg, given intramuscularly, will usually lower the blood pressure for 12 hours or longer. Reserpine, 0.02 mg per kg per day in three to four divided oral doses, may be continued. Diuretics, e.g., hydrochlorothiazide—2 to 4 mg per kg per day—may be helpful. If chlorothiazide is given, do not restrict salt intake. Magnesium sulfate 50%, 0.2 ml per kg intramuscularly every 3 to 4 hours, until the blood pressure is lowered. Also 2 to 3 oz magnesium sulfate may be given orally or rectally, with the dose repeated in 6 to 8 hours. For impending hypertensive encephalopathy, diazoxide, 5 mg per kg, intravenously, every 4 hours, or magnesium sulfate 2%, 100 to 200 ml, given slowly intravenously, should be administered. Although hypertension is only occasionally severe, persistent hypertension is the most serious complication and chief cause of death.
3. Cautious digitalization is begun at the first signs of heart failure. The diminished renal function delays digitalis excretion.

Those patients showing markedly increased BUN and blood pressure and diminished urinary output probably should be treated first for hypertension. This group, of course, is the most difficult to treat, because hypertensive encephalopathy, cardiac failure, and uremia may occur.

Prolonged anuria, persistent hyperkalemia, uremic coma, and serious electrolyte imbalance (which occur rarely) require dialysis.

Course and prognosis

1. Complete clinical healing occurs in the great majority (90 percent) of children, usually in 6 to 12 weeks. However, it is not known whether apparently healed acute glomerulonephritis, after a quiescent period, does or does not contribute to the large number of cases of chronic glomerulonephritis.
2. A small percentage of cases of acute glomerulonephritis progress to subacute (repeated acute exacerbations with progressively worsening kidney function, characterized by a low fixed specific gravity). Death may ensue because of chronic renal failure due to progressive involvement and destruction of active nephrons.
3. Death occurs in a small number of cases and may be attributed to cardiac failure, uremia, infection, or hypertensive encephalopathy.
4. Subclinical cases of this disease occur. This is apparent when serial serum complement levels and urinalyses are made routinely on

either patients with streptococcal infection or on apparently normal household contacts of patients with known streptococcal infection. A number of such individuals are found to have depressed serum complement levels, microscopic hematuria, or both, and renal biopsies reveal typical findings of acute glomerulonephritis.

KIDNEY–FUNCTION TESTS

1. Urinalysis
   a. pH, specific gravity, protein, glucose, acetone, red blood cells, white blood cells, and casts.
   b. Addis count: provides a quantitative determination as to the number of red blood cells, white blood cells, and casts in the urine than is possible from examination of a casual specimen. Method: no fluids are offered after breakfast (dry lunch and dinner): child voids at 8 P.M., then all specimens of urine are collected for the next 12 hours (calculations are made by centrifuging a 10-ml sample for 5 minutes at 3,500 rpm). Normal: the great majority of addis counts reveal no protein when tested by conventional methods. Generally, most 12-hour specimens contain not more than 10 mg; however, over 50 mg is definitely abnormal; casts—5,000 or less; red blood cells—250,000 or less; white blood cells and epithelial cells (counted together)—1 million or less; the specific gravity is normally over 1,025.
   c. Maximal concentrating capacity: an index of the ability of the kidney to excrete a maximal amount of solutes in a minimal volume of water, which is a measure of both glomerular and tubular function. Normal: following a 12-hour period of fluid restriction, the night urine, a specific gravity of 1.026 or more, or osmolar concentration is more than 900 mOsm/kg water.
2. Retention of nitrogenous wastes—elevated BUN and creatinine is indicative of markedly impaired function (more than 50 percent of function must be lost).
3. Clearance tests (clearance = milliliters of plasma that are completely cleared of the test substance each minute): depending on the substance involved, clearance may be primarily related to glomerular function or to both glomerular and tubular function.
   a. Urea clearance: urea is filtered by the glomerulus and partially reabsorbed by the tubules.

C_{urea} (clearance of urea)=

$$\frac{\text{urinary urea (mg/ml)} \times \text{urine vol (ml/min)}}{\text{blood urea (mg/ml)}}$$

Normal urea clearance (ml/min/1.73 sq meter)—60 to 90 ml/min after 1 year of age. (To obtain reliable results, the minimal urinary flow should be 2 ml/min.)

b. Glomerular filtration rate (GFR): obtained by determining the clearance of a substance, e.g., inulin, that is filtered by the glomerulus but is neither secreted nor absorbed by the tubules. Filtration fraction (FF), GFR/RPF (renal plasma flow) is normally 0.2, implying that the volume of glomerular ultra-filtrate formed represents one-fifth of the total volume of plasma perfusing the glomeruli.

Normal GFR (ml/min/1.73 sq meter)—90 to 140 by 1 year of age.

c. Renal blood flow (RBF): Diodrast or para-aminohippurate (PAH) at low plasma levels is practically completely extracted from the renal arterial blood in one passage through the kidney. Hence, from a measure of Diodrast or PAH clearance, the rate at which plasma circulates through the kidney can be obtained. Subsequently the renal blood flow can be obtained from the renal plasma flow (normal, about 700 ml/min/1.73 sq meter) by determining the percentage of plasma in the blood, as obtained by the hematocrit.

d. Transport maximum (*Tm*): when Diodrast or PAH is at high plasma levels, the tubular excretory mechanism is saturated for these substances. The amount filtered by the glomerulus is subtracted from the total (glomeruli and tubules) to give the maximum tubular excretion.

Normal Tm_{PAH} (mg/min/1.73 sq meter)—77.5 after 1 year of age.

4. Dye tests: these, e.g., phenolsulfonphthalein, are primarily tests of tubular function. Normal: excretion of 30 percent of the amount injected in first 20 minutes and 55 percent in first hour for children over 2 years of age.

5. Acidifying capacity following the administration of a standard test dose of ammonium chloride:

	Infant	Children
pH	≲5.0	≲5.0
Titratable acid	45–110 μeq/min/1.73 m²	35–70 μeq/min/1.73 m²
Ammonium	40–80 μeq/min/1.73 m²	45–100 μeq/min/1.73 m²

6. Radioisotopic techniques

a. Renal blood flow scintiphotography

Technetium 99m pertechnetate is used intravenously for renal flow scintiphotography. A bolus of isotope is administered and sequential visualization of the abdominal aorta and vascularization of the kidney is studied.

Applications of this technique are

(1) Patency of the major vessels following renal trauma.
(2) Localization of intrarenal space-occupying lesions.
(3) Renal hypertension; asymmetric renal flow pattern may indicate a correctable unilateral renal disease.

b. Renal scans

(1) 197 Hg-chloromerodrin, a mercurial diuretic that localizes in the renal tubular cells, primarily in the renal cortex, is useful for renal scanning. The chloromerodrin scan is useful to evaluate the size and function of the tubular mass. It can replace the urogram in children with allergy to contrast media and localize the kidney for renal biopsy.
(2) ^{131}I-Hippuran (orthoiodohippurate) can also be used for scanning. This test is useful in detecting unilateral renal disease but is not specific for renovascular disease.

CONDITIONS SIMULATING HEMATURIA

1. Ingestion of certain foods: e.g., beets (anthrocyanin), rhubarb
2. Ingestion of certain drugs: e.g., Pyramidon, Promizole, phenolphthalein, cascara, santonin
3. Hemoglobinuria
4. Porphyria
5. Myoglobinuria
6. Alkaptonuria (urine becomes black upon standing)
7. Extremely concentrated urine
8. Large amounts of bile or uric acid

Dyes may color the urine; for example, methylene blue causes the urine to appear greenish blue.

NEPHROTIC SYNDROME

Pure nephrosis is characterized by massive edema, proteinuria, hypoproteinemia, and hypercholesterolemia unassociated with other systemic disease—such as chronic glomerulonephritis; mercury poisoning; Tridione drug reaction; diabetic nephropathy, e.g., Kimmelstiel-Wilson disease; syphilis; renal amyloidosis; renal vein thrombosis—all of which may also demonstrate these findings.

The cause is unknown, and only by excluding other conditions (listed above) that can also cause the nephrotic syndrome (edema, proteinuria, hypoproteinemia, and hypercholesterolemia) may a diagnosis of nephrosis (pure or lipoid) be made.

The use of percutaneous needle biopsy of the kidney and electron microscopy has been helpful in demonstrating the early pathologic changes that occur in the various diseases that may produce the nephrotic syndrome. Light microscopy demonstrates only minimal glomerular changes, but even early in the disease course electron microscopy demonstrates that nephrosis involves the epithelial cells of the glomeruli ("smudging" of the foot processes is seen).

Clinical features

1. Occurs more frequently in young children, less commonly in older children.
2. Onset is insidious, sometimes without a definite history of preceding infection.
3. Generalized massive edema is the characteristic finding. This may be preceded by hidden edema, causing an unexplained gain in weight. Ascites often predominates, and pleural effusion may be present. Waxy pallor is usually observed.
4. Blood pressure is normal, at least, initially.

Laboratory findings

1. Hypoproteinemia, due mainly to a low albumin level; levels of $alpha_1$ and beta globulins are usually normal, that of $alpha_2$, characteristically, is elevated, and gamma globulin is depressed.
2. Hypercholesterolemia: often 600 mg per 100 ml or more.
3. Urine contains large amounts of protein, many hyaline casts, and lipoid bodies; oliguria occurs frequently.
4. Serum-complement level is normal in the majority of cases, but may be mildly depressed.
5. BUN level and renal-function tests are usually normal.
6. Sedimentation rate is elevated.

Course and prognosis   There is a chronic course extending over a period of years, characterized by spontaneous remission and then by recurrence unless immunosuppressive therapy is initiated. In treated patients recurrences are seen less commonly, and they are usually associated with infection. The role of infection is not clear, since occasionally infection, particularly with rubeola, may initiate a remission. The prognosis for patients not treated as described or those that are steroid-resistant is poor. About two-thirds of such patients will have continued kidney damage and ultimately will develop signs of progressive renal disease—elevated blood pressure, azotemia, diminished urea clearance, and constant hematuria—and will die within a 5-year period.

A number of patients will do well while being treated, but discontinuation of drugs is followed regularly by recurrence of disease. Such steroid-dependent individuals may require very prolonged treatment.

Treatment

1. General measures, including good nursing care, proper psychologic attitudes, and adequate diet, are important (see Chapter 6, "Drugs and Treatment").
2. Normal activity should be permitted and encouraged.
3. Induction of diuresis followed by prolonged intermittent maintenance therapy with large doses of adrenal corticosteroids has reduced mortality to a considerable extent. After routine tuberculin testing, prednisone, 2 mg per kg per day in 3 or 4 doses, will result in complete diuresis in the vast majority of patients within 12 to 21 days.

Five days after the onset of diuresis—but only when complete diuresis occurs—prolonged intermittent maintenance therapy with corticosteroids is begun. One plan is to give three-fourths of the initial dose on three successive days of each week. Antibiotics should be used promptly and more liberally for the nephrotic child following exposure to bacterial infection. After 1 to 2 years therapy is gradually terminated by prolonging the intervals between maintenance courses rather than by decreasing the dose. Other immunosuppressive drugs, e.g., Imuran, have been used for steroid-resistant or steroid-dependent patients, but the role of such drugs has not been established.

4. Paracentesis of the abdomen or thoracentesis occasionally may be necessary if fluid accumulations cause respiratory or cardiac distress.
5. Routine immunizations should not be given because they may cause a recurrence of symptoms.
6. Marked edema may require treatment with diuretics until diuresis can be accomplished by immunosuppressive therapy—HydroDiuril, 2 to 4 mg per kg per day; Aldactone (secondary hyperaldosteronism occurs in nephrosis), 10 to 15 mg per kg per day (HydroDiuril and Aldactone may be used together); or ethacrynic acid, 1 mg per kg per day. Diuresis may also be induced following administration of salt-poor albumin, 0.5 Gm per kg per day for several consecutive days.

ORTHOSTATIC PROTEINURIA (Postural Proteinuria)

Orthostatic (postural) proteinuria is a benign condition characterized by the presence of protein in the urine only when the patient is standing. This condition may be exaggerated when a lordotic position is assumed, and it disappears while the person is reclining. The term "proteinuria" rather than "albuminuria" should be used to designate this condition, as the globulin fraction is excreted also. It may be necessary to perform a percutaneous renal biopsy to demonstrate normal histology and thereby rule out the presence of organic disease, e.g., chronic glomerulonephritis. No specific treatment is available or needed because renal function is not usually impaired. Correction of abnormal posture may diminish the proteinuria. Most cases are discovered after 10 years of age, and many clear spontaneously after age 20.

ACUTE RENAL FAILURE

Acute renal failure is characterized by markedly disturbed tubular function. It may be due to various causes: prerenal, e.g., hemorrhage, burns, dehydration shock; renal, e.g., acute glomerulonephritis; poisons (carbon tetrachloride, diethylene glycol); drugs (sulfa crystals); postrenal, e.g., obstruction of the urinary tract (congenital anomalies, calculi).

Etiology Mechanical, chemical, or hypoxic damage to the tubules which impairs their ability to conserve water results in failure.

Clinical features

1. Low blood pressure and shock are common initially, but high blood pressure may develop later.
2. Oliguria or anuria is characteristic.

Laboratory findings

1. Varying degrees of disturbed renal function, depending on the severity of the renal lesion, e.g., marked elevation of the NPN, hydrogen ion retention
2. Low fixed (1.010) urinary specific gravity
3. Rapidly rising blood-potassium level
4. Proteinuria and a brown urinary sediment containing acid hematin granules
5. Acidosis

Treatment

1. Plasma is helpful when shock is present.
2. Fluid intake should not exceed the urinary output, plus loss of fluid by vomiting or diarrhea, plus insensible water loss (300 to 600 ml per sq meter per day). Fluids should contain glucose 5 to 10% and sodium bicarbonate (10 meq per sq meter per day) to correct existing acidosis or prevent impending acidosis.

3.   Polystyrene sulfate (Kayexalate)—0.5 to 1.5 Gm per kg per day, orally or rectally, for hyperkalemia.
4.   Peritoneal or hemodialysis may be required if anuria persists for more than 7 to 10 days and if electrolyte abnormalities are progressive.

Prognosis   In severe cases death usually occurs within 1 to 2 weeks. Survival beyond this period usually indicates that the patient will recover and kidney function will return to normal. The oliguric phase is followed by a diuretic phase. During this phase large volumes of hypotonic or isotonic (to plasma) urine are formed, and dehydration may occur. Loss of sodium, chloride, and potassium accompany the large volume of urine. Finally well into the recovery phase, urinary volume returns to normal and the ability to produce concentrated urine is restored.

URINARY TRACT INFECTION

Normally urine from the kidney is sterile and remains so until it passes the terminal urethra which contains bacteria on its mucosal surface. Therefore the technique that makes it possible to draw inferences about the bacterial content of bladder urine by study of voided urine is very important.

The anatomical extent and the duration of infection is not readily determined by clinical means. Signs and symptoms may be referable to the lower tract, e.g., urgency or frequency and therefore considered as evidence of urethritis or cystitis, or they may stem from the upper tract, e.g., high fever, chills, back pain and be considered as evidence of pyelitis or pyelonephritis, but in either case the symptoms do not indicate the limits of the infection. The first recognition of infection by either onset of clinical symptoms or positive urinary findings is no assurance that previous infection has not occurred.

Etiology   *E. coli* is the causative agent in about 85 percent of primary infections (those in which no obstruction exists and which have not been previously treated with antibiotics or subjected to instrumentation). If previously treated or instrumented, proteus, pseudomonas, or enterococci are more likely to be found. Other causative organisms include *Aerobacter aerogenes, Streptococcus fecalis,* staphylococcus, hemolytic streptococcus, typhoid, and rarely tubercle bacilli and fungi.

Urinary tract infection may be either the ascending variety or hematogenous in origin. In the newborn the blood-borne type is most common and sepsis is usually present. Both sexes are equally affected. In children, females are much more often affected than males and the retrograde route is the most common. Staphylococcal infection in children is commonly of the hematogenous type.

In chronic cases, congenital malformations of the urinary tract are a frequent predisposing factor by causing obstruction and stasis of urine. Damage to the kidney is likely to cause scarring of the tissue with obstruction of nephrons. Such scarring especially in the renal papillae may predispose to chronic infection.

Reflux of urine from the bladder to the ureters, secondary to either a congenital or an inflammatory lesion, also predisposes to chronic urinary tract infection.

Clinical features   There are two common types of onset:

1. An acute onset, more often seen in infancy, with few if any signs and symptoms referable to the urinary tract. The temperature is high and fluctuates, and the condition of the infant may appear toxic. There may be convulsions or chills and even meningismus, as evidenced by nuchal rigidity. Vomiting and diarrhea may occur commonly. When this type of onset occurs in children, dysuria and frequency may occur.
2. An insidious onset, with localizing urinary tract signs and symptoms, such as pain on micturition (dysuria), frequency of urination, urgency, sometimes abdominal or lumbar pain, recurrence of enuresis, and costovertebral tenderness. There are low-grade fever and little, if any, toxicity. This type of infection is observed principally in older children.

Laboratory findings   The demonstration of significant bacteriuria or pyuria in aseptically collected urine specimens is indicative of infection. (After the genitalia have been washed with surgical soap and an aseptic solution has been applied, a midstream specimen is collected. The first specimen voided in the morning is best; later specimens may yield deceptively low bacterial counts. Voided aseptic specimens can usually be obtained from infants; catheterization or aspiration of urine from the bladder should be performed only when specifically indicated. Bacteriuria* usually precedes and may persist after the pyuria. (Uncentrifuged fresh urine should contain no more than one to two pus cells per low-power field, centrifuged urine, no more than two pus cells per high-power field.) Repeated collections of urine may be necessary to find pyuria. When the patient's temperature is high, there may be blockage of the involved pelvis and ureter, so that pus cells are not draining into the urine and therefore the urine may be normal.

---

* Some bacteria may be found in the urine of patients who do not have pyelonephritis. This may be because of contamination during collection or because of the asymptomatic presence of bacteria in the terminal urethra. The following criteria are indicative of infection: (1) bacteria seen on direct smear of a drop of fresh urine; (2) bacterial colony count of urine culture—more than 100,000 colonies (less than 1,000 colonies is usually not significant, 1,000 to 100,000 colonies is of questionable significance).

Treatment   While awaiting the report on the urine culture, a chemo-therapeutic agent, e.g., sulfa, or an antibiotic, e.g., ampicillin, should be administered. If there has been no response to these drugs, specific antibiotic therapy should be used as indicated by sensitivity tests made with the organism from the culture. Therapy should be continued for a minimal period of 14 to 21 days, and there should be a negative culture before it is discontinued. Several days after therapy is discontinued, another culture should be made. (Recurrences occur most frequently within 1 to 2 weeks after cessation of therapy.) Urinalyses and cultures should be repeated at increasing intervals for a period of 12 months. In addition to antibiotics, chemotherapeutic agents, e.g., nitrofurantoin, can be useful. These may be administered for prolonged periods in chronic or recurrent cases.

In patients who do not respond to treatment promptly, urography including cystometric studies and a voiding cystogram should be performed (if intravenous urography is not satisfactory for diagnosis, cytoscopy and retrograde pyelograms are necessary). In many patients, congenital malformations are found which produce obstruction and require surgery. Persistent reflux of urine with a widely patent ureteral orifice should be corrected surgically.

Prognosis   The prognosis is very good for a single isolated episode of acute infection. For children with recurrent or chronic infection, the prognosis is guarded.

HEMOLYTIC UREMIC SYNDROME

This condition occurs mostly in infants and young children. Hemolytic anemia, thrombocytopenia, and acute renal failure are characteristic. Renal cortical necrosis, renal thrombotic angiopathy, and disseminated thrombotic microangiopathy are the common lesions associated with this condition. The severity of the disease is variable.

Etiology   The etiology is unknown, but various viral infections have been implicated.

Clinical features

1. Gastroenteritis or respiratory tract infection may precede the onset.
2. Fever is variable.
3. Oliguria, the significance of which may not be recognized in a sick infant not feeding well.
4. Pallor develops suddenly.
5. Bleeding—skin or gastrointestinal tract—occurs.
6. Lethargy, irritability, tremors, and convulsions may occur.
7. Hypertension is common.

Laboratory findings

1. Hemolytic anemia and bizarre-shaped red blood cells.
2. Thrombocytopenia, which may be transitory.
3. Oliguria with protein, red blood cells, leukocytes, and red cell or granular casts.
4. BUN and serum bilirubin levels are elevated.
5. Serum potassium level rises and serum bicarbonate falls.

Treatment

1. Fluids should be restricted to cover insensible water loss plus loss by vomiting, urination, and diarrhea.
2. Heparin—rapid injection, intravenously, 50 to 100 units per kg per day every 6 hours or by slow drip, 200 to 400 units per kg per day.
3. Clotting time should be performed daily and maintained at about twice normal.
4. Severe anemia may require transfusion, but further hemolysis may ensue.
5. Cardiac failure, hypervolemia, hyperkalemia, severe acidosis, or continued oliguria may require dialysis.

Prognosis   The prognosis is guarded. Those patients who survive a severe initial phase may develop chronic nephritis.

RENAL VEIN THROMBOSIS

This condition may occur at any age, but the newborn infant, especially one born to a diabetic mother, is particularly prone to develop it. Diarrhea, dehydration, and septicemia are predisposing factors, but the condition may arise with no apparent antecedent.

Clinical features

1. Sudden enlargement of one kidney.
2. Gastrointestinal signs, e.g., vomiting and abdominal distension, are common.
3. Fever may be present.
4. Oliguria or anuria may occur even in unilateral involvement.
5. Generalized edema may occur.
6. Hypertension may be present.

Laboratory findings

1. Hematuria is usually present; it is more commonly gross but may be microscopic.
2. Proteinuria and pyuria may be present.

3. BUN is elevated.
4. Intravenous pyelogram reveals absence of excretion of dye on the affected side.
5. Photoscan of the kidneys reveals no function on the side with the thrombosis.
6. Inferior vena cavagram and renal arteriography with particular attention to the venous phase visualization confirm the diagnosis and extent of involvement.

Treatment

1. Surgical exploration and removal of the clot (in selected cases) or kidney.
2. Some cases may be treated successfully medically, e.g., with supportive treatment and anticoagulant therapy. Too, the condition of the patient may preclude surgical intervention in certain instances.
3. In bilateral cases no surgery is indicated. Anticoagulant therapy is the treatment of choice. Dialysis may be necessary.

Renal artery thrombosis occurs with no predilection for infants. It is characterized by hypertension and cardiac failure. Unilateral involvement is curable by prompt nephrectomy.

RENAL NECROSIS

Necrosis may occur in the cortex or medulla, or it may be isolated in the tubules. The disorder is seen at birth usually following serious illness such as severe anemia or profound hypoxia. Respiratory distress, apnea, flaccidity, and shock are accompanied by anuria or scanty urine containing blood. Blood urea nitrogen and potassium levels rise. After the neonatal period this condition occurs due to sepsis, diarrhea and dehydration, pancreatitis, severe burns, poisoning, and occasionally with no obvious antecedent illness. Treatment consists of combating renal failure. The prognosis is grave. Recovery may be followed by persistent hypertension.

HEREDITARY AND CONGENITAL RENAL DISEASE

The urogenital tract is subject to a greater incidence of anomalies than any other system. They occur in about 10 percent of the population. The largest number of these are gross anatomic abnormalities, e.g., obstruction to the outflow tract or double ureters, and no hereditary factor is known to exist. They are frequently multiple and associated with an increased incidence of other conditions, e.g., oligohydramnios, single umbilical artery, absence of abdominal muscles, anomalies of the lower gastrointestinal tract and genitalia, and external ear anomalies. A second group of conditions which are hereditary consist of syndromes which may represent either dysplasia or an arrest of maturation* involving only the kidney, e.g., cystic disease of the kidney, or several systems, e.g., trisomy D, familial nephritis (Alport's syndrome)—renal, auditory, and ocular, oculocerebrorenal (Lowe's) syndrome. A third group consists of tubular defects which may result in one or more findings, e.g., aminoaciduria, glucosuria, phosphaturia, acidosis, defective concentration of urine. A fourth group of diseases are the result of inborn conditions of other systems, but the kidney is presented with abnormal metabolites and secondarily damaged, e.g., hepatolenticular degeneration, cystinosis.

More than 30 specific inherited renal diseases are now recognized. For simple orientation, these diseases may be classified into two major categories on the basis of structural and functional abnormalities.

I. Structural defects
    1. Nephritis with deafness or ocular abnormalities (Alport's syndrome)
    2. Nephritis with polyneuropathy
    3. Nephritis with hyperprolinemia
    4. Nephritis (without extrarenal manifestations)
    5. Mediterranean fever
    6. Urticaria, deafness, and amyloidosis
    7. Fabry's disease
    8. Infantile polycystic disease
    9. Adult polycystic disease
    10. Cystic disease of the liver and kidney
    11. Medullary cystic disease
    12. Juvenile nephronophthisis
    13. Retinorenal dysplasia
    14. Onychodystrophic renal disease (nail-patella syndrome)
    15. Infantile nephrosis
    16. Unilateral hydronephrosis
    17. Renal agenesis
II. Functional defects
    18. Cystinuria (types I–III)
    19. Hartnup disease

---

*   *Renal agenesis* is the complete absence of identifiable renal tissue. It may be unilateral or bilateral. In the latter case it is often associated with low birth weight and a peculiar facies with low-set ears (Potter's syndrome). The incidence is much higher in males.
Renal aplasia refers to the presence of tissue which is recognizable microscopically but not macroscopically as renal tissue. Multicystic disease is probably a form of aplasia.
Renal hypoplasia describes a kidney which has normal structure but is reduced in size. It may be unilateral or bilateral and must be distinguished from atrophy of a previously normal kidney. Segmental renal hypoplasia occurs and is associated with severe hypertension.
Renal dysplasia is characterized by disorganized morphology (primitive structures and abnormal tissues, e.g., cartilage). It may be unilateral or bilateral, and over 80 percent of patients have associated renal anomalies.

20. Iminoglycinuria
21. Hypercystinuria
22. Dibasic aminoaciduria
23. Glucoglycinuria
24. Renal glycosuria (types A and B)
25. Glucose-galactose malabsorption
26. Idiopathic Fanconi syndrome
27. Oculocerebrorenal syndrome
28. Hypophosphatemic rickets
29. Pseudohypoparathyroidism
30. Proximal renal tubular acidosis
31. Distal renal tubular acidosis
32. Vasopressin-resistant diabetes insipidus

POLYCYSTIC KIDNEY

Polycystic kidney is the result of a congenital developmental defect. It is often associated with cysts of the liver and occasionally those of other organs. Several types have been described. An infantile type occurs in which the kidneys are usually markedly enlarged and death occurs early. More than one child of a sibship may be affected. A second type, which may be a variant of the infantile type, is associated with a more marked degree of fibrosis, and owing to liver involvement, portal hypertension dominates the clinical picture. The adult type frequently presents as a flank mass, proteinuria, and various abnormal formed elements in the urine. Progressive renal failure and its complications, e.g., renal rickets, hypertension, may occur depending on the degree of involvement. This type is transmitted as an autosomal dominant trait.

ECTOPIC KIDNEY

Ectopic kidney is usually asymptomatic unless infection occurs. Diagnosis is made by urography. Surgical correction is frequently impossible because the short blood vessels do not permit the kidney to be moved, and nephrectomy may be indicated.

HORSESHOE KIDNEY

Horseshoe kidney results from a fusion of the lower poles of the kidneys and is usually associated with other anomalies of the tract. The condition may remain asymptomatic, or it may cause infection and calculi formation later in adult life. Treatment is surgical.

STRICTURE OF THE URETER

Strictures of the ureter are characterized by stasis of urine, recurrent infection, and hydronephrosis. Diagnosis is made by urography. Treatment consists of controlling the infection and corrective surgery.

ABERRANT RENAL VESSEL

Aberrant renal vessel frequently causes obstruction of the ureter, resulting in stasis of urine, recurrent infection, and hydronephrosis. Treatment is surgical.

MEGALOURETERS

This condition is characterized by elongation and kinking of the ureters. A slow, progressive destruction of the renal parenchyma occurs owing to stasis of urine and infection. Physical development is usually retarded. Diagnosis is made by urography, cystometrogram, and ureterometrogram. Treatment consists of controlling the infection with antibiotics followed by indicated surgery.

EXSTROPHY OF THE BLADDER

Exstrophy of the bladder involves the urinary tract from the bladder to the external meatus and is more common in males. Plastic repair should be attempted, but at best this condition is difficult to manage, requiring repeated surgical procedures. Urinary diversion is usually indicated.

BIFID PELVIS AND DOUBLE URETER

Bifid pelvis may occur alone or with a double ureter. The condition may be asymptomatic until infection occurs. Diagnosis is made by urography. Treatment is surgical if complications occur.

PERINEPHRITIS AND PERINEPHRIC ABSCESS

Perinephritis is an infection of the soft tissues around the kidney. More than one-half the cases go on to abscess.

Etiology　The cause is most commonly *E. coli,* but staphylococcus is frequently involved. The organism reaches the area by extension from the kidney or by the bloodstream from a distant focus of infection.

Clinical features

1. There is usually an acute onset with fever, chills, and prostration.
2. Pain and tenderness localized in the lumbar region on the affected side are common.
3. Flexion at the thigh with resistance to extension of the leg is observed on the affected side.

Laboratory findings

1. Pyuria may or may not be present.
2. Leukocytosis with polymorphonuclear predominance reflects the inflammatory process.

3. Roentgenograms: distortion or obliteration of the psoas shadow on the affected side, enlarged kidney shadow, lateral curvature of the spine (concavity on affected side).

Treatment

1. Antibiotics and chemotherapy.
2. Surgical drainage if there is abscess formation.

HYDRONEPHROSIS

Hydronephrosis is characterized by dilatation of the kidney pelvis and calyces secondary to obstruction of the urinary outflow tract. Supravesical obstructions, such as ureteral strictures, kinking of a ureter, pressure from an aberrant blood vessel, or ptosis of a kidney, cause hydronephrosis more rapidly than infravesical obstructions. The clinical features are enlarged kidney (movable and fluctuant), secondary infection with symptoms of pyelonephritis, and later renal insufficiency. Intravenous or retrograde pyelography is diagnostic. Surgery is usually indicated to correct the obstruction or remove an irreversibly damaged kidney.

CONDITIONS IN THE FEMALE

VULVOVAGINITIS

Vaginal discharge in children is frequent but is often not reported because of unwarranted shame. Therefore proper psychologic care of these children and their parents is most important.

Vulvovaginitis may be classified as follows:

1. Nonspecific vulvovaginitis: all infections of the vagina and vulva in which no specific etiologic organism can be isolated (repeated cultures usually yield different organisms).
2. Specific vulvovaginitis:
    a. Gonorrhea caused by *Neisseria gonorrhoeae*
    b. Moniliasis, most commonly caused by *Candida albicans*
    c. Trichomoniasis
    d. Pinworm infestation
3. Foreign-body vaginitis: caused by insertion of some foreign body into the vagina.
4. Premenstrual vaginal discharge (a physiologic process).

Procedures necessary for diagnosis

1. Detailed history.
2. Complete physical examination, with special reference to amount, color, odor, and consistency of the vaginal discharge.

3. Determination of the pH of the discharge (nitrazine paper).
4. Direct vaginoscopic examination is used when necessary, e.g., to find foreign body.
5. Rectoabdominal palpation for a foreign body.
6. Microscopic examination of a stained smear of the exudate or of a wet smear if monilia or trichomonas is suspected.
7. Isolation and identification of the organism by culture.

NONSPECIFIC VULVOVAGINITIS

Nonspecific vaginitis is characterized by a moderate amount of thin, watery, light-yellow discharge, which is usually nonirritating but may be foul-smelling. At times the labia may be irritated.

Etiology   The diagnosis of nonspecific vaginitis is made by the exclusion of specific vaginitis. It is usually caused by a combination of organisms. Various strains of streptococcus, staphylococcus, colon bacillus, diphtheroids, or other organisms may be found. The most common predisposing causes are uncleanliness and improper hygiene, specifically improper cleansing after defecation. Other causes are improperly fitted clothing, poor nutrition, chronic skin disease (especially eczema and scabies), worm infestation (secondary to scratching), frequent masturbation, and chronic illness.

Laboratory findings

1. pH of discharge, acid (4.0 to 5.0)
2. Stained exudate showing several organisms other than *N. gonorrhoeae*
3. Culture of organisms

Treatment

1. Removal of predisposing causes.
2. Local hygiene—careful cleansing—should include instructions on proper cleansing of perianal region after defecation, i.e., wiping from vagina toward rectum.
3. For resistant cases, antibiotics and chemotherapy may be tried.
4. The family should be reassured that the condition is common and not of gonorrheal origin.

GONORRHEAL VULVOVAGINITIS

Gonorrheal infection in the female frequently involves first the urinary meatus. As the infection diminishes in the urethral area, the vaginal discharge, characterized by a profuse, thick, yellowish-green mucopurulent exudate, becomes prominent. The mucous membrane of the vulva is usually irritated.

History of the patient may indicate direct contact with someone who has gonorrhea, for example, through sex play or sleeping in the same bed. Actual sexual intercourse may be a cause in older children. Indirect contact, e.g., from toilet seats, is an improbable factor.

Laboratory findings

1. pH of the discharge, alkaline (7.0 to 8.0)
2. Intracellular and extracellular Gram-negative diplococci present in stained smear
3. *Neisseria gonorrhoeae* grown and identified by culture techniques

Treatment

1. Penicillin, orally, is usually sufficient.
2. Tetracycline is also effective.
3. Local therapy consists of providing proper hygiene.
4. Removal of the source of infection.

Treatment should be continued for 1 week after cultures are negative.

Prognosis   Complications are rare. No cases of gonorrheal ophthalmia have been reported, and salpingitis is practically never seen before puberty. Parents and children should be reassured that with adequate treatment the prognosis is excellent.

TRICHOMONAS VULVOVAGINITIS

Trichomonas vulvovaginitis occurs most commonly after adolescence and is characterized by a profuse, thin foamy discharge, punctate vaginitis, and moderate pruritus. The cervix is not involved.

The diagnosis is made by finding the organism in a wet smear of the fresh vaginal secretion.

Treatment

1. Vaginal lavage with a weak lactic acid solution (½ tsp USP lactic acid to 1 pint water).
2. Specific medication (Flagyl—125 mg three times a day, orally, for 10 days) may be tried in stubborn cases.

The patient is considered cured if there is no recurrence for at least 3 months.

Prognosis   The ultimate prognosis is good, but recurrences are common.

MONILIAL VULVOVAGINITIS

Monilial vulvovaginitis is uncommon in children. It is characterized by a white curdy discharge with very little odor, marked inflammation of the vulva, and severe pruritus. A history of antibiotic therapy and diarrhea may precede the onset of the vaginal infection, or this condition may occur early in the course of diabetes.

The diagnosis is established by finding mycelia in the wet smears. (The presence of spores alone is not considered diagnostic.)

Treatment

1. Nystatin vaginal tablets inserted morning and night for 1 month and Nystatin (100,000 units) orally, three times daily for 10 days.
2. Daily vaginal instillation of 1 percent aqueous solution gentian violet preceded by vaginal lavage with sodium bicarbonate solution (1 tsp dissolved in 250 ml of water).

Prognosis   The prognosis is good if the source of the infection, e.g., gastrointestinal tract, is successfully treated.

PINWORM VULVOVAGINITIS

Pinworm vulvovaginitis occurs most frequently in early childhood and is characterized by persistent vaginal discharge and marked pruritus, particularly at night.

Diagnosis is made by macroscopic visualization of the adult pinworm or by finding the ova on perineal, rectal, or vaginal smears.

Treatment   See Chapter 17, "Gastrointestinal Diseases."

Prognosis   The prognosis is excellent.

FOREIGN–BODY VAGINITIS

Foreign-body vaginitis is characterized by a persistent bloody or brownish discharge, which is moderate in amount. It is caused by local irritation of the vaginal mucosa. Secondary nonspecific infection may develop.

Diagnosis

1. History of masturbation or of insertion of objects into the vagina, e.g., balloon, pencil, or coin, may be obtained.
2. Rectal examination may demonstrate a palpable mass.
3. Roentgenogram of the pelvic area will reveal an object if it is radiopaque.
4. Vaginoscopic examination may be necessary and is best done under general anesthesia.

Treatment

1. Removal of foreign body
2. Psychotherapy to prevent recurrence

PREMENSTRUAL DISCHARGE

Premenstrual discharge is characterized by a thick whitish discharge, moderate in amount and neither foul-smelling nor irritating. This discharge is caused by the normal hormonal secretions in girls approaching puberty, usually 6 to 18 months prior to the first menses. The smear is characteristic and reveals epithelial cells with large nuclei. The pH is acid (4.0 to 4.5), and the culture is negative for gonococci.

Treatment   No treatment is necessary. The parent and child should be reassured that this is a normal occurrence and that it will gradually disappear.

LABIAL ADHESIONS

Labial adhesions are characterized by a thin whitish membrane covering the vestibule. They occur most commonly between 2 and 6 years of age and may appear following vaginitis. It is important to differentiate labial adhesions from an absent vaginal orifice.

Treatment

1. No therapy may be necessary because the adhesions invariably disappear later in childhood.
2. Local application of an estrogenic cream, twice a day for 1 to 2 weeks, has been used.
3. Manual separation is effective but rarely necessary.

CONDITIONS IN THE MALE

PHIMOSIS

Phimosis is a narrowing of the preputial orifice so that retraction of the prepuce is either difficult or impossible. If the opening is very small, there may be interference with micturition. If the prepuce cannot be retracted, both adhesions and infection are likely to occur.

Treatment consists of either circumcision or gradual dilatation and good hygiene. A prepuce which appears tight and adherent at birth may, without treatment, become entirely normal by 2 to 3 years of age.

PARAPHIMOSIS

Paraphimosis is characterized by the inability to return the prepuce to its normal position from a retracted position beyond the corona. As soon as possible, manual reduction should be attempted (hyaluronidase may aid in reducing edema). If this is impossible, surgery (dorsal slit) is indicated and should be followed later by circumcision.

CIRCUMCISION

Circumcision is the surgical removal of the prepuce. This operation is indicated in phimosis, paraphimosis, redundant prepuce, and in some cases of balanoposthitis, and it is contraindicated in epispadias and hypospadias. Some investigators believe that it should be performed routinely in newborn males, because thereafter penile cleanliness is simple, and because there is a decreased incidence of penile carcinoma in circumcised individuals.

HYPOSPADIAS AND EPISPADIAS

These are congenital malformations of the urethra with anomalous urethral openings on the penis. In hypospadias, which occurs more commonly than epispadias, the orifice is on the ventral surface of the penis. Severe forms may be confused with hermaphroditism. Epispadias is characterized by a urethral orifice on the dorsal surface of the penis. It may be complicated by extrophy of the bladder. Treatment is plastic surgery, which is best delayed if possible until about 3 years of age.

HYDROCELE

A hydrocele is a collection of fluid within the tunica vaginalis or some part of the peritoneal pouch brought down by the testicle. It may be either congenital or acquired. It is characterized by a tense mass in the scrotum, inguinal canal, or both. It can be transilluminated, no expansile impulse is felt, and it usually cannot be reduced. The congenital type, which may be accompanied by an indirect hernia, usually disappears spontaneously, and only those cases which persist or show progressive enlargement require surgery. Hydrocele of the cord is almost invariably associated with a hernia, and herniorrhaphy with excision of the hydrocele is indicated. Acquired hydrocele is usually a sequela to trauma or epididymitis. This type frequently will also disappear spontaneously, but if there is no regression after several months, surgical excision is the treatment of choice.

REVIEW QUESTIONS

1. The following statements concerning acute glomerulonephritis are true except for one: (a) increase of both systolic and diastolic blood pressure is frequently seen; (b) persistent hypertension is a serious complication and a major cause of death; (c) serum complement activity is elevated; (d) anemia is due to increased blood volume.
2. Normal urea clearance (ml/min/1.73 sq meters) after 1 year of age is (a) 60 to 90; (b) 100 to 120; (c) 150 to 200.
3. Laboratory findings in nephrosis include all but one of the following: (a) elevated gamma globulin; (b) hypercholesterolemia; (c) serum complement is normal or mildly depressed; (d) BUN and renal-function tests are usually normal; (e) sedimentation rate is elevated.

4. In the treatment of nephrosis the following statements are true except for one: (*a*) after routine tuberculin testing, prednisone 2 mg per kg per day in three to four doses is administered; (*b*) routine immunizations may cause a recurrence of symptoms; (*c*) diuretics have no role in the treatment of nephrosis; (*d*) after complete diuresis occurs, prolonged intermittent maintenance therapy with corticosteroids is used; (*e*) salt-poor albumin may be helpful to induce diuresis.

5. The following statements concerning urinary tract infection are true except for one: (*a*) *E. coli* is the causative agent in about 85 percent of primary infections; (*b*) urinary tract infection in the newborn is mostly hematogenous in origin; (*c*) for diagnostic purposes, the first specimen voided in the morning is usually the best; (*d*) in older children, males are more often affected than females.

6. The following statements concerning hemolytic uremic syndrome are true except for one: (*a*) anemia, thrombocytopenia, and acute renal failure are characteristic; (*b*) there is a sudden onset of pallor; (*c*) there are lowered serum potassium levels; (*d*) heparin is used in the treatment.

7. The following statements concerning renal vein thrombosis are true except for one: (*a*) it is prone to develop in infants born to diabetic mothers; (*b*) there is a sudden enlargement of the kidney; (*c*) oliguria is seen only with bilateral involvement; (*d*) photoscan reveals no function on the side of the thrombosis.

8. The following statements concerning genitourinary tract anomalies are true except for one: (*a*) they occur in about 10 percent of the population; (*b*) they are frequently associated with external ear anomalies; (*c*) they play a significant role in chronic urinary tract infection; (*d*) renal agenesis is often associated with low birth weight, peculiar facies, and low-set ears.

9. The pH of the vaginal discharge in nonspecific vulvovaginitis is (*a*) 4 to 5; (*b*) 7 to 8; (*c*) not characteristically affected.

10. Labial adhesions are best treated by (*a*) no therapy; (*b*) surgical incision; (*c*) gradual separation by manual manipulation; (*d*) application of antibiotic ointment.

11. Congenital hydrocele is best treated by (*a*) judicious observation; (*b*) aspiration; (*c*) surgery; (*d*) injection of sclerosing agents.

20 NEUROLOGIC CONDITIONS

It is essential for pediatricians to continually assess the growth and maturation of the nervous system in order to determine subnormal mentation, abnormal behavior, and neurologic or sensory deficit.

CONVULSIVE (Epileptic) DISORDERS

Convulsions are paroxysmal disorders of brain function characterized primarily by changes in consciousness and motor phenomena, either localized or generalized, and less frequently by sensory or behavioral disturbances.

Etiologic factors at different age levels are listed below in order of frequency:

From birth to 6 months

1. Birth injuries (traumatic or hypoxic)
2. Developmental anomalies of the brain
3. Acute infections of the central nervous system: bacterial and viral meningoencephalitides
4. Other less common causes (listed below)

From 6 to 24 months

1. Acute febrile convulsion: for example, at the onset of pneumonia, roseola, pyelitis
2. Acute infections of the central nervous system
3. Residua of birth injuries or developmental anomalies of the brain
4. All other causes (listed below)

From 2 to 6 years of age

1. Acute infections of the central nervous system
2. Residua of cerebral birth injury or developmental anomalies of the brain
3. Idiopathic epilepsy
4. Degenerative diseases of the central nervous system
5. Brain tumor
6. All other causes (listed below)

From 6 to 16 years of age

1. Idiopathic epilepsy
2. Residua of cerebral birth injury or developmental anomalies of the brain
3. Brain tumor
4. Acute infections of the central nervous system
5. Degenerative diseases of the central nervous system
6. All other causes (listed below)

All other causes of convulsions

1. Pathologic brain conditions: including toxoplasmosis; abscess of the brain; and rarities such as (a) tuberous sclerosis—characterized by mental deterioration and skin lesions (adenoma sebaceum), (b) cerebral angiomatosis (Sturge-Weber syndrome—association of a facial nevus with intracranial angiomas on the same side, which may appear calcified on roentgenograms)
2. Kidney: hypertensive encephalopathy of nephritis
3. Cardiovascular: congenital cardiac disease, e.g., cyanotic type with polycythemia predisposing to cerebral thrombosis, aortic stenosis, bacterial endocarditis with cerebral emboli or Stokes-Adams syndrome
4. Blood system: kernicterus, sickle-cell anemia

5. Metabolic: (*a*) carbohydrate disorders causing hypoglycemia, e.g., galactosemia, fructose intolerance, tumor of islet cells of the pancreas, overdosage of insulin in treating a diabetic child (convulsions in the newborn infants of diabetic mothers are usually due to hypoglycemia) hypopituitarism; (*b*) amino acid disorders, e.g., phenylketonuria (deficiency of phenylalanine hydroxylase); (*c*) lipidosis, e.g., complex lipids—sphingolipids (Gaucher's disease, Tay-Sachs disease, Niemann-Pick disease, etc.) accumulate in the cells of the nervous system; (*d*) disorders of metabolism of elements and cations, e.g., copper (hepatolenticular degeneration—Wilson's disease, see p. 156) calcium (hypocalcemia), magnesium (hypomagnesemia); (*e*) vitamin deficiency or dependency, e.g., pyridoxine; (*f*) disturbances of water and electrolyte balance, e.g., hypertonic or hypotonic dehydration.
6. Poisoning: lead, atropine, salicylates, thallium
7. Physical: sensitivity to light intensities

Psychogenic disorders such as hysteria and breath-holding may simulate convulsive disorders.

For purposes of classification the common types of seizures observed are listed below. (In making an etiologic diagnosis too much stress should not be placed on the type of seizure; for example, transient focal signs may appear in grand mal and in no way indicate localization of an organic lesion.)

1. Major motor (grand mal) seizures: generalized involvement usually beginning with a tonic contraction, followed by clonic contractions and associated with loss of consciousness. Tongue-biting and urinary or fecal incontinence may occur. Seizures usually last for several minutes, but a postictal sleep or depression of long duration ensues. The electroencephalogram shows multiple high-voltage spike discharges during a seizure. During an interval of quiescence it shows random, nonspecific spike discharges or a disorganized pattern not consistent with the age of the patient.
2. Petit mal seizures: occur most often between 4 to 7 years of age, consist of transient lapses of consciousness, last 5 to 30 seconds, and usually recur frequently during the day. Slight clonic movements of the eyelids or head may occur. The patient may fall to the floor because of sudden loss of muscular tone (akinetic seizure). A more massive contraction (myoclonic seizure) is less common. Petit mal seizures can usually be precipitated by voluntary hyperventilation. The electroencephalogram typically reveals a three-per-second, bilaterally synchronous spike and wave pattern.
3. Infantile spasm (minor motor seizures): usually occurs between 1 to 12 months of age in the brain-damaged infant with, for example, metabolic disorders, encephalitis, or birth trauma. These seizures usually consist of flexor spasms (jackknife or salaam

seizures) and are of short duration (several seconds), but they may occur often (as many as 100 per day). The electroencephalogram is characterized by random, high-voltage, slow spike and wave forms (hypsarrhythmia). Anticonvulsant drugs are given to control seizures. Specific therapy, e.g., galactose-free diet in galactosemia, should be instituted whenever indicated, and in the remainder of cases ACTH or steroids should be given since they may be effective. Rapid mental deterioration may occur in those patients unaffected by therapy. Infantile spasm usually ceases after 3 to 4 years of age and is replaced by generalized or focal seizures. The vast majority of these children become mildly or severely mentally retarded. About 25 percent die within 3 years.

4. Psychomotor (temporal-lobe) seizures: characterized by semipurposeful movements (also seen in petit mal), e.g., grasping movements of the hand, smacking of the lips; irrelevant speech and inappropriate behavior lasting several minutes and occurring during a period of altered consciousness. The electroencephalogram usually reveals spikes from the temporal area; it may also show nonspecific abnormalities (spikes from other areas, slow waves, or spike-wave discharges); or it may be normal.

5. Focal motor seizures: tonic-clonic movements of the limbs originating from the contralateral frontal motor cortex. "Jacksonian" seizures imply a gradual spread of the convulsive activity reflecting the spread of the cortical epileptic process.

6. Nonconvulsive epileptic equivalents: recurrent episodes of abdominal pain or headache when associated with either an abnormal electroencephalogram or the disappearance of symptoms following administration of anticonvulsive therapy may be of epileptic origin. The electroencephalogram may reveal a 14- and 6-per-second spike pattern.

FEBRILE CONVULSIONS

Febrile convulsions are associated with the sudden onset of acute infections, e.g., pneumonia, exanthems. They occur in about 6 to 8 percent of all children. About half the children having febrile convulsions also have afebrile convulsions.

Clinical features

1. The temperature is elevated [101°F (38.3°C) or more]. Convulsions usually occur with rapid rise of temperature.
2. The child previously has been neurologically normal and is neurologically normal after the convulsions.
3. Age is between 6 months and 4 years.
4. There is frequently a family history of febrile convulsions.
5. Seizures are symmetric and usually last less than 15 minutes.
6. A normal electroencephalogram is obtained about 1 week after the seizure.

Prognosis is good. Convulsions usually disappear by 3 years of age. If they are recurrent, long-term anticonvulsive therapy is given until 4 or 5 years of age. Simple febrile convulsions must be differentiated from epileptic seizures precipitated by fever.

INFANTILE TETANY

Tetany (spasmophilia) is a state of increased neuromuscular irritability dependent on the concentration of the calcium ion, non-protein-bound, in the serum, rather than on the total amount of serum calcium. Serum calcium below 7.0 mg per 100 ml of serum or less, provided that no hypoproteinemia exists, has been suggested to be the critical level to produce tetany. The most common causes in infancy and childhood are rickets, chronic renal insufficiency, steatorrhea (fibrocystic disease of the pancreas, celiac disease), alkalosis (vomiting, hyperventilation), hypoparathyroidism, tetany of the newborn infant (due to high phosphate intake and inability of the neonatal kidney to excrete phosphate), and postacidotic hypocalcemia. Infantile tetany may also be due to hypomagnesemia with or without hypocalcemia.

Clinical features

1. Carpopedal spasm: the thumb is in the cupped palm, hand abducted, wrist flexed, and the fingers positioned as for a vaginal examination. The foot is extended as in talipes equinovarus (clubfoot), with the sole cupped and toes flexed.
2. Laryngismus stridulus (laryngospasm): high-pitched crowing inspiration, greatest danger of tetany in that it may cause suffocation.
3. Generalized convulsions (occasionally unilateral): usually clonic.
4. Latent signs may be elicited even when the more obvious features above are not present: Chvostek's sign—gentle tap where the facial nerve emerges produces a contraction of the facial muscles with movement of the lips and forehead on that side. Erb's sign—contraction of muscles on cathodal opening current of less than 5 milliamperes. Trousseau's sign—firm pressure on the upper arm (to occlude arterial circulation) for 3 minutes produces carpal spasm. Peroneal sign—knee dorsiflexion and abduction of foot when peroneal nerve is tapped just below the head of the fibula.

Treatment

1. Intravenous calcium is the quickest means of raising the blood-calcium level. Calcium gluconate 10% is given. Calcium gluconate 10% has been given intramuscularly; however, this is not recommended because of frequent local reactions with sloughing and calcium-plaque deposits.
2. Intravenous therapy is followed by oral medication. Calcium chloride, 1 to 3 Gm daily in divided doses at concentrations less than

2 percent to avoid gastric irritation, is the drug of choice, but it should be used only for 2 days because it causes hyperchloremic acidosis. Further oral maintenance therapy is provided by administering calcium gluconate or calcium lactate, 0.5 Gm per kg per day.

3. Chronic hypoparathyroidism is treated with vitamin D (calciferol or ergocalciferol 10,000 to 50,000 IU daily for infants and 50,000 to 250,000 IU daily for an older child) and oral calcium.

4. Hypomagnesemia is treated with magnesium sulfate 50 percent, 0.2 ml per kg intramuscularly every 12 hours initially then daily for 7 to 10 days.

LEAD POISONING (Lead Encephalopathy) See p. 115.

IDIOPATHIC EPILEPSY

Idiopathic epilepsy is usually meant when the term "epilepsy" is used. It occurs on a constitutional or hereditary basis. There is no demonstrable pathologic cause. A family history of convulsions is present in one-third of the cases of epilepsy in children.

Epileptic seizures in children manifest themselves in a variety of forms, but usually are either grand mal or petit mal seizures (see Table 20-1). Ninety percent of children with idiopathic convulsive disorders show abnormal EEG tracings, particularly during sleep.

Criteria for diagnosis of idiopathic epilepsy

1. All other etiologic factors, particularly pathologic brain conditions, should be ruled out.

2. Heredity: There may be a history of epilepsy in the family, or there may be asymptomatic members who have abnormal electroencephalograms.

Table 20-1. Therapeutic classification of seizures

Seizure pattern	EEG correlates	Drug therapy
Grand mal and focal motor	Spikes, spike and wave, and sharp waves	Phenobarbital, diphenylhydantoin and primidone
Petit mal	3/sec spike-and-wave	Acetazolamide, ethosuximide, and trimethadione
Psychomotor	Temporal-lobe spikes and sharp waves	Primidone and methosuximide
Minor myoclonic and akinetic	Polyspike-and-wave and 2/sec slow spike-and-wave	Diazepam and primidone
Infantile myoclonic	Hypsarrhythmia	ACTH and diazepam

3. There are repeated characteristic seizures of similar type (disturbance of motor status, behavior, or consciousness).
4. A characteristic electroencephalogram, e.g., paroxysmal generalized three-per-second spike and wave burst, may appear spontaneously or be evoked only with hyperventilation.

Electroencephalography   By means of the electroencephalogram, it is possible to record the electrical waves arising from the cerebrum. Five normal rhythms have been described:

1. Alpha rhythm: regular sinusoidal waves, frequency between 8 and 12 per second, with a voltage of 20 to 60 microvolts
2. Beta rhythm: frequency of 13 to 32 per second, low voltage
3. Delta rhythm: normal until about 2 years of age, frequency of 1 to 3 per second
4. Theta rhythm: dominant rhythm until 7 years of age, tends to disappear by 12 years of age, abnormal in adults, frequency of 4 to 7 per second
5. Gamma rhythm: 33 to 55 per second arising from the frontal lobe, occurs infrequently

Treatment   The convulsion should be controlled as promptly as possible. Convulsions that persist and recur may of themselves produce brain damage. The investigation of the cause of the convulsion should be deferred until later.

1. General measures: clothing should be loosened and the patient protected—body, head, and tongue—from physical injury.
2. Suggested effective methods and medications to stop convulsions that do not subside promptly are intravenous Valium administered slowly over a 2-minute period in a dose of 5 to 10 mg; intravenous barbiturates (5 mg per kg of sodium phenobarbital, sodium Amytal, or Pentothal); intramuscular or subcutaneous sodium phenobarbital or sodium Amytal (10 mg per kg) or paraldehyde (1 ml per year of age).
3. Thereafter appropriate therapy for the cause, e.g., proper insulin dosage for the diabetic child, galactose-free diet in galactosemia, or the indicated anticonvulsant drugs (see below) should be employed to prevent recurring convulsions.
4. Physical hygiene: all abnormalities should be corrected wherever possible and foci of infection removed. Illnesses should be carefully and promptly treated. Regular muscular exercise in the form of supervised play, sports where no bodily contact is involved, and safe, interesting work are helpful. Good daily hygiene should be encouraged and fostered.
5. Psychologic care: mental stress and undue excitement should be avoided. Emotional conflicts between the child and members of the family and the community should be removed wherever possible.

The family and child should be helped to understand the problem and to work toward establishing a feeling of security. The public must be educated to assume a proper attitude toward this illness. As far as possible, the environment and activities should be the same as for a normal child.

6. Long-term drug therapy to prevent seizures: drugs are listed in Table 20-2 for the various types of seizure.

   a. Major motor seizures: Dilantin, phenobarbital, Mebaral, Mysoline, Peganone, bromides, Mesantoin, Gemonil, Valium

   b. Petit mal seizures: Tridione, Paradione, Zarontin, Celontin, Diamox (particularly for cases in which seizures can be precipitated by hyperventilation)

   c. Minor motor seizures: ACTH or adrenal corticosteroids, phenobarbital, Diamox, Valium, bromide

   d. Psychomotor seizures: Dilantin, Mysoline, phenobarbital, Mebaral, Peganone, Mesantoin, Gemonil

   e. Nonconvulsive equivalents: Dilantin, phenobarbital, Mysoline, Diamox

   In most instances, each type of seizure responds to a specific group of drugs, but the single drug most efficacious varies with the individual case; e.g., a child with petit mal may respond to Paradione and not to Tridione. Frequently it is necessary to try several of the drugs, singly or in combination and at various dosage levels, before the optimum therapeutic response is obtained.

7. Dietary therapy: dietary measures, particularly for minor motor seizures, may be used if the drugs are not completely successful. Starvation for a few days with water and salt restriction tends to produce acidosis; a ketogenic diet is then begun and maintained.

With proper care, seizures can usually be well controlled and there is no mental deterioration. Grand mal epilepsy occasionally disappears spontaneously, particularly at puberty. Petit mal tends to disappear at puberty. Psychomotor (behavioral) and minor motor types of epilepsy are often resistant to therapy. Occasionally therapy is ineffective in grand mal, convulsions persist (status epilepticus), and death may occur. Status epilepticus may occur following sudden withdrawal of anticonvulsant drugs.

Idiopathic forms of epilepsy are more amenable to drugs than are forms due to organic brain disease.

Surgery is of no value in idiopathic epilepsy. Where an organic or focal lesion, e.g., tumor or adhesions following hemorrhage, can be demonstrated by physical diagnosis and laboratory tests—roentgenogram, pneumoencephalogram, electroencephalogram—surgery may be helpful for those conditions which cannot be controlled by medical treatment.

Breath-holding spells   These spells usually begin at 6 to 12 months of age and are characterized by voluntary holding of the breath and

Table 20-2. Anticonvulsant preparations, dosages, and more common side effects

Drug	Preparation (Gm)	Average total daily dose for children, mg/kg body weight	Side effects
Phenobarbital	Tablets, 0.016, 0.032, 0.065, 0.1; elixir, 0.02/tsp; injection, 0.12/ml	3–6	Drowsiness, irritability, and hyperactivity
Mephobarbital	Tablets, 0.032, 0.05, 0.1, 0.2	6–12	Same as phenobarbital, but less frequent
Diphenylhydantoin	Tablets, 0.05 Capsules, 0.03, 0.1 Injection, 0.25/5 ml	5–10	Ataxia, gum hyperplasia, rash, and abdominal pain
Primidone	Tablets, 0.05, 0.25	5–20	Drowsiness, ataxia, rash, and anorexia
Acetazolamide*	Tablets, 0.125, 0.25	12–25	Lassitude, paresthesia, and headache
Ethosuximide*	Capsules, 0.25	20–60	Nausea, leukopenia, and rash
Methosuximide*	Capsules, 0.3	20–60	Rash, dizziness, drowsiness, and nausea
Trimethadione*	Tablets, 0.15 Capsules, 0.3 Solution, 0.15/tsp	20–60	Leukopenia, rash, hemeralopia, and nephrosis
Paramethadione*	Capsules, 0.15, 0.3	20–60	Same as trimethadione, but less frequent
Diazepam	Tablets, 0.002, 0.005	0.1–1	Drowsiness and ataxia

* Frequent white cell counts and urinalyses recommended.

509

loss of consciousness. The infant becomes limp or rigid, and a brief generalized convulsion may occur. The electroencephalogram is normal.

Narcolepsy and cataplexy   The uncontrollable desire to sleep (narcolepsy) or sudden transient loss of muscle tone (cataplexy) are seen rarely in children and are disorders of unknown etiology. The electroencephalogram is normal in narcolepsy, and treatment with Dexedrine (2.5 to 5.0 mg, three times a day) or Ritalin (10 mg twice a day) is of value.

MIGRAINE

Migraine is characterized by periodic headache with associated gastrointestinal and visual disturbances. In contrast to adult migraine, children have more frequent attacks, more gastrointestinal symptoms, less cephalgia, and fewer scotomas. The attacks may be psychologic in origin; they occur more often in males and in children whose parents have migraine. The electroencephalogram may reveal dysrhythmia.

Treatment   Aspirin and, if necessary, Cafergot (caffeine 100 mg and Ergotrate 1 mg), 1 tablet repeated in ½ hour for the attack. Some children respond to long-term therapy with antiepileptic drugs. Psychotherapy may be helpful.

SPASMUS NUTANS

Spasmus nutans is characterized by head-nodding, nystagmus, and torticollis and is usually found during the first year of life. The cause is unknown, but keeping an infant in a poorly lighted room may be a factor. This condition may last several months, after which there is spontaneous recovery.

MENTAL RETARDATION

According to the American Association on Mental Deficiency, "mental retardation refers to subaverage general intellectual functioning which originates during the developmental period and is associated with impairment in adaptive behavior." It is estimated that 3 percent of all children may be placed within the classification of mental retardation. Mental retardation is more frequent in boys than in girls.

The association's classification by intelligence is widely used in the field and is as follows:

Degree of retardation	IQ
Borderline	70–84
Mild	55–69
Moderate	40–54
Severe	26–39
Profound	0–25

THE SEVERELY AND PROFOUNDLY RETARDED

Most of these children remain dependent throughout their lifetime and are generally able to achieve only minimum self-care skills. Most of these youngsters are likely to have severe associated sensorimotor handicaps.

THE MODERATELY RETARDED

These children may obtain semi-independent status. Most moderately retarded children can be identified in infancy or early childhood. They show a consistently slow developmental pattern with poor motor coordination and minimum communicative skills.

THE MILDLY RETARDED

With adequate medical and educational programs these children can achieve independent functioning. In contrast to the more severely retarded, the behavior of this group is influenced to a greater degree by psychologic, social, and cultural factors.

Classification   The diagnostic possibilities should be considered under the following scheme:

I. Pathologic classification
    A. Primary cerebrocranial developmental defects
        1. Cerebral malformations: cerebral agenesis, cerebral hypoplasia, cerebral hyperplasia (macrocephaly), hydrocephalus, hydranencephaly
        2. Cranial defects: craniostenosis, hypertelorism
        3. Congenital ectodermoses: tuberous sclerosis, cerebral angiomatosis (Sturge-Weber syndrome), neurofibromatosis
        4. Down's syndrome (trisomy D)
        5. Familial defect (defective or inferior intelligence in one or both parents and in other siblings)
        6. Undifferentiated cerebrocranial defect (primary amentia)
    B. Secondary cerebral malformations
        1. Porencephaly: e.g., from trauma
        2. Hydrocephalus: e.g., following intracranial hemorrhage

associated with birth trauma or hypoxia, infection, or neoplasm

C. Central nervous system abnormalities associated with metabolic defects

1. Abnormal amino acid metabolism: phenylpyruvic oligophrenia, maple syrup urine disease, homocystinuria, histidinemia, prolinemia, etc.
2. Abnormal uric acid metabolism: Lesch-Nyhan syndrome
3. Galactosemia
4. Cretinism (congenital hypothyroidism)
5. Gargoylism (Hurler's, Hunter's, and Sanfilippo's syndromes)
6. Hepatolenticular degeneration (Wilson's disease)
7. Sphingolipidosis: Gaucher's, Niemann-Pick, and Tay-Sachs diseases, metachromatic leukodystrophy, etc.

D. Acquired focal or disseminated central nervous system lesions

1. Posttoxic and infection: lead encephalopathy, viral encephalitis, kernicterus
2. Posttraumatic lesions
3. Posthypoxic

E. Degenerative disorders of the central nervous system (see p. 518)

F. Functional mental retardation (pseudoretardation): emotional disturbances

II. Etiologic classification

A. Prenatal factors

1. Genetically determined: disorders of protein, carbohydrate, and fat metabolism, cerebral demyelinating diseases, gargoylism, cranial anomalies (craniostenosis), congenital ectodermoses (tuberous sclerosis), chromosomal abnormalities (Down's syndrome, Klinefelter's syndrome, triple X syndrome, etc.)
2. Acquired in utero: infection (rubella, herpes, syphilis, toxoplasmosis, cytomegalic inclusion disease), hypoxia, hemorrhage, isoimmunization, endocrine disturbances, roentgen-ray irradiation, drugs

B. Natal factors

1. Hypoxia and hemorrhage
2. Birth trauma
3. Infection

C. Postnatal factors

1. Trauma
2. Infections: meningitis, encephalitis
3. Toxicity: lead, arsenic, coal tar derivatives
4. Vascular accidents: congenital aneurysms, cerebrovascular thrombosis
5. Hypoxia: carbon monoxide
6. Neoplasm
7. Postimmunization encephalopathy: pertussis, smallpox.

The comprehensive evaluation and diagnosis of the child's capacities and limitations are essential to treatment planning. In order to make the most effective use of special facilities and services, such as counseling, education, and rehabilitation, parents have to be informed of their child's condition in detail. The parents can then help in preparing a meaningful plan for the child's present and future care.

Informing the parents After a thorough evaluation of the retarded child, the parents must be given an interpretation of the diagnosis and findings in as clear and detailed a way as possible, but with sensitivity for their feelings. The difficulty that many parents experience in gaining an understanding of their child's handicap, their daily problems in living with him, and their ability to contribute to his well-being are greatly influenced by the kind of professional counsel they receive at this time. The facts should be given frankly and honestly, but without brusqueness or brutality. False reassurances about the child's normality and vagueness in giving information only compound the parents' perplexity and anxiety. On the other hand, the parents' shock and disappointment can be mimimized by giving a total picture—the child's assets and capabilities as well as his deficiencies. One can also attempt to relieve parents' tendency to blame themselves for the child's condition as well as their fears about future pregnancies (if the condition is not hereditary). Recommendations which parents are unready or unable to accept are approached carefully. Even when institutionalization may be an imminent necessity, the physician must anticipate the parents' likely resistance, present the facts about the child's condition and prognosis as well as about institutional care, and then allow the parents to make their own decision in their own time.

The compassionate attitude of the physician, his willingness to give time, understanding, and attention to the parents, and his assurance of continued interest and acceptance of responsibility are essentials that cannot be overstressed.

Treatment There is no specific drug or surgical therapy, except in certain metabolic disorders. The child should be helped by a cooperative team—physician, clinical psychologist, social worker, psychiatrist, educator, special therapist, etc.—to attain his maximum development and live happily in his environment. This can be accomplished by treating the child as a whole: mentally, by providing special training and education; psychologically, by providing good emotional hygiene, with special attention to the need for parental guidance; physically, by correcting defects where possible; and socially, by helping him adjust to his environment.

DOWN'S SYNDROME (Mongolism)

Down's syndrome is one of the common forms of mental retardation. It occurs in all races and nationalities. The brain is small, the convolutional pattern is simple, and the sulci are shallow.

Clinical and laboratory features

1. Most children with this form of mental deficiency are moderately or severely retarded; occasionally some are only mildly retarded.
2. The appearance is characteristic: because of the peculiar maldevelopment of the skull, particularly of the basilar bones, the head is small and flat anteroposteriorly; the face is broad, and the cheek bones are high (mongoloid type), the nose is small (because of hypoplasia of the nasal and facial bones) with a depressed bridge, the eyes are set wide apart and slant upward and outward, strabismus is common, and Brushfield spots are seen in the iris, the palpebral fissures are narrow and the epicanthal folds prominent; the ears are small and may be malformed, the lips are thick, the tongue is large, rough, and fissured, and the permanent teeth show gross abnormalities; the skin is soft, loose, and of good color, with extra folds in the neck.
3. The fifth fingers are short and curve inward (clinodactyly), and the middle and distal phalanges are often rudimentary, as seen on roentgenograms. There are widely spaced first and second digits of short stubby hands and feet, with abnormal plantar and palmar (only one major crease—Simian crease) print.
4. The genitals are small, and there is an absence of mammary tissue in the young infant.
5. Muscular hypotonia and joint hypermobility are present.
6. In a considerable number of cases, there are congenital cardiac defects, e.g., interventricular septal defects, endocardial cushion defect.
7. Infections, particularly respiratory ones, are common. Prior to the advent of antibiotics, infection usually caused death early in life.
8. There may be fairly good growth in height during infancy, but later growth is retarded because of undergrowth of the vertebral bodies and tubular bones in the extremities.
9. Roentgenographically, the sinuses are frequently found to be absent; bone age is normal or moderately delayed; acetabular and iliac angles are smaller than normal.
10. There is a significant increase in the incidence of leukemia, duodenal atresia, and congenital megacolon.
11. Chromosomal studies most often reveal trisomy 21 (see Chapter 8, "Genetics").
12. The following laboratory tests may be abnormal: acid and alkaline phosphatase of white blood cells—elevated; serum serotonin —increased; and glucose-6-phosphate dehydrogenase of red blood cells—increased.

Treatment   There is no specific therapy. Special training, education, and psychologic care of the family and child will help him achieve his maximum potential, but he cannot go beyond a certain level. If home care is impossible, the child may be institutionalized.

HYDROCEPHALUS

Hydrocephalus is an excessive accumulation of cerebrospinal fluid which results from obstruction at any point in the cerebrospinal fluid pathway between the region of principal formation (choroid plexi within the ventricular system) and the point of principal absorption (arachnoid villi in the superior sagittal sinus). It is characterized by a rapid increase in the size of the head, large fontanels, separation of the sutures (papilledema is usually not seen, unless the sutures do not separate rapidly enough), distension of the scalp veins, downward displacement of the eyes with so-called "setting sun" appearance and retarded growth and development. It may result from congenital anomalies of the central nervous system (often associated with other anomalies), following intracranial hemorrhage associated with birth trauma or hypoxia, infection, or neoplasm.

Hydrocephalus may be either obstructive or communicating.

In the obstructive type, the block is within the ventricular system at the various foramina—foramen of Monro, aqueduct of Sylvius, or foramina of Magendie and Luschka.

In the communicating type, the block is in the intracranial sub-arachnoid space, which prevents the fluid from reaching the arach-noidal villi, but the ventricles communicate freely with the spinal subarachnoid space.

Surgery, e.g., arachnoid-ureterostomy, ventriculopleural or ventriculoatrial shunt, is often indicated. Prognosis is guarded. (Subdural hematoma and tumors must always be ruled out.)

CEREBRAL PALSY

Etiology Cerebral palsy (spastic diplegia, Little's disease) may be caused by congenital malformations of the brain or by prenatal, natal, or postnatal cerebral damage. The causative factors which are outlined under Mental Retardation are often identical with those of cerebral palsy.

Clinical features Cerebral palsy comprises those motor and other symptom complexes, e.g., impaired hearing or vision, intellectual deficiency, speech defects, convulsive disorders and psychologic problems caused by a nonprogressive brain lesion (or lesions). The various subtypes may be defined as follows:

1. *Spasticity:* characterized by a lower threshold of the stretch reflex, an enlarged reflexogenic area, augmented responses with clonus. There is a tendency toward greater involvement and contractures affecting the antigravity muscles.
2. *Athetosis:* characterized by involuntary slow, writhing (snakelike), hypertonic movements affecting particularly the peripheral muscles

of the extremities and the mouth, face, and throat muscles. The reflexes are normal.

3. *Rigidity:* a disturbance of the agonist-antagonist relations with resistance to slow passive motion of both agonist and antagonist muscles. If the resistance to passive motion is continuous, it is referred to as "lead-pipe" rigidity; if it is discontinuous, it is called "cog-wheel" rigidity.

4. *Ataxia:* incoordination due to disturbance of kinesthetic sense, or a lesion of the cerebellum.

5. *Tremor:* intentional or constant uncontrollable involuntary motions of a rhythmic, alternating, or pendular pattern due to alternate agonist and antagonist contractions.

6. *Atonia:* lack of tone and failure of muscles to respond to volitional stimulation. The muscle lacks the firmness or turgor of the normal relaxed muscle.

7. *Mixed:* combinations of the above. The term is not used often, as the predominant motor symptoms determine the classification.

Neurologic signs and symptoms change as the nervous system matures, and one must be extremely cautious in making a final descriptive diagnosis in infancy.

Diagnosis   Any infant or child who does not sit up, walk, talk, or develop normally or whose legs cross scissorlike when picked up should be evaluated, particularly with cerebral palsy in mind.

Prognosis   It has been estimated that 7 children per 1,000 born in the United States have cerebral palsies. One dies early; of the remaining six, one has a severe palsy, two have moderate cases, and three have mild cases. Sixty to seventy percent are mentally deficient.

Treatment

1. Reeducation and rehabilitation, consisting of special muscle training, speech training, and physiotherapy.
2. Psychotherapy for the child and his family.
3. Corrective surgery—orthopedic, neurologic, and ocular.
4. Drugs such as meprobamate, Valium, and Robaxin are of value.
5. Anticonvulsive therapy for seizures.

ATAXIA IN CHILDHOOD

Ataxia results from disorders of the cerebellum. In history it may be relatively stationary, with its onset during infancy; progressive and chronic; or acute, with partial or complete recovery. The disorder may be limited to the cerebellum or it may be widespread, involving other areas of the central nervous system.

1. Stationary ataxia: characterized by difficulty in sitting and standing, a delay in walking, and lack of coordination in the use of the arms and legs. Roentgenograms may reveal a shallow posterior fossa demonstrating the basic developmental defect in the cerebellum. There is no treatment.

2. Chronic progressive ataxia

   a. Arnold-Chiari deformity: see p. 207.

   b. Hereditary spinocerebellar ataxia (Friedreich's ataxia): usually has its onset at 7 to 10 years of age. It is transmitted as an autosomal recessive gene and is caused by degeneration of the dorsal and ventral spinocerebellar tracts, the corticospinal tracts, and the posterior columns. Associated anomalies are kyphoscoliosis and pes cavus. It is characterized by dizziness, stumbling, loss of position sense and deep-tendon reflexes, and an abnormal Babinski reflex. Clinical and electrocardiographic findings of myocarditis often are present. Death usually occurs by 30 years of age.

   c. Bassen-Kornzweig syndrome (acanthocytosis): see p. 418.

   d. Hereditary ataxia with myoclonic epilepsy (Ramsay Hunt): probably an inherited disease which has its onset at 7 to 17 years of age and is caused by degeneration of the dentate nuclei. It is characterized by convulsions, myoclonus, intention tremor, and marked incoordination of the arms and legs.

   e. Hereditary cerebellar ataxia: includes a number of clinical pictures in which cerebellar signs occur alone or they are the most prominent findings. The onset is between 3 and 17 years of age. It is characterized by impaired balance, unsteady gait, spasticity of the legs, dysarthria, incoordination of the hands, and optic atrophy.

   f. Ataxia-telangiectasia (Louis-Bar syndrome): transmitted as an autosomal recessive trait. Onset is usually between 1 and 3 years of age with an unsteady, wide-based gait. There is difficulty in coordination of the arms, dysarthria, and nystagmus. Telangiectasia appear at from 4 to 6 years of age on the exposed bulbar conjunctivae, bridge of the nose, ears, and neck. Recurrent ear infections, sinusitis, bronchitis, and pneumonia are common possibly because of immunologic deficiency of serum and secretory IgA. There is also an IgE deficiency and defects in cellular immunity. Death usually occurs before 25 years of age.

   g. Cerebellar tumors: see p. 607.

   h. Multiple sclerosis: multiple sclerosis occurs more often in females and presents a clinical picture similar to that seen in adults. By the nature of the disease process, the variability in the clinical findings is immense. In children, however, just as in adults, weakness of the limbs or incoordination, visual disturbances such as retrobulbar neuritis, diplopia, and nystagmus, abnormalities of speech, and involvement of "posterior-column" sensibilities are present in the majority of instances. The course is likewise variable, and therefore prognosis is difficult to ascertain. During the first episode, the diagnosis may be suspected but, by definition, it cannot be established conclusively. There is no specific treatment.

    i.   Hartnup disease: a rare familial condition associated with an abnormal pattern of amino acid excretion due to diminished renal reabsorption. Clinical symptoms include a "pellegra-like" rash, reversible attacks of cerebellar ataxia, and psychiatric disturbances. Treatment consists of a high-protein diet and oral nicotinamide and oral neomycin during acute attacks. (The normal tryptophan-nicotinic acid pathway is blocked— gastrointestinal bacteria may play a role.) Prognosis is good; improvement occurs with adulthood.

    j.   Refsum's syndrome: see Inherited Disorders of Lipid Metabolism, Chapter 9.

    k.   Cerebral lipidoses: Niemann-Pick disease (see p. 519) and metachromatic leukodystrophy (see p. 520).

3.   Acute ataxia: many of the chronic ataxias may have an acute onset, e.g., multiple sclerosis, encephalitis.

    a.   Acute cerebellar ataxia: a disease of unknown causation— possibly toxic, viral, or allergic in nature—which occurs most commonly in children 2 to 3 years of age. The acute onset of a disturbance in gait is the chief clinical manifestation. Mild tremor, gross rhythmic movements of all parts of the body, nystagmus (especially early in the course), hypotonia, and staccato speech may be present. The peripheral blood, cerebrospinal fluid, roentgenograms of the skull, and electroencephalogram are not diagnostic. Symptoms last for 1 to 2 weeks and are usually completely gone in 2 months; there are most often no residua. Recovery is spontaneous and not altered by drugs. A few cases may have prolonged courses.

    b.   A syndrome similar to acute cerebellar ataxia may occur as a form of encephalitis; intoxication, e.g., Dilantin, tranquilizers, ethyl alcohol; brain tumor; degenerative diseases of the central nervous system, e.g., Friedreich's ataxia; or hysteria.

    c.   Cerebellar tumor or abscess.

    d.   Spinal cord tumor.

    e.   Infectious polyneuropathy (also known as Guillain-Barré syndrome and Landry's paralysis). See Chapter 14, "Infectious Diseases."

    f.   Head injury.

PROGRESSIVE DEGENERATIVE DISEASES OF CHILDHOOD

Diseases affecting gray matter   (The most common findings include convulsions, myoclonus, macular degeneration, and mental deterioration.)

1. Progressive myoclonus (Unverricht-Lundborg syndrome) : a recessive autosomal disease with onset in late childhood or adolescence of seizures and later-developing myoclonus, mental deterioration, and generalized rigidity. The involved neurons contain round inclusion bodies (Lafora) in their cytoplasm. Death occurs in early adulthood.

2. Gangliosidosis

   a. Infantile (Tay-Sachs disease; G_{M2} gangliosidosis, type 1). (See Table 8-2.)

   b. Sandhoff's disease (G_{M2} gangliosidosis, type 2) has almost the same clinical manifestations as Tay-Sachs disease, but occasional lipid-laden histiocytes are found in visceral organs. Hexosaminidase A and B are lacking.

   c. Juvenile amaurotic familial idiocy (G_{M2} gangliosidosis, type 3) ; an inherited disease (autosomal recessive) beginning in childhood and characterized by locomotor ataxia, loss of speech, and progressive spasticity. It is not limited to children of Jewish origin. Progression occurs over a 6- to 10-year period. There is a partial deficiency of hexosaminidase A.

   d. Generalized gangliosidosis (G_{M1} gangliosidosis, type 1) is an autosomal recessive disorder characterized by unusual facial appearance, neurologic symptoms, hepatosplenomegaly, and bone lesions. The disease manifests at birth and leads to death by 2 years of age. There are marked deficiencies of beta galactosidase A, B, and C.

   e. Juvenile type (G_{M2} gangliodosis, type 2) resembles generalized gangliosidosis as regards neurologic symptoms, but hepatosplenomegaly is absent. The disease manifests itself at 6 to 24 months of age, and death occurs by 3 to 10 years. Beta galactosidase B and C are deficient.

3. Niemann-Pick disease (sphingomyelin lipidosis) : an inherited disease (probably autosomal recessive) in which several variants are known. They differ in age of onset, rate of progression, degree of involvement of the central nervous system, the relative excess of sphingomyelin present, and degree of activity of the enzyme sphingomyelinase. Characteristically, cells, primarily reticulum cells, with lipid accumulations (foam cells) infiltrate almost all organs. The diagnosis is suspected when hepatosplenomegaly and abnormal psychomotor development occur together. A cherry-red spot of the macula may be present. Bone-marrow aspiration reveals foam cells. Cholesterol may be increased in the serum. There is no specific treatment. Splenectomy may be helpful for hypersplenism.

4. Gaucher's disease (glycosyl ceramide lipidosis) is inherited as an autosomal recessive disorder in the metabolism of glucosyl ceramide due to an enzymatic defect—glucosyl ceramide hydrolase (glucocerebrosidase), resulting in accumulation of glucosyl ceramide in reticuloendothelial cells. Several variants are known—a slowly progressing chronic or adult type, an acute type with neurologic involvement occurring in infants and rapidly progressing to death,

and a subacute juvenile type in which the neurologic involvement progresses slowly and death occurs in childhood or adolescence. The acute type is characterized by hepatosplenomegaly. There is difficulty in feeding and failure to thrive. The cranial nerve of the midbrain, pons, and medulla are severely involved causing strabismus, dysphagia, and trismus. Most organs demonstrate infiltration by Gaucher cells and may demonstrate signs due to interference with their normal function, e.g., spleen—anemia. Diagnosis is based on clinical features, elevated acid phosphatase, the presence of Gaucher cells in bone-marrow aspirates, and diminished enzyme activity. Death occurs usually due to pulmonary infiltration and recurrent pneumonia.

5. Subacute necrotizing encephalopathy (Leigh's encephalomyelopathy) is probably due to an inborn defect in metabolism beginning at birth to 2 years of age. There is progressive necrosis of gray matter with cavity formation. The infant is quiet and immobile and does not cry. Optic atrophy, seizures, and spasticity are characteristic. Death occurs between 4 months and 4 years of age.

6. Progressive degeneration of cerebral gray matter (Alpers' disease, poliodystrophy) may be transmitted by an autosomal recessive gene. The onset may appear shortly after birth or anytime until 2 years of age. There is marked loss of neurons, which are replaced by astrocytes. The condition is characterized by seizures, generalized spasticity, dementia, blindness, and deafness. Death occurs in several years.

7. Wolman's disease is a generalized xanthomatosis characterized by diarrhea, forceful vomiting with marked abdominal distension, hepatosplenomegaly, failure to thrive, neurologic symptoms, and adrenal calcification. Almost all organs contain foam cells loaded with cholesterol and glycerides.

8. Mucopolysaccharidoses 1 to 3 (see p. 539).

Diseases affecting white matter

Progressive paralytic dementias of children are associated with a hereditary defect in myelin or an acquired degeneration of cerebral white matter. Clinically, these leukodystrophies are characterized by spasticity, ataxia, optic atrophy, and involvement of peripheral nerves.

1. Metachromatic* leukodystrophy (sulfatide lipidosis) is inherited as an autosomal recessive condition due to arylsulfatase A deficiency resulting in an accumulation of sulfatide. There are several types, with the late infantile being the most common. The onset occurs at between 12 to 18 months of age with flaccidity which progresses to spastic paralysis. Mental regression, optic

---

*   Metachromatic refers to the capacity of some dyes to change color in the presence of certain chemicals. Biologic substances (chromotropes) possessing the ability to affect dyes include sulfatides.

atrophy, and ataxia occur. Terminally, there are decerebrate posture and bulbar paralysis.

2. Globoid cell leukodystrophy (Krabbe's disease) is inherited as an autosomal recessive condition with an onset at 3 to 6 months of age with progressive retardation, spells of incessant screaming, spastic quadriparesis, blindness, and deafness. Cerebrospinal fluid protein is elevated. Death occurs by 2 years of age. Globoid cells are found in the white matter. There is a severe deficiency in the activity of the enzyme galactocerebroside β-galactosidase.

3. Leukodystrophy with spongy degeneration is inherited as an autosomal recessive trait and characterized by widespread demyelination. It is more common in Jews. The onset is from birth to 2 months of age. There is an arrest of psychomotor development, flaccidity progressing to decerebrate rigidity, and optic atrophy. Macrocephaly occurs which may be confused with hydrocephalus. Death occurs by 18 months of age.

4. Pelizaeus-Merzbacher disease is inherited as a sex-linked recessive trait. The onset is in infancy or early childhood with nystagmus and cerebellar signs. The condition is progressive, but at about 6 years of age the rate of progression may slow markedly and patients may live well into adulthood. Gradual development of spasticity, dementia, ataxia, and seizures late in the course is characteristic.

5. Sudanophilic leukodystrophy is characterized by extensive symmetric demyelinization in cerebral and cerebellar white matter. It is a progressive disease occurring in late childhood with signs of progressive pyramidal tract and cerebellar involvement. One variety is inherited as a sex-linked recessive trait associated with Addison's disease.

6. Cerebrohepatorenal syndrome (see p. 174).

FAMILIAL DYSAUTONOMIA

Familial dysautonomia (familial autonomic dysfunction, Riley-Day syndrome) is a disorder of the central nervous system occurring mostly in Jewish families. It is characterized by defective lacrimation, absence of tastebud papillae of the tongue, skin blotching, excessive perspiration, drooling, emotional instability, episodic hypertension, and feeding problems during infancy, e.g., vomiting. There may be hyporeflexia, relative indifference to pain, corneal hypesthesia and ulceration, stunted growth, occasionally mental retardation, motor incoordination, and characteristically abnormal speech. Frequent respiratory tract infections are common. An inborn error of catecholamine metabolism has been suggested to be the cause. The cornea is treated with methylcellulose 0.33% drops in the daytime, bland ointment at night. Tarsorrhaphy may be required. There is no specific treatment; intramuscular chlorpromazine is used for vomiting, and electrolyte balance should be preserved. Congenital analgesia (recessive trait disease), with injuries and burns of the limbs from insensitivity to pain, may need to be differentiated from familial dysautonomia.

REVIEW QUESTIONS

1. The most common etiologic factor of convulsive disorders from 6 to 24 months is (a) residua of birth injuries; (b) acute infection of the central nervous system; (c) acute febrile convulsions; (d) idiopathic epilepsy.
2. The following conditions are associated with convulsions except for (a) galactosemia; (b) Stokes-Adams syndrome; (c) elevated serum magnesium level; (d) Wilson's disease.
3. Column I lists several types of seizures; column II contains some statements concerning these seizures. Match the two:

	I			II
A.	Major motor (grand mal) _____		(a)	Transient lapses of consciousness lasting 5 to 30 seconds.
B.	Petit mal _____		(b)	EEG shows high-voltage spike discharges.
C.	Minor motor _____		(c)	Originates from the contralateral frontal motor cortex.
D.	Psychomotor _____		(d)	EEG usually reveals spikes from the temporal area.
E.	Focal motor _____		(e)	EEG shows random, high-voltage slow spike and wave form.

4. Febrile convulsions occur in (a) 1 to 3 percent; (b) 6 to 8 percent; (c) 10 to 12 percent; (d) 15 to 20 percent of all children.
5. The following statements about febrile convulsions are true except (a) family history of febrile convulsions is rarely obtained; (b) the child is neurologically normal before and after the convulsions; (c) seizures are symmetrical and usually last less than 15 minutes; (d) a normal electroencephalogram is obtained after 1 week.
6. The critical level for serum calcium below which tetany may occur is (a) 9 mg per 100 ml; (b) 7 mg per 100 ml; (c) 6 mg per 100 ml; (d) 5 mg per 100 ml.
7. The following conditions may lead to the hypocalcemic type of tetany except for (a) rickets; (b) hyperparathyroidism; (c) chronic renal insufficiency; (d) hypomagnesemia.
8. The treatment of choice to correct infantile tetany is (a) intravenous calcium gluconate; (b) intravenous calcium chloride; (c) oral calcium gluconate; (d) intramuscular calcium chloride.
9. Column I lists several types of convulsive seizures; column II lists some drugs used in the treatment of these seizures. Match the two:

	I		II
A.	Major motor _____	(a)	ACTH, Diamox, Valium
B.	Petit mal _____	(b)	Tridione, Zarontin, Celontin
C.	Minor motor _____	(c)	Dilantin, Mysoline, Mesantoin

10. Ataxia, gum hyperplasia, abdominal pain, and rash are frequently seen as side effects in therapy with (a) phenobarbital; (b) diphenylhydantoin; (c) diazepam; (d) bromide.

11. All the following are features of breath-holding spells except (a) they begin at 6 to 12 months of age; (b) there is loss of consciousness; (c) a brief generalized convulsion may occur; (d) there is a characteristic abnormal EEG pattern; (e) they are difficult to differentiate from true convulsions.

12. The following statements concerning spasmus nutans are true except for (a) it is characterized by head-nodding, torticollis, and nystagmus; (b) the condition may last several months followed by spontaneous recovery; (c) some patients respond to long-term therapy with antiepileptic drugs; (d) it usually occurs during the first year of life.

13. Mental retardation occurs in approximately (a) 1 percent; (b) 3 percent; (c) 6 percent; (d) 9 percent of all children.

14. The following are features of Down's syndrome except for (a) the fifth finger is short and curves inward; (b) there is increased muscle tone; (c) patients frequently have associated congenital cardiac abnormalities; (d) trisomy 21 is the most frequent chromosomal pattern; (e) an increased incidence of duodenal atresia is noted.

15. The following are true for cerebral palsy except (a) antigravity muscles more commonly involved; (b) 60 to 70 percent are mentally retarded; (c) it occurs in 7 per 1,000 live births; (d) it may be caused by congenital anomalies of the brain; (e) it is associated with increased incidence of chronic myelogenous leukemia.

21

DISEASES OF THE SKELETAL SYSTEM

COLLAGEN DISEASES

Collagen diseases, i.e., rheumatic fever, rheumatoid arthritis, dermato-myositis, scleroderma, disseminated lupus erythematosus, polyarteritis nodosa, anaphylactoid purpura, purpura fulminans, erythema multiforme exudativum (Stevens-Johnson syndrome), morphea (focal sclero-derma), are considered as a group because they have the common property of producing destructive, degenerative, and proliferative changes in connective tissue. The causation of these diseases is unknown, but allergy is a conspicuous feature. For example, some cases of periarteritis nodosa, anaphylactoid purpura, and Stevens-Johnson syndrome are related to hypersensitivity to drugs; rheumatic fever is related to hypersensitivity to streptococci. It is of interest, also, to note that this group of diseases responds favorably to treatment with adrenal corticosteroids, and that there is an increased incidence within families.

RHEUMATIC FEVER

This condition is presented in Chapter 16, "Heart Diseases."

RHEUMATOID ARTHRITIS

Rheumatoid arthritis is a chronic disease of unknown etiology. Several factors such as constitutional susceptibility, tissue sensitization, infection, and trauma appear to play roles but require further evaluation. It is more common in females. Onset is rare under 1 year of age but not infrequent before 5 years. There may be a history of an upper respiratory tract infection or infection elsewhere in the body preceding the onset.

Clinical features

1. The onset varies from insidious, with few constitutional manifestations, to acute, with spiking temperature and toxicity, which precedes the joint pain by days to weeks. An evanescent, small macular rash (salmon pink with pale centers) often appears with the fever and then disappears rapidly. The fever is often of the intermittent or septic type.
2. Generalized lymphadenopathy may be present, especially in the early stage. The nodes are nontender and well circumscribed.
3. Pain and stiffness of joints often precede swelling. Knees, ankles, feet, wrists, and fingers are frequently involved at the onset. Early in the course up to 50 percent of patients have mono- or pauci-articular involvement which may then persist for years. The joint involvement is frequently symmetric in patients with polyarthritis. The affected joints are swollen and warm but without erythema. Spindling of fingers is seen often even in young children. The cervical spine is frequently involved with neck stiffness and pain.
4. Finally there are involvement of many joints and marked muscle atrophy, resulting in deformities and ankylosis.
5. Splenomegaly may accompany the chronic arthritis (Still's disease). Hepatomegaly is rare.
6. Iridocyclitis may occur and precede the onset of joint pains or follow arthritis by several years. It is most frequent in patients with mono- or pauci-articular disease.
7. Subcutaneous nodules, nontender, may occasionally be seen.
8. Pericarditis (chest pain, cardiac enlargement, and electrocardiographic abnormalities) is frequently seen. Myocarditis is uncommon.
9. Nonspecific abdominal pain occurs in 25 percent of these children.

Laboratory findings

1. Sedimentation rate is usually increased, and leukocyte count may be elevated with an associated anemia, often severe.
2. Tests for rheumatoid factor (latex, sensitized sheep-cell agglutination and bentonite particle tests) are positive in only a small percent of children with rheumatoid arthritis.
3. C-reactive protein is frequently positive.
4. Antistreptolysin O titer may be elevated.
5. Serum proteins may be altered—albumin, decreased; alpha$_2$ globulin, increased; gamma globulin, increased.
6. LE cells may be observed in up to 5 percent of patients.
7. Roentgenograms reveal soft-tissue swelling, demineralization (particularly juxta-articular), and alteration of the joint spaces (narrowing) and articular surfaces. Cervical spine changes (narrowing and fusion of apophyseal joints) are characteristic.

Treatment

1. Salicylates constitute the main therapeutic modality and are helpful to relieve pain. The usual dose is 100 mg per kg per day, divided in 4 to 6 doses. A blood level of 25 mg per 100 ml is desirable. Indomethacin may be tried in cases not responding to salicylates.
2. Iridocyclitis should be treated with local corticosteroids and systemically if necessary.
3. Corticosteroids may be effective in severe cases which do not respond to salicylates.
4. Monoarticular synovitis with effusion which does not respond to medical treatment may be treated by removal of the synovial membrane.
5. Physical therapy, orthopedic care to prevent deformities, and corrective surgery are important in rehabilitation. As in any chronic disease, psychologic care is of prime importance.

Prognosis With individualized management, the prognosis for life in juvenile rheumatoid arthritis is excellent, and many patients recover without severe sequelae. Complications: amyloidosis is rare.

ANAPHYLACTOID PURPURA (See p. 588)

DERMATOMYOSITIS

Dermatomyositis is a rare chronic inflammatory disease involving the skin, striated muscles, and associated vascular structures. The onset is usually prior to 10 years of age. The coexistence of malignancies observed in adults is not seen in children.

Clinical and laboratory features

1. The onset is extremely insidious, with weakness or easy fatigability, especially in the legs and shoulder girdle. Fever and malaise herald active disease. Involvement of the muscles of respiration and of the palate may be a cause of death. The disease is more common in females.
2. Induration of the muscles and the subcutaneous tissues occur with calcinosis present in 50 to 60 percent of children. Muscle pain may be prominent. Later, the muscles may become atrophied and contracted.
3. Dermatitis: A pathognomonic symmetric erythema occurs over the extensor surfaces of the joints, especially the knuckles, elbows, and knees. A butterfly rash may also be present. The upper eyelids assume a pathognomonic violaceous discoloration (heliotrope eyelids).
4. Other systems, e.g., eye, heart, kidney, small intestine, may be involved.
5. Eosinophilia may be present, the sedimentation rate is usually elevated, and creatinuria may be present. Muscle enzymes, e.g., creatine phosphokinase (CPK), glutamic oxaloacetic transaminase (SGOT), aldolase and lactic dehydrogenase (LDH) are elevated.
6. Biopsy of the skin and muscle are helpful in confirming the diagnosis.
7. Electromyography is useful in distinguishing myopathy from neuropathy and in selecting the site for biopsy.

Prognosis   The prognosis is guarded, since even with recovery, contractures are common.

Treatment   Adrenal corticosteroids, especially if given early, may relieve the symptoms and induce a remission. Early in the course the pain requires relief; later the prevention of contractions and rehabilitation are of prime importance.

SCLERODERMA AND MORPHEA

This condition—very rare in children—may occur as a localized form (morphea), or it may be generalized. It affects females more often and may begin anytime during childhood. In the generalized form (the fingers and toes are usually affected—sclerodactylia), not only the skin and subcutaneous tissues but also the muscles, bones, and internal organs (gastrointestinal tract, kidney, and lung) may be involved. The skin at first is firm and edematous; then it is smooth, hard, and taut; and finally there is atrophy. Entire extremities may become withered and lacking in soft tissue. Pigmentary changes (hyper- or depigmentation) occur in 50 percent of patients. Adrenal corticosteroids have been used without much beneficial effect. The prognosis in morphea is good, but in the generalized type of scleroderma, the prognosis is grave.

DISSEMINATED LUPUS ERYTHEMATOSUS

This condition is uncommon in young children. The vast majority of cases occurs in females between adolescence and the menopause. It is characterized by irregular and intermittent fever; weight loss, weakness, and easy fatigability; synovial and serous-membrane involvement, e.g., polyarthritis, pericarditis; vascular changes in the kidney (wire-loop lesion), retina, skin (erythematous rash in a butterfly distribution over the nose and cheeks); and various disturbances of the central nervous system (e.g., psychoses, hemiplegia, and convulsions). Hepatomegaly, splenomegaly, and generalized lymphadeonopathy are common.

Laboratory findings

1. The finding of lupus erythematosus cells (polymorphonuclear leukocytes with engulfed amorphous material) in the blood is diagnostic of lupus erythematosus in 95 percent of the cases. Antinuclear antibodies are present in the great majority of patients.
2. Anemia, leukopenia, and thrombocytopenia (hemorrhagic phenomena) are common. Coombs' test may be positive.
3. Serum-complement level is low; sedimentation rate is very much elevated.
4. Hematuria and albuminuria are commonly found. Renal insufficiency, the most serious aspect of the disease, is manifested by elevation of BUN and abnormal renal function tests.
5. Elevated levels of gamma globulin are present.
6. False-positive serologic tests for syphilis can occur.
7. Skin and renal biopsy are helpful. Using immunofluorescent technique, gamma globulin and complement can be demonstrated in glomeruli and skin.

Treatment   The recommended treatment is adrenal corticosteroids in large dosages for prolonged periods of time. The disease is chronic and subject to remissions, which makes it difficult to evaluate the long-term effects of adrenal corticosteroids. However, such therapy appears to retard progression of or even reverse some renal lesions. Immunosuppressive drugs, e.g., Imuran, may be used in conjunction with adrenal corticosteroids or alone when steroids are contraindicated. Sunlight should be avoided since it may cause an acute exacerbation of the disease. The prognosis is guarded. The largest number of deaths is due to renal failure.

DRUG–INDUCED LUPUS ERYTHEMATOSUS

A number of children have had clinical and laboratory findings consistent with lupus apparently following the use of drugs, e.g., long-acting sulfonamides, tridione, hydralazine. In a number of these patients the classic Stevens-Johnson syndrome was present at the onset. In most instances patients make a complete recovery when the drug is withdrawn, although fatalities have occurred.

PURPURA FULMINANS (See p. 589)

ERYTHEMA MULTIFORME EXUDATIVUM
(Stevens–Johnson Syndrome) (See p. 683)

POLYARTERITIS NODOSA (Periarteritis Nodosa)

This disease is a panarteritis involving chiefly the medium-sized and small arteries. It is rare during childhood, and males are affected more often than females.

Clinical features   Symptoms depend chiefly on the location of the obstructed or ulcerated vessels. There may be vague abdominal complaints, arthritis, neuritis, myositis, edema, purpura, hypertension, cough and wheezing, tachycardia, and convulsions. Hepatosplenomegaly is common. Signs of systemic illness, e.g., fever, anorexia, lethargy, are usually present. Nodules occur along small and medium-sized arteries in only about 20 percent of cases. Polyarteritis occurring in infants is characterized mainly by involvement of the coronary arteries.

Laboratory findings   These findings are nonspecific. Anemia is common. Eosinophilia may be present and is usually marked in cases with pulmonary involvement. The sedimentation rate may be elevated, and tests for acute-phase reactants may be positive. Renal function studies may be abnormal. Hematuria, proteinuria, and cylindruria are common.

Treatment   There is no specific therapy. Adrenal corticosteroids relieve symptoms and may favorably influence the course of the disease.

Prognosis   The prognosis is poor.

MUSCLE DISEASES

CONGENITAL MUSCLE DISEASES

Absence   The muscles most commonly involved are the pectoral muscles (in combination with syndactyly—Poland's syndrome). Such absence does not result in abnormal function of the antagonist with resultant contractures. (For Congenital Deficiency of the Abdominal Muscles, see p. 209.)

Contractures

1. Torticollis in the newborn has been described in Chapter 12, "Diseases of the Newborn." Torticollis (wryneck) may also result from disorders of muscles, e.g., myositis of the trapezius muscle; nerves, e.g., tumors of the central nervous system, poliomyelitis with involvement of the spinal accessory nerve; bone, e.g., rotatory subluxation of the atlantoaxial joint (usually follows a sore throat and is precipitated by a sudden turning of the head), tumors, tuberculous cervical spondylitis, congenital malformation of the cervical spine; and soft tissue, e.g., mumps and cervical lymphadenitis. Treatment is directed toward the primary cause. Children with hearing or visual defects or with tics may assume a position simulating that of torticollis.
2. Clubfoot (see p. 546).

MUSCULAR DYSTROPHY

The term "muscular dystrophy" refers to a group of primary degenerative diseases of skeletal muscle which are genetically determined and have a progressive course. They are characterized by weakness and wasting of muscle groups. The primary lesion is in the muscle, especially the proximal segments. The disease occurs more frequently in males, in whom it also tends to be more severe and to progress more rapidly. It appears in early childhood when transmission is sex-linked or autosomal recessive. In cases of dominant transmission onset occurs later in life. The earlier its onset and the more generalized its involvement, the more rapid is the progress of the disease. Those types with limited involvement may be arrested after progressing to a certain point.

Pseudohypertrophic muscular dystrophy (Duchenne type) is the commonest form of progressive muscular dystrophy. It is inherited as a sex-linked recessive trait and is found mostly in males from 2 to 10 years of age. Death usually occurs in the middle or late teens.

There is pseudohypertrophy of the muscles, especially of the calves. Symmetric progressive weakness of the muscles of the pelvis, abdomen, and thigh renders the patient unable to walk and causes him to fall easily and then to have trouble in getting up. Lordosis, waddling gait, and deformities develop. When the patient attempts to rise from a sitting position, he "climbs up on himself" (Bower's sign). The deep-tendon reflexes, but not the superficial reflexes, are gradually lost. There are no sensory changes. Cardiac involvement can occur and is a common cause of death. The urinary creatine-creatinine ratio is disturbed, with excessive urinary excretion of creatin and decreased excretion of creatinine. Creatine phosphokinase (CPK) is always elevated. The transaminases, too, are elevated.

Biopsy of the involved muscles shows the characteristic degenerative changes (disappearance of muscle fibers with increase in connective tissue and fat cells; marked variation in the size of fibers; sarco-lemma nuclei are larger and increased numerically, or are centrally placed).

A less common form of Duchenne-type dystrophy occurs in both sexes and has a later onset and slower progression.

Among other less-common muscular dystrophies are facioscapulo-humeral type, inherited as an autosomal dominant trait; limb-girdle type, inherited as an autosomal recessive trait; myotonic dystrophy, inherited as an autosomal dominant trait and characterized by myo-tonia, cataracts, gonadal atrophy, alopecia, mental retardation, hyperos-tosis frontalis and cardiac abnormalities; and congenital muscular dystrophy, which resembles the Duchenne type but has its onset in the neonatal period.

Treatment   There is no specific therapy for any form of muscular dystrophy. Relief from myotonia in myotonic dystrophy may be achieved to a degree by drugs (see Myotonia Congenita, p. 535). Pro-gression of Duchenne type is associated with involvement of the muscles of respiration which may require tracheostomy and assisted ventilation. Genetic counseling is important. In Duchenne-type muscu-lar dystrophy, female carriers can frequently be identified by elevated levels of CPK.

MYOSITIS

Myositis is a primary, localized, or diffuse inflammatory disorder of muscles. It may be acute or chronic. Etiologically, it may be infectious, for example, viral (Coxsackie, group B), bacterial (staphylococcus or streptococcus, usually associated with septicemia or extension from a joint), fungal (actinomycosis), protozoan (toxoplasmosis), or para-sitic (trichinosis), or it may be associated with primary disorders of connective tissue, for example, dermatomyositis. Adrenal corticoster-oids are used, but their effect is questionable.

METABOLIC DISEASES

Glycogen-storage disease (see pp. 167–169)

Disorders of potassium metabolism   Muscle weakness can occur in a variety of conditions, e.g., diarrhea causing hypokalemia, diabetic acidosis, renal tubular acidosis, and thyrotoxic hypokalemia. There are several conditions in which potassium disturbances are due to intrinsic muscle disorders, and serum potassium level during an attack may be low, normal, or elevated. For the most part, these conditions are transmitted as autosomal dominant traits.

Paramyotonia congenita begins during infancy or early childhood and may be a variant of hyperkalemic periodic paralysis. It is characterized

Table 21-1. Disorders of potassium metabolism

	Hypokalemic (familial periodic paralysis)	Hyperkalemic (adynamia episodica hereditaria)	Normokalemic
Age at onset	7 to 21 years	Before 10	Before 10
Duration of attacks	Usually several hours	Less than 1 hour	Several days to weeks
Precipitating factors	Rest after exertion, excessive carbohydrate ingestion, stress, drugs, e.g., epinephrine, ACTH, steroids	Rest after exertion	Rest after exertion
Muscular involvement	Frequently complete but sparing face, respiratory, and deglutition muscles; ECG is characteristic of hypokalemia	Usually mild local weakness	Often complete with loss of cough reflex
Prophylactic measures	Spironolactone, low-sodium diet, chlorothiazide, Diamox	Gradual cessation of exercise, frequent carbohydrate feedings, Diamox, chlorothiazide	Gradual cessation of exercise, Diamox, fluorohydrocortisone
Treatment	KCl, 0.2 Gm per kg	Calcium gluconate, 10%, 10 ml intravenously or epinephrine, subcutaneously	NaCl

by episodic attacks of weakness in the proximal muscles. Myotonia is present in the lingual muscles, eyelids, facial muscles, and the extremities primarily when the patient is exposed to cold. Symptoms improve with age.

MYOPATHY ASSOCIATED WITH ENDOCRINE ABNORMALITIES

Muscular weakness may be seen in hyperthyroidism, hypothyroidism, hyperparathyroidism, and hyperadrenocorticism. It may occur also during adrenocorticosteroid therapy in which case it subsides after cessation of the drug.

MYOGLOBINURIA

Myoglobinuria may complicate muscular dystrophy, occur after excessive muscle trauma, or be caused by ingestion of poisoned fish (Haff disease). Hereditary (autosomal recessive) metabolic myopathy with paroxysmal myoglobinuria, due to abnormal glycolysis, is characterized by repeated episodes of muscle cramping with passing of red urine precipitated by exercise. Hypertrophy of the calf muscles occurs early. The course is chronic with exacerbations and remissions. A high serum activity of muscle enzymes and the presence of myoglobin in the urine support the diagnosis. Treatment consists of avoidance of physical exertion.

DISORDERS OF NEUROMUSCULAR TRANSMISSION

Myasthenias The etiology of these disorders is unknown, but the cases can be divided into three groups:

1. Myasthenia neonatorum: present in newborn infants of myasthenic mothers. There are generalized weakness, immobile face, ocular palsies, dysphagia, and respiratory distress. Complete recovery occurs in less than 1 month. Treatment: neostigmine bromide (3.75 to 7.5 mg orally) is given with each feeding.
2. Myasthenia congenita: a familial condition causing ocular muscle weakness, ptosis, weak cry, and dysphagia.
3. Myasthenia gravis juvenilis: onset is usually after 2 years of age, and there is a marked familial incidence. It is more frequent in females. Ptosis, unilateral or bilateral, is a common symptom. Weakness of the extremities and dysphagia occur later. There may be remissions with arrest of the condition, or it may become progressively worse. The muscular weakness is best demonstrated after repetitive contractions. Rest or sleep is followed by improvement. The neostigmine test (neostigmine methyl sulfate 0.04 mg per kg intramuscularly, followed by improvement in 20 minutes);

repetitive electric stimulation of the nerves with resultant progressive failure (myasthenic reaction) ; and a characteristic electromyogram are diagnostic. Treatment: neostigmine methyl sulfate, intramuscularly, or neostigmine bromide 3.75 to 7.5 mg, orally or pyridostigmine bromide 15 to 20 mg orally three times a day (prolonged-action or slow-release tablets can be used for nights). Thymectomy has been reported to be helpful in some cases. Myasthenic crisis is characterized by sudden increase in the severity of symptoms culminating in respiratory arrest.

Myotonias   These conditions are characterized by myotonus and their autosomal dominant mode of transmission.

1. Myotonic dystrophy (see p. 532).
2. Myotonia congenita (Thomsen's disease) is a rare disease usually transmitted by an autosomal dominant gene. There are also some cases with recessive transmission. In the dominant type the symptoms begin in early infancy and are generalized, whereas in the recessive type they start at 4 to 6 years in the legs. There are muscle hypertonicity and contraction, with difficulty of relaxation, as shown by the hand-grasp test. Characteristically, after a "warm-up" period of some activity, this hypertonicity is relieved. The muscles are somewhat hypertrophic and do not degenerate. The myotonia is present in most of the voluntary muscles and is nonprogressive. In treatment, quinine, 0.3 to 0.6 Gm three times a day, is effective. Adrenal corticosteroids, acetazolamide, and chlorothiazide may also be used.

Myopathies (unclassified)

1. Central core disease is a nonprogressive myopathy which is transmitted as an autosomal dominant trait, causing proximal muscle weakness, a delay in walking, and retarded motor development. The presence of a hyaline mass as a central core in many muscle fibers is characteristic. Absence of an oxidative enzyme is believed to be responsible for the condition.
2. Nemaline myopathy resembles central core disease clinically, but on histologic examination characteristic irregular threadlike bands are found in affected muscle fibers.
3. There are several other conditions characterized by muscular weakness and wasting and named according to their characteristic histologic abnormalities, including myotubular myopathy and myopathy with giant abnormal mitochondria.

THE FLOPPY INFANT

A "floppy infant" is an infant with decreased resistance to passive movements, variable amounts of muscle mass, hyperextensibility of joints, and deep tendon reflexes which may vary from normal to absent.

The symptoms may be present at birth, in which case there is usually a delay in reaching motor milestones, or they may become obvious in late infancy or childhood. The causes of this syndrome are multiple (see Table 21-2).

The hypotonia may be associated with paralysis in some conditions, of which infantile spinal muscular atrophy (Werdnig-Hoffmann disease) is encountered most frequently. It is characterized by progressive hypotonia and wasting of skeletal muscles as a result of degeneration of motor neurons. The condition usually leads to death at an early age, but more benign variants exist.

Common causes of hypotonia not associated with paralysis are benign congenital hypotonia, in which muscular weakness and hypotonia are present from birth but subside completely or partially over a period of years, and hypotonia with mental retardation.

Diagnostic studies of a floppy infant include: assessment of the developmental level of the infant, determinations of urinary creatine and creatinine excretion, and serum enzyme concentration, measurement of nerve conduction time, electromyography, and muscle biopsy.

GENERALIZED CONGENITAL ABNORMALITIES OF BONE

OSTEOGENESIS IMPERFECTA

Osteogenesis imperfecta is a hereditary defect (pleiotropic dominant gene with incomplete penetrance and variable expressivity; sporadic cases occur) of bone matrix; calicification of the matrix that is formed proceeds normally. There are two clinical varieties of this disease: osteogenesis imperfecta congenita—the severe form in which multiple fractures occur in utero and during birth and the infants are often stillborn or die shortly after birth (often transmitted as an autosomal recessive trait), and osteogenesis imperfecta tarda—in which blue sclera, arcus juvenilis (opacity in the periphery of the cornea), and excessive joint mobility are found. Minor trauma often causes fractures, which usually occur after 1 year of age and become rare after puberty. Deafness occurs later in life. Laboratory findings are within normal limits except alkaline phosphatase, which may be elevated. Roentgenograms show slender bones with thin cortices and fractures in various stages of healing. Wormian bones are found in the skull. Orthopedic treatment consists of staged osteotomies and intramedullary rodding. Medical treatment, consisting of sodium fluoride and calcitonin, has been used with good results in some patients.

OSTEOPETROSIS

Osteopetrosis (Albers-Schönberg disease, marble bones) is a rare disorder characterized by a homogeneous opacity of the bones, obliteration of the marrow cavities, and abnormal fragility of bone. An accom-

Table 21-2.   Causes of the floppy infant

1. Diseases of the central nervous system
   Congenital malformations
   Cerebral birth injury
   Cerebral damage from hypoxia or intracranial hemorrhage
   Nonspecific mental deficiency
   Hypotonic cerebral palsy
   Metabolic disorders (see metabolic and endocrine disorders below)
   Mongolism, trisomy 13 syndrome, chromosome 18q-syndrome
   Kernicterus
   Familial dysautonomia
2. Diseases of the spinal cord and peripheral nerves
   Infantile spinal muscular atrophy (Werdnig-Hoffmann disease and benign variants)
   Intraspinal tumor
   Spinal cord trauma
   Intoxications
   Poliomyelitis
   Polyneuritis
   Neuropathic arthrogryposis multiplex congenita
3. Congenital myopathies
   Central core disease
   Nemaline myopathy
   Myotubular myopathy
   Mitochondrial abnormalities
   Myopathic arthrogryposis multiplex congenita
4. Other neuromuscular disorders
   Muscular dystrophy
   Peripheral neuropathies
   Myasthenia gravis, dystrophia
   Myotonica, periodic paralysis
5. Metabolic and endocrine disorders
   Mucopolysaccharidosis
   Lipidosis (leukodystrophies)
   Glycogenosis
   Galactosemia
   Renal tubular acidosis
   Rickets
   Celiac disease
   Hypothyroidism
6. Connective tissue disorders
   Congenital laxity of ligaments
   Ehlers-Danlos syndrome
   Marfan's syndrome
   Osteogenesis imperfecta
7. Acute illness
8. Miscellaneous
   Congenital heart disease
   Prader-Willi syndrome
   Cerebro-hepato-renal syndrome
   Oculo-cerebro-renal syndrome
   Tanatophoric dwarfism
9. Essential hypotonia (benign congenital hypotonia)

panying myelophthisic anemia is the rule. In addition optic atrophy, deafness, and facial or ocular palsy are often found. Osteomyelitis is a frequent complication. General growth is retarded and some patients are dwarfed. The prognosis is poor. No specific treatment is available. The transmission is probably autosomal recessive.

PYKNODYSOSTOSIS

Pyknodysostosis is a type of osteosclerosis associated with peculiar face, open sutures and fontanels, and dwarfism. There is no associated anemia.

ELLIS–VAN CREVELD SYNDROME

Ellis-van Creveld syndrome (chondroectodermal dysplasia) is characterized by a shortening of the extremities that is more pronounced distally, underdeveloped teeth and nails (ectodermal dysplasia), polydactyl, and frequently a congenital heart defect. The condition is transmitted by a recessive gene.

OSTEOCHONDRODYSPLASIAS

1. Achondroplasia (chondrodystrophy) produces a dwarfing characterized by short extremities and a comparatively large trunk, lumbar lordosis, protruding abdomen, and prominent buttocks. The head is large. The mentality is normal, and such persons are able to procreate. Roentgen findings: The long bones appear short and thick, with the shortening involving mainly the proximal bones (the humerus is more shortened than the radius and the ulna). A deformity (ball-and-socket type) is seen at the epiphyseal-metaphyseal junction. The defect consists of a disturbance of endochondral ossification. The disorder is transmitted by an autosomal dominant gene, but sporadic cases occur frequently.
2. Hypochondroplasia causes dwarfism with short limbs and a normal skull. The transmission is autosomal dominant.
3. Ollier's dyschondroplasia is characterized by the presence of nonossified cartilage in the metaphyses and adjacent diaphyses of long bones. The disorder is usually unilateral and leads to shortening of the limbs and limitation of movement.
4. Hereditary multiple exostoses is transmitted by an autosomal dominant gene and is characterized by irregular prominences in the region of the metaphyses. The exostoses are usually bilateral and often symmetric. Surgical intervention may be required for limitation of movement or relief of pressure symptoms.
5. Morquio's disease (see Mucopolysaccharidosis).
6. Chondrodystrophia calcificans congenita (Conradi's disease, stippled epiphyses) may be recognized at birth. It causes dwarfing because of short extremities. Associated findings are flexion of joints with limitation of motion, general weakness, failure to

thrive, bilateral congenital cataracts, and mental retardation. Roentgenographically the epiphyseal centers in the long bones, the small bones, and the epiphyseal strips may show multiple foci of ossification which usually fuse into a single mass during the first year of life. There is no known treatment. Many patients die in early infancy.

HEREDITARY DISORDERS AFFECTING MULTIPLE ORGAN SYSTEMS INCLUDING THE SKELETON

MUCOPOLYSACCHARIDOSES

A group of disorders which have in common an inherited disturbance in the metabolism of mucopolysaccharides (see Table 21-3). They are characterized by abnormal deposition in tissues and/or excretion in the urine of acid mucopolysaccharides.

Marfan's syndrome   Marfan's syndrome (arachnodactyly) is transmitted by an autosomal dominant gene, but sporadic cases, due to new mutations, do occur.

Clinical manifestations include anomalies in the skeletal, ocular, and cardiovascular systems. The patients have long, thin extremities and long fingers (spider fingers). The pelvis-to-sole measurement is in excess of the pubis-to-vertex measurement, and the arm span is greater than the height. The muscles are flaccid and the joints are hyperextensible. The commonest ocular defect is dislocation of the lens. There is an inborn weakness of the media of the aorta and the main pulmonary artery. Dissecting aneurysms are common. Other congenital heart defects may also be present (valvular deformities, patent ductus arteriosus). The prognosis depends chiefly upon the cardiac lesions.

Ehlers-Danlos syndrome   Ehlers-Danlos syndrome (cutis hyperelastica) is inherited as an autosomal dominant trait. It is characterized by hyperelasticity of the skin and hypermobility of the joints. The skin is extremely fragile so that even minor trauma causes excessive bleeding and gaping wounds, and characteristic "cigarette-paper" scars develop at the site of the trauma. Associated anomalies include those of the heart, gastrointestinal, respiratory, and genitourinary tract. Microscopically there is an abnormality of the collagen fibers and a questionable excess of elastic fibers.

METABOLIC BONE DISEASES

Generalized bone disorders due to metabolic disturbances include alterations in either bone deposition or bone resorption, or both. Bone deposition involves osteoblastic formation of organic matrix and calcification of the matrix. Bone resorption involves osteoclastic removal of

Table 21-3. The mucopolysaccharidoses

Disease	Clinical characteristics	Biochemical findings	Genetic transmission
Hurler's syndrome; mucopolysaccharidosis I; gargoylism	Severe mental retardation, dwarfism with skeletal deformities, e.g., malformed skull, delayed closure of anterior fontanel, short neck, kyphosis, limited extension of joints, clawlike hands; corneal opacities; hepatosplenomegaly; absence of sexual maturation	Dermatan sulfate and heparan sulfate in urine and tissues; dermatan sulfate in fibroblasts; increased gangliosides in brain; decreased beta-galactosidase in tissues	Autosomal recessive
Hunter's syndrome; mucopolysaccharidosis II	Similar to Hurler's but less severe; moderate mental retardation; early deafness. No corneal clouding	Dermatan sulfate and heparan sulfate in urine and tissues; dermatan sulfate in fibroblasts; increased gangliosides in brain; decreased beta-galactosidase in tissues	Sex-linked recessive
Sanfilippo's syndrome; mucopolysaccharidosis III	Severe mental retardation; mild skeletal changes, corneal clouding questionable	Heparan sulfate in urine and tissues; dermatan sulfate in fibroblasts; decreased beta-galactosidase in tissues	Autosomal recessive
Morquio's syndrome; mucopolysaccharidosis IV	Severe skeletal deformities marked spondyloepiphyseal dysplasia; no mental retardation; corneal opacities may occur	Keratan sulfate and chondroitin—4/6—sulfate in urine	Autosomal recessive
Scheie's syndrome; mucopolysaccharidosis V	Mild skeletal changes; no mental retardation; severe corneal opacities	Dermatan sulfate in urine	Autosomal recessive
Maroteaux-Lamy syndrome; mucopolysaccharidosis VI	Severe skeletal deformities; gross corneal opacity, no mental retardation	Dermatan sulfate in urine	Autosomal recessive

formed bone and the release of bone mineral. Some metabolic disorders (rickets) affect calcification of the matrix, whereas others (scurvy, osteoporosis) affect osteoblastic formation of matrix (decreasing it) or osteoclastic bone resorption (increasing it).

For the most frequent metabolic disturbances causing generalized bone disorders see Table 21-4.

LOCALIZED CONGENITAL ANOMALIES OF BONE

LACUNAR SKULL

Lacunar skull is a congenital malformation and is characterized by rarefactions or lacunae with interlacing ridges of density in the cranial vault, usually associated with meningocele and hydrocephalus, in which case the prognosis is poor. There is no treatment.

CRANIOSTENOSIS (Premature Synostosis)

Premature synostosis of the sutures of the skull is a developmental malformation. Because the skull is held rigid at the sites of the pre-

Table 21-4.   Metabolic causes of generalized bone disorders

1. Nutritional
   Scurvy
   Protein deficiency
   Caloric deficiency
   Malabsorptive states (celiac disease, cystic fibrosis, biliary atresia)
   Vitamin D–deficient rickets
2. Endocrine
   Pituitary dysfunction
   Hypothyroidism
   Hyperthyroidism
   Hyperadrenalism (Cushing's syndrome)
   Side effects of adrenal corticosteroid therapy
   Hypoparathyroidism
   Hyperparathyroidism
   Pseudohypoparathyroidism (also a failure of bone to respond to parathyroid hormone)
3. Renal
   Renal tubular diseases
   Chronic renal insufficiency
4. Metabolic and genetic
   Osteoporosis of disuse
   Hypophosphatasia
   Hyperphosphatasia
   Mucopolysaccharidoses
   Gaucher's disease
   Osteogenesis imperfecta
   Chondrodysplasias

mature synostoses, localized expansion of the growing skull is prevented or limited in a direction perpendicular to the long axis of the obliterated suture, and compensatory overgrowth of the skull occurs in other directions: closure of the coronal suture—brachycephaly; sagittal—dolichocephaly (scaphocephaly); all sutures—oxycephaly if the top of the skull is conical, acrocephaly if it is high or rounded. If one side of the suture is obliterated, plagiocephaly occurs. Brain damage and blindness may result from compression. Roentgenograms show premature closure of the sutures, convolutional atrophy, and shallow orbits. A suture that will close prematurely is very narrow, with dense bone margins. (Craniostenosis must be differentiated from microcephaly, due to cerebral agenesis, in which the sutures are open.)

Craniectomy with insertion of polyethylene film to relieve cerebral compression and correct deformity is indicated as early as possible, preferably before 6 months of age in cases of complete synostosis. Where synostosis is incomplete, cosmetic improvement may follow surgery, but the effect on the central nervous system is uncertain.

Acrocephalosyndactyly (Apert's syndrome) consists of acrocephaly and syndactyly (usually of only the hands). Acrocephaly is also present in Crouzon's disease (craniofacial dysostosis).

HYPERTELORISM

Hypertelorism is caused by a defective development of the sphenoid bone, with the lesser wings larger than the greater wings. The eyes are very wide apart and are separated by a broad nose with an especially wide, flat bridge. There may be other anomalies of the face. Hypertelorism is often associated with mental retardation, but it occurs in otherwise normal children.

CONGENITAL CLEIDAL DYSOSTOSIS

Congenital cleidal dysostosis is characterized by absence or aplasia of the clavicles, usually bilateral and causing extraordinary mobility of the shoulders with anterior approximation. Often the cranium, too, is poorly ossified and brachycephalic (cleidocranial dysostosis); the sutures and fontanels may remain wide open even as late as 16 years of age. The majority of children with this condition are small in stature, and the mentality is usually normal. It is usually transmitted as a dominant trait. There is no specific treatment.

KLIPPEL–FEIL SYNDROME

Klippel-Feil syndrome is a reduced number of cervical vertebrae or fused hemivertebrae formation, producing a short, immobile neck and lowered hairline. This may be associated with Sprengel's deformity, in which one or both of the scapulae are in a congenitally high position, with the lower angle turned toward the spine and with the arm on the affected side unable to be raised above a right angle with the body.

CONGENITAL FUNNEL CHEST AND PIGEON BREAST

These are deformities of the anterior chest wall—a depression deformity (funnel chest, pectus excavatum, familial chonechondrosternon), which may be due to a short central tendon of the diaphragm and which is present in newborn or young infants; it may also be caused by rickets; and a protrusion deformity (pigeon breast, pectus carinatum) which is due to disproportionate rib growth, with some ribs growing longer than others. This is not clinically apparent until 6 years of age. Surgical treatment may be indicated primarily for psychologic and cosmetic reasons and to prevent possible potential cardiorespiratory embarrassment.

DEFORMITIES OF THE SPINE

Scoliosis (lateral curvature of the spine) may be structural (fixed, irreversible) or functional (reversible). In the first case it is caused by congenital abnormalities of the vertebral column (hemivertebrae), fusion of the ribs, paralysis of muscles, etc. In the second case it is caused by muscle spasm secondary to trauma or inflammation or to lower limb length discrepancy. The functional type has a definite familial incidence. It tends to occur during three specific age groups— birth to 3 years (more common in males), between 4 to 9 years, and during adolescence (the latter is more common in females). Scoliosis is recognized clinically by the curvature and rotation that it produces. The rotation is most noticeable when the child bends forward. The scoliosis increases with growth so that treatment (exercise, bracing, and surgery) is prescribed depending on age of the child as well as degree of severity of the deformity.

SPINA BIFIDA (See Chapter 12, "Diseases of the Newborn")

CONGENITAL DISLOCATION OF THE HIP

Congenital dislocation of the hip is a displacement of the femoral head out of the acetabular socket and is accompanied by abnormal development of the acetabulum. In dislocation, the femoral head is completely outside the socket. In subluxation, it is at the edge of the acetabulum and is usually reduced when the hip is flexed and abducted. The condition is more common in females (8:1) and is often bilateral. Two types exist:

Teratologic—characterized by gross developmental defects of the joint and frequently associated with spina bifida.
Typical—characterized by postnatal appearance in usually otherwise normal infants.

Clinical and roentgenographic features

1. With the thigh at right angles to the body, abduction is painful and limited on the affected side.
2. Skin folds of the thigh in the ipsilateral limb are frequently different in depth and number. This situation may also be present in normal persons.
3. An early clinical sign is the palpable and occasionally audible click as the femoral head enters and dislocates from the socket when the flexed hip is abducted and adducted (Ortolani test).
4. The involved extremity (in unilateral conditions) appears shorter.
5. Standing on the abnormal leg causes the pelvis to drop on the normal side (Trendelenburg test).
6. The earliest roentgenographic sign is a small undeveloped acetabulum. The epiphyseal center of the femoral head is small and delayed in development, and the acetabular index is greater than normal (30°). The femoral head is displaced outward and upward.
7. As the child grows old enough to walk, a limp ("going downstairs" limp) is noted in unilateral involvement and a "duck waddle" gait in bilateral dislocation.

Treatment   The diagnosis should be made as early as possible for optimum results. When the condition is recognized in early infancy (before 3 months of age), a position of abduction and flexion is maintained by abduction splints or the use of a pillow between the thighs. Between 3 and 18 months a closed reduction is carried out after a preliminary period of traction on the hip. The reduced hip is maintained in a position of marked flexion and moderate abduction in a hip spica cast for many months. Between 18 months and 5 years open reduction is often indicated.

BOWLEGS

Bowlegs (genu varum) is an increased distance between the knees when the legs are extended and the ankles are brought together. Infants usually have some degree of bowlegs for the first few years due to a combination of factors—internal torsion and varus of the tibia and external torsion of the femur—which are probably due to intrauterine position. If the condition persists and worsens, it may require nighttime splinting. Marked bowing may be due to disease, e.g., rickets, tibia vara.

KNOCK–KNEES

Knock-knees (genu valgum) is an increased distance between the ankles when the legs are extended and the knees are brought together. The normal genu varum of the infant gradually changes to a mild valgum with growth. Severe degrees of valgum may be due to disease. In all but extreme cases surgical correction is unnecessary.

TIBIAL TORSION

The tibia may be twisted either in an inward or outward position. With the leg extended and the patella facing anteriorly, the foot will turn inward or outward depending on the direction of tibial torsion. Internal tibial torsion is the most common cause of toeing in as seen in young children. Treatment of internal tibial torsion in the infant consists of the use of a Denis-Browne splint. Untreated tibial torsion which is marked may require osteotomy in the older child.

DISORDERS OF THE HANDS AND FEET

Normally the foot of the infant and preschool child may resemble flat-foot, because the longitudinal arch is overlaid with fat, the muscles are elastic, and the foot may even be slightly everted.

FLATFOOT, OR PRONATED FEET

If pronation and eversion of the foot are so pronounced that a straight line down the back of the leg is medial to the os calcis, correction is necessary, because sooner or later pain and fatigue will result from the poor mechanical alignment.

Treatment A corrective shoe with wedging of the medial border of a Thomas heel, ⅛ in., and a scaphoid pad should be worn.

PIGEON TOE

Normally, slight toeing in of the foot is desirable, as it tends to produce good mechanical alignment. If the toeing in is marked, the lateral aspect of the heel can be wedged. Toeing in of the foot may be caused by

1. Metatarsus adductus: adduction of the forefoot with no deformity of the hindfoot. It is the most common of the congenital foot deformities and requires passive stretching, reversing shoes, or casting.
2. Inward tibial torsion—frequently associated with metatarsus adductus.
3. Inward femoral torsion: with the child in a supine position the inward rotation of the leg at the hip is exaggerated and outward rotation is almost nonexistent. Usually no treatment is required.

SYNDACTYLY

Syndactyly is a congenital union of the fingers or toes. There may be actual fusion of the bones or only webbing of the skin (zygodactyly). It occurs as an isolated anomaly or in combination with other congenital defects, e.g., acrocephalosyndactyly. Most commonly it involves the third and fourth fingers and the second and third toes. Where possible, corrective surgery is recommended.

POLYDACTYLY

Supernumerary fingers or toes may occur sporadically or as an inherited, dominant trait. Extra digits occur about seven times more frequently in blacks than in whites. It may occur as a component of inherited syndromes, e.g., Laurence-Moon-Biedl. Surgical correction is usually indicated.

ABSENCE OF EXTREMITIES

There may be complete absence of all extremities (amelia) or of one extremity (ectromelia). The proximal part of the extremity may be defective, with a hand or foot arising directly from the trunk (phocomelia). Individual bones may be absent, and this anomaly may be associated with other skeletal malformations, e.g., absence of the radius with a clubhand. Sirenomelia (mermaid fetus) consists of more or less complete fusion of the lower limbs to form a single extremity. It is usually accompanied by severe dysplasia of the urinary tract. Monomelia—the presence of a single lower extremity that shows no indication of having occurred from fusion of two lower limbs—is very rare. Thalidomide when taken early in the course of pregnancy has caused anomalies mainly of the extremities and gastrointestinal tract.

CLUBFOOT (Talipes)

Congenital clubfoot, which is quite common (2 per 1,000 live births), affects boys twice as often as girls and is bilateral in 50 percent of affected children.

The most frequent deformity is equinovarus, in which the foot is in plantar flexion and deviates medially.

In calcanevalgus (rare) the foot is dorsiflexed and deviated laterally.

Clubfoot cannot be passively overcorrected and requires orthopedic treatment.

DISSEMINATED BONE DISORDERS OF UNKNOWN ETIOLOGY

INFANTILE CORTICAL HYPEROSTOSIS (Caffey's Disease)

This disease is found in young infants and is more common in males. The onset may occur from the last month in utero to 6 months of age. It is characterized by hyperplasia of the subperiosteal bone with tender, indurated swelling of soft tissue, brawny discoloration of the skin, irritability, pallor, anorexia, and some fever. Roentgenograms reveal the hyperostosis nearly always in the mandible and commonly in the clavicle, calvarium, and long bones. This may persist for several months after the soft-tissue swelling has disappeared. The sedimentation rate and serum-alkaline phosphatase level are usually increased. The signs and symptoms may last from weeks to months but usually disappear eventually. The clinical symptoms subside before the radiographic findings disappear. Adrenal corticosteroids may be used in treatment and probably hasten resolution.

OSTEOCHONDROSES

Osteochondroses are usually seen between 3 and 10 years and affect boys more frequently than girls. Also the lower limbs are more frequently involved than the upper limbs. In 15 percent of involved children osteochondrosis of a given epiphysis is bilateral.

Coxa plana   Osteochondrosis of the femoral capital epiphysis (Legg-Calvé-Perthes disease) is most often unilateral. It is found usually in males from 4 to 9 years of age. It is characterized by symptoms of hip-joint irritation (protective limp, pain on forced motion, muscular guarding against motion, and restricted motion). Abduction and internal rotation are characteristically limited and the hip is held in flexion. The pain is frequently referred to the knee. Roentgenograms differ according to the stage of the disease.

In the first stage (incipient) there is swelling of the capsular shadow, widening of the joint space, and demineralization of the femoral metaphysis. In the second stage (aseptic necrosis) there are signs of the first stage associated with an increase in density of the femoral head. In the third stage (regenerative), revitalization of the head is taking place as evidenced by the presence of radiolucent areas. Widening of the femoral neck also may be evident.

Treatment   Weight-bearing in abduction plaster casts or some type of abduction brace in indicated. Surgical intervention has been used successfully in older children.

Osgood-Schlatter disease   This is an osteochondrosis of the tibial tubercle. There are tenderness and swelling in the region of the tibial tubercle. Usually the onset is from 10 to 15 years of age. Roentgenograms show irregular areas of bone deposition and bone resorption in the proximal part of the tibial tubercle. The disease is usually self-limiting but may require treatment.

Kohler's disease   Osteochondrosis of the navicular bone causes a slight limp and soreness in the foot. Roentgenograms show increased density and fragmentation of the bone. Treatment consists of casting the foot to protect against weight bearing.

Scheuermann's disease   Osteochondrosis of the spine begins usually at puberty, causes kyphosis, and affects both sexes. It commonly involves the epiphyseal plates of three or four adjoining vertebral bodies in the midthoracic region.

FIBROUS DYSPLASIA OF BONE

Polyostatic fibrous dysplasia: This condition is characterized by replacement of bone by fibrous tissue, leading to deformities and fractures. The bone lesions may be associated with brown pigmentation of the skin and precocious puberty (more common in females), the McCune-Albright syndrome.

RETICULOENDOTHELIOSIS (see p. 624)

DISORDERS OF EPIPHYSEAL GROWTH

SLIPPED FEMORAL EPIPHYSIS

Slipped femoral epiphysis occurs during adolescence (10 to 17 years of age), usually in obese boys, and is of unknown etiology but may be associated with some endocrine abnormality. There is pain in the hip or referred pain in the knee, with limitation of motion in internal rotation and abduction, and a limp of gradually increasing severity. Roentgenograms show the head of the femur slipped backward and downward (on lateral projection). About one-third of cases are bilateral. Surgery with pin fixation often is necessary.

BLOUNT'S DISEASE

Blount's disease (tibia vara) is characterized by a progressive bowleg. It is more common in girls and becomes manifest at the age of 2 years. It is thought to present a localized form of epiphyseal dysplasia. Radiographically there is defective ossification of the medial portion of the upper tibial epiphysis.

MADELUNG'S DEFORMITY

This growth disturbance of the medial side of the distal radial epiphysis causes distortion and limitation of motion of the wrist. It is more common in females and usually is bilateral. Surgical correction is usually indicated.

SCOLIOSIS (See Structural Scoliosis, p. 543)

INFECTIONS OF BONE

ACUTE HEMATOGENOUS OSTEOMYELITIS

Etiology and pathogenesis   In infancy and childhood *Staphylococcus aureus* is most often the causative organism. The portal of entry is not always obvious; it may be an abrasion of the skin, a furuncle, tonsillitis, etc. The epiphyseal end of the metaphysis of long bones is vulnerable to infection and development of the osteomyelitis. Bacteria are trapped in small terminal capillaries, with resultant thrombosis, ischemia, necrosis, and abscess formation. Extension may occur toward the medullary canal or toward the overlying cortical bone. The disease occurs more frequently in boys (4:1) and is more often in the lower extremities than in the upper. In children with sickle-cell anemia salmonella is often the causative organism.

Clinical and laboratory features

1. There is usually high temperature and marked toxicity.
2. Pain and localized tenderness followed by swelling and redness are found over the involved bone, with limitation of adjoining joint motion.
3. Blood cultures may reveal the causative organism.
4. There is a marked polymorphonuclear leukocytosis.
5. Roentgenograms may be negative for the first week or 10 days. After 10 days there are small areas of diminished density and elevation of the periosteum; in 2 to 3 weeks the involucrum appears, followed by sequestration.

Treatment

1. Specific antibiotics and chemotherapy for the causative organism continued for 4 to 6 weeks.
2. Surgery is indicated for drainage when there is abscess formation.

BONE AND JOINT TUBERCULOSIS

Tuberculosis of bones and joints has become rare. It occurs mostly in the spine (Pott's disease) and the hip, and in infants the fingers and toes may be involved.

It is always secondary to a tuberculous lesion elsewhere in the body (usually a pulmonary lesion). The pathologic process begins usually in the metaphyseal portion of the epiphyses and leads to bone destruction. The necrotic process may invade the surrounding tissues and form cold abscesses which often appear at points far from their sources. The destruction may involve only the bone, but often the lesion extends through the epiphysis into the capsule of the joint. (See Tuberculosis, Chapter 14.)

CHRONIC GRANULOMATOUS DISEASE OF UNDETERMINED ETIOLOGY

Sarcoidosis Sarcoidosis is rare in children under 10 years and is characterized by mediastinal or superficial lymphadenopathy, hepatosplenomegaly, uveitis, enlargement of the salivary or lacrimal glands, cystic bone lesions of the hands or feet, polyarticular arthritis, lung infiltrations, granulomatous skin lesions, and cardiac involvement. The pathologic abnormalities are similar to those observed in chronic granulomatous diseases, especially tuberculosis, but caseation is absent.

Laboratory findings Abnormal findings include hyperproteinemia, hyperglobulinemia, hypercalcemia, hypercalcinuria, leukopenia, and eosinophilia. Liver function tests may also be abnormal.

The Nickerson-Kveim test (formation of a granuloma several weeks after intradermal injection of material from a sarcoid lesion), organ biopsy, and x-rays of the lungs help in making a diagnosis. The classical bone lesion is a sharply defined punched-out area of rarefaction in the phalanges. Adrenal corticosteroids are of value in suppressing the acute manifestations of sarcoidosis and decreasing the severity of organ involvement. The disease usually progresses slowly with remissions and relapses and ultimate quiescence.

REVIEW QUESTIONS

1. Rheumatoid arthritis occurs most frequently (a) in females; (b) in males; (c) with the same frequency in both sexes.
2. Hypersensitivity to drugs is associated with some cases of periarteritis nodosa, anaphylactoid purpura, and (a) rheumatic fever; (b) sarcoidosis; (c) Stevens-Johnson syndrome; (d) osteogenesis imperfecta.
3. All the following apply to rheumatoid arthritis except for one: (a) cervical spine is involved with neck stiffness and pain; (b) the affected joints are erythematous; (c) spindling of fingers; (d) pericarditis; (e) iridocyclitis.
4. Laboratory findings in juvenile rheumatoid arthritis include all the following except one: (a) latex-fixation test is often positive; (b) elevated sedimentation rate; (c) C-reactive protein is frequently positive; (d) antistreptolysin-0 titer may be elevated.
5. In the treatment of rheumatoid arthritis a blood salicylate level of (a) 10 mg per 100 ml; (b) 25 mg per 100 ml; (c) 50 mg per 100 ml; (d) 75 mg per 100 ml is desirable.
6. All the following apply to disseminated lupus erythematosus except for one: (a) polyarthritis and pericarditis; (b) "wire-loop lesion" in the kidney; (c) most cases occur in males; (d) hepatomegaly, splenomegaly, and lymphadenopathy; (e) personality changes.
7. Laboratory findings in disseminated lupus erythematosus include all the following except for one: (a) Coombs' test may be positive; (b) the use of immunofluorescent technique with skin and renal biopsies reveals deposition of gamma globulin and serum complement; (c) antinuclear antibodies are present in most patients; (d) serum-complement activity is high.
8. The following statements concerning pseudohypertrophic muscular dystrophy (Duchenne type) are true except for one: (a) this is the commonest type of progressive muscular dystrophy; (b) it is a sex-linked trait; (c) males from 2 to 10 years of age are most frequently affected; (d) creatine phosphokinase (CPK) is reduced.
9. Muscular weakness may be seen in the following endocrine abnormalities ex-

cept for one: (*a*) hyperthyroidism; (*b*) hypoparathyroidism; (*c*) hyperparathyroidism; (*d*) precocious puberty.

10. All the following statements concerning osteogenesis imperfecta are true except for one: (*a*) it may be transmitted as an autosomal recessive trait; (*b*) fractures from minor trauma are rare after puberty; (*c*) alkaline phosphatase is low, but laboratory findings are otherwise within normal limits; (*d*) wormian bones are found in the skull.

11. All the following statements concerning Marfan's syndrome are true except for one: (*a*) height is greater than the arm span; (*b*) pelvis-to-sole measurement is greater than pubis to vertex measurement; (*c*) joints are hyperextensible; (*d*) long, thin extremities and spider fingers.

The following questions are of the matching type. In each blank in column I insert the letter corresponding to the word or phrase in column II which is associated most appropriately:

I		II	
12.	Congenital dislocation of the hip	(*a*)	Bilateral in 50 percent of affected cases
13.	Internal tibial torsion	(*b*)	Mandible most frequently affected
14.	Congenital clubfoot	(*c*)	Ortolani test
15.	Infantile cortical hyperostosis	(*d*)	Osteochondrosis of the tibial tubercle
16.	Osgood-Schlatter disease	(*e*)	Most common cause of toeing in as seen in young children
17.	Slipped femoral epiphysis	(*f*)	Usually occurs in obese males

22 BLOOD DISORDERS

The hematopoietic system of infants and children differs from that of adults in its relative size, nutritional requirements, and its response to stimuli and noxious agents. As a result, disorders of the blood in infants and children, whether they involve the erythron, the white blood cells, the platelets, or the components of the hemostatic mechanism, have qualities and characteristics that set them apart from similar disorders in older persons.

DISORDERS OF THE RED BLOOD CELLS

Anemia is a lowering of the hemoglobin concentration, red cell count, or both below the normal values. Polycythemia, an absolute increase above normal in both the red cell count and the hemoglobin concentration, is rare in infants and children and is encountered principally as a compensatory reaction (secondary polycythemia) to states of chronic hypoxia, e.g., cyanotic congenital heart disease.

There is a considerable physiologic variation in the red cell count and hemoglobin concentration during the first year of life (Table 22-1), which should always be considered before a diagnosis of anemia is made.

Anemia may be caused by any of the following four fundamental disturbances of normal red blood cell equilibrium:

1. A lack of blood production: aplastic or hypoplastic anemia
2. An arrest of erythrocyte maturation: iron-deficiency or megaloblastic anemia
3. A shortened erythrocyte survival time: hemolytic anemia
4. A loss of blood: hemorrhage

The following is a clinically useful classification of the more common anemias of infancy and childhood, grouped according to relative frequency at different age periods:

1. Anemias of the neonatal period
    a. Acute hemorrhage: external bleeding, e.g., from umbilical cord (loose tie), prepuce (postcircumcision), gastrointestinal (hemorrhagic disease of the newborn); internal bleeding, e.g., cephalhematoma, subdural hematoma, ruptured viscus (spleen), bleeding of one twin into the circulation of the other or from fetus to mother (transplacental hemorrhage)
    b. Hemolytic disease of the newborn: erythroblastosis fetalis (Rh and other secondary blood group factors) and icterus praecox (ABO blood group incompatibility)
    c. Acquired hemolytic anemia: infections, particularly septicemia or toxins, e.g., naphthalene
    d. Congenital transplacental disseminated infection: syphilis, toxoplasmosis, cytomegalic inclusion body disease, histoplasmosis, rubella
    e. Myelophthisic anemia: rare, e.g., leukemia
2. Anemias of infancy
    a. Physiologic "anemia": a moderate postnatal reduction in hemoglobin and red blood count which occurs in all normal infants and is believed due to an "overshoot" reaction of feedback control to adjustment to a postuterine environment
    b. Anemia of prematurity: probably an accentuation of factors causing physiologic anemia
    c. Iron-deficiency anemia: from poor antenatal storage of iron due to iron deficiency of the mother, inadequate diet, infection, or chronic bleeding
    d. Acquired hemolytic anemia: from infections, drugs, poisons

   e. Hereditary chronic hemolytic anemias: Mediterranean (Cooley's) anemia, sickle-cell anemia, congenital hemolytic jaundice, glucose-6-phosphate dehydrogenase deficiency and glycolytic pathway enzyme defects

   f. Megaloblastic anemia of infancy: folic acid deficiency from inadequate diet, infection, or protracted diarrhea; congenital vitamin B_{12} disorders

   g. Aplastic anemias: congenital aplastic anemia, aplastic anemia secondary to drugs or poisons, congenital pure red blood cell anemia

   h. Myelophthisic anemia: leukemia, neuroblastoma, Letterer-Siewe disease

3. Anemias of childhood

   a. Iron-deficiency anemia: from inadequate diet, chronic bleeding, intestinal parasites

   b. Chronic normochromic anemia: from chronic infection, e.g., rheumatic fever, tuberculosis, or from renal insufficiency or hypothyroidism

   c. Acute hemorrhage: postoperative, trauma, hemorrhagic diathesis

   d. Hereditary chronic hemolytic anemias

   e. Hemolytic anemia: e.g., acquired acute or chronic, autoimmune

   f. Myelophthisic anemia: secondary to leukemia, neuroblastoma, miliary tuberculosis, reticuloendothelioses (Gaucher's, Niemann-Pick, or Hand-Schüller-Christian disease)

   g. Rare anemias: aplastic anemia (usually secondary to drugs, infection), congestive splenomegaly (Banti's syndrome), juvenile pernicious anemia (due to vitamin B_{12} deficiency secondary to congenital lack of gastric intrinsic factor excretion or a defect in absorption of vitamin B_{12} in the ileum)

ANEMIA OF ACUTE HEMORRHAGE

This anemia is due to the acute loss of a considerable quantity of blood from the peripheral circulation. A blood loss that would be quantitatively insignificant to an adult is a serious loss to a child. A hemorrhage of 95 ml in a 7-lb newborn infant, whose total blood volume is 280 ml, will reduce the hemoglobin concentration from 18 Gm per 100 ml to 12 Gm per 100 ml, or about one-third its former value. In an adult with a total blood volume between 5,000 and 6,000 ml, this would be equivalent to a hemorrhage of 1,700 to 2,000 ml.

Clinical features

1. Symptoms are usually proportional to the degree and rapidity of the blood loss. The most common are lethargy, irritability, and loss of appetite or willingness to nurse. If the blood loss is not too rapid or severe, there may be surprisingly few symptoms.

2. The principal physical findings are pallor of the skin and mucous membranes.
3. Jaundice may occur if the lost blood is retained within the body in such regions as the peritoneal cavity or beneath the scalp (cephalhematoma) because of the breakdown of retained hemoglobin.
4. Very rapid and profound bleeding is characterized by signs of cardiovascular collapse and shock.
5. The chief laboratory findings are a normocytic, normochromic anemia, accompanied by a reticulocytosis that rises and remains elevated for several days to a week after the hemorrhage has ceased.

Course   The course is uneventful when the anemia is not severe. If the nutrition and iron stores are adequate, the red cell count and hemoglobin concentration return to normal levels within 4 to 8 weeks. A hypochromic anemia is the most frequent delayed complication, particularly when the hemorrhage is in the neonatal period or early infancy.

Treatment   Treatment depends on the rapidity of the hemorrhage and the severity of the anemia. With rapid blood loss to hemoglobin levels of 5 to 6 Gm per 100 ml, transfusion is urgent. The amount of blood given is usually not more than 7.5 ml per lb at any one transfusion, provided that the acute blood loss has stopped, in order not to overload the cardiovascular system and produce pulmonary edema or acute cardiac dilatation with resultant heart failure. If the blood loss is continuing, a transfusion of a larger quantity of blood may be required. If the bleeding has been controlled, the patient's general condition is good, and the hemoglobin concentration has not fallen below 8 to 9 Gm per 100 ml, transfusion may be withheld. In such cases, oral iron medication sufficient to provide 75 to 100 mg elemental iron daily will speed blood regeneration.

ACQUIRED HEMOLYTIC ANEMIA

This disorder is characterized by increased intravascular or extravascular destruction of blood. It may be acute or chronic.

Etiology   The cause is often obscure. In infants and young children, an acute form frequently occurs in association with infection, particularly septicemia; autohemagglutinins and autohemolysins are occasionally demonstrable. In older children, household poisons such as benzol derivatives and naphthalene (moth balls) act as hemolytic agents. Antimalarial drugs (such as primaquin), sulfonamides, or ingestion of the beans or inhalation of the pollen of the fava plant may

Table 22-1. Average blood cell values during infancy and childhood*

Cells	Birth	2 days	2 weeks	3 months	1 year	5 years	10 years
Red blood cells, millions per cu mm	4.9-5.5	5.3-6.5	4.5-5.5	3.9-4.8	4.5-5.0	4.7-5.1	4.8-5.2
Hemoglobin, Gm per 100 ml	16-20	18-22	14-17	10.5-11.5	12-13	12.5-13.5	12.5-14.5
Reticulocytes, %	3-5	1-5	1-2	0.1-0.5	0.1-1.5	0.1-1.5	0.1-1.5
Nucleated red blood cells, per 100 white cells	2-10	0-5	0-2	0	0	0	0
White blood cells, thousands per cu mm	10-20	12-22	8-12	5-9	6-10	6-10	6-10
Neutrophils, %	45-55	50-65	30-45	30-40	35-45	40-50	45-55
Lymphocytes, %	45-30	40-20	55-45	65-50	60-50	55-45	50-45
Others, % (monocytes, eosinophils, basophils)	10-15	10-15	15-10	5-10	5	5	5
	Occasional myelocytes						
Platelets, thousands per cu mm	200-300	450	350	200-300	250-350	250-350	250-350

* Determination of the peripheral red cell count or hemoglobin reflects the true size of the circulating red blood cell mass only when the blood volume is normal. In dehydration, for example, when the plasma volume is greatly reduced, peripheral measurements give falsely high values. In brisk hemorrhage, on the other hand, while plasma and red blood cell volumes are being proportionately reduced, early peripheral measurements do not reflect the true reduction of total red blood cell mass. After the bleeding has slowed or stopped and plasma volume has been restored from the extravascular fluids, red cell and hemoglobin concentrations indicate the change in size of the circulating red blood cell mass. In chronic anemia, the total blood volume is usually unchanged; the total circulating red blood cell mass is reflected by the peripheral values. Several hours after birth, the total erythrocyte, plasma, and blood volume increases by as much as 20 percent and remains elevated for about 2 weeks.

557

cause an acute hemolytic anemia in individuals with a congenital deficiency of erythrocyte glucose-6-phosphate dehydrogenase (G-6-PD) of the African (A-) type. Other G-6-PD variants (B- type), which occur more often among Caucasians, are usually associated with a chronic nonspherocytic hemolytic anemia (see below).

A rarer cause of the disorder is exposure to cold and rewarming in individuals with the Donath-Landsteiner cold hemolysin (paroxysmal "cold" hemoglobinuria). The hemolysin attaches to the cells only in the cold; acute intravascular hemolysis and hemoglobinuria follows return to warmer temperatures. In individuals with congenital syphilis, a circulating "cold" hemolysin may be lifelong. When it arises in association with other infections, it may disappear after a few months or years. Increased phagocytic activity of the splenic reticuloendothelial system (hypersplenism) may produce a chronic hemolytic anemia.

Clinical features

1. The principal clinical manifestations of the mild acute or chronic types of acquired hemolytic anemia are jaundice and moderate splenomegaly. The urine is usually darker than normal because of increased urobilinogen. Pallor is frequently masked by the icterus.
2. In the severe acute types, pallor is commonly the first symptom, with jaundice not appearing until 8 to 24 hours later. In such instances, when the blood destruction is massive, circulatory collapse and death from severe anemia may occur before treatment can be instituted. The urine in such cases is port-wine-colored, owing to the marked hemoglobinuria.

Laboratory findings   Anemia, elevated serum-bilirubin level, chiefly of the indirect or protein-bound type, increased urine urobilinogen (but absence of bilirubin), and greatly increased stool urobilinogen are found. Hemoglobinuria occurs with rapid and extensive blood destruction. Occasionally circulating antibodies or sensitized red blood cells (positive direct Coombs' test) may be demonstrable. The increased blood production that always accompanies hemolytic anemia is also accompanied by nucleated red blood cells and increased reticulocytes in the peripheral blood and a normoblastic hyperplasia in the bone marrow. A deficiency of erythrocyte G-6-PD may be demonstrated.

Treatment   Treatment is directed toward removing the possible cause, with replacement of blood when the anemia is severe. Antibiotics are indicated if infection is present. Splenectomy is usually reserved for the chronic cases or those in which a diagnosis of hypersplenism can be established. Certain chronic cases may respond to ACTH or adrenal corticosteroid therapy, which may be required for years to maintain reasonable hemoglobin levels.

Prognosis   In general, the prognosis is good in the acute cases but poor in the chronic cases.

HEMOLYTIC DISEASE OF THE NEWBORN
(Erythroblastosis Fetalis)

Erythroblastosis fetalis is a self-limited hemolytic anemia of late fetal or early postnatal life due to transplacental isoimmunization to the Rh or certain other erythrocyte antigens. A sufficiently large amount of Rh-positive antigen of the red blood cells of the fetus usually gains access to the mother's circulation during delivery of the products of her first pregnancy (fetus of 20 weeks or older) through tears in the placental villae, resulting in initial sensitization in the 5 percent of Rh-negative women who are sensitizable. In the circulation, the Rh-positive antigen stimulates the production of antibodies in the Rh-negative mother. In subsequent pregnancies there is passive transfer of the anti-Rh antibodies from the mother back through the placenta to the fetus, where they become attached to the infant's Rh-positive red blood cells. Small amounts of Rh-positive fetal cells which gain access to the mother's circulation from minute tears in the normal placenta during the course of a subsequent pregnancy may stimulate a further increase of Rh antibodies by an anemnestic response. Once sensitized, an Rh-negative individual continues to produce Rh antibodies for many years without further stimulation. The sensitized erythrocytes in the infant with erythroblastosis fetalis are removed from the circulation by increased reticuloendothelial phagocytosis rather than by intravascular hemolysis.

The disease occurs in from 1 in 250 to 1 in 500 births in Caucasians, less frequently in Negroes and Asiatics. Only 1 of 20 Rh-negative women married to Rh-positive men has an infant with erythroblastosis fetalis. It does not occur during the first pregnancy unless the mother has been immunized by a prior transfusion or injection of Rh-positive blood. Succeeding newborn Rh-positive infants are usually more severely affected. (Rh-negative infants born to sensitized mothers are unaffected.)

Immunization to the Rh factor through transfusion or the intramuscular injection of Rh-positive blood into Rh-negative persons is becoming less frequent, as Rh typing prior to transfusion is now universally performed.

The antigens   The principal antigen causing erythroblastosis fetalis is the $Rh_0(D)$ factor of the Rh system, resulting in approximately 90 percent of Rh isoimmunization. The next most common factor is the hr′ (c) factor (3 to 5 percent). Less commonly the blood group antigens in the following order may result in isoimmunization and erythroblastosis fetalis: rh″ (E), K (Kell), rh_w (C_w), rh′ (C), k (allele of Kell), hr″ (e), Jk^a (Kidd), S, Fy^a (Duffy).

The antibody   There are two general varieties of Rh antibodies—complete and incomplete. The complete antibodies (IgM), or 19S antibodies of Svedberg ultracentrifuge designation, do not traverse the placenta. They are readily detected in saline dilutions of the serum.

The incomplete antibodies (IgG), or 7S antibodies, do not cause agglutination in saline dilutions of the serum but require special techniques for their detection. (These special techniques include adding serum albumin or other hydrophilic colloid to the solution, modifications of the test cell by exposure to a 0.1 percent solution of the enzyme trypsin, or the use of antiglobulin antibody (Coombs' serum) to cause agglutination of the unagglutinated but antibody-coated Rh-positive test cells.) The IgG variety occurs more commonly than the IgM variety and traverses the placenta readily because of its smaller size. Any Rh-antibody titer is significant; even a titer of 1:2 in the mother may cause erythroblastosis fetalis in her Rh-positive infant, but the disease is more likely to be clinically mild.

Pathologic physiology in infants   Most of physiologic and clinical characteristics of erythroblastosis fetalis can be related to increased red blood cell destruction and increased red blood cell regeneration superimposed on the poor liver function characteristic of the newborn infant and the infant's ability to compensate for their deleterious effects. There is no evidence that the Rh antibody has any effect on tissues other than the red blood cells. Anemia occurs after birth not because there is an increase in the hemolytic process, which is probably most severe at term, but because the infant's ability to continue markedly increased red blood cell production begins to lag after birth.

The jaundice in infants with erythroblastosis fetalis is due to two factors:

1.   There is an increased amount of hemoglobin presented to the reticuloendothelial system for metabolism because of the hemolytic process. The pigment part of hemoglobin is normally broken from the rest of the molecule and converted to bilirubin, which is then excreted through the biliary system.
2.   The infant's ability to conjugate and excrete bilirubin (as bilirubin glucuronide, which is soluble and "direct" reacting in the van den Bergh reaction) during the first few days of life is not so efficient as it is later. Liver enzyme "glucuronyl-transferase," necessary for conjugation, is low during the first few days of life.

Clinical features   Symptoms vary widely, from infants who are stillborn to those who are apparently normal and have only a very mild anemia that requires no treatment. Although there is much overlapping, three clinical forms are differentiated:

1.   Hydrops fetalis (approximately 3 percent): The infants have generalized edema, severe pallor, moderate jaundice, and striking enlargement of the liver and spleen. The placenta is also enlarged. Frequently the fetuses are stillborn.
2.   Icterus gravis (approximately 27 percent): The infants usually

appear normal at birth. Within a few hours, however, jaundice appears and soon becomes intense. The anemia and enlargement of the spleen may not be pronounced. Kernicterus is most common in this group.

3. Hemolytic anemia of the newborn (approximately 70 percent): The infants with this form are also normal at birth. Mild jaundice may be noted on the second day of life. This frequently is considered an early physiologic icterus but may become moderately intense on succeeding days. The anemia is minimal at first, and pallor may not be observed clinically until the jaundice subsides toward the end of the first week. Occasionally the anemia may be so slow in developing that it is not noted until the second to fourth weeks of life. The degree of hepatomegaly and splenomegaly may vary from minimal to moderate enlargement.

Laboratory findings   The principal laboratory findings are summarized in Table 22-2. The diagnosis is most accurately established immunologically by the demonstration of antibody-coated red blood cells (positive direct Coombs' test) in a newborn infant whose mother's serum contains anti-Rh or similar blood group antibodies for the infant's red blood cells.

Differential diagnosis   Icterus praecox, delayed initiation of hepatic bilirubin-conjugating mechanisms, or acquired hemolytic anemia associated with sepsis are the most common conditions to be differentiated. Also, increased hemolysis due to administration of synthetic vitamin K to infant or mother during labor may result in neonatal hyperbilirubinemia. More rarely, cytomegalic inclusion body disease, congenital obstruction of the bile ducts, congenital syphilis, congenital toxoplasmosis, G-6-PD or glutathione reductase deficiency, congenital hemolytic jaundice, Crigler-Najjar syndrome, and occasionally hereditary nonspherocytic anemia due to a variety of red cell enzyme defects may simulate erythroblastosis fetalis.

Complications

1. Kernicterus is the most serious complication of the disease, and it tends to occur in those infants who are severely jaundiced. A factor that may play a role in increasing the incidence of kernicterus is acidosis. Classically, the basal ganglions of the brainstem are grossly icteric and may show degeneration of the nerve cells. Occasionally the basal ganglions are spared, and there may be degenerative changes in the higher centers. Clinically the early manifestations are poor feeding, spasticity, convulsions, and opisthotonos. Later, athetosis and mental retardation may become manifest.

2. Residual hepatosplenomegaly, which may occasionally persist for many months.

Table 22-2. Summary of anemias of infancy and childhood

Disorder	Clinical features	Red blood cell morphology	Reticulocytes	Nucleated red blood cells
Anemia of acute hemorrhage	Pallor, rapid pulse, shock	Normal	Increased after few days	May be present
Acquired hemolytic anemia: Acute	Pallor, tachycardia, anorexia early, jaundice later	Normal or fragmented	Increased moderately	Frequently present
Chronic	Pallor, jaundice, splenomegaly	Normal	Increased moderately to markedly	Rarely present
Erythroblastosis fetalis: Rh	Pallor, jaundice, hepatosplenomegaly, kernicterus	Normal, occasional macrocytes	Increased	Usually many present
Iron-deficiency anemia	Pallor, usually slight to moderate splenomegaly	Hypochromia, microcytosis, anisocytosis, and slight poikilocytosis	Normal	Rare
Megaloblastic anemia	Pallor, anorexia, lethargy, hepatomegaly, splenomegaly, petechiae, infections	Normochromic, anisocytosis, marked poikilocytosis, macrocytosis unusual	Normal or slightly increased	Few usually present
Cooley's anemia, thalassemia major or Mediterranean anemia	Pallor, jaundice, hepatosplenomegaly, characteristic facies, retarded growth, Mediterranean ancestry	Marked hypochromia, striking variation in size and shape, polychromatophilia, target cells	Increased	Usually many present
Sickle-cell anemia	Pallor, periodic crises, splenomegaly early, shrunken spleen later, asthenic habitus	Moderate hypochromia, moderate to marked variation in size and shape, target cells	Increased	Increased, especially following crisis
Hereditary spherocytosis (congenital hemolytic jaundice)	Pallor, splenomegaly, jaundice with hemolytic crisis	Spherocytes	Increased, especially following crisis	May be present
Aplastic anemia	Pallor, petechiae, secondary infections	Normal	Very low or absent	Absent
Chronic hypoplastic anemia	Pallor	Normochromic, normocytic	Absent	Absent
Myelophthisic anemia	Pallor, purpura, and symptoms and signs of primary disease	Normochromic, normocytic	Decreased	Few usually present

White blood cells	Platelets	Bone marrow	Special examinations	Treatment
Slight leukocytosis, moderate shift to left	Usually increased	Normal early; normoblastic hyperplasia later		Transfusion if severe; iron if mild
Usually slight leukocytosis with shift to left	Normal or increased	Moderate normoblastic hyperplasia in a few hours	If drug- or toxin-induced: erythrocyte glucose-6-phosphate dehydrogenase frequently decreased, Heinz bodies increased. If severe, hemoglobinuria. Serum "free" bilirubin rises after 1–2 days	Offending agent removed; tranfusion if severe
Usually normal	Usually normal	Moderate normoblastic hyperplasia	Serum-"free" bilirubin, urine and stool urobilinogen increased. Occasionally positive direct Coombs' test	Splenectomy or adrenal corticosteroids beneficial in selected cases
Moderate leukocytosis with shift to left	Normal	Marked normoblastic hyperplasia	Direct Coombs' test always positive	Exchange transfusion if severe, simple transfusions for mild cases (compatible Rh-negative blood)
Normal or slight leukopenia	Normal	Normoblastic hyperplasia with pronormoblast increase, stainable iron decreased or absent	Low serum-iron content (<60 μg%) and elevated serum–iron-binding capacity (>370 μg%)	Iron in mild and moderate cases, transfusion plus iron in severe cases
Usually leukopenia, neutropenia, hypersegmented polymorphonuclears	Normal or decreased	Erythroid hyperplasia with megaloblastic pattern in erythroid, myeloid, and megakaryocytic cells	Folic acid deficiency: elevated urine FIGLU* after histidine, low serum folic acid; vitamin B_{12} deficiency: low serum vitamin B_{12}, elevated urine MMA**	Folic acid or vitamin B_{12} as indicated
Moderate leukocytosis with shift to left	Normal or decreased	Striking erythroblastic hyperplasia, stainable iron increased in older children	Increased resistance to hypotonic saline solution, increased fetal hemoglobin	Periodic transfusions for anemia; splenectomy in selected cases where erythrocyte survival time is greatly reduced
Normal, slight leukocytosis following crisis	Normal	Moderate to marked normoblastic hyperplasia	Red blood cells "sickle" under appropriate conditions, hemoglobin electrophoresis characteristic of hemoglobin S	Transfusion usually recommended when hemoglobin falls below 5.5 Gm/100 ml
Normal, slight leukocytosis following crisis	Normal	Moderate to marked normoblastic hyperplasia	Increased fragility to hypotonic saline solution	Splenectomy after 2 yr of age
Leukopenia	Decreased	Hypoplastic for all elements		Transfusion; toxic cause removed if known
Normal	Normal	Very hypoplastic for erythroid cells (0.5–3%) only	Increased urinary anthranilic acid in some cases	Periodic transfusions
Neutropenia with a relative lymphocytosis and occasional myelocytes	Decreased	May reveal a primary disease, i.e., leukemia, neuroblastoma, tumor cells, Gaucher's cells, etc.	Roentgenograms of the bones; biopsy of lymph nodes or spleen	Transfusions; primary disease treated

* Formimino glutamic acid.
** Methylmalonic acid.

3.   Obstructive jaundice, which may persist for weeks (see Chapter 12, "Diseases of the Newborn").
4.   Greenish staining of deciduous teeth.

Prognosis   The criteria for assessing prognosis have been carefully developed with relation to the immediate postnatal period. Outlook for survival decreases in direct proportion to the cord blood hemoglobin. A cord blood hemoglobin of 8 Gm per 100 ml is associated with a 50 percent mortality. A hemoglobin of 13.5 Gm or more per 100 ml is associated with 2 to 3 percent mortality.

Severe kernicterus is more likely to occur in infants whose serum-bilirubin level reaches 20 mg or more per 100 ml during the first few days of life. However, mild kernicterus and later mental retardation may occur with bilirubin levels as low as 12 mg per 100 ml. Therefore, bilirubin values below 20 mg per 100 ml are not an absolute assurance against the effects of bilirubin-encephalopathy. Kernicterus is unknown during the first 12 to 18 hours. Infants with cord serum-bilirubin levels of 4 mg or more per 100 ml are most likely to develop serum-bilirubin levels of 20 mg or more during the first few postnatal days unless treated by exchange transfusion. Development of kernicterus is also associated with the state of maturity of the infant's central nervous system. It is more common at the same level of hyperbilirubinemia in premature infants than in full-term infants. Prematurity predisposes to hyperbilirubinemia and kernicterus, whatever the causation.

Antenatal prediction of severity   Severity of the disease often increases with succeeding pregnancies, but not invariably. A history of previous siblings with severe erythroblastosis fetalis is therefore associated with a greater likelihood of severe disease for the patient. High maternal titers of Rh antibody are more frequently associated with severe erythroblastosis fetalis in the infant, although there is no direct correlation between the antibody titer and the severity of the disease. However, a titer of 1 : 64 or more is usually associated with moderate to severe erythroblastosis fetalis. Conversely, maternal anti-Rh titers of 1 : 16 or less are often, although not invariably, associated with infants having mild disease. A rapidly rising maternal antibody titer, particularly an increase of fourfold or more, is usually associated with infants having moderate to severe erythroblastosis fetalis.

Determination of the level and pattern of change of a bilirubin-related pigment in the amniotic fluid between 28 and 36 weeks of gestation is a parameter used to assess the severity of erythroblastosis fetalis of a fetus in utero. Amniotic fluid may be obtained for analysis by needle amniocentesis with relatively little danger to mother or fetus. Based upon such analyses, criteria have been developed for early interruption of pregnancy or for intrauterine transfusion of a severely affected fetus to forestall severe anemia which may result in a fatality before the infant can be delivered.

Treatment Exchange transfusion is performed to alleviate the anemia and hyperbilirubinemia. It diminishes hyperbilirubinemia by removing the infant's blood, which contains elevated amounts of bilirubin, and replacing it with normal blood. Anemia is corrected by exchange transfusion using donor blood with a higher hematocrit than that of the infant's blood. (Severe anemia can be corrected to a greater extent by giving packed or sedimented cells instead of whole blood.) An exchange also removes circulating antibodies and Rh-positive cells and substitutes Rh-negative cells which, because they are not rapidly destroyed, serve to lessen hyperbilirubinemia and anemia during the early neonatal period.

Indications for exchange transfusion within a few hours of birth
1. Positive Coombs' test
2. Cord blood hemoglobin of 12.5 Gm or less per 100 ml or cord serum bilirubin of 4.5 mg or more per 100 ml
3. History of severe erythroblastosis fetalis in previous siblings, particularly if the infants were stillborn or had hydrops fetalis
4. Prematurity

See page 247 for comments on the use of phototherapy.

Indications for later or repeat exchange transfusions
1. Increasing jaundice: serum bilirubin of 6 mg per 100 ml at 6 hours, 10 mg per 100 ml at 12 hours, or 20 mg per 100 ml at any time up to 5 days
2. Progressive anemia: hemoglobin of 11.5 Gm per 100 ml or less within the first 24 hours, 10 Gm per 100 ml at 24 to 48 hours, 9 Gm per 100 ml at 48 to 96 hours
3. Progressive abnormal physical findings: edema, hypotonia, hepatomegaly (3 cm or more), irregular respiration, or spasticity

Prophylaxis Specific Rh_0 antibody is administered intramuscularly to the Rh-negative woman within 72 hours of the delivery of her first Rh_0-positive infant. The antibody coats the Rh_0-positive cells of the infant which have gained entrance into the mother's circulation in relatively large numbers through tears and compression of the placenta during delivery and prevents them from being antigenic. Prophylaxis by avoiding sensitization of Rh-negative women by transfusion of accurately typed Rh-negative blood is also very important.

Teamwork between the obstetrician and pediatrician to assess the probable severity of erythroblastosis fetalis in the fetus of a pregnant mother before delivery, so that preparations can be made for prompt treatment of the newborn infant, greatly reduces the mortality and morbidity in this disease. The assessment of intrauterine severity of erythroblastosis in the fetus has been aided by the measurement of bilirubin pigments in amniotic fluid obtained antepartum by amniocentesis. If the disease is judged to be advanced, early induction of labor may be instituted to prevent further exposure of the infant to maternal Rh antibody.

Early induction of labor in an immunized Rh-negative woman may also be considered after the thirty-seventh week of gestation if there has been a fourfold rise in the Rh-antibody titer. In reaching this decision, the hazards of prematurity must be weighed against those of further exposure to maternal Rh antibody. To prevent the intrauterine death of a severely anemic infant who is too premature for delivery, transfusion of the fetus in utero has been done. This is accomplished via a trochar and plastic catheter through the abdominal wall and uterine musculature of the mother into the peritoneal cavity of the fetus. The transfused cells enter the circulation of the fetus by diapedesis.

ICTERUS PRAECOX

This is a form of hemolytic disease of the newborn due to ABO blood group incompatibility between the mother and infant. The anti-A or anti-B antibodies of a mother of blood group O, B, or A may cross the placenta and sensitize the red blood cells of an A, B, or AB infant. This disorder is more frequent than erythroblastosis due to the Rh factors. In contrast to erythroblastosis, icterus praecox usually affects firstborn infants. Clinically, the disease is usually milder than Rh erythroblastosis fetalis and is characterized by early jaundice, usually beginning within the first 24 hours (in contrast to "physiologic," jaundice which begins after 24 hours of age). There is a gradual development of a mild anemia which often does not become apparent until several weeks postnatally. The liver and spleen become only slightly enlarged if at all. The laboratory findings usually show evidence of a mild hemolytic process including moderate reticulocytosis, increased osmotic fragility, and spherocytosis. The direct Coombs' test result is usually negative, occasionally 1 to 2+. Kernicterus has been reported in rare instances.

Treatment   The treatment is similar to that for erythroblastosis fetalis. Exchange transfusion is indicated if the serum bilirubin reaches levels similar to those described for the infant with erythroblastosis fetalis— 10 mg or more per 100 ml before 12 hours of age, 20 mg or more per 100 ml within the first few neonatal days. Donor blood is usually group O in which the anti-A and anti-B agglutinins have been neutralized with soluble A and B (Witebsky) substance. Prematurity and anemia are additional indications for exchange transfusion when present, as in erythroblastosis fetalis. It is sometimes possible to predict the occurrence of icterus praecox prenatally by demonstrating a high titer of IgG (hyperimmune) type ABO isoagglutinins, which are resistant to inhibition by group-specific substance.

Prognosis   The prognosis for survival in icterus praecox is much better than in Rh erythroblastosis fetalis. Death is usually due to a complicating kernicterus.

Prophylaxis   No practical procedures are currently available.

PHYSIOLOGIC ANEMIA OF INFANCY

Physiologic anemia is not a true anemia (see Fig. 22-1). The red blood cells and hemoglobin, normally at mild polycythemia levels at birth, drop sharply during the first 2 weeks of life and more gradually thereafter, reaching a low point averaging about 4 million red blood cells and 11 Gm hemoglobin at about the third month of life. They rise very slowly thereafter during the balance of the first year, but a slight hypochromia and microcytosis persist. The etiology and pathogenesis of this condition are not completely understood. It is probably due to a temporary hypofunction of the bone marrow as a result of a "feedback" arrest occurring during the adjustment to an extrauterine existence. It does not respond to iron, liver extract, folic acid, or other medication. There are no clinical symptoms, and no treatment is indicated.

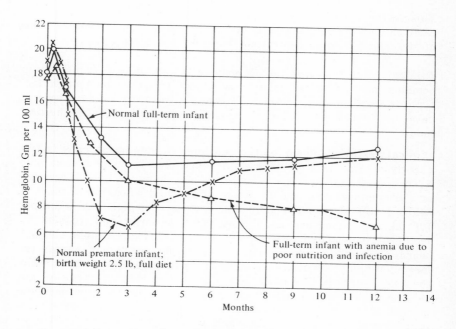

Figure 22-1. The normal course of hemoglobin concentration in the blood during the first year in a full-term infant weighing 7 lb at birth and a premature infant whose birth weight was 2½ lb. The continuation of the early "physiologic anemia" as the result of inadequate diet and infection is shown in the third curve.

ANEMIA OF PREMATURITY

This is a normochromic, slightly microcytic anemia which develops during the first 4 to 10 weeks of postnatal life in premature infants. The etiology and pathogenesis are obscure. It appears to be an accentuation of the same process that results in the physiologic "anemia" of full-term infants. The early anemia of prematurity occurs in the presence of a relative excess of iron; later there is an iron deficit. The premature infant usually does not get sufficient iron in his early diet and by the eighth to tenth week should get 15 to 30 mg elemental iron per day to satisfy requirements for hemoglobin synthesis and for storage. When the hemoglobin falls below 7 Gm per 100 ml before the third month, transfusion is the only efficacious treatment, since there is poor response to iron or other antianemic medication until after the third month. Hypochromic anemia after this time will usually respond promptly to iron medication by mouth in the dosage recommended for the treatment of iron-deficiency anemia, especially if a low serum-iron level is demonstrated.

IRON–DEFICIENCY ANEMIA

This is the most commonly encountered anemia of late infancy and early childhood and is characterized by a greater proportional lowering of the hemoglobin concentration than of the red cell count.

Etiology The following factors may act singly or more commonly in combination: poor antenatal storage of iron (most common single factor), inadequate diet, infection, chronic hemorrhage, e.g., intestinal parasites (hookworm), or acute hemorrhage, particularly in the first months of life (see p. 40).

Clinical features Pallor of the skin and mucous membranes is frequently all that is seen, even with hemoglobin levels as low as 5 to 6 Gm per 100 ml. The child usually has good appetite, normal activity, and adequate growth and development. A child whose blood count is below 3 million per cubic milimeter, with a hemoglobin of 5 Gm per 100 ml, may have anorexia, irritability or lethargy, and frequent infections. The heart rate may be increased, with a soft systolic murmur heard precordially, and not infrequently the heart may appear enlarged on roentgenogram. The spleen is often palpable 1 to 2 cm below the costal margin. The chief laboratory features of the disorder are outlined in Table 22-2. Diagnosis is made by establishing each of the laboratory features, particularly the severe hypochromia, low serum-iron level (less than 50 micrograms per 100 ml), and elevated iron-binding capacity (over 350 micrograms per 100 ml) and a low saturation of the transferrin protein (less than 16 percent).

Treatment

1. Correct the anemia by transfusion and the iron deficiency by iron medication.
2. Eliminate associated etiologic factors.

Indications for transfusion Severe anemia or associated medical complications requires transfusion. If the hemoglobin is less than 6 Gm per 100 ml, transfusion may be given. Infection, anorexia, or other medical complications would make the indications for transfusion more immediate. The very anemic child should receive no more than 5 ml per lb as total volume at any one transfusion. If a rapid increase of the hemoglobin concentration is important, packed cells may be used. If infection is present, whole blood would be preferable for the antibody content of the plasma. Red blood cells provide a readily utilizable source of iron, approximately 0.5 mg elemental iron per milliliter of whole blood. However, the iron content of a whole blood transfusion is insufficient to overcome the iron deficit and to provide a store for future growth in a moderately or severely anemic infant. Supplementation with medicinal iron is indicated.

Iron medications and their indications Iron medication may be administered orally, intramuscularly, or intravenously. Oral medication is the treatment of choice if there are no medical contraindications. The minimal dosage of elemental iron for oral therapy in infancy is 90 to 150 mg per day. The most effective oral iron medication is ferrous sulfate, which is available both in a drop and in teaspoon dosage forms. The teaspoon of the liquid preparations contains approximately 40 mg elemental iron per 5 ml. Drop preparations are more concentrated; they contain 25 mg elemental iron per milliliter. The standard 3 gr (0.2 Gm) ferrous sulfate tablet contains 65 mg elemental iron. Iron medications are best given with citrus or tomato juice approximately 1 hour before meals. Ascorbic acid–containing juices aid in the absorption of iron from the gastrointestinal tract. Under these conditions as much as 25 percent of an orally administered dose may be absorbed in a severely anemic individual. Milk and solid foods containing phosphates and phytates form insoluble or poorly dissociated iron compounds which interfere with the absorption of the elemental iron. Ferrous gluconate preparations are about half and iron ammonium citrate preparations about one-quarter as effective as the sulfate of the same weight. Iron chelate preparations containing higher concentrations of iron than the usual sulfate preparations are also available for oral use but they have no advantage.

Parenteral iron preparations include saccharated iron compounds, which may be administered either intramuscularly or intravenously. (Dosage is determined by the hemoglobin level and the desired rise of this level.) Indications for their use are (1) when more rapid blood regeneration is desired than obtainable by the oral preparations, (2) when oral preparations are not tolerated, and (3) when it is doubted that the oral preparation will be continuously and faithfully administered over the required therapeutic period. A disadvantage of parenteral iron medications is that they usually require 5 to 10 dosage administrations; occasionally this may present a technical problem and be an inconvenience for the patient being treated on an ambulatory care basis. Maculopapular rashes as well as local abscesses have been reported following intramuscular administration of iron.

The degree and rapidity of hemoglobin response to iron medication is directly proportional to the severity of the anemia; with a hemoglobin level of 5 to 7 Gm per 100 ml, the best that can be expected from adequate oral medication is a hemoglobin rise of approximately 1 to 1.5 Gm per 100 ml per week. A rise of 2 Gm per 100 ml per week can be obtained initially following intravenous or intramuscular iron administration. Iron medication should be continued beyond the time that the blood levels reach normal in order to saturate the body iron stores that have been depleted. With oral medication this may require 12 to 16 weeks of continuous therapy.

Prognosis With adequate therapy, prognosis for nutritional iron-deficiency anemia is invariably good. Truly refractory iron-deficiency anemia in infancy and childhood is uncommon. When it allegedly occurs, it most often is due to inadequate therapy; other deficiencies, e.g., folic acid, B_{12}, pyridoxine; or associated chronic disease, e.g., tuberculosis, and chronic nephritis.

IRON–DEFICIENCY ANEMIA ASSOCIATED WITH HYPOCUPREMIA AND HYPOPROTEINEMIA

This is a syndrome of unknown etiology found in older infants and young children. It is characterized by a severe iron-deficiency anemia associated with a low plasma-copper level and a lower plasma-protein level, chiefly hypoalbuminemia. Serum-protein levels may fall to 2 Gm per 100 ml, and severe pitting edema of the extremities may be present. The anemia responds to treatment with iron preparations, which usually contain sufficient copper as a contaminant, to correct the associated copper deficiency. Indications for transfusion are the same as those for iron-deficiency anemia. Administration of copper alone does not correct the condition.

MEGALOBLASTIC ANEMIAS

Megaloblastic anemia usually results from a deficiency of folic acid or vitamin B_{12}. In rare instances, it may occur as a result of a hereditary defect of pyrimidine metabolism, which results in a folic acid and vitamin B_{12}–resistant megaloblastic anemia and in increased orotic acid excretion in the urine. Recently another rare type has been reported which responds only to pharmacological doses of thiamine (vitamin B_1).

Differences between folic acid and vitamin B_{12} account for the differences in the causation of megaloblastic anemia due to a deficiency of one or another of these two vitamins. The minimum daily requirement for folic acid for an infant is 40 to 50 micrograms; the requirement for vitamin B_{12} is 0.1 to 0.2 microgram per day. Folic acid is found in both plant and animal foods while vitamin B_{12} is found only in animal foods.

Liver, red meat, and egg yolks are good sources of both. Cow's milk (50 micrograms of folic acid per liter) and fowl are borderline sources of folic acid. Goat milk (10 to 20 micrograms of folic acid per liter) is an inadequate source. Orange juice (but not other citrus fruits) is a rich source of folic acid (45 micrograms per 3 oz). Cow's milk is a rich source of vitamin B_{12} (5 micrograms per liter).

Folic acid has a biological half-life in man of about 3 to 4 weeks; the half-life of vitamin B_{12} is 1 to 1½ years. With no further intake and no increase of requirement, an individual's store of folic acid would be down to less than 1 percent (deficiency levels) in about 5 to 7 months; vitamin B_{12} stores would last 7 to 10 years under similar circumstances. This explains why nutritional folic acid deficiency is generally so common, whereas nutritional vitamin B_{12} deficiency is unknown except in individuals who are consistently strict vegetarians (not lactovegetarians) for many years.

Folic acid, in addition, is readily destroyed by heating, light, and storage at room temperature, whereas vitamin B_{12} is stable to autoclaving, light, and room temperature storage. Thus much folic acid is lost by overcooking. Ascorbic acid protects against cooking and storage loss and explains the value of adding ascorbic acid to milk prior to preparation as a powder.

Folic acid is absorbed throughout the small intestine, and, although there is an active transport mechanism for physiological amounts, there are few blocks to absorption even in disorders such as celiac disease. (A rare hereditary syndrome, congenital malabsorption of folic acid is characterized by mental retardation, spasticity, and convulsions.) Vitamin B_{12} is absorbed in a limited portion of the small intestine (ileum) and requires the elaboration of a gastric "intrinsic factor" to protect food vitamin B_{12} on the way down to the ileum and to mediate its absorption there.

Folic acid and vitamin B_{12} are required for the normal growth of all tissues, including all the elements of the hematopoietic system. Effects of deficiency are most readily observed in tissues with a rapid turnover time, such as the hematopoietic cell and gastrointestinal mucous membrane. Therefore, effects of deficiency in infants include, besides anemia, leukopenia (chiefly neutropenia), thrombocytopenia, reduced serum proteins (edema), decreased antibody formation, glossitis, and growth failure.

MEGALOBLASTIC ANEMIA OF INFANCY

This is the second (after iron deficiency) most common nutritional anemia of infants. The age range of greatest occurrence in the United States is 2 to 18 months.

Etiology   The cause is limited to folic acid deficiency in most parts of the world (except in India, where strict vegetarianism is widely practiced, and infants are breast fed by mothers who are vitamin B_{12} deficient). Although folic acid deficiency may occur because of an inadequate nutritional intake (goat milk feeding), it usually results when, in addition to an inadequate dietary intake, there is an increased requirement generated by severe or repeated infection. In the case of protracted gastroenteritis, three factors may operate to produce folic acid deficiency: poor dietary intake, increased loss, and increased requirement due to the underlying infection.

Clinical features

1.   Pallor, splenomegaly, and frequently hepatomegaly are the most common findings.
2.   Petechial hemorrhages (practically unknown in iron-deficiency anemia) are frequent. Purpura and bleeding may occasionally be the presenting complaint.
3.   Anorexia, weight loss, irritability, and infection (often of the respiratory system or gastroenteritis) are common.
4.   Central nervous system disorder is unknown in nutritional folic acid deficiency. When due to vitamin B_{12} deficiency, irritability is the principal manifestation.

Laboratory features   The chief laboratory findings are summarized in Table 22-2. Since a deficiency of folic acid or vitamin B_{12} can result in identical morphological change, one must resort to biochemical tests to differentiate between the two.

Prognosis   Patients with nutritional megaloblastic anemia are potentially more seriously ill than those with iron deficiency. In the former, resistance to infection is extremely poor because of neutropenia and reduced antibody formation. The danger of intracranial hemorrhage is always present when thrombocytopenia exists. However, the prognosis is excellent with specific treatment. After correction of the diet and elimination of precipitating factors, recurrence is unknown.

Treatment   For folic acid deficiency, 5 to 10 micrograms is given daily, either parenterally or by mouth, for 10 to 14 days. For vitamin B_{12} deficiency, 5 to 10 micrograms is given daily, intramuscularly.

Blood transfusion may be indicated when the initial hemoglobin level is below 3 Gm per 100 ml. Treatment by transfusion alone, however, may mask the true nature of the disorder by making the morphologic changes in the blood and bone marrow more difficult to recognize, thus permitting the disorder to progress to a dangerous thrombocytopenia or leukopenia because specific therapy is withheld.

VITAMIN B_{12}-RESPONSIVE MEGALOBLASTIC ANEMIA

Several disorders exist in infants and children which give rise to a nondietary vitamin B_{12} deficiency and megaloblastic anemia. Laboratory findings are summarized in Table 22-2.

Infections with the fish tapeworm *Diphillobothrium latum,* which leads to vitamin B_{12} deficiency due to competition between host and worm for dietary vitamin B_{12}, is rare in infants and children. Although vitamin B_{12} deficiency is common in tropical sprue in adults, it is rare in celiac disease.

Surgical resection of the terminal ileum may lead to vitamin B_{12} deficiency after several years because the area of gastrointestinal tract required for absorption of dietary vitamin B_{12} gastric intrinsic factor complex has been removed.

Juvenile pernicious anemia is a condition in which there is a congenital absence of gastric intrinsic factor excretion. Clinical symptoms rarely occur before 2 years of age. A specific vitamin B_{12} malabsorption syndrome which is associated with proteinuria has also been described.

Treatment   Since the more common vitamin B_{12}-responsive anemias above have some form of interference with the intestinal absorption of vitamin B_{12}, therapy is almost invariably parenteral. Because vitamin B_{12} has a long biological half-life and is retained avidly in the liver, the interval between dose administrations for these conditions can be long. Cyanacobalamin, 20 to 50 micrograms, intramuscularly, monthly, is the usual dose.

Prognosis   This depends upon the underlying condition but is generally good with an appropriate vitamin B_{12} treatment regimen.

CHRONIC HEREDITARY ANEMIAS

The principal chronic hereditary anemias are thalassemia major (Cooley's anemia), sickle-cell anemia, congenital spherocytosis, and nonspherocytic chronic hemolytic anemia. In each there is a congenital defect of the red blood cell or of hemoglobin synthesis. The many clinical features they have in common stem from the fact that in each there is a shortened survival time of the erythrocytes, with a compensatory marrow and extramedullary erythroid hyperplasia. The salient features of these chronic hereditary anemias are compared in Table 22-3.

ABNORMAL HEMOGLOBINS AND HEMOGLOBINOPATHIES

Several chronic hereditary anemias have been described in association with an abnormal type of hemoglobin. More than 75 different varieties of hemoglobin have been described to date which have slightly different physical, chemical, or electrophoretic properties and can be differentiated from one another by such procedures as paper or agar electrophoresis, differential solubility, and resistance to denaturation by strong alkali.

Normal adult hemoglobin has been designated hemoglobin A. The hemoglobin that forms a large portion of the blood of newborn infants differs from normal adult hemoglobin and has been designated as fetal hemoglobin or hemoglobin F. In sickle-cell disease an abnormal adult hemoglobin has been found and designated as hemoglobin S. Two previously unclassified chronic hereditary anemias occurring in Negroes and in which there is a large percentage of target cells, but no sickling, have been found to be associated with two additional abnormal hemoglobins designated as hemoglobin C and hemoglobin D. By the cellulose acetate electrophoresis technique now used in most clinical laboratories, hemoglobin A travels the fastest and is followed in order by hemoglobin F, hemoglobin S (hemoglobin D has an identical speed with hemoglobin S), and hemoglobin C. Hemoglobin D may be differentiated from hemoglobin S by the fact that cells containing hemoglobin D do not sickle when exposed to reducing agents or decreased oxygen tension.*

Fetal hemoglobin is not produced by a gene at the same locus as hemoglobin A or any of the abnormal hemoglobins discussed above. As a result the production of fetal hemoglobin may go on simultaneously with, and independent of, the production of hemoglobin A or any of the other abnormal hemoglobins. In late fetal life the fetal hemoglobin may comprise 50 to 90 percent of the circulating hemoglobin. By the end of the first year this gradually diminishes to a level of 2 percent or less. Amounts greater than 2 percent after 2 years of age are usually abnormal. A small amount of fetal hemoglobin, however,

---

* Genetically, these various types of hemoglobin are determined by genes which occur at the same locus as hemoglobin A. Because these hemoglobin characteristics are determined by a pair of genes occurring as alleles on the same chromosome, the condition existing when both genes are similar is referred to as homozygous and when these genes are dissimilar as heterozygous. The heterozygous condition in which hemoglobin A is present in conjunction with one of the abnormal hemoglobins usually does not result in clinical anemia. Most of the severe clinical anemias occur in those situations in which there is homozygosity for an abnormal hemoglobin such as in sickle-cell anemia where both hemoglobin determining genes are S or in hemoglobin C disease where both hemoglobin determining genes are C. The occurrence of two different abnormal hemoglobin genes in the same individual such as S and C results in a hemolytic anemia which has many of the characteristics of sickle-cell anemia. This is usually referred to as S-C disease.

Table 22-3. Comparison of the chronic hereditary anemias

	Thalassemia major	Sickle-cell anemia	Congenital spherocytosis	Nonspherocytic chronic hemolytic anemia
Racial incidence	Chiefly Mediterranean	Chiefly Negro	Chiefly Caucasian	Various, chiefly Caucasian
Red blood cell morphology	Thin macrocytes, microcytes, and target cells	Elongate (sickle) at reduced O_2 tension	Smaller, wider cells (spherocytes)	Normal to moderate poikilocytosis
Degree of anemia in case of average severity	6 Gm per 100 ml	8 Gm per 100 ml	10 Gm per 100 ml	8–10 Gm per 100 ml
Frequency of reticulocytes and nucleated red blood cells in peripheral blood	Moderate to marked constant reticulocytosis and normoblastosis	Constant slight reticulocytosis occasional normoblastosis; marked increase following hemolytic crisis	Slight constant reticulocytosis; marked reticulocytosis and normoblastosis following hemolytic crisis	Constant, mild reticulocytosis; occasional nucleated RBC
Fragility of red blood cells to hypotonic saline solutions (normal range, begin–complete hemolysis: 0.46–0.30%)	Decreased fragility, 0.40–0.16%	Decreased fragility, 0.42–0.20%	Increased fragility, 0.70–0.40%	No marked change
Degree of clinical jaundice	Constant slight to moderate	Medium to marked following hemolytic crisis, absent to slight at other times	Moderate to marked following hemolytic crisis, absent to slight at other times	Slight to moderate following hemolytic crisis; usually none at other times
Degree of hepatosplenomegaly	Moderate to marked liver and spleen enlargement; gradual constant increase	Slight to moderate splenic enlargement, early; atrophy later; liver enlargement absent to slight	Slight to moderate splenic enlargement; liver enlargement rare	Slight to moderate splenic enlargement, liver enlargement uncommon
Bone changes seen by x-ray: thinning of cortices, thickening of trabeculations, widening of medullary cavities	Moderate to marked changes involving all bones (hair-on-end skull bones)	Slight to moderate changes, chiefly in skull; rare in tubular bones	Slight changes, chiefly in frontal and parietal bones	None to slight changes
Effect on physical growth and development	Marked retardation	Moderate retardation	Mild retardation	Mild retardation
Prognosis	Poor	Fair	Good	Good to fair
Treatment	Repeated periodic transfusions Splenectomy for hypersplenism or greatly enlarged spleen	Transfusions usually following anemic crisis, otherwise infrequently needed	Splenectomy very helpful Transfusions usually following anemic crisis	Splenectomy helpful in occasional case, transfusion if hemoglobin is low or following anemic crisis
Hereditary defect	Failure to produce hemoglobin β chains; hemoglobin A markedly reduced; compensation by marked increase of fetal hemoglobin	Production of abnormal hemoglobin β chains (sickle-cell type): Hemoglobin S 75–98%, fetal hemoglobin 2–25%	Hemoglobin A, but spherocytes have poorly defined membrane and intrinsic enzyme defect	Hemoglobin A; various intra-erythrocyte enzyme defects, frequently of the glycolytic or the G-6-PD and glutathione pathways

575

is apparently present in all adult blood. Severe chronic hemolytic anemia may be associated with a compensatory increase in fetal hemoglobin, e.g., Cooley's anemia, sickle-cell anemia. Patients with thalassemia major may have as much as 50 to 95 percent fetal hemoglobin; sickle-cell anemia patients, 10 to 15 percent.

Individuals having normal and abnormal types of adult hemoglobin in their blood are also referred to as having a "trait condition" for the abnormal hemoglobin. For example, if both hemoglobins A and S are present, it is referred to as sickle-cell trait. In thalassemia minor (Cooley's anemia trait) there is an increase in hemoglobin A_2, another type of normal adult hemoglobin, usually comprising about 2.5 percent of the total. Hemoglobin A_2 is best identified by starch block electrophoresis. Its increased occurrence in thalassemia minor aids in identifying that condition.

Thalassemia major   Thalassemia major (Cooley's or Mediterranean anemia) is a hereditary, chronic hemolytic anemia, characterized by pallor, jaundice, and extramedullary hematopoiesis in the bones, liver, and spleen. It occurs most commonly in persons of Italian or Greek ancestry, although it has been observed in others of Mediterranean ancestry. Frequently, both parents have a similar but milder condition, thalassemia minor (see below). A summary of the features of this disease is found in Tables 22-2 and 22-3. The basic genetic defect in classic thalassemia major is apparently an inability to manufacture the beta chain of hemoglobin A due to a problem at a still undetermined site. As a compensatory mechanism, the amount of hemoglobin F is increased.

Thalassemia intermedia is a mild form of the disease, in which the red blood cell defect is not as pronounced. It presently includes several forms less well defined than classical beta thalassemia. The clinical features are correspondingly less severe, the anemia is milder, and the prognosis for life is much better.

Thalassemia minor is the trait condition of beta thalassemia usually present in the parents of children with thalassemia major. Red blood cell changes are minimal, but there are increased basophilic stippling and hemoglobin A_2. Usually there is no or only minimal anemia. Prognosis for life is excellent.

Sickle-cell anemia   This is a chronic hereditary anemia, characterized by a constant pallor and by periodic crises of pain in the abdomen and extremities or by increased anemia and jaundice. It occurs primarily in black individuals, but on rare occasions it has been observed in other races. A summary of the features of this disease is found in Tables 22-2 and 22-3.

Sicklemia, or sickle-cell trait, is the heterozygous condition in which a mixture of hemoglobins S and A is present. Such red blood cells will also assume the sickle form under conditions of reduced oxygen tension. It is hereditary and has the same racial distribution as sickle-cell anemia, but no anemia is present. Persons with the trait are essentially symptom-free and require no treatment but may develop sickling and splenic infarcts when exposed to an environment with low oxygen tension, e.g., when flying at high altitude.

Sickle-cell trait may also occur as a double-trait condition with thalassemia, hemoglobin C, or hemoglobin D.

Sickle-cell hemoglobin C disease Next to sickle-cell anemia this is the most common cause of chronic hemolytic anemia in blacks. Since sickling occurs in this condition, it is frequently confused with sickle-cell anemia. However, certain important features differentiate it from sickle-cell anemia, both clinically as well as in its laboratory findings. The anemia is rarely as severe, and hemoglobin averages 9.5 to 10.5 Gm per 100 ml. There is striking splenomegaly throughout life, in contrast to sickle-cell anemia, in which the spleen is palpable only in young children and atrophies in the older child and adult. There are crises of bone pain very similar to those in sickle-cell anemia. (Adult women patients with sickle-cell hemoglobin C disease are more likely to have crises during pregnancy than are those with sickle-cell anemia. The prognosis for the fetus of a woman with sickle-cell hemoglobin C double trait is poorer than that for a woman with sickle-cell anemia.)

Electrophoresis reveals that the hemoglobin is a mixture of hemoglobin S and C. The life expectancy of the person with hemoglobin S-C disease is almost normal. Transfusions are necessary only during an anemic crisis.

Congenital spherocytosis This is a chronic hereditary anemia in which the erythrocytes are spherocytic. (Certain enzymes concerned with glucose metabolism are believed to be absent, and the erythrocyte survival time is diminished because the spherocytes are more susceptible to destruction in the spleen.) It is characterized in infants and children by a moderate chronic anemia and periodic crises in which the anemia worsens and jaundice appears. The defect is inherited as a Mendelian dominant or may appear de novo as a mutant. A summary of this disease is found in Tables 22-2 and 22-3.

CRISES IN CHRONIC HEREDITARY ANEMIAS

In thalassemia major, sickle-cell anemia, and congenital hemolytic anemia, anemic crises may occur; they are usually associated with stress, e.g., infection. The crises may be "aplastic" (e.g., erythroid hypoplasia in the marrow and a peripheral reticulocytopenia) or "megaloblastic" (e.g., megaloblastosis in the marrow and a peripheral macrocytosis). The so-called hyperhemolytic crisis, in which there is increased hemolysis, is much less frequent than was formerly believed. More commonly, a "sequestration" crisis occurs in which there is an increased anemia (without increased jaundice) due to an increase in the abdominal splanchnic bed in which large amounts of blood are sequestered from the general circulation with resulting peripheral anemia. The aplastic, hemolytic, and sequestration crises are usually self-limiting. Transfusion is recommended if the hemoglobin level falls to 5 Gm per 100 ml or less. The "megaloblastic" crisis is usually due to folic acid deficiency and responds well to oral therapy—synthetic folic acid, 5 to 10 mg twice a day. The more common crises of fever and pain in sickle-cell anemia are usually not associated with an intensified anemia or jaundice.

A "functional asplenia" has been identified in sickle-cell anemia as a result of infection and may account in part for the decreased ability of such individuals to control infections, giving rise to frequent pneumonia and osteomyelitis ("hand-foot" syndrome).

Hereditary elliptocytosis   Hereditary elliptocytosis is characterized by a high percentage of cigar-shaped erythrocytes. Some cases are associated with a mild chronic hemolytic anemia; however, there is no clinical disease in most cases.

Hereditary chronic nonspherocytic hemolytic anemia   This is a group of rare familial disorders in which a compensated chronic hemolytic anemia is the common feature. At birth, many present with hyperbilirubinemia. Kernicterus has been reported. The degree of anemia is variable. Splenomegaly is present to a greater or lesser degree. The red cell morphology also varies from minimally to considerably distorted cells. Other clinical and laboratory findings are summarized in Table 22-3.

Many of these disorders have an erythrocyte enzyme deficiency of either the glycolytic pathway (pyruvate kinase; 2,3 diphosphoglycerate mutase; and others) or the oxidation-reduction, glutathione-related pathway (glucose-6-phosphate dehydrogenase, glutathione synthetase, glutathione reductase, or 6-phosphogluconate dehydrogenase). In many, no enzyme abnormality has been identified.

When G-6-PD deficiency is found, it is due to a variant (B⁻), different from the type (A⁻) commonly found in blacks. In the latter, anemia is mild or nonexistent unless challenged by a hemolysis-precipitating drug or infection. The B⁻ type occurs more frequently in Caucasians. Their disease is less well compensated, and anemia, which may vary from 6 to 11.5 Gm percent, is always present. It may slowly increase in some patients.

At birth, measures to reduce hyperbilirubinemia when present (exchange transfusion, phototherapy) are important to avoid neurological complications. Later, transfusions are given as necessary to maintain adequate hemoglobin levels and permit normal growth or to raise the level if it remains below 5 Gm per 100 ml after hemolytic crisis. Although splenectomy does not "cure" these children as it does in congenital spherocytosis, many are benefited by lower transfusion requirements.

APLASTIC ANEMIA

Aplastic anemia is a rare disorder in which there is a reduction in all the cellular elements of the peripheral blood. It may be congenital, may follow the ingestion of sulfonamides, chloramphenicol, benzol derivatives, or other drugs, or may occur at the end stage of chronic hookworm disease. Aplastic anemia may be associated with multiple congenital anomalies, e.g., microcephaly, bone anomalies, and pigmentation of the skin (Fanconi's anemia). A summary of the features is given in Table 22-2.

CHRONIC HYPOPLASTIC ANEMIA

This is a rare form of hyporegenerative anemia in which only the red blood cell–producing tissue is involved. It is of unknown causation, but is probably congenital. A summary of the clinical features is found in Table 22-2.

There is an abnormality of tryptophan metabolism with increased anthranilic acid and occasionally increased xanthurenic acid in the urine in some of these patients.

MYELOPHTHISIC ANEMIA

This syndrome in which leukopenia and thrombocytopenia accompany the anemia is secondary to infiltration of the marrow hematopoietic tissue, by foreign cells, e.g., abnormal blood cells (leukemia), reticulum cells (Gaucher's disease), granulomatous processes (tuberculosis and congenital syphilis), tumor tissue (neuroblastoma) or by parasitic (toxoplasmosis), viral (rubella), or mycostic (histoplasmosis, torula) disease. The latter group is most frequently encountered as a transplacentally transmitted infection. A summary of the clinical features is found in Table 22-2.

HYPERSPLENISM

Hypersplenism is a disorder due to overactivity of the spleen, in which anemia, leukopenia, or thrombocytopenia (or any combination of these conditions) may result. There is evidence that the spleen in this disorder removes cells from the peripheral blood, either by phagocytosis or by sequestration, faster than they are supplied by the bone marrow. When there is no primary disease of the spleen, the condition is called idiopathic hypersplenism. When there is a primary disease of the spleen, e.g., Hodgkin's disease, leukemia, sarcoidosis, or congestive fibrosis (Banti's disease), there may also be splenic hyperactivity (secondary hypersplenism).

The clinical features depend on which cellular elements are involved. The anemia may resemble a hemolytic anemia, with jaundice, peripheral blood reticulocytosis, and marrow erythroid hyperplasia. On the other hand purpura may be the primary clinical feature, or the disease may resemble agranulocytosis or an aplastic anemia. The degree of splenic enlargement has no direct relationship to the severity of the condition. The laboratory examinations, in addition to the findings outlined above, may reveal the cause of the underlying process. Splenectomy may be of great value in idiopathic hypersplenism. The advisability of splenectomy for secondary hypersplenism must be weighed against the possible effect on the primary disease. Adrenal corticosteroids are of only temporary benefit. Prognosis in idiopathic hypersplenism is often good; in secondary hypersplenism it is poor.

SPLENOMEGALY AND SPLENECTOMY

Some of the more common causes of enlargement of the spleen are listed below and classified in relation to splenectomy. Splenectomy is indicated in congenital hemolytic jaundice; chronic idiopathic thrombocytopenic purpura (ITP) or acute ITP with severe hemorrhage which cannot be controlled by medical means; congestive splenomegaly (portal hypertension); hypersplenism; cysts and hemangiomas of the spleen; rupture of the spleen; and any condition in which the spleen, owing to its size, e.g., in Cooley's anemia, Gaucher's disease, produces symptoms and in which splenectomy is not contraindicated. Splenectomy is of doubtful value in sickle-cell anemia, cirrhosis, and tuberculosis of the spleen. Splenectomy is contraindicated in polycythemia vera, leukemia, Hodgkin's disease, rheumatoid arthritis, Hand-Schüller-Christian disease, Niemann-Pick disease, histoplasmosis, malaria, and subacute bacterial endocarditis.

Splenectomized persons may be more subject to overwhelming bacterial infections that are difficult to control. Infections in the splenectomized patient should be treated promptly and vigorously.

DISORDERS OF THE WHITE BLOOD CELLS

The white blood cells, like the erythyroid cells, vary physiologically during the first year of life (Table 22-1). Polymorphonuclear leukocytes are predominant in the differential count at birth but decrease by the second to third week, so that they make up less than 50 percent of the total number of cells throughout the remainder of the first year of life and early childhood. Some of the more frequent causes for white cell changes in the blood during infancy and childhood are the following:

1. Neutrophilic leukocytosis
   a. Acute infections: pyogenic; certain virus infections, early in

the course; some spirochetal diseases, e.g., Weil's disease; collagen diseases, e.g., rheumatic fever, rheumatoid arthritis, and periarteritis nodosa

b. Acute hemorrhage or intravascular blood hemolysis

c. Rapid breakdown of body tissue or parenteral administration of protein materials

d. Stress reactions: convulsions, prolonged vomiting, dehydration, and acidosis

2. Eosinophilia
   a. Allergic disorders: eczema, hay fever, asthma, Loeffler's syndrome
   b. Parasitic infestations that invade tissue: trichinosis, hydatid disease (echinococciasis), ascariasis, visceral larva migrans, and hookworm disease
   c. In the recovery stage of certain diseases: scarlet fever, tuberculosis, acute infectious lymphocytosis
   d. Neoplasm: Hodgkin's disease, chronic myelocytic leukemia
   e. Others: tropical eosinophilia, familial eosinophilia, periarteritis nodosa

3. Leukopenia (with lymphocytic predominance)
   a. Certain infections: viral, e.g., measles, exanthem subitum, rubella, infectious hepatitis; bacillary, e.g., typhoid, brucellosis; protozoal, e.g., malaria
   b. Drugs and poisons: sulfathiazole, Dilantin, Tridione, Mesantoin, thiouracil, aminopyrine, benzol derivatives, chloramphenicol, DDT
   c. Hematologic disorders: agranulocytosis, aplastic anemia, leukemia, megaloblastic anemia, myelophthisic anemia, splenic neutropenia (hypersplenism), congestive splenomegaly (Banti's disease)
   d. End stages of overwhelming infections and cachectic conditions: tuberculosis, pneumonia, septicemia
   e. Serum sickness

4. Lymphocytosis
   a. Certain infections: bacillary, e.g., pertussis; or viral, e.g., infectious mononucleosis and acute infectious lymphocytosis
   b. Physiologic lymphocytic predominance of infancy and childhood
   c. Convalescent stage of acute infections and healing stage of chronic infections: tuberculosis, syphilis
   d. Leukemia

5. Monocytosis
   a. Certain infections: bacterial, e.g., tuberculosis, subacute bacterial endocarditis, typhus, typhoid fever; protozoal, e.g., malaria, kala-azar
   b. Recovery phase of acute infections or agranulocytosis
   c. Certain drugs: tetrachlorethylene
   d. Hodgkin's disease, Niemann-Pick disease

LEUKEMOID REACTIONS

Leukemoid reactions are not uncommon in infancy and childhood because of the great lability of the hematopoietic system during this age period. The blood picture resembles that in leukemia, either because of the height of the total white cell count and/or the immaturity of some of the cells. The immaturity of the cells (resembling "blast" cells or early myeloid cells) is the most important distinguishing feature of the "leukemoid" reaction. High white cell counts without a significant number of immature cells resembling those found in leukemia is best referred to as a leukocytosis. In such different conditions as severe septicemia, meningococcemia, pneumonia, diphtheria, and an occasional case of erythroblastosis fetalis, the blood picture may simulate that of myeloblastic or myelocytic leukemia. In whooping cough, infectious mononucleosis, and infectious lymphocytosis, the blood picture may resemble that in lymphatic leukemia. Leukemoid reactions can usually be differentiated from true leukemia by correlating the clinical picture with the complete blood and marrow pattern. (See Leukemia, in Chapter 23.)

AGRANULOCYTOSIS

Agranulocytosis is a disorder in which there is a striking reduction in the total number of circulating neutrophils. It is usually, but not always, associated with leukopenia.

Etiology   Agranulocytosis is usually due to such drugs as are listed under leukopenia (above), certain infections, or in rare instances, to unknown causes. Either there is an arrest of maturation of neutrophils in the bone marrow at the level of promyelocytes and myelocytes, or the spleen removes them from the circulation more rapidly than they are supplied (splenic neutropenia).

Clinical features   Symptoms may vary from slight fever, malaise, and irritability to the clinical features of severe infections. Severe infections may occur secondary to the neutropenia—ulcerations of the oropharyngeal mucous membranes, skin abscesses, pneumonia, or septicemia. The physical findings are those of the primary and complicating conditions. The laboratory finding of diagnostic importance is the demonstration of an absolute severe neutropenia in the peripheral blood. There is usually a myeloid arrest of maturation in the bone marrow. If the spleen is overactive, there is a compensatory myeloid hyperplasia in the bone marrow. In the recovery phase of agranulocytosis associated with a myeloid-maturation arrest, a transient monocytosis and slight leukocytosis are commonly observed.

Treatment   The treatment is directed toward removing the offending agent, if known, and the prevention or treatment of secondary infection. Adrenal corticosteroids are helpful in those cases where an immunologic mechanism may be partially responsible for neutropenia. Splenectomy is helpful in those cases due to hypersplenism. Antibiotics, by preventing fatal secondary infection, have improved the prognosis greatly.

ACUTE INFECTIOUS LYMPHOCYTOSIS

This disease is characterized by an increase in the total number of circulating lymphocytes in the blood. It has been found chiefly in infants and children. The etiologic agent is probably a virus, and the disease is moderately contagious. The incubation period is probably 12 to 21 days. The disease is much less prevalent now than it was during the past two decades. It frequently occurred in epidemics among children in institutions for the mentally retarded.

Clinical symptoms and signs are conspicuously absent. Occasionally there may be a low-grade fever, rarely above 101°F (38.3°C), and transient abdominal pain. There is hardly ever any clinically detectable enlargement of the lymph nodes, liver, or spleen. The disease is usually discovered by the physician in making a blood count for unrelated complaints.

The diagnosis is made entirely from laboratory findings of an increase in the absolute number of apparently normal small to medium-size lymphocytes in the blood in the presence of a normal marrow picture. The total leukocyte count may vary from 20,000 to 120,000 per cubic millimeter, with lymphocyte percentages from 60 to 95. There is no anemia or thrombocytopenia. The sedimentation rate and heterophile antibody titer are not increased. The absolute blood lymphocytosis rises, reaches a peak for several days, and then gradually descends over a period of 3 to 6 weeks, occasionally 10 weeks. Characteristically, as the lymphocytosis is waning, the eosinophils increase in total numbers to a height of 3,000 to 5,000 per cubic millimeter (10 to 25 percent in the differential count) and slowly recede to normal levels during a period of 2 to 3 weeks. No treatment is required, and the prognosis is invariably excellent.

INFECTIOUS MONONUCLEOSIS

This is an acute infectious disease in which the most constant characteristic is the appearance of abnormal mononuclear cells in the peripheral blood. It is probably of viral etiology and, although infectious, is of low-grade contagiousness. Besides the abnormal mononuclear cells in the blood, there is a mononuclear cell infiltration of many of the organs of the body, principally perivascular, which accounts for the variable clinical picture of the disease. The incubation period is considered to be 4 to 14 days. The condition may occur at any age but is rare during infancy.

The clinical features are protean and include fever, generalized malaise, and the symptoms of an upper respiratory infection. The onset may be insidious or quite sudden. There may be an inflamed or ulcerated pharynx with a tonsillar or pharyngeal membrane. There is some generalized lymph node enlargement and splenomegaly; either the lymph nodes or the spleen may occasionally be large. Pressure by enlarged lymph nodes on adjacent structures may cause compression symptoms, such as cough and respiratory obstruction when the paratracheal and mediastinal lymph nodes are enlarged. Skin rashes occur and may be morbilliform, scarlatiniform, or petechial in nature. Jaundice may be present. Central nervous system manifestations such as headache, nuchal rigidity, blurring of vision, mental confusion, and convulsions have been observed. The spinal fluid, when central nervous system symptoms are present, may be normal or may show an increase in the number of cells and amount of protein.

The most important laboratory aid in diagnosis is the blood smear, which shows a large number of abnormal mononuclear cells. There is usually a leukocytosis, occasionally a thrombocytopenia, but rarely an anemia. Several types of abnormal mononuclear cells occur in this disease. There are moderate-sized cells with basophilic cytoplasm and irregularly shaped nuclei. The variation among the mononuclear cells themselves is one of the characteristics of the blood picture of this disease. The bone marrow pattern in essentially normal. (This is often crucial in the differential diagnosis from acute leukemia.)

The heterophile antibody titer is usually positive by the tenth day and may remain elevated for several months. Titers of 1:112 or above are significant. Antibody absorption techniques add to the specificity and accuracy of the titer as a diagnostic procedure. Exposure of the patient's serum to a guinea pig kidney emulsion does not cause absorption of the heterophil antibody associated with infectious mononucleosis but removes nonspecific heterophil antibodies due to other causes. Exposure of the patient's serum to ox erythrocytes causes complete absorption of the infectious mononucleosis heterophile antibody. These differential immunologic tests are most important when the heterophile antibody titer is below 1:112. With titers as low as 1:14, failure of absorption (lowering of the titer) after exposure of the serum to guinea pig kidney emulsion is significant of infectious mononucleosis.

However, 20 to 40 percent of these patients never develop a significant heterophile antibody titer. The cytologic diagnosis of infectious mononucleosis is therefore more dependable than the serologic diagnosis in infants and children.

The disease usually runs a course of 2 to 4 weeks. It rarely recurs, but occasionally chronic cases of reinfections have been observed. There is no specific treatment.

THE HEMORRHAGIC DISORDERS

Hemorrhage results from a disturbance of the normal function of the capillaries, the platelets, or the clotting elements of the plasma. These factors may be congenitally deficient or, more often, secondarily injured or defective.

The normal physiologic processes of hemostasis may be summarized as follows: an arteriole-sized blood vessel, when injured, quickly contracts. Platelets adhere to the injured epithelial surface and form a platelet thrombus, which initially slows or stops the flow of blood. The disintegration of platelets at the bleeding site also releases both a powerful vasoconstrictor, which further aids in stemming the flow of blood, and a platelet "enzyme," which participates in initiating blood clotting. This results in the formation of a strong plug, which prevents further hemorrhage.

A simplified outline of the blood coagulation and lytic processes follows:

I. Phase I—thromboplastin formation:[1]
    A. Plasma

$$HF^2 + PTA^3 + PTC^4 + AHG^5 + Stuart^6 +$$
$$labile\ factor^7 \xrightarrow[Ca^{++}]{platelet\ factor\ 3^8} activated\ (plasma)\ thromboplastin$$

    B. Tissue

$$Tissue\ thromboplastin + stable\ factor^9 +$$
$$Stuart^6 + labile\ factor^7$$
$$\downarrow$$
$$activated\ (tissue)\ thromboplastin$$

II. Phase II—thrombin formation:

$$Prothrombin + activated\ thromboplastin \xrightarrow[labile\ factor\ +\ SPCA^{10}]{Ca^{++}}$$
$$thrombin$$

III. Phase III—fibrin formation:
    Fibrinogen + thrombin $\longrightarrow$ fibrin
$$\downarrow Factor\ XIII^{11}$$

IV. Phase IV—fibrinolysis: fibrin clot
$$Plasminogen \xrightarrow{(activators)} plasmin \longrightarrow \downarrow$$
fibrin split
products and
clot lysis

1. Activated thromboplastin is now believed to arise from plasma and tissue precursors.
2. HF: Hageman factor, factor XII, surface contact factor first factor involved in coagulation process.
3. PTA: plasma thromboplastin antecedent, factor XI, is activated by "activated" HF.
4. PTC: plasma thromboplastin component, factor IX.
5. AHG: antihemophilic globulin, factor VIII.
6. Stuart: Stuart-Prower factor, factor X.
7. Labile factor: factor V.
8. Platelet factor 3: formerly "thromboplastinogenase." Other platelet factors are concerned with capillary contraction and clot retraction.
9. Stable factor: factor VII is important in conversion of the precursor of tissue thromboplastin to the active form and appears to play no significant role in conversion of plasma thromboplastin precursors, although it is found in plasma.
10. SPCA: serum prothrombin conversion accelerator, activated factor VII (stable factor). This plus factor V influences the speed of thrombin formation.
11. Factor XIII: aids lateral bonding between fibrin strands to form a stable clot.

A severe deficiency or absence of any factor will retard or prevent the coagulation of the blood. A balance between the coagulation and the anticoagulation processes normally maintains the blood fluidity. Heparin-like substances, present in plasma, prevent in vivo clot formation. Small clots that may be formed are rapidly dissolved by fibrinolysin. Fibrinolysin occurs normally in plasma as inactive profibrinolysin. The latter requires an intermediate or "activator" to be converted into activated fibrinolysin. Hemorrhagic states may occasionally result from an abnormal increase of circulating anticoagulants. An increase in fibrinogenolysins, which act directly upon fibrinogen rather than on fibrin, may result in an acquired hypofibrinogenemia, and when severe, in hemorrhagic phenomena.

The following classification of the hemorrhagic diseases according to the principal part of the hemostatic system affected aids in the understanding, diagnosis, and treatment of these conditions.

I. Vascular dysfunction (nonthrombocytopenic purpura)
    A. Mechanical trauma
    B. Infection: meningococcemia, rickettsial diseases, typhoid fever
    C. Allergy or anaphylaxis: Henoch-Schönlein purpura, serum sickness
    D. Emboli: subacute bacterial endocarditis
    E. Drugs: atropine, mercurials, iodides, procaine penicillin, hypnotics

    F.   Metabolic disturbance: anoxia, avitaminosis C

    G.   Hereditary capillary fragility (von Willebrand's pseudo-hemophilia)

    H.   Hereditary hemorrhagic telangiectasis (Osler-Rendu-Weber disease)

    I.   Congenital cutis hyperelastica (Ehlers-Danlos syndrome)

II. Platelet dysfunction

    A.   Thrombocytopenic purpura

       1. Unknown cause: idiopathic thrombocytopenic purpura (ITP, Werlhof's disease), hemolytic-uremic syndrome (see p. 488), Wiskott-Aldrich syndrome

       2. Autoimmune thrombocytopenic purpura associated with platelet agglutinins

       3. Infection: septicemia, measles, and transplacentally transmitted congenital infections: e.g., rubella, syphilis, toxoplasmosis, and cytomegalic inclusion disease

       4. Drugs: sulfonamides, benzol derivatives, DDT, chloramphenicol

       5. Hypersplenism: idiopathic, congestive splenomegaly (Banti's syndrome), splenic infiltration due to Hodgkin's disease, leukemia, thalassemia major, or kala-azar

       6. Myelophthisis (amegakaryocytic): leukemia, granulomatous infections (tuberculosis) or tumors metastatic to the marrow (neuroblastoma), aplastic anemia

       7. Thrombocytopenic purpura of the newborn, e.g., from intrauterine passive transfer of an isoimmune (non-thrombocytopenic mother) or an autoimmune (thrombocytopenic mother) platelet agglutinin

       8. Megaloblastic anemia due either to folic acid or vitamin B_{12} deficiency

    B.   Thrombocytopathic purpura: thrombasthenia of unknown cause, e.g., Glanzmann's pseudohemophilia

III. Dysfunction of the plasma factors affecting coagulation

    A.   Hypoprothrombinemia: vitamin K deficiency, e.g., celiac disease, obstructive jaundice, liver disease, from Dicumarol and salicylates

    B.   Multiple factor deficiency: hemorrhagic disease of the newborn, consumption coagulopathy (disseminated intravascular coagulation—DIC)

    C.   Hemophilia and hemophilia-like conditions:

       1. Congenital AHG (factor VIII) deficiency

       2. Congenital deficiency of PTC (Christmas factor or factor IX)

       3. PTA (factor XI) deficiency, usually congenital

       4. Vascular purpura with AHG (factor VIII) deficiency, congenital

       5. Fibrinogenopenia: congenital deficiency, acquired—severe liver disease, scarlet fever, fibrinogenolysins

6. Labile factor (factor V) deficiency, acquired and congenital
7. Stable factor (factor VII) deficiency, acquired and congenital
8. Stuart factor (factor X) deficiency, congenital and acquired
9. Hageman factor (factor XII) deficiency, congenital

ANAPHYLACTOID PURPURA

Anaphylactoid purpura (Henoch-Schönlein purpura, allergic capillary purpura) is a nonthrombocytopenic purpura that results from increased capillary permeability.

Etiology This is possibly of allergic origin through sensitization to certain bacteria, drugs, or foods or following infection often of the upper respiratory tract. In most cases the precipitating factor is not apparent.

Clinical features This disease is a common form of purpura during early childhood. The majority of cases occur between 2 and 4 years of age and in the spring and fall of the year. The classical clinical triad is involvement of the skin, the gastrointestinal tract, and the joints. These may be affected individually, in combination, or in sequence. Occasionally the renal glomerular capillaries are involved.

1. The purpura usually begins about the buttocks and spreads to involve the posterior aspect of the thighs and legs. It may later involve the other extremities or the trunk. The rash may be petechial or a blotchy macular type. Often it is a slightly raised (occasionally urticarial) hemorrhagic rash; the rash is pleomorphic and frequently becomes coalescent; ecchymoses are uncommon.
2. The visceral manifestations are melena or hematuria and abdominal pain, sometimes simulating an acute surgical condition of the abdomen, e.g., appendicitis, intussusception.
3. The synovial manifestations result in painful and swollen joints. The knee and ankle joints are most commonly affected. The joint pain may remit and recur spontaneously, its migrating character often resembles that in rheumatic fever.
4. There may be general systemic manifestations such as fever, anorexia, malaise, and vomiting.
5. The principal laboratory findings are listed in Table 22-4 (p. 592). There is frequently also a slight polymorphonuclear leukocytosis and occasionally a slight eosinophilia.

Prognosis The course of the disease is usually self-limiting. Its duration may be 2 to 4 weeks. Recurrences are common during the first few months after recovery. Long-term recurrences are rare. Although there may be considerable morbidity, the outcome is usually without sequelae. Renal involvement may appear several days or several weeks after initial symptoms. If manifestations of an acute glomerulonephritis develop, prognosis is more guarded since some children go on to a chronic glomerulonephritis.

Treatment   The treatment is chiefly symptomatic. Infections should be treated with the indicated antibiotics. In severe cases adrenal corticosteroids are helpful in relieving symptoms but do not influence the course of the disease. It is not certain whether they favorably influence the complicating nephritis. Once started, adrenal corticosteroid therapy should be continued for at least 10 to 14 days.

PURPURA FULMINANS

This is a rare but serious disorder occurring in infants and older children. It is characterized by hemorrhagic bullous lesions usually arising initially on the skin of the extremities which go on to involvement of the underlying tissue with gangrene. Extremities may be lost as a result of the gangrenous process.

The disease is often characterized by incoagulability of the blood which may be associated with severe hypofibrinogenemia and thrombocytopenia. Other plasma coagulation factors may also be reduced. Death occurs because of hemorrhage, renal glomerular and tubular obstruction by fibrin plugs, or other less well-defined factors.

The etiology of the disease is obscure; its pathogenesis is believed to be related to a Schwartzman-like phenomenon initiated by infection.

Treatment is not satisfactory. If the progression of the disease is spontaneously arrested, recovery is complete. Occasionally, amputation of an affected extremity will arrest the disease. Recently beneficial results have been reported with the use of parenteral heparin, which presumably counteracts a circulating coagulation-initiating factor.

HEREDITARY HEMORRHAGIC TELANGIECTASIS

Hereditary capillary telangiectasis (Osler-Rendu-Weber disease) is a non-sex-linked hereditary disease exhibiting telangiectatic lesions consisting of thin-walled dilated capillaries. These may be located on the skin or mucous membranes (often at the mucocutaneous junction) or in the viscera and may bleed from slight trauma. There is no specific treatment, and prognosis depends on the amount and frequency of bleeding that occurs.

IDIOPATHIC THROMBOCYTOPENIC PURPURA (ITP)

Etiology and pathogenesis   In this disease, also known as Werlhof's disease, there is a deficiency of platelets in the peripheral blood. As a result, the bleeding time is prolonged because injured blood vessels do not contract well and platelet plugs are poorly formed. The blood clot is soft and does not retract. In addition, there is apparently a capillary dysfunction, which is poorly understood.

In most cases the principal defect is an arrest of production from the megakaryocytes. Occasionally, platelet production by these cells may be hyperactive, and recent studies indicate that the spleen removes the platelets from the circulation faster than the marrow produces them. In the latter instance a platelet agglutinin often may be demonstrated. The platelet antibody may affect the megakaryocyte and prevent normal platelet formation.

Clinical and laboratory features

1.   ITP may occur at any age but is most frequent between the ages of 3 and 6 years. A history of the presence of or recovery from a recent URI or contagious disease of childhood is common.
2.   There are petechiae in the skin and mucous membranes; ecchymoses are present, particularly over bony prominences such as the tibiae, the superior iliac crests, and the scapulae.
3.   Epistaxis, melena, and hematuria are not uncommon.
4.   The spleen is somewhat enlarged. If it is greatly increased in size, the thrombocytopenia is secondary to other diseases.
5.   The laboratory features are summarized in Table 22-4. The bone marrow is normal for myeloid and erythroid cells and usually contains normal or increased numbers of megakaryocytes.
6.   In the differential diagnosis of idiopathic thrombocytopenic purpura, the other causes for thrombocytopenia listed in the classification should be ruled out (see p. 586).

Course   In childhood, the course is usually relatively benign. The duration is customarily 2 to 10 weeks, with spontaneous recovery reputed to occur in about 80 percent of the cases. Exsanguinating epistaxis, melena, or intracranial hemorrhage are infrequent but dread complications. In about 20 percent, the thrombocytopenia persists for months or years.

Treatment   There is no specific therapy. Bacterial infection, when present, should be combated vigorously with appropriate antibiotics. Severe bleeding can frequently be controlled by fresh blood transfusion or platelet concentrates.

Adrenal corticosteroids promptly and regularly raise the platelet count to normal levels and cause a cessation of the hemorrhagic phenomena in the great majority of cases. The latter usually occurs within 24 to 48 hours and is a result of an effect on the capillary bed. The platelet count may not rise to significant levels before 72 to 96 hours after corticosteroid therapy is commenced. Dosage must be adequate: Prednisone, 2 to 4 mg per kg body weight (20 to 80 mg per day) in three or four divided doses, orally, depending on age and weight of patient. Because it is not possible to predict in any individual patient, at the onset of an episode of ITP, whether this patient will have a spontaneous remission or go on to chronicity, and since corticosteroid therapy is rapid and essentially safe, it is recommended that corticosteroid therapy be given as soon as the diagnosis of the first episode of ITP is made if the platelet count is below 90,000 per cu mm. In order to prevent a post-therapy relapse, corticosteroid therapy, once begun, should not be discontinued when the platelet count has risen to normal levels (usually in 7 to 10 days) but should be continued for a minimum of 3 weeks and then discontinued gradually over a period of 2 to 3 weeks.

Splenectomy is done infrequently for this disorder in childhood. The indications for splenectomy are either chronicity of the disease (usually lasting 6 months or more) or a fulminating course, with severe hemorrhage that is difficult to control by medical means. Splenectomy is not always curative; the best results are obtained in those cases where the marrow is actively producing platelets. For chronic ITP not responsive to splenectomy, adrenal corticosteroids (and occasionally other immunosuppressive agents) will control bleeding either by strengthening the capillary bed or raising the platelet count, as long as corticosteroids are continued. The drawbacks are the well-known side effects of long-term corticosteroid therapy.

HEMOPHILIA

Classic hemophilia is a sex-linked recessive hereditary bleeding disorder occurring in the male and transmitted by the female. It is now recognized that this disease is caused by a deficiency of one of two plasma factors required in the first stage of the coagulation process for thromboplastin formation. The majority of hemophilia, 75 to 85 percent, is due to a congenital deficiency of the antihemophilic globulin (AHG, or factor VIII); the remaining 15 to 25 percent, to a deficiency of plasma thromboplastin component (PTC, or factor IX).

Clinical features

1. The disorder is present at birth (bleeding in the average severe case may occur following circumcision) but in mild cases may not become clinically manifest until late infancy or early childhood.
2. There is a lifelong susceptibility to hemorrhage; bleeding may occur following minor trauma.
3. Hemarthroses occur following minor trauma and may result in severe disability because of damage to the synovial membrane from repeated episodes.

Table 22-4.   Summary of the hemorrhagic disorders

Disorder	Clinical features	Normal values			
		Platelet count 150,000–400,000 per mm³	Tourniquet test (Rumple-Leed) 3–4/cm²	Bleeding time <1.5 min	Clot retraction 4+ in 2 hr
Anaphylactoid or allergic capillary purpura (Henoch-Schönlein)	Petechiae, pleomorphic rash, abdominal and joint pain, glomerulonephritis	Normal	Positive in 25–30% of patients	Normal	Normal
Vitamin C deficiency	Petechiae, mucous-membrane hemorrhages, bone pain and tenderness (subperiosteal hemorrhage)	Normal	Positive	Normal or slightly prolonged	Normal
Idiopathic thrombocytopenic purpura (ITP)	Petechiae, ecchymoses, easy bruising, slight splenomegaly	Decreased	Strikingly positive	Prolonged	Poor
Pseudohemophilia	Petechiae, easy bruising, mouth hemorrhages, epistaxis	Normal	Positive in 50% of cases	Strikingly or only slightly prolonged	Poor
Hypoprothrombinemia	Petechiae, ecchymoses, easy bruising, melena	Normal	May be positive	May be prolonged	Normal
Hemophilia: factor VIII or factor IX deficiencies	Ecchymoses, abnormal bleeding from minor cuts, hemarthroses	Normal	Normal	Normal if puncture wound not too deep	Normal
Congenital afibrinogenemia	Abnormal bleeding from minor cuts or following surgery	Normal	Normal	Normal if puncture wound not too deep	Usually small clot which may be missed

Laboratory findings   The findings are summarized in Table 22-4. Coagulation-time tests should be done on venous blood by the Lee-White test-tube method; studies using the capillary-tube techniques are subject to many errors and are not recommended. The prothrombin-consumption test, which measures the completeness of the conversion of prothrombin to thrombin during the coagulation process, is more dependable than coagulation-time tests in establishing the diagnosis. The thromboplastin generation test is the most reliable but is more complicated to perform. The most practical test with which to follow the patient's coagulation activity is the partial thromboplastin time. Differentiation of AHG from PTC deficiency is accomplished by "cross-correction" tests. The blood of patients with AHG deficiency will correct the clotting defect in the blood of patients having PTC deficiency.

Coagulation time (Lee-White) <13 min	One-stage prothrombin time <14 sec	*Normal values* Prothrombin consumption >28 sec	Partial thrombo-plastin time <45 sec	Fibrinogen 150–300 mg %	Treatment
Normal	Normal	Normal (80–100% consumed)	Normal	Normal	Symptomatic, elimination of cause (cortico-steroids in severe cases)
Normal	Normal	Normal	Normal	Normal	Ascorbic acid
Normal	Normal	Poor (40–60%)	Normal	Normal	Adrenal cortico-steroids if severe, splenectomy in chronic cases
Usually normal, occasionally slightly pro-longed	Normal	Normal, poor if com-bined AHG deficiency	Vascular type—normal; AHG defi-ciency—prolonged	Normal	No satisfactory treatment for purely vascular type, AHG, if this deficiency coexists
Usually nor-mal	Prolonged	Normal	Prolonged	Normal	Vitamin K trans-fusion of plasma or whole blood
Prolonged	Normal	Poor (5–20%)	Prolonged	Normal	Fresh frozen plasma or whole blood transfusion
Normal if clot large enough to be seen	Normal if not too se-vere, other-wise spuriously prolonged	Normal	Normal if not too se-vere, other-wise spuriously prolonged	Decreased	Cryoprecipitate or other AHG concentrate for factor VIII de-ficiency (80% of cases) or PTC concentrate for factor IX defi-ciency

Specific identification of the deficiency requires the demonstration that the clotting defect can be corrected (in vivo or in the test tube) by a purified sample of the missing factor and that the patient's plasma does not correct the defect in a known case of the deficiency.

Course and prognosis   These depend on the severity of the disease, which varies considerably, but in general the prognosis is poor. The principal complications are exsanguinating hemorrhage or chronic joint disability due to the hemarthroses. With modern scientific and supportive therapy, however, the outlook for long-term survival with minimal disability has improved considerably.

In classic hemophiliacs, the plasma level of factor VIII varies from unmeasurable to 5 to 10 percent of normal. With factor VIII levels of 20 percent or more, spontaneous bleeding is rare. With current techniques to assay factor VIII, patients with AHG levels of 20 to 40 percent have been identified. These patients only bleed from extensive tissue trauma where mechanical hemostasis is difficult to apply, such as after prostatectomy or crushing injuries. These individuals are mild hemophiliacs.

Current assay techniques have also permitted the identification of low factor VIII levels (45 to 65 percent) in some female carriers of hemophilia. This permits the specific identification of such carriers for genetic counseling and also forewarns them of possible hemorrhagic phenomena. Thus it no longer is correct to say that hemophilia does not occur in the female. Some females, heterozygous for the hemophiliac gene, may have sufficiently low factor VIII levels to bleed after extensive trauma.

Treatment The therapy of an acute bleeding episode consists of

1. Local control of bleeding by the application of cold compresses or pressure, if possible, and rest.
2. Swollen or tender joints should be immobilized. Aspiration, under very strict aseptic conditions, of the blood from a joint after restoring and maintaining normal coagulability with AHG or PTC concentrates is now practiced with good long-term results in relation to preventing disabling hemarthrotic joints. After the acute episode, motion should be begun and physical therapy employed to prevent contractures.
3. Normal coagulability of the blood should be restored by the intravenous administration of thawed fresh-frozen plasma, 5 to 10 ml per kg body weight, fresh whole blood, or a concentrate of antihemophilic globulin (factor VIII or IX as indicated).

Factor VIII precipitates from plasma in the cold ($-20°C$); the other coagulation factors do not. Although easy to prepare, the cryoprecipitated concentrates vary in potency. A lyophilized commercial AHG preparation, not cold precipitated, is available which, when reconstituted in a 10 ml volume, contains 250 AHG units (1 unit = amount of AHG in 1 ml normal plasma). Eighty units will raise the plasma factor VIII level of a 20 kg child about 10 percent. The half-life of AHG is approximately 4 to 6 hours. Thus to maintain hemostatic levels, intravenous injections of concentrate are required every 6 to 8 hours, depending upon the level initially established. Availability of such concentrates has greatly facilitated the treatment of hemophilia.

Another recently available lyophilized commercial coagulation factor concentrate contains, when reconstituted, a mixture of factor IX (500 units per 30 ml), factor II (300 units per 30 ml), and factors VII and X (only assayed upon request). Thus five types of congenital coagulation factor deficiencies can now be treated with small volumes of a concentrate of the missing factor.

Preventive treatment consists of avoiding injury. In severe cases biweekly prophylactic intravenous injections of concentrates of factor VIII or IX are helpful but require further evaluation regarding long-term benefit. Good psychologic care of the child and family is important, as in all handicapping conditions.

PLASMA THROMBOPLASTIN ANTECEDENT (Factor XI) DEFICIENCY

This is a clinically mild, congenital, hemorrhagic disease, usually not causing symptoms until the patient undergoes a surgical procedure, e.g., tonsillectomy or tooth extraction. Both males and females are equally affected. It is characterized by a prolonged clotting time, a normal prothrombin time, but an abnormal prothrombin consumption. It is differentiated from AHG and PTC deficiency by appropriate "cross-correction" tests (see above).

VASCULAR PURPURA WITH AHG (Factor VIII) DEFICIENCY (Subtype of von Willebrand's Pseudohemophilia)

Characterized by prolonged bleeding time, prolonged clotting time, and poor thromboplastin consumption, this condition is due to a combination of congenital AHG deficiency and vascular purpura. It occurs in both sexes. Hemarthroses usually do not occur. Treatment of acute bleeding episode: fresh whole blood, fresh-frozen plasma, or purified concentrates of antihemophilic globulin (cryoprecipitate).

STUART FACTOR (Factor X) DEFICIENCY

This is a bleeding disorder resulting from a deficiency of the Stuart factor, which is concerned chiefly with thromboplastin formation. A temporary deficiency of this factor plays a role in hemorrhagic disease of the newborn. A decrease of factor X also occurs with vitamin K deficiency and after surgery. A congenital deficiency results in a mild bleeding disorder in either males or females.

HAGEMAN FACTOR (Factor XII) DEFICIENCY

This is the first factor involved in thromboplastin formation and is activated by contact with a foreign surface. Only patients in whom a congenital deficiency occurred have been described. This congenital abnormality is characterized by prolonged coagulation time and deficient prothrombin consumption. There are, however, no symptoms, and patients have been operated upon without extensive bleeding.

LABILE FACTOR (Factor V) DEFICIENCY

Labile factor deficiency is most frequently acquired, occurring following operations or with extensive liver disease. The congenital variety is characterized by epistaxis, ecchymoses in the skin, but no hemarthroses. It occurs in either sex. There may be a family history, but sporadic cases are common. It is characterized by a prolonged prothrombin time, prolonged clotting time, and poor prothrombin consumption. The deficiency is corrected only by fresh plasma or blood.

STABLE FACTOR (Factor VII) DEFICIENCY

Stable factor deficiency results most commonly from therapy with an anticoagulant, such as Dicumarol, which reduces the stable factor as well as the prothrombin. The congenital variety is characterized by epistaxis, ecchymoses, melena, and occasionally mild hemarthroses. There is no sex predilection. The clotting time is only slightly prolonged, the prothrombin time and prothrombin consumption are abnormal, but the thromboplastin generation test most clearly identifies the clotting defect.

FACTOR XIII DEFICIENCY

This recently recognized inherited bleeding disorder is characterized by bleeding after separation of the umbilical cord stump or by gastrointestinal, intracranial, or intra-articular hemorrhages. Standard coagulation tests are normal. Deficiency of factor XIII (fibrin-stabilizing factor) is diagnosed by abnormal solubility of the clot in 5 M urea and by a short euglobulin lysis time.

PSEUDOHEMOPHILIA

This is a group of rare bleeding disorders in which the most constant feature is a prolonged bleeding time. The disorder may be due to a capillary or a platelet dysfunction or both with and without an associated factor VIII deficiency. In von Willebrand's type (hereditary capillary fragility) platelet function is normal but the capillaries of the nail beds and the conjunctivas are elongated and tortuous. In some of these patients there is an associated congenital deficiency of AHG These patients show considerable response to treatment with fresh-frozen plasma or factor VIII concentrates. In Glanzmann's type (thrombocytopathic purpura), clot retraction is frequently poor. The principal laboratory features of this group of disorders are outlined in Table 22-4. The course is chronic. No satisfactory treatment is known when the capillary or platelet disorder is the principal defect. The prognosis is variable because of a wide range of clinical severity.

CONGENITAL AFIBRINOGENEMIA

This rare bleeding disorder, characterized by incoagulable blood, is due to very low or essentially absent levels of fibrinogen. Other coagulation factors are normal but require addition of fibrinogen to the standard tests for their assay in the plasma of these patients. Spontaneous hemorrhages or hemarthroses are rarely seen in this disease, but trauma or surgery may be followed by severe bleeding. Coagulability of the blood can be restored by intravenous infusion of fibrinogen concentrates. Because the half-life of fibronogen is about 5 days, fibrinogen concentrate transfusions are required less frequently than are the comparable factor VIII transfusions for hemophilia. The risk of developing serum hepatitis following fibrinogen concentrates is greater than following factor VIII concentrates.

Genetically, congenital afibrinogenemia is characterized by the homozygous presence of autosomal recessive gene.

CONSUMPTION COAGULOPATHIES AND DISSEMINATED INTRAVASCULAR COAGULATION (DIC)

These terms are applied to a group of recently recognized acquired bleeding disorders which occur in a variety of disease states in childhood. When fully developed, DIC is a serious hemorrhagic condition, difficult to control and with a high associated mortality.

The pathologic characteristics of these intravascular coagulation states are due to the presence of the following clotting mechanism abnormalities and the degree of their interaction:

1. Activation of coagulation versus clearance of activated coagulation factors
2. Deposition of fibrin versus lysis of fibrin deposits by the fibrinolytic mechanism
3. Consumption of coagulation factors and inactivation of plasmin versus production of coagulation factors and plasminogen

The five principal intravascular coagulation disturbances which have thus far been recognized and the main disease states which give rise to them are:

1. Activated coagulation with blockade of the reticuloendothelial system (RES) or reduced rate of blood flow: This may occur, particularly in infants, with severe bacterial or viral infections or following circulatory shock in severe gastroenteritis. Despite markedly increased levels of the coagulation factors induced by endotoxin, DIC does not occur unless there is blockade of the RES or the rate of blood flow is markedly diminished.
2. Activation of coagulation factors with intravascular coagulation compensated by activation of fibrinolysis and increased production of the clotting factors: This may occur in children with granulocytic leukemia and solid tumors and some children with acute glomerulonephritis. It also occurs in occasional children with cyanotic heart disease, especially during extracorporeal circulation.
3. Intravascular coagulation associated with increased fibrinolysis but not compensated by increased production of clotting factors:

This type is seen following Gram-negative septicemia and shock, massive viral infections in the newborn, purpura fulminans, giant hemangioma, in patients with the Goodpasture's syndrome, and in membranoproliferative glomerulonephritis.

4. Activation of coagulation compensated by increased production of clotting factors but not by sufficiently increased fibrinolytic activity: Under these circumstances there may be local deposition of fibrin in various tissues, such as may be seen in histologic sections of the kidney. This type of coagulopathy is seen in the hemolytic-uremic syndrome and in some patients with purpura fulminans. High levels of fibrin degradation products are seen in the serum and urine because they are not lysed by increased plasmin activity. There is evidence, that in many cases with this situation, administration of anticoagulants, such as heparin, early in the disease, may be beneficial.

5. Intravascular coagulation uncompensated by increased production of coagulation factors or by activation of fibrinolysis: This situation is not commonly encountered in pediatrics but may occur in some cases of acute promyelocytic leukemia.

The laboratory findings in consumption coagulopathy will vary with the type and severity of the disturbance. There is often depletion of fibrinogen, prothrombin, labile factor, and factor VIII. Platelets may also often be reduced. The detection of increased levels of fibrin split products in serum or urine is sometimes helpful in differentiating the types and severity of disseminated intravascular coagulation.

The disease is often self-limiting. Treatment is principally elimination of the precipitating factors, if possible. Anticoagulants may be helpful in certain circumstances, as noted in item 4 above.

HEMORRHAGIC DISEASE OF THE NEWBORN
(See Chapter 12, "Diseases of the Newborn")

REVIEW QUESTIONS

1. Criteria for performing an exchange transfusion within a few hours of birth include cord serum bilirubin levels. The lowest level to warrant this is (*a*) 2.5 mg or more per 100 ml; (*b*) 4.5 mg or more per 100 ml; (*c*) 6.5 mg or more per 100 ml; (*d*) 8.5 mg or more per 100 ml.

2. The minimal dosage of elemental iron for oral therapy of iron-deficiency anemia in infancy is (*a*) 25 to 50 mg per day; (*b*) 50 to 75 mg per day; (*c*) 75 to 90 mg per day; (*d*) 90 to 150 mg per day.

3. The minimal daily requirement of folic acid for an infant is (*a*) 10 to 20 micrograms; (*b*) 40 to 50 micrograms; (*c*) 75 to 100 micrograms; (*d*) 200 to 400 micrograms.

4. The best test to screen the state of a patient's coagulation activity in hemophilia and to follow the results of therapy is (*a*) partial thromboplastin time; (*b*) prothrombin time; (*c*) prothrombin consumption time; (*d*) clotting time.

5. A 9-year-old boy is bleeding profusely from the nose following slight trauma. Three years previously he had prolonged oozing after extraction of a tooth. His left elbow joint showed decreased mobility. There are no petechiae or ecchymoses. The following laboratory data are reported: Hgb: 13 Gm percent; RBC: 4,300,000; WBC: 12,000, differential count reveals shift to the left, reticulocytes: 3.5 percent. A maternal uncle was a "bleeder." What is the most probable diagnosis: (*a*) idiopathic thrombocytopenic purpura; (*b*) Henoch-Schönlein disease; (*c*) hemophilia; (*d*) chronic leukemia; (*e*) Hageman factor deficiency.

The following questions are of the matching type. In each blank in column I, insert the letter corresponding to the word or phrase in column II which is associated most appropriately.

I	II
6. Red blood cell fragility is increased _____	(*a*) Iron-deficiency anemia
7. Type S hemoglobin predominates _____	(*b*) Cooley's anemia
	(*c*) Congenital hemolytic jaundice
8. Folic acid is treatment of choice _____	(*d*) Sickle-cell anemia
9. Roentgenogram of skull shows "hair-on-end" appearance _____	(*e*) Megaloblastic anemia of infancy

10. Megaloblastic anemia of infancy is characterized by the following except (*a*) recurrent respiratory infections and diarrhea; (*b*) hepatosplenomegaly; (*c*) goat's milk diet; (*d*) transfusion is the preferred form of therapy.

11. Sickle-cell disease is associated with the following except (*a*) a small amount of hemoglobin S present at birth; (*b*) hematuria; (*c*) splenomegaly in adulthood; (*d*) hemoglobin level lower than in patients with sickle-cell hemoglobin C disease.

12. Treatment for acute bleeding into a joint in a patient with hemophilia includes (*a*) AHG; (*b*) application of cold; (*c*) immobilization; (*d*) aspiration of blood from the joint; (*e*) adrenal corticosteroids.

13. Splenectomy may be indicated in the following conditions except (*a*) congenital hemolytic jaundice; (*b*) chronic idiopathic thrombocytopenic purpura; (*c*) congestive splenomegaly; (*d*) acute myeloblastic leukemia.

14. A low-grade fever and white blood count of 25,000 per cu mm for 4 weeks, followed by an eosinophilia in a child who has little or no symptomatology is characteristic of (*a*) infectious mononucleosis; (*b*) infectious lymphocytosis; (*c*) infectious hepatitis; (*d*) early leukemia.

23

Tumors may occur in the fetus, during the neonatal period, and in childhood. Benign tumors are more common than malignant tumors. In children between the ages of 1 and 15 years, cancer is the leading cause of death due to disease. It accounts for 12 percent of childhood deaths. Only accidents take a greater toll in this age group.

LOCATION OF MALIGNANT TUMORS

The ten most common types of malignant tumors seen in children less than 15 years of age, listed in order of decreasing frequency, are as follows: leukemia (about 50 percent), central nervous system (20 percent), lymphoma, neuroblastoma, Wilms's tumor, bone tumors, rhabdomyosarcoma, liver tumors, retinoblastoma, and teratoma. Other cancers which rarely appear in childhood are of the thyroid and ovary.

PREVENTION

Prevention of disease including cancer is most important. Few preventive measures to control cancer in children are known today. They consist of the following:

1. The least amount of exposure to radiation as is possible and necessary in the interest of the patient is important.
    (*a*)   Dental x-rays
    (*b*)   No radiation therapy for benign ailments, e.g., radiation therapy to the thyroid area has been established to have a causal relationship to thyroid cancer.
    (*c*)   The people exposed to the atom bomb in Hiroshima and Nagasaki have a higher incidence of leukemia than the population in other parts of the world.
    (*d*)   Children who drink milk contaminated with strontium 90 develop bone cancer in greater frequencies than the rest of the population.
2. Genetic counseling should be given in those instances of inherited tumors (see p. 151).
3. Drugs and chemicals either as medication or food preservatives should be used with caution. Certain of these have caused concern because of animal experiments or clinical observation as being carcinogenic, e.g., cyclamates and diethylstilbestrol administered during pregnancy.
4. Recent research has indicated that some human milk contains viruslike particles similar to murine mammary tumor virus. This has led to a suspicion that breast-fed infants may develop breast cancer with increased frequency. Epidemiologic studies have not supported this theory. Further investigation is required before an evaluation can be made.

Age incidence   In the early diagnosis of childhood cancer peak age incidence is important to know since part of the insidiousness of cancer is that it simulates many common nonmalignant conditions. Before the age of 5, leukemia, neuroblastoma, Wilms's tumor, embryonal rhabdomyosarcoma, hepatoblastoma, and retinoblastoma are common, and the incidence of brain tumors, bone tumors, and lymphoma and Hodgkin's disease starts to rise around the age of 8 years.

Etiology   In an attempt to elucidate the etiology of malignancy, increased emphasis is being placed on conditions which are frequently associated with benign and malignant tumors. Evidence exists for a relationship between autoimmune diseases and malignant disease and even more broadly between immunity and malignant disease. Certain tumors are inherited as autosomal dominant traits, yet others are associated with congenital anomalies. The following conditions are associated with an increased incidence of tumor formation:

Leukemia
    Down's syndrome
    Ataxia telangiectasia (Louis-Bar syndrome)
    Bloom's syndrome
    Fanconi's anemia
    Marfan's syndrome
    Treacher Collins syndrome
    Ollier's disease
    Osteogenesis imperfecta
    Irradiation in utero
Wilms's tumor
    Aniridia
    Hemihypertrophy   } Also adrenal cortical carcinoma
    Beckwith's syndrome } and carcinoma of the liver
    Urinary tract anomalies
Pheochromocytoma
    Neurofibromatosis
    Hippel-Lindau disease
    Thyroid cancer
Thyroid carcinoma
    Irradiation of head, neck, or chest early in life.
Lymphoma and lymphosarcoma
    Ataxia telangiectasia
    Wiskott-Aldrich syndrome
    Agammaglobulinemia
    Chédiak-Higashi syndrome
Melanoma
    Epidermolysis bullosa
    Xeroderma pigmentosum
Glioma
    Tuberous sclerosis
    Hereditary polyposis
    Tetralogy of Fallot
Medulloblastema
    Cleidocranial dysostosis
Osteosarcoma
    Irradiation for retinoblastoma
    Irradiation for Wilms's tumor or } Also
    Neuroblastoma early in childhood } osteochondroma
Carcinoma of the liver
    Giant-cell hepatitis
Gonadal tumors
    Sex anomalies

Undescended testes
Maffucci's syndrome—also chondroma and angioma
Hamartoma
Turner's syndrome ⎱ Also neurogenic
Noonan's syndrome ⎰ tumors
Strong hereditary aspect and may be inherited as
Autosomal dominant trait
Neurofibromatosis
Retinoblastoma
Gardner's syndrome
Nevoid basal-cell carcinoma syndrome
Adenoma sebaceum

GENERAL PRINCIPLES IN TREATMENT OF NEOPLASMS

1. The treatment modalities depend upon the tumor type and consist of single or combined therapy provided by surgery, radiation therapy, and chemotherapy.
2. All masses should be considered malignant until histologic study has proved them otherwise.
3. In palpation and examination of the tumor mass for diagnosis, unnecessary manipulation should be avoided.
4. Chemotherapy with the broad spectrum of drugs may be indicated. The drugs commonly employed at the present time fall into six major categories according to their mechanism or action—(*a*) antimetabolites, (*b*) alkylating agents, (*c*) anticancer antibiotics, (*d*) enzymes, (*e*) vinca alkaloids, (*f*) hormones, and (*g*) miscellaneous compounds.
5. Psychologic care of the patient and family is of great importance.
6. Treatment is best accomplished by a team approach—pediatrician, psychiatrist, radiation therapist, surgeon, and pharmacologist.

PROGNOSIS

The cures which occur in childhood cancer (and adult cancer) occur with early detection followed by prompt treatment. The prognosis for survival is often age related.

LEUKEMIA

Leukemia is a neoplasm in which there is a proliferation of abnormal white blood cells. It may occur at any age, the highest incidence being from 3 to 6 years. It is the most common neoplastic disease in individuals under 15 years of age, accounting for about 45 percent of deaths from malignant disease. In Caucasians, the death rate from leukemia is 3 to 5 per 100,000 children under 15 years of age; in blacks, 1 to 2 per 100,000.

The disease is best classified according to cell type rather than duration. The cells may be lymphoblasts, myeloblasts, monoblasts, myelocytes, or promyelocytes. In most cases, however, the abnormal blast cell cannot be easily classified and is referred to simply as a stem cell.

Leukemia is also classified as acute or chronic, depending upon its duration. In the past, the blast-cell types of leukemia usually were "acute" and of short duration. With modern methods of treatment, however, these terms have lost some of their significance as the duration of many cases of what formerly was acute leukemia may now exceed that of chronic leukemia. Acute leukemia, the more fulminating disease, usually causes the death of the patient within 6 months if no treatment in instituted. Over 95 percent of leukemia in childhood is of this variety. Chronic myelocytic leukemia, a more benign disease, usually averages 2 to 4 years in duration before the patient succumbs. Chronic lymphatic leukemia, such as occurs in adults, is unknown in children.

The pathologic disturbances are essentially due to the infiltration of the bone marrow, lymph nodes, liver, spleen, and other organs by the neoplastic cells. The crowding out of the normal erythroid, myeloid, and megakaryocyte tissues from the marrow and the other organs or tissue invasion by the leukemic cells results in characteristic signs and symptoms.

Clinical features   Any or all the following may be present:

1. Pallor and hemorrhagic phenomena such as easy bruising, petechiae, epistaxis, and on rare occasions intracranial bleeding due to interference with hematopoiesis.
2. Anorexia, easy fatigability, and weight loss due to the presence of a generalized disease.
3. Reduced resistance to infection, so that respiratory tract infections, septicemia, abscess formation, and unexplained fever are common complications.
4. Pressure symptoms due to leukemic infiltration of tissues and organs, e.g., bone and joint pain. The latter are particularly common symptoms in childhood and may resemble rheumatic fever. Cough and respiratory difficulty resulting from tracheal compression by enlarged mediastinal nodes are rare manifestations. Occasionally infiltrations in the retroorbital region (exophthalmos) or localized swelling about the cranium or a rib (chloroma) may be the presenting complaint. Neurologic manifestations which simulate an acute meningitis occur at times, as well as those due to spinal cord compression.
5. In the majority of children with acute leukemia, only minimal or moderate enlargement of the spleen, liver, and lymph nodes is

found when the disease is first recognized. In chronic leukemia, however, the liver and spleen may be greatly enlarged.

Laboratory findings   The chief diagnostic finding is the presence of the abnormal white cells characteristic of leukemia, either in the peripheral blood or bone marrow. The marrow may be examined either by aspiration or by surgical biopsy. If these are not satisfactory, a biopsy of an enlarged superficial lymph node may establish the diagnosis.

The total white cell count may vary from leukopenic levels of 2,000 or less per cubic millimeter to a leukocythemia of 500,000 or more per cubic millimeter. The majority of patients have total white cell counts between 4,000 and 20,000 per cubic millimeter.

The anemia is normochromic and normocytic; reticulocytes are few, but nucleated red blood cells may be present. Platelets, which may be normal in number early in the disease, become reduced, except in chronic myelogenous leukemia, where they are normal or even increased in number until the terminal stages.

Roentgenograms of the long bones or skull may show pinpoint areas of decreased density or larger areas of rarefaction, which occasionally become cystlike.

Treatment

1.   Specific for acute leukemia
     a.   To induce a remission—prednisone (1 to 2 mg per kg per day) plus an alkylating agent, e.g., cyclophosphamide (Cytoxan), 2.0 to 3.0 mg per kg per day orally; or a vinca alkaloid, e.g., vincristine (Oncovin), 0.05 to 0.1 mg per kg intravenously once weekly for 3 to 4 weeks; 6-mercaptopurine (Purinethol), 2.5 to 3.0 mg per kg per day orally; or amethopterin (methotrexate), 2.5 to 3.0 mg per day orally. Recently, the combination of two drugs, thioguanine and cytosine arabinoside, have been demonstrated to induce remissions. In the acutely ill patient with severe hemorrhagic phenomena, e.g., internal organs, adrenal corticosteroids are given intravenously. Remission is judged by the extent of elimination of the leukemic cells from the blood and marrow. When maximum effect is achieved, usually in 3 to 6 weeks, prednisone is tapered and discontinued. This regimen induces remissions in 80 to 95 percent of children with acute "stem cell" leukemia.

     L-asparaginase (100 to 1,000 units per kg per day or once or twice a week) is a recently introduced mode of therapy. It is based upon the fact that many malignant cells cannot synthesize the amino acid L-asparagine, which is essential for their continued survival. L-asparaginase presumably destroys this amino acid in the circulation, thus depriving the malignant cells of their supply. Acute lymphatic leukemia responds best to L-asparaginase therapy. Used alone, however, remissions of only several weeks to several months occur. The ideal way to use this modality, probably in conjunction with other antileukemic medications, is still under study. Toxic effects include anaphylactic shock, hepatitis, diarrhea, neuropathy, and alopecia.

b. To maintain a remission, a drug of the above group not previously used, e.g., 6-mercaptopurine, amethopterin, or cyclophosphamide is given in full therapeutic dosage, unless serious side effects occur (mouth ulcerations, alopecia, hemorrhagic cystitis, abdominal pain, and diarrhea). They usually recede or disappear when the dosage is reduced or the medication discontinued. The maintenance agent is changed every 3 to 4 months, and the rotation among them in sequence is continued as long as remission persists. If relapse occurs, induction therapy is reinstituted and the cycle repeated.

Immunotherapy for acute leukemia has recently been introduced. It may be active, passive, or supportive. Although benefit is claimed, its role in the induction and maintenance of remission is still to be assessed.

Chronic myelocytic leukemia responds temporarily to roentgen therapy; sulfonyloxybutane (Myeleran), 2 to 6 mg per day; or to 6-mercaptopurine, in the same dosage as for acute leukemia.

2. Supportive measures include transfusion with whole blood or packed red cells for anemia, platelet concentrates for thrombocytopenic hemorrhage, and antibiotics and leukocyte concentrates (when leukopenia is severe) to combat infection. Hyperuricemia is treated by adequate hydration and allopurinol. Psychologic guidance of the child and family is very important.

3. Current prophylactic treatment of the brain and spinal cord with radiation and intrathecal methotrexate holds promise for improved prognosis and possible cure.

Prognosis With sequential cyclic therapy, the average survival has been extended from 1 5–2 years to 2.5–3.5 years, with a small percentage surviving 5 to 8 years or longer. Spontaneous remissions of several weeks to months occur in 5 to 10 percent of patients following severe infections or stress. Survival in chronic myelocytic leukemia, as in adults, is 3 to 5 years.

INTRACRANIAL TUMORS

The incidence of brain tumors increases in children with age to a maximum between the ages of 5 to 8 years. The sex distribution shows brain tumors slightly more common in boys. Approximately 55 percent of brain tumors are infratentorial, located in the posterior fossa, and 45 percent are supratentorial.

Since there are no lymphatics draining the central nervous system, distant metastases are uncommon. Because of the blood brain barrier, the malignant tumors of the brain do not spread into the bloodstream and metastasize. An occasional malignant brain tumor seeds itself down the spinal cord. This occurs more frequently after surgical procedures are performed to relieve obstructive hydrocephalus produced by a tumor which cannot be removed.

In the 1800s and early 1900s 50 percent of intracranial tumors in infants and children were tuberculomas. At the present time this lesion is rare due to the excellent medical and public health measures in the United States.

The two most common brain tumors seen in childhood are the benign cystic astrocytoma (glioma) and the malignant medulloblastoma.

Clinical and laboratory features

1. In general, the symptoms, course, and neurologic findings vary with the type of tumor, the location, and the rapidity of growth.
2. Increased intracranial pressure is most frequently manifested by increase in head circumference, the presence of papilledema and vomiting (projectile or nonprojectile). The nausea and vomiting are intermittent, usually with no relation to meals, and frequently may occur on arising.
3. Headache is often present in older children.
4. There is usually an insidious and subtle onset of abnormalities of behavior, of intellect, or of actual motor or sensory function.
5. Signs and symptoms depend upon the location of the tumor.
   a. Posterior fossa lesions: ataxia, stiffness of the neck, spasm of the neck muscles, nystagmus, suboccipital tenderness, dysmetria, adiadochokinesis, paralysis of the cranial nerves, hypotonia, hyporeflexia, and tonic seizures.
   b. Brainstem lesions: bilateral cranial nerve abnormalities and pyramidal tract signs.
   c. Parasellar lesions: disturbance of vision, abnormalities of water or carbohydrate metabolism, autonomic or pituitary dysfunction.
   d. Cerebral hemisphere lesions: alteration of speech or visual perception; motor weakness usually noted by the family as a failure to use an extremity as well as before; reflex abnormalities and seizures.
6. Roentgenographic visualization of brain tumors is possible only if there are positive shadows, e.g., teratoma, calcified hemangioma, or craniopharyngioma. Indirect roentgenographic evidence of tumor involves signs of increased intracranial pressure, e.g., widening of the suture lines, increased vascular markings in the skull, and the thinning of overlying bone.

7. Brain scanning following the use of radioactive isotopes is most helpful.
8. Arteriography can be performed in children of any age and is valuable in locating the tumor.
9. Electroencephalography may be of value in localizing the lesion.
10. Air studies may be helpful when there is suspicion of a focal lesion. If there is no evidence of increased intracranial pressure, a pneumoencephalogram may be performed. In the presence of increased intracranial pressure, a ventriculogram is performed.
11. Spinal taps, if performed, should be done with caution. Increased intracranial pressure may cause herniation of the medulla into the spinal column when there is a sudden release of pressure below the block.
12. Ultrasound scanning is useful in deep-seated lesions.

MEDULLOBLASTOMA

Medulloblastomas occur in children from 1 month to 13 years of age, with the majority occurring at 3 to 6 years of age. They constitute 20 percent of intracranial tumors. In general they are located in the midline in the cerebellum in the posterior fossa. This is one of the few brain tumors that tends to seed to distant points in the meninges. It also has a tendency to rapid growth.

Clinical and laboratory features

1. Increased intracranial pressure (see p. 608).
2. Posterior fossa features (see p. 608).
3. Ventriculogram—symmetric dilation of the lateral and third ventricles. The fourth ventricle is not usually seen because it is blocked by the tumor.
4. Isotope scans are usually positive.

Treatment   The treatment is palliative.

1. Surgery—at surgery the tumor is distinguished from other posterior fossa tumors. The borders of the tumor are difficult to distinguish from normal brain tissue, consequently complete surgical extirpation is not accomplished.
2. Radiation—following surgery the entire cerebrospinal axis is treated.
3. Recurrences are treated with radiation or by intrathecal methotrexate or radioactive gold. Tumor recurrence is determined by spinal fluid protein of over 100 mg per 100 ml or by the presence of tumor cells.

Prognosis   No cures have occurred. Most patients die within 2 years after the diagnosis is made. Some prolonged survivals do occur.

GLIOMA

All tumors of glial origin are called *gliomas*. Some of these tumors are malignant (second most common malignant brain tumor) and others are benign (grade I cystic astrocytoma constitutes 50 percent of all intracranial tumors found in childhood and 25 percent of all intracranial lesions). Included in this group are the four grades of astrocytoma (grade IV is known as a glioblastoma), mixed gliomas including oligodendriglioma, optic nerve glioma, and ependymoma (benign).

GLIOMA OF THE BRAINSTEM

The peak incidence of this tumor is in children from 5 to 8 years of age. It constitutes 10 percent of the intracranial tumors in children. Many are mixed gliomas.

Clinical and laboratory features

1. Brainstem features (see p. 608). Cranial nerves 5 to 9 and especially 6 are involved.
2. Mimics encephalitis, meningitis, and cerebrovascular disorders.
3. Increased intracranial pressure occurs very late, usually just prior to death. Because of the lack of increased intracranial pressure, lumbar puncture may be carried out without danger. There may be no cells or a pleocytosis up to 20 to 30 white blood cells. If the spinal fluid protein is high, it indicates that the tumor is pressing on the subarachnoid cerebrospinal fluid pathways.
4. The best diagnostic method to locate the tumor is by positive-contrast ventriculography.

Treatment The usual treatment is radiation of the brainstem (surgical removal is usually impossible).

Prognosis The prognosis is poor. The average patient lives less than 1 year.

GLIOMAS OF THE CEREBRAL HEMISPHERES

Gliomas of the cerebral hemispheres occur in about 10 to 15 percent of children with intracranial tumors. The malignant astrocytomas (grades II and III and the glioblastomas) are the third most common brain tumor in children. They occur in up to 8 percent of patients with brain tumors. These tumors are seen in children from the ages of 6 to 9 years.

Treatment

1. Surgical removal of as much tumor tissue as possible.
2. Radiation following surgery.

3. Recurrence is treated by radiation and sometimes in conjunction with chemotherapy.

Prognosis These tumors are fatal. Usual life expectancy is 1 to 2 years, although occasionally patients with posterior fossa solid astrocytomas may survive many years.

OLIGODENDRIGLIOMA

This is a rare tumor, usually supratentorial, which is slow growing. Surgery followed by radiation is the preferred treatment. Since they grow slowly, repeat surgery is feasible. Average survival is about 5 years; occasionally survival may be as long as 30 years.

CEREBELLAR SARCOMA

This tumor is located in the midline in the posterior fossa. It is highly malignant and behaves as does the medulloblastoma. The treatment and prognosis is like that of the medulloblastoma.

INTRACRANIAL TERATOMA

Intracranial teratomas may be either malignant or benign (see p. 623). In general these tumors tend to occur in surgically inaccessible areas of the brain, most often in the third ventricle. If the tumor can be completely removed surgically, the patient can be cured. If surgical removal is not possible, the average survival in these cases is about 3 years.

RHABDOMYOSARCOMA

Rhabdomyosarcoma, a malignant tumor, may occur in the orbit. It arises from one of the extraocular muscles. Radical surgery, radiation therapy, and chemotherapy are employed as therapy.

RETINOBLASTOMA

Retinoblastoma, a malignant tumor of the retina, is transmitted as an autosomal dominant disease with a varying degree of penetrance. Often parents note a white spot (cat's eye reflex) in the pupil of the eye. Other presenting signs are strabismus, head tilt, enlarging globe and dilated pupil. The tumor is bilateral in one-third of the cases. The tumor spreads locally within the eye or by extention to surrounding areas and distally via the emissary veins or along the optic nerve.
    Treatment depends upon prompt diagnosis and proper staging (I to V) and includes radiation therapy and chemotherapy (stages IV and V). Enuncleation is reserved for a tumor with extensive retinal involvement. Chemotherapy consists of triethylenemelamine or Cytoxan. The overall mortality rate is 15 percent.

METASTATIC BRAIN TUMORS

Most common is the leukemic involvement of the central nervous system. It is the meninges which are involved with leukemic infiltrates. Of children with acute leukemia, about half will develop signs referable to the central nervous system (CNS). This may be present at the time of the initial diagnosis or develop at a later time. The spinal fluid may show from 5,000 to 7,000 blast cells per mm, a normal or low sugar content, and protein level ranging from normal to over 500 mg per 100 ml. With the exception of the adrenal corticosteroids, the other anticancer drugs employed in the treatment of acute leukemia do not pass into the cerebrospinal fluid in doses high enough to produce remissions of the meningeal disease. CNS leukemia is generally treated with intrathecal methotrexate, 0.25 to 0.5 mg per kg every 3 to 5 days. One final dose is administered after the pleocytosis in the cerebrospinal fluid has returned to normal. In general three doses are sufficient, but occasionally up to eight may be necessary.

The methotrexate may be mixed with the cerebrospinal fluid for intrathecal administration. Oral and intravenous methotrexate are not given during the intrathecal therapy. Remissions of CNS leukemia following intrathecal methotrexate may last for an average of 4 months. When relapse occurs radiation therapy to the whole brain and cord may produce remission lasting on the average for 2 months. Prednisone, orally, provides remissions in CNS leukemia lasting on the average for 4 to 6 weeks.

Other metastatic tumors seen in the brain in a small percent of children are neuroblastoma, Hodgkin's disease, lymphomas, and Wilms's tumor. Surgery is indicated for the Wilms's tumor metastatic lesion if it is a solitary and accessible one. The other tumors are treated by radiation therapy and chemotherapy.

BENIGN BRAIN TUMORS

The most common of the benign brain tumors to occur in childhood is the cystic astrocytoma (see p. 610). The peak incidence is from 5 to 8 years of age. Generally it is located in the cerebellum.

Clinical and laboratory features

1. Increased intracranial pressure occurs (see p. 608).
2. Posterior fossa features occur.
3. X-ray may reveal signs of increased intracranial pressure (see p. 608 and occasionally calcification in the tumor. Ventriculography reveals symmetric dilation of the lateral and third ventricles.
4. Brain scans frequently show outlines of the cystic tumor.

Treatment   Surgery is the treatment of choice for the grade I cystic astrocytoma. By evacuating the astrocytoma cyst patients may be asymptomatic for long periods of time. Frequently the tumor can be completely removed.

Prognosis   This brain tumor has the best prognosis of any.

CRANIOPHARYNGIOMA

This is the second most common benign tumor of the brain and constitutes somewhat less than 10 percent of intracranial tumors in children. It arises from two sources of epithelium, one from the buccal epithelium of Rathke's pouch and two from squamous-cell rests which lie in the region of the hypophyseal stalk. The continued growth of this epithelium forms masses and cysts filled with cellular debris and cholesterol ester crystals. Although its histologic picture is benign, it frequently behaves as a malignant tumor.

Clinical and laboratory features   See Chapter 24, "Endocrine Diseases," for pituitary adenomas.

Treatment   Surgery is the treatment of choice. An attempt is made to completely excise the tumor. When this cannot be done, the cyst is aspirated and biopsied. This is followed by a spinal fluid shunt operation or radiation therapy. Since the advent of the use of adrenal corticosteroids, the surgical results have improved because these drugs decrease the complications that occur when surgery is involved near the area of the pituitary and hypothalamus.

Prognosis   Most patients with this tumor survive 5 to 10 years. An occasional patient has lived longer.

EPENDYMOMA

The ependymomas, of glial origin, are histologically benign tumors but behave as malignant tumors. In general they occur in the fourth ventricle. They are seen in children from 2 months to 12 years of age. They occur more often above the tentorium. The signs and symptoms include increased intracranial pressure and stiffness and spasm of the neck and shoulder area (the lesion spreads down the cervical canal). Because of their location they cannot be completely removed surgically, hence they are generally treated by radiation therapy. The average survival of patients with this tumor is about 3 years.

OPTIC NERVE GLIOMA

Optic nerve gliomas are also benign tumors which occur in children and constitute about 4 percent of intracranial lesions. It is a slow-growing tumor. When it is confined to the optic nerve, it is surgically curable; however, when it extends into the hypothalamus, it is inoperable.

CHOROID PLEXUS PAPILLOMA

Choroid plexus papillomas occurs in infants in 3 percent of the intracranial lesions. It usually occurs in children under 2 years of age and produces hypersecretion of cerebrospinal fluid and hydrocephalus. The major sign which occurs is separation of the cranial sutures. The cerebrospinal fluid pressure is high. Air contrast studies reveal dilatation of the ventricular system. Treatment of this lesion consists of total excision. Patients with tumors in the lateral ventricle do well following surgical excision. Occasionally some degree of neurologic deficit occurs especially visual, hemiparesis, and convulsions.

ACOUSTIC NEURINOMA

The acoustic neurinoma involves the acoustic nerve and is usually a neurofibroma. Many of these children have evidence of von Recklinghausen's disease (neurofibromatosis) elsewhere in the body. Usually these tumors are removed surgically.

PINEALOMA

Pinealomas are generally seen in adolescent males and rarely occur in children under 12 years of age. They press upon the posterior portion of the third ventricle and aqueduct of Sylvius to produce hydrocephalus. Pinealomas are associated with sexual precocity due either to a secretory product of the tumor (melotonin) or to pressure on the hypothalamus. In addition they press upon the quadrigeminal plate area to alter pupillary and extraocular muscle function. Ventriculograms will usually demonstrate a mass in the third ventricle. Surgery in this area is hazardous. Generally a ventriculoatrial shunt is performed to relieve the hydrocephalus. This is followed by deep radiation therapy. Remissions last many years.

Other benign intracranial lesions which occur in children and are exceedingly rare include colloid cysts (attached to the choroid plexus of the third ventricle), chordoma, and pituitary adenomas other than craniopharyngioma (see Chapter 24, "Endocrine Diseases").

PSEUDOTUMOR CEREBRI

Pseudotumor cerebri is a syndrome in which there is an excessive amount of spinal fluid in the subarachnoid space. The fluid itself is otherwise normal. The symptoms are those of an intracranial space-occupying lesion or hydrocephalus. The condition is mostly benign with the exception of possible loss of visual acuity due to persistent increased intracranial pressure. The increased intracranial pressure is probably due to interference with absorption of cerebrospinal fluid. The syndrome may be due to known causes, e.g., obstruction of intracranial venous drainage due to inflammatory reaction of adjacent structures (mastoiditis), vitamin A intoxication or deficiency, hypoparathyroidism, tetracycline therapy, certain systemic diseases (roseola infantum), head trauma, or it may be due to unknown causes. Where a known cause exists, it should be removed. In other instances spontaneous cure will usually occur. If not, and vision is affected, decrease of pressure may be accomplished by repeated spinal taps or, in a few instances, by a shunting procedure.

TUMORS OF THE SKULL AND MENINGES

TERATOMA AND DERMOID

Teratoma and dermoids (see p. 623) may occur in the scalp or within the skull. The tumor mass frequently is large.

RETICULOENDOTHELIOSIS

The skull as well as other bones may be involved by the reticuloendothelioses (see p. 624).

FIBROUS DYSPLASIA OF BONE (See p. 622)

OSTEOMA

These are slow-growing benign tumors which arise in the face and skull and frequently project into the orbit and paranasal sinuses. (In association with multiple soft-tissue tumors and gastrointestinal polyps, they constitute Gardner's syndrome.) Excisional surgery is the therapy of choice.

MENINGIOMA

Meningioma is the most frequent tumor arising from the meninges. Although common in adults, it is rare in children. Surgical removal is the recommended treatment.

Other rare tumors include leptomeningeal sarcoma, malignant melanoma of the meninges, and fibrosarcoma of the dura. Benign brain lesions that mimic tumors include hematoma, abscess, and pseudotumor cerebri.

INTRASPINAL TUMORS

These tumors are uncommon and generally similar in type to the intracranial tumors.

Clinical and laboratory features

1. Abnormalities of posture and gait—these may be present prior to obvious neurologic deficit.

616   SURVEY OF CLINICAL PEDIATRICS

2. Weakness—either generalized, e.g., easy fatigability, or localized in a limb.
3. Pain—frequently aggravated by increasing cerebrospinal fluid pressure, e.g., straining, or by certain postural changes.
4. Reflexes—depending on the site (hyperactive below the lesion) and the presence of "spinal shock" (absent deep-tendon reflexes).
5. Bladder and bowel function—loss of control.
6. Sensory changes may occur below the level of the tumor.
7. Skin lesions—certain tumors, e.g., dermoid, may be associated with overlying lesions, e.g., dimple, tuft of hair.
8. X-rays—bony changes are seen in a majority of cases. Myelography can definitely locate and define the tumor.
9. Cerebrospinal fluid may reveal alterations in pressure, color (xanthochromia), cell count, and protein content. Sugar content may be low (metastases).

Treatment   Surgical removal, decompressive laminectomy, and radiation as well as chemotherapy are employed.

NEUROFIBROMATOSIS

Neurofibromatosis (von Recklinghausen's disease) is hereditary (autosomal dominant with variable expressivity) and is characterized by café au lait spots on the skin and flat or pedunculated tumors (skin or subcutaneous tissue) which are nontender, nodular, and associated with peripheral nerves. Similar tumors may be found in the brain, cranial nerves, or spinal nerves. In any one patient, the tumors tend to occur either peripherally or within the bony confines of the central nervous system. Ocasionally neurofibromatosis is associated with mental deficiency. Treatment is surgical, with removal of major symptomatic lesions. A nonaggressive attitude is recommended. As in any other disease transmitted in this manner, supportive psychologic aid is extremely important.

MALIGNANCIES OF LYMPHOID TISSUE

LYMPHOSARCOMA

This is a rare malignant disorder in which the lymphoid tissue becomes infiltrated with "immature" mononuclear cells; this infiltration increases the size of the glands and destroys their architecture.

Clinical features   Local pressure effects may be present. These effects may cause tracheal compression, intestinal obstruction, bone pain, spinal cord signs, etc. As the disease becomes widespread, anorexia, weight loss, and pallor occur. There are local (chiefly cervical) and generalized lymph node enlargement and hepatosplenomegaly. There may be fever, easy fatigability, and bleeding phenomena when the marrow and peripheral blood are involved.

Laboratory findings There may be little change in the blood in the early stages, except for a normochromic anemia. Later, especially if the marrow becomes involved, anemia and thrombocytopenia occur. In some cases the lymphosarcoma cell appears in the peripheral circulation; such cases are difficult to distinguish from acute lymphatic leukemia. When marrow invasion occurs, roentgenographic changes in the bones are similar to those in acute leukemia.

Diagnosis The diagnosis is made by correlating the histologic examination of the biopsied lymph node or tumor with the clinical features.

Course Progression of the disease varies considerably. Some cases are fulminating and resemble acute leukemia; others are slowly progressive, and the patient may live for several years. Death results from compression or invasion of vital organs, e.g., spinal cord, secondary infection, cachexia, and hemorrhage.

Treatment and prognosis See Hodgkin's Disease, below.

HODGKIN'S DISEASE

This is an uncommon neoplasm in childhood in which the lymphoid tissue of the lymph nodes, spleen, and later other organs is replaced by an infiltration of lymphocytes, giant multinucleated reticuloendothelial cells (Reed-Sternberg), and eosinophils. The disease is extremely rare before 8 years of age. It is usually slowly progressive, with the average duration varying from 2 to 7 years. Occasionally a fulminating form is encountered that differs little from acute leukemia. The cause is unknown.

Clinical features The disease often begins insidiously with the swelling of localized groups of lymph nodes frequently in the supraclavicular region. These are usually discrete, firm, and nontender. Pressure symptoms may be present; their nature depends on whether cervical, mediastinal, or abdominal lymph nodes are most involved. There may be engorgement of the neck vessels, cough, respiratory difficulty, ascites, or obstructive jaundice. Constitutional symptoms such as anorexia, fatigue, irritability, or fluctuating fever (Pel-Ebstein) may occur. Splenomegaly is moderate to marked, and slight hepatomegaly may be present. Hemolytic anemia, jaundice, and bleeding phenomena occur when the bone marrow becomes massively infiltrated. Eventually, all the lymphoid structures in the body become involved.

Laboratory findings In the early stages, the blood shows a rapid sedimentation rate but little change in the cellular elements. The white cell count varies from 4,000 to 20,000. Later, there are anemia, thrombocytopenia, and leukopenia. The number of monocytes and eosinophils may be increased.

Diagnosis Diagnosis is made by histologic examination of biopsy material from an involved lymph node or the spleen. Bone marrow aspirates occasionally show the characteristic Reed-Sternberg cells.

Treatment

1. Treatment depends on staging (I to IV) which connotes the location and extent of the disease at the time of diagnosis.
2. Radiation therapy is the primary form of treatment. The disease varies considerably in susceptibility; recurrences are re-treated, but eventually the disease becomes resistant to the treatment.
3. In addition to radiation, the drugs employed systemically in the advanced stages (III and IV) of these tumors are nitrogen mustard, the ethyleneimine compounds, chlorambucil (Leukeran), cyclophosphamide (Cytoxan), methotrexate, Velban, vincristine, procarbazine (Matutane), and adrenal corticosteroids.

Prognosis Chemotherapy can produce complete or partial remissions in the majority of cases with lymphoma or Hodgkin's disease. The remissions will last for months to years. Some patients have had remissions from drug therapy alone lasting more than 20 years.

Survival depends upon the degree of malignancy of the tumor. The least malignant tumors are associated with 50 to 85 percent survival for 5 years.

ABDOMINAL TUMORS

NEUROBLASTOMA

Neuroblastoma originates from the neuroblasts that form the adrenal medulla or any of the sympathetic ganglions. It accounts for 4 to 6 percent of all cancer in childhood.

Clinical features

1. A firm, solid abdominal mass is the most common presenting feature.
2. Metastases occur early (present in 70 percent of patients at time of initial diagnosis), so that presenting findings may be due to orbital involvement, with exophthalmos and periorbital ecchymoses; bone involvement, producing limp and pain (here the lesions may

be bilaterally symmetric); or liver involvement, producing hepato-megaly (but jaundice is rare).
3. Fever and anorexia may be present.
4. Roentgenography may demonstrate that the mass is retroperi-toneal, not associated with the kidney, and often calcified; the long bones may reveal metastases.
5. Diagnosis is made by histopathologic study of the main lesions or of a peripheral lymph node. If marrow metastases have occurred, bone marrow aspiration smears occasionally reveal the character-istic pseudorosette of tumor cells.
6. Increased secretion of catecholamines may occur, causing symp-toms (see p. 654) and increased output.

Differential diagnosis Neuroblastoma is one of the most frequent abdominal tumors of infancy and childhood. Sometimes only laparotomy can differentiate neuroblastoma from the following:

1. Wilms's tumor
2. Hydronephrosis
3. Retroperitoneal sarcoma
4. Liver tumor: hemangiomas and hepatomas
5. Mesenteric, omental, and choledochal cysts—usually large, soft, freely movable
6. Ovarian tumor

Treatment

1. Surgical extirpation if possible, followed by irradiation and de-pendent on staging (I to IV).
2. Irradiation to the metastases.
3. Chemotherapy: vinca alkaloids and cyclophosphamide. Methotrex-ate and antitumor antibiotics have also provided remissions.

Prognosis The prognosis is grave, the disease being fatal usually within 2 years. About 25 percent of patients have survived 3 to 8 years after treatment. Neuroblastomas have been reported on occasion to mature to a benign form (ganglioneuroma) or even to disappear com-pletely, probably as the result of hemorrhage or infarction of the tumor.

WILMS'S TUMOR (Embryonal Adenomyosarcoma of the Kidney)

Clinical features

1. The majority of cases of this tumor occur during the first 2 to 5 years of life. The tumor is bilateral in 7 percent of cases.
2. An abdominal swelling, firm, nontender, smooth, or nodular, is

frequently the only presenting sign. Sometimes it appears suddenly or increases rapidly in size in a short time; this is usually because of hemorrhage within the tumor.

3. Fever may be present; hypertension is not uncommon; and hematuria is rare.
4. Metastasis is usually to the lung, practically never to bone.
5. Roentgenographic findings: a pyelogram may reveal distortion of the renal pelvis with little or no displacement of the kidney. (Neuroblastoma shows displacement of the kidney out of proportion to distortion of the renal pelvis.)

Treatment   Treatment consists of immediate nephrectomy followed by irradiation and chemotherapy dependent on staging (I to V). If the tumor is of such a size as to make removal mechanically impossible, preoperative radiation may be necessary. Otherwise radiation is usually postponed until after surgery. Chemotherapy: actinomycin D (0.015 mg per kg for 5 days) acts synergistically when used concomitantly with radiation and is continued at 1- to 2-monthly intervals for 1½ to 2 years. Other drugs, e.g., cyclophosphamide and vincristine, are used when the latter treatment fails.

Prognosis   The prognosis is grave, but cures have been reported. The best prognosis is for infants when the tumor is discovered during the first year of life. Recurrences, when they occur, usually take place within 2 years.

BONE TUMORS

These may cause pain, swelling, fever, and impaired function. Diagnosis depends on history, roentgenograms, and biopsy. Bone sarcomas account for 5 to 10 percent of childhood malignancies.

EWING'S SARCOMA (Endothelioma)

Ewing's sarcoma is a malignant tumor occurring during childhood and early adulthood. Although the involved bones in Ewing's sarcoma are the same as in osteogenic sarcoma, in the former the neoplastic process usually begins in the diaphysis, while in osteogenic sarcoma it begins in the metaphysis.

Clinical and laboratory features

1. A history of trauma is frequently elicited.
2. Fever may be present.
3. Pain is a most constant finding.
4. Roentgenographic findings: there is an early widening of the medullary canal and thickening of the cortex. Later there is the

typical onionskin appearance due to destruction of the cortex, with areas of thickening which are lamellated.
5. Ewing's sarcoma, clinically and roentgenographically, may simulate chronic osteomyelitis. (With the advent of the antibiotics, chronic sclerosing osteomyelitis that resembles the various bone neoplasms has become much less common. When diagnosis is in doubt, a biopsy should always be made.)

Treatment   Treatment consists of radiation in combination with chemotherapy. Radiation can produce marked palliation. Chemotherapeutic drugs, e.g., nitrogen mustard, actinomycin D, and vincristine can produce remissions.

Prognosis   The prognosis is poor.

OSTEOGENIC SARCOMA

Osteogenic sarcoma is a highly malignant tumor occurring most frequently about the time of puberty. Any bone may be involved, but the most common sites are the distal ends of the shafts of the femur and the proximal ends of the shafts of the tibia or humerus.

Clinical and laboratory features

1. Pain, which may be intermittent and worse at night.
2. Fever is occasionally present.
3. Roentgenograms reveal localized rarefaction and sclerosis; later the typical sunburst pattern with invasion and penetration of the cortex and surrounding tumor formation is seen.
4. Metastases occur most commonly to the lung, less often to viscera and bone.
5. Calcium level and alkaline phosphatase may be elevated.

Treatment

1. If the diagnosis is suggested by the clinical and roentgenographic findings, a biopsy should be performed.
2. After histologic confirmation of the diagnosis, resection of the tumor or amputation of the extremity should be done as soon as possible.
3. Radiation is sometimes administered preoperatively. Metastases are treated with radiation, nitrogen mustard, actinomycin D, or vincristine, but these have only slight beneficial effect.

Prognosis   The prognosis is poor.

METASTATIC BONE TUMORS

The most frequently seen metastatic bone tumors are those due to acute leukemia and neuroblastoma.

BENIGN BONE TUMORS

CHONDROMATOSIS

Chondromas are benign and are the most common tumors of bone. They are derived from the proliferating cells of the epiphyseal cartilage, and their growth pattern is similar to that of normal cartilage in that they stop growing when normal growth stops. Exostoses (external chondromatosis) grow away from the bone and are found most frequently at the distal ends of the long bones; when they are multiple, the condition is usually familial. In internal chondromatosis (Ollier's disease), multiple enchondromas grow within the shaft of the bone, usually unilateral, most commonly in the small bones of the hands and feet. There may be associated vascular malformations (Maffucci's syndrome). These tumors require treatment only if they are producing pressure symptoms or signs. Malignant degeneration is rare.

GIANT–CELL TUMOR

This is a benign destructive neoplasm of bone which is rare under the age of 20. Roentgenographically it may appear similar to a unilocular bone cyst. The unilocular cyst is more common and does not invade the epiphysis. Giant-cell tumors characteristically involve both metaphysis and epiphysis. Treatment is surgical removal of the tumor. The incidence of malignant degeneration is low, about 10 to 15 percent.

UNILOCULAR BONE CYST

This is a benign cyst and must be differentiated from giant-cell tumor, osteoid osteoma, and eosinophilic granuloma. The benign cyst occurs at the epiphyseal end of the metaphysis. Roentgenograms reveal the cystic mass, which frequently causes thinning and distension of the cortex and only rarely penetrates it. Occasionally pathologic fractures occur. Treatment of choice is surgery.

OSTEODYSTROPHY FIBROSA

Osteodystrophy fibrosa (fibrous dysplasia of bone) is characterized by fibroblastic tissue replacing the marrow and the cancellous part in a single bone (monostotic) or a number of bones (polyostotic), usually unilateral. Clinically there may be swelling or a fracture in the involved area. The blood chemistry is normal, except for an increased serum-phosphatase level. Roentgenograms may show osteoporosis, sclerosis, and evidence of fractures.

Polyostotic bone changes are often associated with unilateral hyperpigmentation of the skin; there may be precocious puberty (Albright's syndrome, see p. 644), usually in females.

There is no specific treatment.

SOFT–TISSUE TUMORS

Soft-tissue sarcoma accounts for approximately 10 percent of all cancer in children.

RHABDOMYOSARCOMA

Of the soft-tissue sarcomas the embryonal rhabdomyosarcoma is the most common. It arises out of striated muscle. The presenting sign is usually a mass.

Treatment consists of surgical excision. If complete excision is not possible, radiation therapy and chemotherapy are given. The drugs of choice are actinomycin D, cyclophosphamide, or vincristine. These drugs may be given postoperatively with radiation treatment. Metastatic disease is treated with radiation and the anticancer drugs to produce temporary remissions. Some patients have been cured.

TERATOMA, DERMOID, AND HAMARTOMA

Teratomas are collections of embryonal cells which apparently retain their ability to differentiate into various types of tissue. The simplest form is a dermoid, which is lined by membrane resembling skin and may contain hair, sebaceous glands, and occasionally teeth. More complex teratomas may contain any kind of tissue, e.g., bone, nervous tissue. These tumors arise predominately at or near the midline and frequently just anterior to the spinal column. Hamartomas are tumors of multiple tissues, foreign to the organ in which it is found, and demonstrating a degree of disorganized growth.

Teratoma is the third most frequent retroperitoneal tumor. It is discovered either as a palpable mass or because it encroaches on an adjacent organ and interferes with its function. The most frequent teratoma occurs in the sacrococcygeal region. Teratomas are most often benign, but malignancy does occur. Surgery is the treatment of choice. In incompletely removed tumors radiation therapy and chemotherapy, usually actinomycin D, are given. Nitrogen mustard or vincristine may also be employed if the tumor is malignant.

RARE TUMORS OF CHILDHOOD

The rare tumors seen in childhood include those of the thyroid, testis, liver, and ovary.

PAPILLARY CARCINOMA OF THE THYROID

This occurs in children and young adults and more frequently in females. (Thyroid carcinoma appears to be increasing in frequency.)

There is a hard, stony mass in the thyroid region and lateral aspect of the neck which must be differentiated from benign thyroid adenomas, lymphomas, branchial-cleft and thyroglossal-duct cysts, inflammatory masses, Hodgkin's disease, lymphosarcoma, and leukemia. Growth is slow, and metastasis takes place late. Treatment is surgical removal of all thyroid tumor masses; when malignant, the entire lobe is removed and a radical neck dissection is performed. This should be followed by roentgen-ray therapy or radioactive iodine.

TUMORS OF THE OVARY

Tumors of the ovary are uncommon and usually occur in the 6- to 12-year age group. They may be benign (including teratomas, dermoids, or simple cysts) or malignant (including adenocarcinoma, granulosa cell carcinoma, dysgerminoma, and malignant teratoma). The clinical features are abdominal pain and discomfort and lower abdominal mass on rectal examination. Twisting of the pedicle may produce acute abdominal distress resembling other acute abdominal conditions. Granulosa cell carcinoma may cause sexual precocity and uterine bleeding in a preadolescent girl. The treatment is surgical excision. In cases where the entire tumor cannot be removed, radiation and alkylating agents are employed. The prognosis is good for benign lesions and granulosa cell tumors, which metastasize late, and poor for malignant tumors.

TUMOR OF THE TESTIS

Testicular tumors include teratomas, embryonal carcinoma, and interstitial cell tumor (the latter may produce precocious puberty). A scrotal mass is frequently the first clinical finding.

Treatment is surgical excision.

TUMORS OF THE LIVER

These tumors are uncommon and occur usually in the first 2 years of life. The benign tumors are hemangiomas, hamartomas, and angioendotheliomas. Malignant lesions are usually carcinomas of hepatic cell origin. Clinically the first manifestation is an enlarging abdomen followed by weight loss, fever, jaundice, and portal venous obstruction. Treatment is resection of the tumor, and even lobectomy may be performed. Hamartomas are usually successfully resected, x-ray therapy may be used for hemangiomas. Prognosis is good for benign tumors and very poor for malignant tumors.

RETICULOENDOTHELIOSES

The reticuloendothelioses are a group of rare diseases of unknown cause that are characterized by proliferation of the cells of the reticuloendothelial system at one or more sites of the body, e.g., the lymph nodes, spleen, liver, lungs, skin, and bone marrow.

LETTERER–SIWE DISEASE

This disease, also called acute disseminated histioreticuloendotheliosis, develops during the first year of life and is a much more acute process than Hand-Schüller-Christian disease or eosinophilic granuloma. A very high familial incidence exists. There is a diffuse, generalized invasion of affected organs with histiocytes and occasional eosinophils. This condition can be considered identical with histiocytic leukemia. These large mononuclear cells with a basophilic-staining cytoplasm usually do not contain lipid. The clinical features are fever; eczematoid, xanthomatous, and purpuric skin lesions; progressive splenomegaly; hepatomegaly; and anemia. The lymph nodes may enlarge considerably. Skeletal and lung infiltration may be visualized on roentgenographic examination as radiolucent areas in the ribs, skull, and long bones, and as diffuse densities of the lung. The diagnosis is based on the demonstration of the abnormal reticulum cell hyperplasia in biopsy or aspiration material from lymph nodes, spleen, or bone marrow. The course of the disease is rapid and prognosis is poor, but adrenal corticosteroids in large doses and maintained for long periods often have a favorable effect. Nitrogen mustard and other alkylating agents such as cyclophosphamide and chlorambucil may also be beneficial. More recently vinca alkaloids, e.g., Velban and vincristine, have been advocated. Small doses of radiation therapy are palliative. Spontaneous change of the condition to a more chronic form has been reported, as has apparent spontaneous cure.

HAND–SCHÜLLER–CHRISTIAN DISEASE

This disease occurs in older children or young adults and has a protracted course. It is believed that this disorder is a more benign form of reticuloendotheliosis than Letterer-Siwe disease and that there has therefore been time for lipoid (cholesterol) deposition in the reticulum cells. In the more chronic cases, fibroblastic tissue and occasional eosinophilic infiltration begin to appear in addition to the fat-laden reticulum cells. The classic triad consists of punched-out lesions in the skull, bilateral exophthalmos, and diabetes insipidus. Almost all organs are involved. Commonly, chronic bilateral otitis media is a presenting symptom. The blood may show anemia, leukopenia, and thrombocytopenia. The serum-cholesterol level is normal, despite the large cholesterol deposits in the reticuloendothelial cells. Diagnosis is confirmed by biopsy, which demonstrates reticulohistiocytic hyperplasia, with cholesterol-containing cells.

The disease may run a course of many years. Spontaneous remissions occur occasionally. The osseous and soft-tissue lesions may be benefited by roentgen-ray, adrenal corticosteroid, antifolic acid drug, or occasionally nitrogen mustard therapy. The diabetes insipidus responds poorly to any of the foregoing but may be controlled to some extent by pitressin.

EOSINOPHILIC GRANULOMA

Eosinophilic granuloma is believed to be the most benign variant of the preceding group of reticuloendothelioses. The lesions are limited chiefly to the skeleton and may occur as a solitary xanthoma (eosinophilic granuloma) of one bone or may involve several bones. Roentgenographically, they appear as localized areas of rarefaction or cysts. There may be no symptoms, or there may be pain, swelling, spontaneous fractures of the affected bones, and a low-grade fever. Occasionally a moderate blood eosinophilia is present. Treatment consists of surgery preferably or roentgen-ray therapy in cases with multiple bone involvement. Either treatment usually results in a cure of the local lesion, but the prognosis is guarded because of the possibility of lesions appearing elsewhere.

TUMORS OF VASCULAR AND LYMPHATIC ORIGIN

KAPOSIS SARCOMA

Kaposis sarcoma is seen more commonly in children in Africa than in the United States. In the majority of cases this tumor arises as bluish-toned nodules in the skin of the lower extremities. Histologically it is characterized by anastomosing capillaries and proliferation of endothelial cells and fibroblasts. Irradiation and chemotherapy are the treatment of choice. Regression of the disease may be achieved with the use of cyclophosphamide; if resistance occurs, vincristine combined with methotrexate and eventually cytosine arabinoside may be used. Some cures do occur.

Hemangioma (See Chapter 26, "Skin Disorders")

CYSTIC HYGROMA

Cystic hygroma is a benign, multilocular, soft cystic tumor of lymphatic origin usually seen in infants. It may be found in the deep fascia of the neck, in the axilla, or over the sacrum. Growth of the tumor is progressive and may cause symptoms from pressure on the trachea, pharynx, blood vessels, or nerves. Diagnosis is made by the flabby consistency of the tumor, its location, and its ill-defined borders. Treatment is complete surgical excision as early as possible, since the tumor becomes very large and may become infected, making surgical removal extremely difficult.

SKIN TUMORS

MELANOMA

Malignant melanoma is rare before puberty but may be present at birth. They may arise from giant nevi and are almost always fatal. Other melanomas in children have a somewhat better prognosis. The juvenile melanoma, seen in childhood, is a benign tumor which has a malignant appearance microscopically.

NEVI (See Chapter 26, "Skin Disorders")

XANTHOMAS

Xanthomas are yellow, café au lait, or orange nodules in the skin. Histologically, intracellular lipoid material in abnormal quantities can be demonstrated (Sudan stain). Xanthomas may be divided into those associated with a normal serum-cholesterol level and those with an elevated serum-cholesterol level.

Xanthomas with normal serum-lipid level:

1. Xanthomas can be found in the following reticuloendothelioses: Letterer-Siwe disease and Hand-Schüller-Christian disease.
2. Familial xanthomas without hyperlipidemia—these conditions may be variants of reticuloendothelioses.

Xanthomas with elevated serum-lipid level:

1. Familial hyperlipoproteinemia (see Inherited Diseases of Lipid Metabolism, Chapter 9).
2. Secondary xanthomas are occasionally found in nephrosis, diabetes mellitus, hypothyroidism, certain types of pancreatitis, and glycogen-storage disease.

KELOIDS

Keloids are composed of dense fibrous tissue which forms in scars, usually of black-skinned people. It appears to develop in certain families and may be considered hereditary. The best method of therapy is excisional surgery followed by postoperative radiotherapy.

REVIEW QUESTIONS

1. Acute leukemia occurs most frequently in the following age groups: (*a*) 0 to 3 years; (*b*) 3 to 6 years; (*c*) 8 to 10 years; (*d*) 10 to 15 years.
2. Over 95 percent of leukemia in childhood is (*a*) chronic myelocytic; (*b*) chronic lymphatic; (*c*) acute stem cell.

3. The greatest incidence of brain tumors occur in children between the ages of
    (*a*) 3 to 5 years; (*b*) 5 to 8 years; (*c*) 8 to 10 years; (*d*) 10 to 12 years.
4. The following conditions are associated with an increased incidence of leu-
    kemia except (*a*) osteogenesis imperfecta; (*b*) Down's syndrome; (*c*) Ollier's
    disease; (*d*) Beckwith's syndrome.
5. The most common benign brain tumor in childhood is (*a*) cystic astrocytoma;
    (*b*) ependymoma; (*c*) craniopharyngioma; (*d*) medulloblastoma.
6. A malignant tumor of childhood that metastasizes to bone most often is
    (*a*) Wilms's tumor; (*b*) astrocytoma; (*c*) adenocarcinoma of the adrenal gland;
    (*d*) granulosa cell tumor of the ovary; (*e*) neuroblastoma.
7. A pyelogram that reveals distortion of the renal pelvis out of proportion to
    displacement of the kidney is suggestive of (*a*) neuroblastoma; (*b*) Wilms's
    tumor; (*c*) neither (*a*) nor (*b*); (*d*) mesenteric cyst.
8. In osteogenic sarcoma the neoplastic process usually begins in (*a*) diaphysis;
    (*b*) metaphysis; (*c*) midshaft; (*d*) epiphysis.
9. In Hand-Schüller-Christian disease, the bone lesions are usually found in
    (*a*) hands and feet; (*b*) vertebrae; (*c*) pelvis; (*d*) ribs; (*e*) skull.
10. The younger the child at the time of onset the better the prognosis except for
    (*a*) Wilms's tumor; (*b*) acute leukemia; (*c*) neuroblastoma.
11. Remission in leukemia is judged best by (*a*) weight gain; (*b*) absence of fever;
    (*c*) elimination of leukemic cells from blood and marrow; (*d*) sedimentation
    rate; (*e*) none of the above.
12. To induce a remission in leukemia the best therapy is (*a*) prednisone; (*b*)
    prednisone plus an alkylating agent; (*c*) alkylating agent; (*d*) alkylating agent
    plus an antimetabolite.
13. Distant metastasis from brain tumors commonly include those to (*a*) bone;
    (*b*) lung; (*c*) abdominal viscera; (*d*) none.
14. Pseudotumor cerebri may be caused by the following except (*a*) vitamin A
    intoxication; (*b*) vitamin A deficiency; (*c*) tetracycline therapy; (*d*) head
    trauma; (*e*) dehydration.

The following questions are the matching type. In each blank in column I
insert the letter corresponding to the word or phrase in column II which is
associated most appropriately.

I		II	
15.	Hand-Schüller-Christian disease _____	(*a*)	Bone cysts
16.	Eosinophilic granuloma _____	(*b*)	Increased production of urine
17.	Letterer-Siwe disease _____	(*c*)	Eczema
18.	Teratoma _____	(*d*)	Hands and feet
19.	Ollier's disease _____	(*e*)	Sebaceous glands

24

ENDO-CRINE DISEASES

Hormones probably exert their effects on the body by accelerating or inhibiting enzyme systems. The synthesis of hormones from their precursors depends upon enzyme systems within the endocrine glands. Some endocrine disorders are caused by inborn errors of metabolism affecting these enzyme systems.

PITUITARY GLAND AND HYPOTHALAMUS

The pituitary gland (hypophysis) is a complex structure lying in a bony walled cavity, the sella turcica, in the sphenoid bone. The sella

EDITORS' NOTE: The section on Diabetes was prepared by Harold S. Cole.

turcica is separated superiorly from the cranial cavity by a tough reflection of dura mater, the diaphragma sella, through which the pituitary stalk and its attendant blood vessels reach the main body of the gland. The pituitary gland is formed by two distinct parts, an anterior portion and a posterior portion.

ANTERIOR PITUITARY (Adenohypophysis)

This portion of the pituitary gland originates from the buccal cavity (Rathke's pouch) and constitutes 75 percent of the total weight of the gland. The adenohypophysis acts as a control center for most of the endocrine system. It is in turn regulated both through the nervous system and by the level of circulating hormones of the "target" glands (thyroid gland, adrenal cortex, and gonads). The nervous system influences the rate of secretion of the pituitary tropic hormones through release of neurohumoral factors. These secretions, which contain tropin-releasing factors, originate in the hypothalamus and pass through the portal vessels to the adenohypophysis, where they cause the release of the tropic hormones. Hypothalamic releasing factors have been described for corticotropin (ACTH), thyrotropin, and gonadotropic hormones.

Seven hormones are known to be secreted by the anterior pituitary:

1. Thyrotropin (TSH): stimulates thyroid gland activity.
2. Adrenocorticotropin (ACTH): controls gluconeogenic and androgenic hormones of the adrenal cortex.
3. Follicle-stimulating hormone (FSH): causes maturation of graafian follicles in females and development of seminiferous tubules in males.
4. Luteinizing hormone (LH): causes ovulation and formation of the corpus luteum in females. In males (may be called interstitial cell–stimulating hormone—ICSH) it controls androgen secretion of the testicles.
5. Prolactin or luteotropic hormone (LTH): maintains the corpus luteum and initiates lactation; has no known function in the male.
6. Melanocyte-stimulating hormone (MSH): stimulates pigment formation.
7. Growth hormone (somatotropic hormone—STH): causes growth of tissues, increases protein anabolism, and increases mobilization of fatty acids from adipose tissue.

POSTERIOR PITUITARY (Neurohypophysis)

This part of the pituitary gland originates from the floor of the diencephalon. It is now generally accepted that the neurohypophyseal hormones originate in the supraoptic and paraventricular nuclei of the anterior hypothalamus. The hormones then migrate within and along the axons of the supraopticohypophyseal tract to the axon terminals within the posterior pituitary, which functions as a storage-release center rather than as a gland of internal secretion. The neurohypophyseal hormones are:

1. Oxytocin: stimulates uterine contraction and participates in the regulation of lactation.
2. Vasopressin (antidiuretic hormone—ADH): promotes renal tubular water reabsorption and stimulates smooth-muscle contraction of the blood vessels and gastrointestinal tract.

Pituitary gland diseases and brain lesions in the area of the hypothalamus give rise to a number of clinical syndromes in which certain similar manifestations occur.

PITUITARY ADENOMAS

Craniopharyngioma (suprasellar cyst) This adenoma arises from the craniopharyngeal duct and usually lies above the sella. In a majority of cases, a roentgenogram of the skull reveals areas of calcification, destruction of clinoid processes, and a flat sella turcica.

Clinical findings
1. Onset is usually before 15 years of age.
2. Visual symptoms, e.g., diplopia, and neurologic signs, e.g., papilledema are common.
3. Involvement of the hypothalamic center causes obesity, which may or may not be associated with diabetes insipidus and sexual infantilism (Froehlich's syndrome or dystrophia adiposogenitalis). Diabetes insipidus may occur alone, or obesity may be the only symptom. In other cases, there may be signs only of deficiency of anterior pituitary function, such as hypopituitary dwarfism and sexual infantilism.
4. Simmond's disease with pituitary cachexia has resulted from craniopharyngiomas.
5. Prolonged somnolence and disturbance of temperature regulation have been described.

Treatment The treatment is surgical removal of the tumor, which is difficult because of its location. (Craniopharyngiomas are resistant to radiation.)

Pseudofroehlich's syndrome In obese prepuberal boys, the pubic fat pad covers the genitalia, giving a false impression that the penis is small. These boys require only reassurance since they grow normally and have no lesion of the pituitary or hypothalamic glands.

Eosinophilic (acidophilic) adenoma Increased growth-hormone production by the tumor causes either gigantism (if it occurs before epiphyseal fusion has taken place) or acromegaly (if it takes place after fusion). It is very rare during childhood, and the onset of excessive growth usually occurs during adolescence. Eosinophilic adenomas rarely attain a sufficiently large size during childhood to compress the optic chiasma. Accordingly, defects in the visual fields usually are not found. Serum growth hormone levels are high and not suppressed following administration of glucose. Serum-phosphorus level is elevated.

Treatment   Surgical removal is difficult and is accompanied by a high mortality rate. Irradiation has been used with some success.

Basophilic adenoma   This may be associated with Cushing's syndrome. However, it is frequently found on postmortem examination in individuals with no evidence of Cushing's disease. Basophilic adenomas are usually small and do not cause enlargement of the sella or ophthalmologic symptoms.

Chromophobe adenoma   This is rare in childhood. The tumor grows upward, compressing the optic chiasma and extending into the third ventricle. The tumor may destroy the adjacent portion of the gland. Accordingly, it may cause visual (bitemporal hemianopsia), hypothalamic, and endocrine disturbances. Chromophobe adenomas have been associated with Cushing's syndrome and acromegaly and have occurred following adrenalectomy for Cushing's syndrome.

SIMMONDS' DISEASE (Panhypopituitarism)

This condition is due to a destructive lesion of the anterior pituitary gland. The disease is associated with a deficiency in thyroid, adrenocortical, and gonadal function and is characterized by asthenia, loss of weight, intolerance to cold, amenorrhea in females, loss of libido and impotence in males, loss of axillary and pubic hair, hypotension, and hypoglycemia.

Treatment   Treatment is directed toward the relief of signs and symptoms—cortisone, thyroid hormone, and sex steroids have been recommended. Salt-retaining hormones are usually not necessary.

Prognosis   The prognosis is good.

PINEAL TUMORS (See Chapter 23, "Tumors of Infancy and Childhood")

ENCEPHALITIS AND MENINGITIS

These conditions have been known to cause various hypothalamic symptoms, e.g., sexual precocity or infantilism.

CONGENITAL DEFECTS OF THE HYPOTHALAMUS

Such defects may cause various symptoms, depending on their location.

LAURENCE–MOON–BIEDL SYNDROME

This is a rare heredofamilial syndrome transmitted as an autosomal recessive trait and characterized by obesity, hypogonadism, acrocephaly, mental deficiency, retinitis pigmentosa, and syndactyly or polydactyly. Incomplete forms may occur. There is no treatment.

ALBRIGHT'S SYNDROME (McCune-Albright Syndrome)

This condition is characterized by unilateral skin pigmentation, polyostotic fibrous dysplasia, and sexual precocity. It occurs more commonly in females and is probably due to a congenital anomaly of the hypothalamus. There is no treatment.

PITUITARY DWARFISM

See Dwarfism, below.

DIABETES INSIPIDUS

Diabetes insipidus is caused by a deficiency of vasopressin (antidiuretic hormone—ADH, see p. 631). There are three types:

1. Organic: transient postoperative; posttrauma; postinfectious, e.g., encephalitis; tumors, e.g., neoplasm arising from the third ventricle; xanthomatosis, e.g., Hand-Schüller-Christian disease
2. Nephrogenic: failure of the renal tubule to respond to normally secreted ADH (caused by sex-linked dominant gene; may be associated with mental retardation)
3. Idiopathic

Clinical features

1. Polyuria (enuresis may be the first symptom).
2. Polydipsia.
3. Fatigue, irritability, sleep disturbance.
4. In infants there may be excessive crying, dehydration, and circulatory collapse.

This condition must be differentiated from renal diseases, e.g., polycystic kidney; psychogenic polydipsia; salt-losing adrenogenital syndrome; and diabetes mellitus.

Laboratory findings

1. Increased 24-hour urine volume (5 to 10 liters), low specific gravity (1.001 to 1.007).

2. Levels of serum sodium and chlorine may be elevated.
3. Hypertonic saline infusion test: sodium chloride 2.5% is given intravenously (Hicky-Hare test). In normal persons or in those with psychogenic polydipsia there is marked reduction of urine volume; there is no response in the patient with true diabetes insipidus or nephrogenic diabetes insipidus.
4. Pitressin test: aqueous pitressin 0.1 unit is given intravenously. In the patient with diabetes insipidus there is a reduction of urinary volume and increased specific gravity in half an hour. Patients with the renal type of diabetes insipidus do not respond to the pitressin test.

Treatment   In organic diabetes insipidus, pitressin tannate in oil (0.5 to 1.0 ml) is given intramuscularly, every 2 to 3 days to control polyuria. Lysine vasopressin is available as a nasal spray. Overdose with pitressin causes water intoxication with restlessness, mental confusion, poor muscle coordination, nausea, vomiting, and convulsions. Death may result.

Adequate amounts of water should be given to those with nephrogenic and idiopathic types of diabetes insipidus.

THYROID DISORDERS

Hypothyroidism is far more frequent during childhood than hyperthyroidism, and it is the endocrine disorder most commonly observed in childhood.

Ingested iodine is transported in the blood as iodide anion, which is converted back to iodine by an oxidase in the thyroid gland. The iodine combines with tyrosine to form monoiodotyrosine and diiodotyrosine, which become, through the action of a coupling enzyme, triiodothyronine (T_3) and thyroxin (tetraiodothyronine). Thyroxin, when bound to globulin, forms thyroglobulin (colloid), which is stored in the thyroid gland. Proteolytic enzymes in the thyroid gland act on the large thyroglobulin molecules to form thyroxin, which is secreted. The plasma thyroxin is bound to several carrier proteins. The primary carrier is a specific inter-alpha globulin glycoprotein.

Thyroid gland activity is stimulated by thyrotropic hormone (TSH) secreted by the anterior pituitary gland, which in turn is regulated by the amount of circulating thyroid hormone. TSH is not normally transmitted through the placenta, while the passage of thyroxin is slow and incomplete. Iodides and antithyroid drugs (thiouracil derivatives) are transmitted to the fetus and could be a cause of congenital goiter. Antithyroid drugs may also be secreted in the milk.

Hypothyroidism may be either congenital or acquired.

CONGENITAL HYPOTHYROIDISM (Congenital Cretinism)

1. Agenesis or dysgenesis of the thyroid gland (athyreotic cretinism). (Some cases may be due to maternal autoimmunization.)
2. Defective hormonogenesis:
   a. Inborn enzymatic defect.
   b. Lack of maternal dietary iodine (endemic cretinism).
   c. Congenital goiter, due to maternal ingestion of goitrogens.

ACQUIRED HYPOTHYROIDISM

1. "Idiopathic"—possibly due to autoimmunization.
2. Thyroidectomy for thyrotoxicosis, lingual thyroid, or carcinoma. Thyroid carcinoma may follow x-ray irradiation of the thymus or tonsils during infancy and early childhood. Any hard irregular nodule of the thyroid in a child must be considered malignant until proved otherwise by microscopic examination. These tumors metastasize to the cervical lymph nodes, lungs, and bones.
3. Thyroiditis or other infiltrative process: chronic lymphocytic thyroiditis or Hashimoto's disease is the most common type of thyroiditis and occurs frequently in childhood. It may be related to autoimmunization.
4. Ingestion of antithyroid agent.
5. TSH deficiency: either isolated or due to panhypopituitarism.

Clinical features

1. Cretinism may not become apparent clinically until 2 or 3 months after birth, because the mother's thyroid hormone has been supplied to the infant until birth.
2. Physical findings: dry, cool, thick (myxedema of subcutaneous tissue) skin that appears mottled; coarse, brittle hair that grows down onto the forehead; seborrhea of the scalp; stunted growth; delayed and defective dentition; infantile facial configuration and infantile skeletal proportions; lordosis; coxa vera; protruding abdomen and poor muscle tone (constipation and umbilical hernia are common); poor peripheral circulation and subnormal body temperature with intolerance to cold; moderate overweight; prolonged relaxation phase of tendon reflexes (hung-up reflex).
3. Retarded growth, both developmental and emotional, which may not be severe in early infancy.
4. Mental retardation—if thyroid deficiency begins after 6 years of age, mental development is not retarded although reactions may be sluggish.

Differential diagnosis   The disease should be differentiated from mongolism and other causes of mental or physical retardation, e.g., pituitary dwarfism, osteogenesis imperfecta, achondroplasia; amyotonia congenita; lipodystrophy (Hurler's syndrome); and glycogen-storage disease.

Laboratory findings

1. Bone development: roentgenograms reveal late appearance of the ossification centers, with punctate epiphyseal dysgenesis and late closure of the fontanels. A delay in the appearance of ossification centers may be caused by other factors, e.g., nutritional deficiency or pituitary dwarfism. The finding of epiphyseal dysgenesis is therefore an additional significant finding. On roentgenograms, either several foci of ossification are seen at the epiphysis instead of the usual single center, or if these several foci have coalesced, they have a moth-eaten appearance instead of the normal smooth outline (a roentgenographic picture similar to that seen in osteochondritis or chondrodystrophy). In early infancy, these changes are seen best in the cuboid bone or at the epiphyseal centers near the knee joint.

2. Serum-cholesterol level: usually elevated (275 to 600 mg per 100 ml) but may be normal, particularly in infants.

3. Urinary creatine to creatinine ratio is decreased, alkaline phosphatase level is decreased, fasting blood-sugar level is low, and plasma-carotene level is increased (abnormality in conversion of carotene to vitamin A).

4. Protein-bound iodine (PBI): measures organic as well as inorganic iodine in the blood. Normal PBI levels are 4.0 to 8.0 micrograms per 100 ml. During the first 2 months of life the PBI level may be much higher (5.6 to 14.0 micrograms per 100 ml). PBI is low in hypothyroidism.

    Butanol-extractable iodine (BEI): measures only organic iodine compounds in the blood. (Normal BEI level is 3.5 to 7 micrograms per 100 ml.) The level is low in hypothyroidism. This test is not influenced by ingestion of inorganic iodides, but it is affected by contamination with exogenous organic iodine.

5. Serum thyroxine (T_4): values (normal—4 to 11 micrograms per 100 ml) are not influenced by substances of clinical importance.

6. Radioactive iodine (I^{131}) uptake and conversion ratio are of value in studying the enzyme deficiency type of hypothyroidism (I^{131} uptake is substantial or increased in all types of defective hormonogenesis except that due to enzymatic inability of the gland to trap iodide) and in differentiating primary hypothyroidism from secondary hypothyroidism of pituitary origin (by determination of I^{131} uptake before and after TSH stimulation). In normal persons, 10 to 40 percent of the administered dose (I^{131} dose is 0.5 to 1.0 microcuries per kg body weight) is retained by the thyroid at the end of 24 hours. Uptake is low or absent in the "athyrotic" type of hypothyroidism.

7. Erythrocyte uptake of radioactive triiodothyronine is a reliable

test in the absence of nephrosis. Normal uptake of triiodothyronine is 16.5 percent. In hypothyroidism, triiodothyronine uptake is less than 13 percent.

When the diagnosis is difficult to make, a therapeutic test is helpful. If the child has hypothyroidism, there should be rapid clinical improvement when thyroid hormone is administered. The serum-cholesterol level is decreased, and creatinuria is increased. In 2 to 4 months accelerated bone growth should be evident. Withdrawal of the therapy causes a regression and rise of serum cholesterol to high levels in 2 weeks to 2 months.

Treatment   Thyroid hormone—substitution therapy using desiccated thyroid extract, starting with ¼ gr (15 mg) once a day for infants and ½ gr (30 mg) once a day for older children. The dosage is increased on the basis of PBI or BEI determinations about every 3 weeks. Cretins under 2 years of age often require 1 to 2 gr (0.06 to 0.12 Gm) a day, older children, 2 to 3 gr (0.12 to 0.18 Gm) a day. Sodium L-thyroxin (0.1 mg is equivalent to 100 mg desiccated thyroid) may also be used; triiodothyronine is started at 25 micrograms daily and may be increased at weekly intervals to 75 to 100 micrograms. Triiodothyronine is used for acquired hypothyroidism.

The effectiveness of treatment is judged clinically by:

1.   The disappearance of the clinical deficiency pattern.
2.   Increased growth as evidenced by measurement of height and appearance of new ossification centers.
3.   Laboratory determinations of BEI (should be kept at 5 to 7 micrograms per 100 ml levels) or PBI (kept at 4.5 to 8 micrograms per 100 ml with desiccated thyroid, 10 to 15 micrograms per 100 ml with sodium L-thyroxin; but with triiodothyronine, patients may be euthyroid at 2 to 3 micrograms per 100 ml).

Overdosage is indicated by:

1.   Marked excitability and insomnia
2.   Polyuria
3.   Tachycardia
4.   Hypertension
5.   Abdominal symptoms: vomiting, diarrhea, and pain

Prognosis   For physical growth and development, prognosis is usually good when therapy is begun early. It is guarded for mental development even when treatment is started early; if started after 12 months of age, most cretins will not reach normal intelligence. In acquired hypothyroidism, there is an excellent prognosis for mental development.

HYPERTHYROIDISM

Hyperfunction is due to:

1. Toxic adenoma: increased hormone production by tumor tissue, rare before 20 years of age and usually without exophthalmos (Plummer's disease)
2. Diffuse toxic goiter: increased production of hormone due to an overactive thyroid gland and frequently associated with exophthalmos (Graves's disease)

The cause of thyrotoxic goiter remains unknown. TSH levels in the plasma are generally normal, while plasma levels of a long-acting, TSH-like substance (long-acting thyroid stimulator, or LATS) may be increased. The plasma titer of LATS (extrapituitary in origin) correlates more closely with the degree of exophthalmos than with the severity of the thyrotoxicosis. In children, hyperthyroidism is more common during early adolescence, and there is often spontaneous regression following this period of rapid growth and stress. Females are affected more often than males.

Clinical features

1. Young children are not likely to complain of subjective symptoms, e.g., palpitation, heat intolerance, weakness, or tremor.
2. The most common early findings are excessive activity and emotional instability.
3. Fine tremors of the hands, which are noticeable when fingers are extended.
4. Tachycardia; increased systolic pressure with increased pulse pressure; flushing of the cheeks; warm, moist skin, especially of the palms.
5. Diffuse, firm enlargement of the thyroid; bruits and thrills over the gland.
6. Exophthalmos: may be unilateral or bilateral. Malignant exophthalmos is very rare.
7. Accelerated growth, weight loss even though appetite is good. Vomiting and diarrhea in one-third of cases.
8. Thyroid crisis (less common than in adults): high fever, vomiting. diarrhea, restlessness, prostration, and sometimes death.

Laboratory findings

1. Elevated BMR: higher than +20.
2. Increased creatinuria and increased creatine-to-creatinine ratio.
3. Low serum-cholesterol level.
4. PBI (most reliable and specific if patient is not given iodine previously), BEI, and T_4—elevated.

5. I^{131} uptake—rapid; administration of triiodothyronine fails to suppress I^{131} uptake.
6. Erythrocyte uptake of radioactive triiodothyronine is over 20 percent.

Differential diagnosis Hyperthyroidism must be differentiated from chorea and from rheumatic heart disease.

Treatment

1. Medical treatment consisting of antithyroid drugs, e.g., propylthiouracil, Tapazole, or potassium perchlorate, should be tried and will result in a permanent remission in a majority of patients. Treatment with propylthiouracil is begun with 300 mg per day (100 mg three times a day). When the patient becomes euthyroid (2 to 4 months), the dosage of propylthiouracil is reduced gradually to 100 mg per day (50 mg twice a day) as maintenance therapy for a period of at least 2 years. Patients should be examined frequently for drug reactions, e.g., rash, unexplained fever, lymphadenopathy, splenomegaly, and leukopenia. Unless the drug reactions are severe, treatment is continued, and usually the reactions subside in several weeks. Granulocytopenia and buccal ulcerations usually respond well to treatment with adrenal corticosteroids. During drug therapy the thyroid gland may become progressively enlarged. Desiccated thyroid (2 to 3 gr per day), in addition to the propylthiouracil, will cause a rapid decrease in its size.
2. Surgical treatment: in severe cases surgery is usually necessary. Preoperactive preparation is carried out with iodine (Lugol's solution, gtt 5 to 10 per day) and antithyroid drugs. Following surgery, patients should be observed for signs and symptoms of hypothyroidism.
3. Radioactive iodine treatment is not used in children because of its possible carcinogenic effect.

DWARFISM

A child is a dwarf if he is 5 cm or more shorter than 90 percent of children of the same chronologic age.

Etiology

1. Nutritional disorders: chronic malnutrition secondary to chronic infection, celiac syndrome, chronic renal disease
2. Metabolic disorders: Hurler's disease, glycogen-storage disease, galactosemia, idiopathic infantile hypercalcemia
3. Disorders resulting in chronic hypoxia: congenital heart disease

with cyanosis, chronic pulmonary disease interfering with oxygenation of the blood, chronic hemolytic anemias
4. Bone disorders: chondrodystrophies, rickets, tuberculosis of the spine, and osteogenesis imperfecta
5. Endocrine disorders: hypothyroidism, sexual precocity with early epiphyseal fusion, hypopituitarism, gonadal dysgenesis with stunted growth
6. Genetic: familial, sporadic (primordial dwarf)
7. Dwarfism associated with brain damage and severe mental retardation
8. Delayed adolescence and its associated growth spurt
9. Unknown causes: progeria

All these causes except the following have been discussed under the primary condition.

DELAYED ADOLESCENCE AND ASSOCIATED GROWTH SPURT

This is the most frequent cause of dwarfism and is probably due to a delay in the activation of the pituitary-gonadal-adrenal system. Although these patients usually have normal birth weights, they fail to show the normal spurt of growth and sexual development at the usual time during early teens. Epiphyseal development is delayed 2 to 4 years. However, there is no specific defect of any gland, and such patients eventually mature normally. No treatment is necessary except emotional support during the period of growth delay.

PRIMORDIAL DWARFISM

Genetically transmitted, this condition is more often sporadic than familial.

Clinical features

1. Infants are small at birth.
2. Growth is slow from infancy.
3. Skeletal proportions are normal.
4. Facial features are mature.
5. Sexual development is normal.

Laboratory findings

1. PBI and urinary excretion of 17-hydroxycorticoids, 17-ketosteroids, and FSH are normal.
2. Epiphyseal ossification and fusion are in keeping with the chronologic age. (Not infrequently there is wide "scattering" of the development of the different epiphyseal centers.)

Treatment There is none available. Prognosis for offspring is good, since they may be normal.

PITUITARY DWARFISM

This type of dwarfism is difficult to diagnose during childhood.

Etiology

1. Organic lesions of the pituitary gland: rarely dwarfism may be caused by a tumor, e.g., craniopharyngioma or optic chiasm glioma
2. Hormonal deficiency without a demonstrable anatomic lesion: deficiency of growth hormone, either isolated or associated with a deficiency of other pituitary hormones

Clinical features

1. Normal size at birth; growth normal during the first year, then continuing at a very slow rate.
2. Skeletal proportions are normal.
3. Normal thyroid function unless associated with TSH deficiency.
4. Possible hypoglycemic attacks because of a deficiency of gluconeogenetic factors of the adrenal.
5. Absence of sexual hair as the child grows older because of a deficiency of adrenal androgens.
6. Failure of sexual development and absence of secondary sex characteristics because of FSH deficiency.
7. Immature features and poor musculature.

Laboratory findings

1. Roentgenogram reveals delay in appearance of ossification centers and epiphyseal fusion (epiphyseal line may remain open indefinitely); delayed calcification of ossification centers.
2. Decreased urinary excretion of 17-hydroxycorticosteroids and 17-ketosteroids (less than 2 mg per 24 hours—significant after 12 years of age). Response to Metopirone (adrenal blocking test) may be defective. However, true Addisonian symptoms with evidence of failure of the electrolyte-regulating factors are not encountered.
3. FSH decreased in the urine (less than 6 mouse units per 24 hours —excretion significant after 12 years of age).
4. Low PBI, increased blood-cholesterol level, and diminished I^{131} uptake if there is a TSH deficiency.
5. Buccal smear: a normal sex chromatin body pattern differentiates this condition from gonadal dysgenesis during the early years of life.
6. Increased insulin sensitivity and low serum growth hormone level which does not increase during insulin hypoglycemia. (Insulintolerance test should be performed with caution using a maximum

of 0.05 unit per kg of body weight and with intravenous glucose readily available—see p. 666.)

Treatment   The treatment of dwarfism depends upon its cause.

1. In the constitutional pattern of slow growth and delayed adolescence, the subjects mature into normal adults without therapy. If onset of puberty has not occurred by the age of 14, acceleration of the process may be obtained with chorionic gonadotropin (2,000 to 4,000 units twice weekly for 3 to 6 months). The use of chorionic gonadotropin is not recommended in females because it causes cystic changes in the ovaries.
2. In pituitary dwarfism the administration of human growth hormone has resulted in significant acceleration of growth. Androgenic steroids may also accelerate growth in these subjects. However, because of premature epiphyseal closure, they may decrease the height these patients would ultimately have attained. Androgenic steroids are nevertheless of value in male subjects after they have reached the age when virilization is desirable. Methyltestosterone, 10 to 20 mg per day, orally, or long-acting testosterone cyclopentylpropionate by injection once a month should be given. In females, estrogens (stilbestrol, 1 mg daily) as well as androgens should be administered.

PROGERIA

A rare, nonfamilial syndrome of unknown causation, progeria starts in infancy or early childhood; growth ceases and the epiphyses fuse. The condition is manifested by premature aging, absence of hair, large head size, birdlike facies, severe mental retardation, arteriosclerosis, and early death. No treatment is available.

SEXUAL INFANTILISM

Sexual infantilism should be differentiated from delayed adolescence (the start of adolescence normally may be delayed until 17 years of age).

Etiology

1. Hypothalamic (neurogenic) (see Froehlich's Syndrome)
2. Pituitary (see Pituitary Dwarfism, above)
3. Gonadal: gonadal dysgenesis (Turner's syndrome), testicular dysgenesis (Klinefelter's syndrome), prepuberal castration

GONADAL DYSGENESIS (Turner's Syndrome)

Dwarfism with a congenital dysgenesis of the gonads may be associated with other congenital malformations, such as webneck, coarctation of the aorta, deafness, eye-muscle defects, shieldlike chest, cubitus valgus, lymphedema of the extremities (Bonnevie-Ulrich type), and mental retardation. Other features include failure to develop secondary sex characteristics except sexual hair (which develops normally), and infertility. Most of these patients have a female phenotype.

Laboratory findings

1. Epiphyseal ossification and fusion are usually slightly delayed.
2. FSH excretion in the urine is high after the age of puberty.
3. The majority of these subjects have a chromatin-negative nuclear pattern. Chromosomal count of cells from tissue culture usually reveals 45 chromosomes, the sex chromosome pattern being XO rather than XY (see p. 124). Mosaicism is occasionally encountered. A small number of subjects have positive sex chromatin smears. In this group, the congenital defects are much less obvious and less frequent.

There have been a number of reports of phenotypic males with somatic anomalies of Turner's syndrome and XY karyotypes. Usually testicular development and function are normal, but occasionally there is some type of testicular dysgenesis.

Treatment After 16 years of age, stilbestrol (1 mg per day) for 3 weeks of each month; during the third week, progesterone should also be given (10 to 30 mg per day) in an attempt to stimulate a normal ovarian cycle. No therapy is given during the fourth week.

KLINEFELTER'S SYNDROME

Clinical features

1. Eunuchoidism and obesity
2. Gynecomastia, reduced facial and abdominal hair
3. Small testicles, small prostate, azospermia, variable sexual hair, variable libido, and infertility
4. Mental retardation

Laboratory findings

1. Increased urinary FSH excretion.
2. Moderately low urinary 17-ketosteroid excretion.
3. Testicular biopsy reveals fibrosis, disappearance of Sertoli cells, and hyalinization of the seminiferous tubules. Leydig cells are well preserved.
4. Buccal smear for chromatin pattern: 80 percent of cases have positive chromatin pattern and 20 percent have negative chromatin pattern.

Chromosome count of cells from tissue cultures reveals 47 chromosomes with an XXY sex chromosome constitution or in some persons mosaicism.

Treatment   Androgen therapy should be directed toward developing male secondary sex characteristics. Psychologic support may be necessary.

SEXUAL PRECOCITY

Etiology

1. Idiopathic or constitutional: premature activation of the pituitary
2. Neurogenic: brain tumor, encephalitis, hamartoma of the tuber cinereum, or congenital defect of hypothalamus (McCune-Albright syndrome)
3. Gonadal: ovarian neoplasms (granulosa-cell tumors, luteomas or thecomas, teratomas, chorioepitheliomas) and endocrine tumors of the testes (Leydig cell tumors, teratomas)
4. Adrenal
5. Hepatomas: secretion of gonadotropic hormones by the tumor
6. Premature pubarche (sexual hair) and premature thelarche (breasts)

In the constitutional and neurogenic types, the precocious sexual development is always complete and resembles normal sexual development. In the adrenal and gonadal types, the sexual precocity is always incomplete, e.g., spermatogenesis or ovulation does not occur.

IDIOPATHIC OR CONSTITUTIONAL SEXUAL PRECOCITY

The vast majority of cases of sexual precocity are of this type.

Etiology   The etiology is unknown; probably related to premature activation of the pituitary gland. Genetic factors may be involved.

Clinical features

1. Sexual development is normal but starts early in life; procreation is possible.
2. Libido is present early, but the mental development is equal to the chronologic age.
3. Children with this disorder are tall in childhood but eventually are short adults because their epiphyses fuse early.

Laboratory findings

1. Spermatogenesis and ovulation occur.
2. Sex hormones are secreted in normal adolescent amounts; FSH is present in the urine.

3. Vaginal smear reveals estrinization of cells.
4. Roentgenograms show moderately advanced bone age.

Treatment   No treatment is necessary; the prognosis is excellent.

NEUROGENIC SEXUAL PRECOCITY

This is due to lesions of the hypothalamus, e.g., tumor (pineal), hamartoma of the tuber cinereum, congenital defect, cyst of the third ventricle, encephalitis. In addition to the precocious sexual development, there are neurologic symptoms and signs. Prognosis and treatment are unsatisfactory.

ADRENAL SEXUAL PRECOCITY

This is discussed further on in this chapter under Adrenogenital Syndrome.

GONADAL SEXUAL PRECOCITY

Precocious puberty of gonadal origin is usually due to a neoplasm.

Females

1. Granulosa-cell tumor of the ovary: there is a palpable abdominal tumor, premature sexual hair, and advanced osseous development and height; uterine bleeding may occur without ovulation, urinary estrogens are increased, and vaginal smear reveals estrinization of epithelium. Urinary FSH is usually absent. This tumor is of low-grade malignancy. Treatment is removal of the tumor; there may be recurrences.
2. Teratoma of the ovary.
3. Chorionepithelioma, luteoma, and thecoma are very rare.

Males

1. Interstitial-cell adenoma
2. Teratoma of the testicle

These tumors are manifested by unilateral testicular enlargement, premature sexual hair, advanced height and bone age, increase in urinary 17-ketosteroid excretion; there is no spermatogenesis, and urinary FSH is absent.

Treatment   Treatment consists of removal of the tumor.

PREMATURE THELARCHE

This refers to early development of the breasts without other secondary sex characteristics and may represent an end organ sensitivity to minute amounts of estrogenic hormones. In premature thelarche the nipples and areolae do not develop prematurely.

PREMATURE PUBARCHE

Development of sexual hair without other secondary sex characteristics may represent an end organ hypersensitivity to normal amounts of androgens. The only positive laboratory finding is slightly increased 17-ketosteroid excretion in the urine.

ABNORMAL SEX DIFFERENTIATION

In patients with abnormal sex differentiation, the gonads and external genitalia and/or the secondary sex characteristics are discordant. Such conditions may be classified as:

1. Congenital abnormal sex differentiation
2. Postnatal abnormal sex differentiation

Congenital types

1. True hermaphroditism: individuals with mixed gonads—the pattern of chromosomal constitution may be female (XX), male (XY), or mosaic.
2. Male pseudohermaphroditism: the gonads are testicles. External genitalia may resemble the male or the female; in the latter case, the condition is known as testicular feminization syndrome. Chromosomal constitution is usually male (XY).
3. Female pseudohermaphroditism: may be associated with adrenal hyperplasia and increased 17-ketosteroid excretion (see Adrenogenital Syndromes below) or following administration of androgenic agents to the mother during pregnancy. Chromosomal constitution is usually female (XX).

CRYPTORCHISM

Cryptorchism (undescended testes) is the arrest of one or both testes in their descent into the scrotum. (When bilateral, abnormal sex differentiation should be excluded.) The testes may descend spontaneously at any time until puberty. If descent does not occur, the involved testicle or testicles will become atrophic, sterile, and subject to malignant change. The treatment for cryptorchism varies in different clinics.

Some institute medical treatment early (3 to 6 years) for fear that delay may result in irreversible damage; others start later (just before puberty); and still others delay therapy in the hope that descent might occur spontaneously. (This happens not infrequently.) According to the latter group, orchiopexy occasions many needless operations, particularly in instances in which spontaneous descent would eventually occur. In addition, it is uncertain whether allowing the testes to remain undescended until early puberty constitutes a greater risk than the possibility of surgical injury. In any event, human chorionic gonadotropin (HCG) can be used to determine which testes will fail to descend because of anatomic obstructions. The usual dosage of HCG is 1,000 IU in two to three doses a week for 6 to 8 weeks or 4,000 IU three times a week for 2 to 3 weeks. Evidence of sexual precociousness is an indication for the immediate withdrawal of treatment. After regression of undue development, a reduced dosage regime may be resumed. If this is unsuccessful, surgery is indicated. When cryptorchism is complicated by hernia, early surgery should be performed.

ADRENAL CORTEX

The adrenal gland is composed of two parts: the medulla, which is ectodermal in origin and secretes epinephrine and norepinephrine; and the cortex, which is mesothelial in origin and arranged in three zones —zona glomerulosa, zona fasciculata, and zona reticularis (the zona reticularis is related to the fetal zone).

The functional level of the adrenal cortex is under the direct influence of the anterior pituitary hormone, adrenocorticotropin (ACTH). An increase in the level of adrenal corticosteroids results in a decreased ACTH secretion, and a decrease in adrenal hormones results in increased secretion of ACTH ("negative-feedback" mechanism). In addition to this mechanism, the adrenals are capable of responding to nervous stimuli. Stressful stimuli acting through the hypothalamus and pituitary gland cause the release of ACTH and subsequent secretion of adrenal steroids. It is of interest that large amounts of exogenous corticosteroids do not prevent the outpouring of ACTH as a result of surgical stress. Thus, under stress stimuli the pituitary-adrenal system acts independently of the negative-feedback mechanism. There is also a diurnal rhythm in adrenocortical secretion of hydrocortisone associated with diurnal release of ACTH. Plasma corticoids reach a maximum at about 6 or 8 A.M., after which there is a gradual decline to the lowest level between early evening and midnight.

Cortical hormones

1. Electrolyte-regulating hormone: aldosterone acts on the distal renal tubules to cause sodium retention and potassium loss. Desoxycorticosterone (DOCA) and 9-alpha-fluorohydrocortisone are synthetic products, and their actions are similar to those of aldosterone.
2. Carbohydrate-regulating steroids (21-carbon steroids) : hydrocortisone (17-hydroxycorticosterone, cortisol, or compound F) is the principal hormone secreted by the adrenal cortex; cortisone (11-dehydro-17-hydroxycorticosterone, or compound E), which is not secreted by the adrenal but is produced peripherally from cortisol,

has a similar action. These hormones cause deamination of amino acids and their conversion into carbohydrate (gluconeogenesis), thus sparing liver glycogen; decreased carbohydrate utilization; decreased protein anabolism; and retention of sodium and potassium loss. They also have anti-inflammatory effects which include lympholysis of lymphoid tissue and thymus, lowering of blood eosinophils and lymphocytes, suppression of inflammatory response to mechanical and chemical injury and to bacterial infection, and protection against the damage of antigen-antibody combination to body cells.

3. Androgens (19-carbon steroids, testosterone, androstenedione, dehydroepiandrosterone, adrenosterone) : cause the growth of sexual hair, increased protein anabolism, accelerated growth and osseous development, and hirsutism. Androgens are excreted as 17-ketosteroids.

Evaluation of the functional status of the adrenal cortex involves the use of a number of tests.

Water and electrolyte regulation

1. Serum electrolytes: adrenal insufficiency associated with a low sodium (<130 meq liter), high potassium (>6 meq liter) and low carbon dioxide (<20 meq liter). In hyperadrenocorticism or hyperaldosteronism there is retention of sodium and loss of potassium with the development of hypokalemic alkalosis. Electrocardiographic changes may reflect the serum-potassium level.
2. Sodium-potassium ratio in the urine, sweat, and saliva: on a fixed sodium and potassium intake, a high Na/K ratio (normal—32, expressed in milliequivalents) is suggestive of adrenal insufficiency.
3. Urinary sodium loss or low sodium intake: excessive loss of sodium, with a negative balance and a high Na/K ratio is diagnostic of adrenal insufficiency. A low-sodium diet may precipitate an adrenal crisis.

Glucocorticoid function

1. Carbohydrate metabolism: there is a tendency for low blood sugar in adrenal insufficiency associated with an increased sensitivity to insulin. The insulin-tolerance test, however, is dangerous and should not be used. In hyperadrenocorticism of the Cushing type a diabetic glucose-tolerance curve is frequently, but not always, found.
2. Water-load test: in adrenal insufficiency there is a delay in diuresis. Administration of cortisol corrects this defect.
3. Plasma and urinary 17-hydroxycorticoids (17-OHCS): normal— plasma, 10 to 15 micrograms per 100 ml; urine, 3.1 ± 1.1 mg per

24 hours per sq meter; cortisol secretory rate, 12 ± 2 mg per 24 hours per sq meter. ACTH stimulation test: 25 mg ACTH intravenously over 8 hours results in an increase in plasma 17-OHCS to 40 ± 6 micrograms per 100 ml at the eighth hour. In Addison's disease (adrenal insufficiency) there is no response to ACTH stimulation; in secondary hypoadrenalism due to pituitary insufficiency, ACTH stimulation will cause an increase in corticosteroid output.

4. Metopirone (adrenal blocking test) (see pp. 109, 641): 300 mg per sq meter orally every 4 hours for 24 hours normally results in an increase in urinary 17-OHCS to 2.5 to 6 times the resting level. In instances of secondary hypoadrenalism due to pituitary insufficiency there is no increase in urinary 17-OHCS.

5. Dexamethasone suppression test: administration of 1.25 mg per 100 lb of body weight reduces the urinary 17-OHCS to low levels in 3 days in normal subjects but not in Cushing's syndrome (adrenal hyperplasia or tumor). However, the daily administration of 3.75 mg of dexamethasone per 100 lb of body weight will suppress the urinary 17-OHCS excretion in Cushing's syndrome due to adrenal hyperplasia but not due to adrenal carcinoma.

ACUTE ADRENAL INSUFFICIENCY

More common than the chronic form in children. It may occur during the course of any severe septicemia or overwhelming infection, e.g., meningococcemia or diphtheria, following the abrupt withdrawal of adrenal corticosteroid therapy, as a result of congenital hypoplastic adrenal glands or congenital adrenogenital syndrome, or following adrenalectomy. (Adrenal hemorrhage in the newborn infant has been discussed in Chapter 12, "Diseases of the Newborn.")

Clinical features

1. Cold moist skin, often with purpuric or ecchymotic rash
2. Cyanosis
3. Rapid, thready pulse and a falling blood pressure
4. Rapid, labored respirations
5. Coma and possibly death

Laboratory findings

1. Decreased serum-sodium and serum-chloride levels
2. Increased serum-potassium level
3. Hypoglycemia

Treatment

1. Antibiotics and chemotherapy for the infection
2. Transfusion
3. Oxygen

4. Infusions (glucose 5% in saline solution) plus *l*-norepinephrine (Levophed), 4 ml to 1 liter
5. Hydrocortisone (intravenously)

Prognosis   The prognosis is grave.

CHRONIC ADRENAL INSUFFICIENCY (Addison's Disease)

This disease is rare in children.

Etiology   The cause is unknown in most cases. It may be due to tuberculosis or generalized fungous infections, or nontuberculous adrenal atrophy (? autoimmune disease).

Clinical features

1. Insidious onset, with anorexia, weight loss, asthenia, and general debility; or acute onset, with profuse diarrhea, abdominal pain, vomiting, convulsions and coma
2. Generalized pigmentation of the skin and mucous membranes
3. Hypotension and decreased heart size

Laboratory findings

1. Serum-sodium and -chloride levels are decreased and serum-potassium level is increased (ECG changes of hyperpotassemia).
2. Acidosis, increased hematocrit, and elevated blood–urea nitrogen level.
3. Water-load test: if it is negative, Addison's disease is unlikely.
4. ACTH-stimulation test: 17-hydroxycorticosteroid level does not rise following ACTH administration.
5. Blood and urinary 17-hydroxycorticosteroids: low.
6. Hypoglycemia and flat glucose-tolerance curve.
7. Roentgenogram of the abdomen may reveal calcified areas in the region of the adrenal glands.

Treatment

1. The acute abdominal episodes are treated in the same manner as acute adrenal insufficiency.
2. Chronic insufficiency is treated with a maintenance dose of cortisone acetate, 25 to 37.5 mg daily (20 to 25 mg daily hydrocortisone) in two divided doses; 9-fluorocortisol (Florinef), 0.05 to 0.2 mg once a day; and normal daily sodium intake (3 to 6 Gm). During periods of stress the cortisone dosage should be increased to 50 to 100 mg daily, (Overdose with adrenal corticosteroids may result in excessive sodium retention, edema, hypertension, convulsion, cardiac failure, and muscle weakness due to hypokalemia.)

Prognosis   Good.

SECONDARY ADRENAL INSUFFICIENCY DUE TO HYPOPITUITARISM

This condition may be differentiated from primary hypoadrenalism by ACTH stimulation test (see Chronic Adrenal Insufficiency).

This type of adrenal insufficiency is usually associated with deficiencies of other tropic hormones, e.g., TSH, FSH.

HYPERACTIVITY OF THE ADRENAL CORTEX

1. Adrenogenital syndrome
2. Cushing's syndrome
3. Primary hyperaldosteronism
4. Feminizing adrenal tumors

Adrenogenital syndrome   The postnatal type may be due to adrenal hyperplasia or tumor. The congenital type is due to bilateral hyperplasia of the adrenal cortex and is strongly familial. It is probably inherited as an autosomal recessive trait.

Pathogenesis of the various types of adrenogenital syndrome   Congenital adrenogenital syndrome is due to one of several enzymatic defects in the biosynthesis of hydrocortisone. Associated with the impaired production of hydrocortisone there occurs an excessive accumulation of various of its precursors, many of which are androgenic and result in virilism. In a compensatory attempt to supply the physiologic requirements of hydrocortisone, the pituitary secretes large amounts of ACTH. Stimulation by ACTH brings about adrenal hyperplasia, but also increases the production of androgen and other steroids such as 17α-hydroxyprogesterone (excreted in urine as pregnanetriol), and in some patients it causes hyperpigmentation similar to that in Addison's disease. The most common cause of virilizing adrenal hyperplasia is due to a C-21-hydroxylase defect. Approximately one-third of this group have a salt-losing syndrome associated with vascular collapse and early death, unless vigorously treated with mineralocorticoids and hydrocortisone. The salt-losing defect is due to an associated defect in aldosterone biosynthesis. C-11-hydroxylase defect is characterized, in addition to virilism, by an increase in 11-desoxycortisol (compound S), which has little biologic effect, and 11-desoxycorticosterone, which is a potent mineralocorticoid and leads to hypertension.

3β-hydroxysteroid dehydrogenase defect is a rare cause of adrenal virilism. There is profound adrenocortical insufficiency with sodium loss, collapse, and early death. Other rare enzyme defects include congenital lipoid adrenal hyperplasia and 17-hydroxylase deficiency.

The clinical features differ in males and females:

Females with congenital adrenogenital syndrome (pseudohermaphroditism)

1. Abnormal genitalia at birth: enlarged clitoris, labioscrotal fusion, urogenital sinus

2. Internal genitalia: normal ovaries, fallopian tubes, and uterus
3. Accelerated growth, osseous development, early epiphyseal fusion
4. Precocious appearance of sexual hair, masculine muscular development, deep voice, small or absent breasts, and in untreated cases primary amenorrhea
5. Failure to thrive, dehydration, and acute adrenal crisis during early infancy associated with salt-losing crisis

Postnatal adrenal hyperplasia or tumor causes virilism. This is associated with an enlarged clitoris but without urogenital abnormalities.

Women taking progesterone, synthetic progestins, or testosterone during their pregnancy may give birth to a female with an enlarged clitoris. It does not continue to grow abnormally, however, and these infants do not have increased 17-ketosteroid excretion.

Males with congenital adrenogenital syndrome (macrogenitosomia praecox)
1. At birth the male infants usually show no obvious abnormalities except for occasional Addisonian-like pigmentation. Later there is a large penis with frequent erections and a large prostate gland; the testes remain of normal prepuberal size.
2. Precocious development of secondary sex characteristics: acne, deep voice, sexual hair.
3. Accelerated growth and osseous development, well-developed muscles, early epiphyseal fusion.
4. Salt-losing type: same as in females (see above).

Laboratory findings (male and female)
1. Urinary 17-ketosteroids: increased.
2. ACTH-stimulation test: no response of 17-hydroxycorticosteroids (C-21-hydroxylase defect).
3. Buccal smear is helpful in determining the genetic sex of the individual.
4. Increased urinary pregnanetriol in congenital adrenogenital syndrome, increased dehydroepiandrosterone in adrenal tumors.
5. Roentgenograms reveal advanced bone age.
6. In salt-losing type, decreased serum-sodium level, serum-chloride level, and plasma-CO_2 content, increased serum-potassium level.
7. Therapeutic test: Dexamethasone, 3.75 mg per 100 lb body weight, daily for 7 days, causes a marked fall in urinary 17-ketosteroids in congenital adrenal hyperplasia. No response is found in adrenal tumors.

Treatment
1. For adrenocortical tumor producing virilism—surgical removal.
2. For congenital adrenal hyperplasia—cortisone in small maintenance doses to suppress the oversecretion of ACTH by the pituitary gland. The urinary excretion of 17-ketosteroids is decreased and

the level may be used as a guide to the individual child's dosage requirement.
3. In females, plastic surgery of the genitalia (best performed by 5 years of age) may be necessary.
4. In the salt-losing type, 9α-fluorocortisol (Florinef) and salt are added. Later, salt-retaining hormones may not be necessary as the child ingests normal quantities of salt. However, the salt-losing defect persists indefinitely.
5. Psychologic care and guidance for the child and family.

Prognosis The prognosis is good if treatment is begun early.
If treatment is begun sufficiently early (before 2 to 3 years of age), no secondary sex characteristics appear until the usual age.

Cushing's syndrome This is due to hypersecretion of hydrocortisone by the adrenal cortex associated with adrenal hyperplasia or tumor (adenoma or carcinoma).

Clinical features Symptoms vary, depending on the type of adrenal hormones that are being produced in excessive amounts.

1. Hypersecretion of gluconeogenic hormones causes decreased protein anabolism, osteoporosis, muscle weakness, capillary fragility (red striae), retarded growth, obesity, moon facies, buffalo hump, and diabetic glucose tolerance.
2. Hypersecretion of electrolyte-regulating hormones causes hypertension, increased blood volume, increased serum sodium and decreased serum potassium.
3. Hypersecretion of androgen causes hirsutism and acne. Severe virilism is usually associated with adrenal carcinoma.

Laboratory findings
1. Urinary 17-hydroxycorticosteroid excretion is increased whether due to tumor or to hyperplasia. Urinary 17-ketosteroid excretion is moderately increased in adrenal hyperplasia, low in adrenal adenoma, and markedly increased in adrenal carcinoma.
2. Daily administration of 3.75 mg dexamethasone per 100 pounds body weight suppresses elevated levels of urinary 17-OHCS in adrenal hyperplasia but not in adrenal tumor.
3. Diabetic glucose-tolerance curve and insulin resistance. Increased serum-sodium, decreased serum-potassium levels.
4. Roentgenograms reveal osteoporosis.

Treatment Surgical removal of the tumor. In the treatment of Cushing's syndrome with adrenal hyperplasia, pituitary irradiation may be used. If there is no response, bilateral adrenalectomy is performed. Pituitary tumor occasionally develops after this procedure. o,p'-DDD shows promise as an antiadrenal agent in nontumorous Cushing's syndrome.

Primary aldosteronism (Conn's disease)   Aldosterone is the main electrolyte-regulating hormone of the adrenal cortex. Secretion of aldosterone is not regulated by the pituitary gland, but rather by sodium intake, serum-potassium level, and blood volume. (Normal secretory rate of aldosterone in the adult is 50 to 150 micrograms daily.) Increased aldosterone secretion is found in primary and secondary hyperaldosteronism. Secondary hyperaldosteronism occurs in conditions such as nephrosis, hepatic failure, cardiac failure with edema, and hypopotassemic periodic familial paralysis.

Primary aldosteronism is generally due to an adrenal tumor.

Symptoms are muscle weakness, paresthesias, periodic paralysis, hypertension, edema (usually not present despite hypernatremia), and tetany due to alkalosis.

Laboratory findings
1. Increased serum-sodium level, decreased serum-potassium level, metabolic alkalosis
2. Increased secretory rate and urinary excretion of aldosterone associated with a low or absent plasma renin titer (plasma renin activity is increased in secondary hyperaldosteronism)

Treatment   Treatment is surgical removal for tumor or hyperplasia.

Feminizing adrenal tumors   These tumors excrete excessive estrogen, which causes gynecomastia in males. It is very rare in children and is treated by surgical removal.

SURGICAL REMOVAL OF THE ADRENAL GLAND

If one adrenal gland is removed because of a tumor, an acute adrenal insufficiency may result postoperatively. In these cases the contralateral gland is usually atrophic or its activity has been suppressed by the excessive hormone production of the tumor. Preoperative preparation and intensive postoperative treatment—salt, proper fluid balance, glucose, and hormone replacement therapy (cortisone)—are important to prevent or overcome such a crisis.

PHEOCHROMOCYTOMA

Pheochromocytoma is a tumor of the adrenal medulla and/or other chromaffin tissue located along the aorta, in the organ of Zuckerkandl or the carotid body. It is very rare in children and is usually benign but may become malignant. Pheochromocytoma may be associated with neurofibromatosis of von Recklinghausen. Epinephrine and norepinephrine are produced in large quantities by the chromaffin cells of this tumor. The clinical picture is that of persistent hypertension or paroxysmal attacks of hyperadrenalism, e.g., palpitation, sweating, elevated blood pressure, tachycardia, heart failure, and pulmonary edema.

There is increased concentration of pressor (catechol) amines in the blood (normal plasma norepinephrine, 3 to 6 micrograms per liter; epinephrine, less than 1 microgram per liter) or urine. The basal metabolic rate is usually markedly elevated and the glucose tolerance decreased. Urinary excretion of vanilmandelic acid (VMA)—the principal product derived from metabolism of epinephrine and norepinephrine—is increased and may be detected by colorimetry. Another test which may be used during the hypertensive phase is the injection of adrenolytic agents, e.g., benzodioxane, Regitine, which results in a fall of the blood pressure. (The patient should be prone during the test.)

The treatment is surgical, and the prognosis is grave.

OBESITY

Obesity may be:

1. Exogenous—due to emotional factors
2. Endogenous—e.g., Cushing's syndrome, Laurence-Moon-Biedl syndrome, or Froehlich's syndrome

Exogenous obesity has been discussed in Chapter 5, "Psychologic Problems."

Endogenous obesity is extremely rare. Cushing's disease and lesions around the hypothalamus may produce obesity. Hypothyroidism never results in true obesity, but rather in myxedema. The prognosis of endogenous obesity is usually guarded. Treatment is directed toward the primary disease.

PARATHYROID DISORDERS

Parathyroid hormone has two actions:

1. Production of a phosphorus diuresis by decreasing renal tubular reabsorption of phosphorus
2. Mobilization of calcium from bone into the blood

HYPERPARATHYROIDISM

Hyperfunction of the parathyroids

1. Primary—due to adenoma or idiopathic hyperplasia
2. Secondary—due to chronic renal insufficiency with retention of phosphates, e.g., chronic glomerulonephritis or congenital polycystic kidneys

Primary hyperparathyroidism   This is rare in children.

Clinical findings
1. Weakness, hypotonicity, hyperextensible joints, anorexia, nausea and vomiting, constipation, and weight loss
2. Bradycardia and irregularities of cardiac rhythm
3. Polyuria, polydipsia, nocturia, renal colic, and hematuria
4. Bone tenderness
5. Keratitis

Laboratory findings
1. Hypercalcemia (more than 10.5 mg per 100 ml) resulting in metastatic calcification of soft tissue, e.g., kidney (nephrocalcinosis), eye, ligaments, cartilage; hypophosphatemia and increased amount of serum alkaline phosphatase.
2. Increased urinary excretion of calcium (more than 200 mg per 24 hours on a low-calcium diet) and increased urinary phosphorus.
3. Increased plasma parathyroid hormone level with no change during calcium infusion.
4. Skeletal changes, as evidenced by roentgenograms, showing cyst-like areas of decalcification, thinning of the cortex, and lack of calcification at the ends of bones (osteitis fibrosa cystica); a high calcium (milk) and high vitamin D intake may make these changes less evident.
5. Tubular reabsorption of phosphate (TRP = phosphorus clearance divided by creatinine clearance): normal TRP values range from 78 to 93 percent; in hyperparathyroidism TRP is decreased below 78 percent.
6. Cortisone test: adrenal corticosteroids (prednisolone, 20 to 40 mg per day for 2 weeks) reduce elevated serum-calcium levels resulting from causes other than hyperparathyroidism. There is no response in hyperparathyroidism.

Differential diagnosis   The disease should be differentiated from idiopathic hypercalcemia of infancy, vitamin D intoxication, hypercalcemia of disuse (prolonged bed rest), malignancies with bone metastasis, sarcoidosis, multiple myeloma, hypercalcemia due to alkalosis or to diet rich in milk, and secondary hyperparathyroidism.

Treatment   Surgical removal if a parathyroid adenoma is present and subtotal resection for hyperplasia are the treatments of choice.

Prognosis   The prognosis depends on the extent of damage to the kidney and other soft tissues prior to surgery.

Secondary hyperparathyroidism   This is discussed under Renal Rickets in Chapter 3, "Vitamins and Metabolism."

HYPOPARATHYROIDISM

Hypofunction of the parathyroid may be

1. Acute—usually the result of accidental surgical removal or trauma during thyroid surgery.
2. Tetany of the newborn (see Chapter 12, "Diseases of the Newborn").
3. Chronic hypoparathyroidism: of unknown causation. It is relatively rare during childhood and may be associated with Addison's disease or generalized moniliasis.

Clinical features

1. Tetany (usually the only symptom in the acute hypofunction)—irritability, carpopedal spasm, and convulsions
2. Trophic changes in the teeth, skin, hair, and nails
3. Recurrent diarrhea and steatorrhea
4. Photophobia, blepharospasm, conjunctivitis, and lenticular opacities
5. Mental retardation, eventually, if untreated

Laboratory findings

1. Serum-calcium level is low, serum-phosphorus level is high, and serum–alkaline phosphatase activity is normal.
2. Urinary excretion of calcium and phosphorus is low.
3. Roentgenograms of the skull may show symmetric calcification in the region of the basal ganglions.
4. Abnormal EEG and ECG (prolonged Q-T interval) findings.
5. Tubular reabsorption of phosphorus (TRP) test: more than 93 percent.
6. Ellsworth-Howard test: intravenous administration of parathyroid hormone causes increased urinary phosphorus, increased serum-calcium level, and decreased serum-phosphorus level.

Differential diagnosis Hypocalcemia of rickets, celiac syndrome, pseudohypoparathyroidism, and pseudopseudohypoparathyroidism are possible diagnoses.

PSEUDOHYPOPARATHYROIDISM (Seabright-Bantam Syndrome)

This is a congenital, X-linked dominant disorder that resembles idiopathic hypoparathyroidism but does not respond to parathyroid extract. It is due to an end organ resistance, with the renal tubules failing to respond to parathormone. The patients usually have a round face, short stature, dyschondroplasia, and abnormalities of some metacarpal and metatarsal bones because of early epiphyseal closure. Roentgenograms reveal metastatic calcification of subcutaneous tissue. Blood and urine chemistry is similar to that of hypoparathyroidism. There is excessive secretion of parathyroid hormone and hyperplasia of the gland.

Dihydrotachysterol (A.T. 10) or large doses of vitamin D and calcium corrects the disorder (see Treatment below).

PSEUDOPSEUDOHYPOPARATHYROIDISM
(Brachymetacarpal Dwarfism)

This condition is found in relatives of individuals with pseudohypoparathyroidism. It has skeletal and developmental features similar to those of Seabright-Bantam syndrome, without any abnormalities of calcium or phosphorus metabolism.

Treatment

1. For tetany—discussed in Chapter 20, "Neurologic Conditions."
2. Calcium lactate, 5 to 10 Gm per day, orally, in mild chronic cases.
3. Low-phosphorus diet: aluminum hydroxide may be added to reduce phosphorus absorption from the gastrointestinal tract.
4. Vitamin D_2: 50,000 to 125,000 units per day; calcium should be maintained at 9 to 11 mg per 100 ml (hypercalcemia and hypercalcinuria must be avoided). A.T. 10, 1 to 2 ml per day, may be used in addition to vitamin D_2 if response to vitamin D is inadequate.

Prognosis   The prognosis is good in early mild cases but guarded in the more severe cases.

DIABETES MELLITUS

Diabetes mellitus is a disorder of carbohydrate, fat, and protein metabolism due to the lack of sufficient, available, effective insulin. It is manifested by glycosuria, hyperglycemia, and frequently acidosis.

Diabetes is probably transmitted as a recessive trait which has varying degrees of penetrance. In about 5 percent of patients diabetes begins before the age of 15. They are juvenile diabetics, who most often manifest the growth-onset type of diabetes characterized by being both insulin-requiring and insulin-sensitive. They are prone to develop ketoacidosis. Growth hormone, adrenal corticosteroids, thyroid hormone, epinephrine, and glucagon all act as insulin antagonists. Glucagon, in addition, causes an increase in insulin secretion.

Pathogenesis   The mechanism of insulin action is the removal of a barrier to glucose entry into the tissues, primarily muscle and adipose. In muscles, glucose is converted to glycogen and amino acids are converted to protein. In adipose tissue, glucose is converted to lipids, and there is inhibition of free fatty acid release. Insulin increases gluco-kinase activity in the liver, resulting in both increased uptake of glucose and its storage as glycogen. A decline in the concentration of insulin initiates a series of events opposite to the above. Adipose tissue releases free fatty acid, muscle releases amino acids from its stored protein and liver glycogen is mobilized as glucose. In the liver the amino acids are deaminated and the process of gluconeogenesis produces more glucose. The energy source of the liver is the free fatty acids which are oxidized to ketone bodies. The blood ketones are produced in excess of the capacity of the peripheral tissues to metabolize them and consequently are excreted in the urine. Fixed base is used by the kidney to excrete these organic acids, thus further increasing the degree of acidosis. Osmotic diuresis, characterized by polyuria and polydipsia, is produced by the large volume of solute in the form of glucose presented for renal tubular reabsorption. Electrolytes, urea, and ketones also play a role in the elevation of osmolarity. Dehydration occurs. In the presence of infection, diabetic patients are even more likely to develop dehydration and acidosis. If the condition is untreated, coma and subsequently death may occur.

Clinical features

1. Polyuria, polyphagia, and polydipsia are the classic symptoms.
2. Weight loss in spite of adequate or excessive food intake.
3. The onset is usually sudden and frequently ushered in by an infection. The average duration of symptoms prior to the development of overt diabetes or even acidosis in children is about 1 month.

Laboratory findings

1. Glycosuria and hyperglycemia are the most constant findings. The normal maximum values for the standard glucose-tolerance test using venous blood measured by the Somogyi-Nelson method are:

    Fasting—100 mg percent
    30 minute—160 mg percent
    60 minute—145 mg percent
    90 minute—125 mg percent
    120 minute—110 mg percent
    180 minute—105 mg percent

2. Capillary blood can also be used in children after oral glucose loading. Standards for this method are presently available.
3. A 2-hour postprandial level of blood glucose of more than 140 mg percent suggests a presumptive diagnosis of diabetes mellitus.
4. The blood-cholesterol and -lipid levels are elevated in uncontrolled cases.
5. In diabetic acidosis there is ketonemia and ketonuria and a pro-

gressive lowering of the plasma-CO_2 content. The plasma-sodium level falls, and in severe acidosis there is impairment of kidney function, resulting in changes in the blood chemistry, e.g., an elevated urea-nitrogen level.

Treatment   The treatment may be divided into several phases.

Diet   The diet must be adequate to supply the calories, proteins, vitamins, and other essentials for normal growth as well as for the daily activity. Many diets have been recommended. They range from strict control to a more practical, so-called "free" diet with a calculated amount of calories served at regular intervals and no food restrictions except on overindulgence in candy, cake, jelly, etc. Several simple rules may be used as guides if a calculated diet is desired.

Children's diets are based upon age and nutrition. Carbohydrate should constitute 40%, fat 40%, and protein 20% of the total number of calories. A diet of 1000 Cal is prescribed for a child 1 year of age, and an additional 100 Cal is added for each additional year of age. Thus, a 5-year-old child receives 1400 calories. If a child is obese, several hundred calories are subtracted from the daily diet; if underweight, several hundred are added. During peak growth periods, adolescent girls require 2400 to 2700 and adolescent boys, 3100 to 3600 Cal per day. One-fifth of the total calories is given for breakfast, two-fifths for lunch, and two-fifths for dinner. From the total daily calories which have been calculated, three 50 to 150 Cal snacks are substracted and offered midmorning, midafternoon, and at bedtime. The amount of carbohydrates necessary is calculated by dividing the total daily calories by 10, giving the number of grams of carbohydrate for the daily diet.

A simple way of calculating the amount of fat required is to divide the carbohydrate requirement (in grams) in half. The grams of protein in the diet are determined exactly as the fat content.

Example: 10-year-old child requires 1900 Cal

$$\frac{1900}{10} = 190 \text{ Gm carbohydrate}$$

$$\frac{190}{2} = 95 \text{ Gm fat}$$

$$\frac{190}{2} = 95 \text{ Gm protein}$$

The diet should be varied and readily accepted and conform as much as possible to the diet of other members of the family.

Insulin   When insulin requirements are being determined, the patient should be allowed normal activity. This is particularly true if regulation is being carried out in the hospital. The starting dose of insulin is ¼ unit per pound. With any degree of ketonuria the beginning dose should be ½ unit per pound. An intermediate-acting insulin (NPH or lente) may be given before breakfast, or regular insulin may be given before each meal. Regular insulin can also be mixed with NPH or lente insulin to achieve better control. Changes in the dosage of insulin may vary from ½ to 10 units. Changes when indicated are best made at about 2- to 3-day intervals. The urinalysis one day governs the insulin dose on the following day.

The urine should be free from acetone at all times, and over any 24-hour period it should not contain more than 10 percent of the carbohydrate intake as determined by quantitative glucose testing.

Exogenous insulin is subject to a binding action by the proteins of the blood (mainly gamma globulins). This may represent an antigen-antibody response and may account for the phenomenon of insulin resistance. Patients with insulin resistance require 200 units or more daily. The insulin-binding capacity of serum can be measured (marked increase in serum-gamma globulin level) and counteracted by adrenal corticosteroids.

Table 24-1. Approximate time of activity of single large doses of various types of insulin

Type of insulin	Action demonstrable, hr	Peak action, hr	Duration of effect, hr
Short or rapid-acting:			
Regular	½–1	2–4	6–8
Semilente	½–1	5–7	12–18
Intermediate-acting:			
Globin	2–4	8–14	24
NPH	1–2	7–11	24–28
Lente	1–2	14–18	28–32
Long-acting:			
Protamine zinc	6–8	16–24	24–72
Ultralente	5–8	22–26	36–96

Psychologic care As in any chronic disease, it is most important for the patient to accept his disability and learn to adjust to his environment. Frequently at 8 years of age, children can be taught to test their own urine and inject themselves. This is a major step in building security because they no longer depend on others for a substance which they soon learn is vital. Diabetic children should be encouraged to lead as normal a life as possible, and this can be accomplished only with the full cooperation of the patient, his parents, and the physician. Another important parameter in the treatment of the juvenile diabetic is the education of the parents (and the child if sufficiently mature). At the time of diagnosis the child must be admitted to the hospital. The parent is given instructions for urine testing; administration of insulin; diet; recognition, prevention, and treatment of hypoglycemic attacks; and also treatment of the child during acute infections.

Oral sulfonylurea and other drugs that are said to increase the production of endogenous insulin are being used principally in adults; they have little or no value in diabetic children.

Complications

1. Neuropathies and gangrene are rare in childhood.
2. Hepatomegaly: may be associated with persistent acidosis.
3. Xanthomatous skin lesions: associated with hyperlipemia.
4. Arteriosclerosis: nephrosclerosis, retinal changes, and hypertension may be found when diabetes has been present for longer than 10 to 12 years. Arteriosclerosis is the most important single factor in determining life expectancy of the diabetic patient. Glomerulosclerosis is the leading cause of death in juvenile diabetes.

Prognosis

For juvenile diabetic patients, good. They can expect to live two-thirds to three-quarters of the normal lifespan if their diabetes is controlled. Control is best judged by the following standards:

1. Freedom from symptoms
2. Adequate nutrition
3. Normal weight gain and growth
4. No disturbance by hypoglycemic reactions
5. Potential for normal activity

Minimal diurnal glycosuria and hyperglycemia are preferable to repeated hypoglycemic reactions.

Diabetic coma and insulin shock are major problems in the management of diabetic children. Children are likely to develop these complications because of:

1. Variable amount of exercise performed from day to day (activity decreases blood sugar).
2. Difficulty in maintaining a prescribed diet—increased or decreased intake.
3. Increased frequency of infection. Most cases of diabetic coma are associated with infections of the respiratory tract or failure to administer prescribed insulin.

DIABETIC ACIDOSIS AND COMA

Treatment

1. Correction of acidosis and dehydration is of primary importance and has been discussed in Chapter 7, "Fluid and Electrolyte Balance." As soon as possible fluids are given by mouth, and intravenous therapy is discontinued.

2. Insulin administration: regular insulin only should be used—2 to 4 units per kg immediately—half intravenously and half intramuscularly. The blood-sugar level should be determined again after 2 hours. For rising blood sugar insulin should be given in amounts equal to, or as much as double the initial dose. For falling blood sugar no further insulin should be given until the result of blood sugar at 4 hours after the initial dose is known.

    The blood-sugar level at 4 hours after the initial insulin dosage is a reasonable, accurate guide to its maximal effectiveness. One-quarter to one-half the total insulin of the first hour should be given if the blood glucose still exceeds 300 mg percent and is greater than one-half the pretreatment level. No insulin is necessary at this time if the clinical condition is improving and the blood glucose has fallen below 300 mg percent or to less than half the pretreatment level. Occasionally additional regular insulin may be necessary because of failure of the clinical condition to improve even with falling blood glucose.

    From the sixth to the twenty-fourth hour of treatment regular insulin dosage may be adjusted according to urine tests every 2 to 4 hours if the fall in blood sugar has been satisfactory. For a child 10 years of age or older:

    If test is 4+: regular insulin—10 units
    If test is 3+: regular insulin—8 units
    If test is 2+: regular insulin—6 units
    If test is negative or 1+: no insulin

    For a child less than 10 years of age give half of the above dosage.
3. Gastric lavage is advisable to avert gastric atony and dilatation and subsequent vomiting. It will shorten the time until oral intake can begin.
4. The precipitating infection should be determined and treated with antibiotics and chemotherapy.
5. Potassium should be given as soon as the blood glucose level falls (3 to 6 hours) and renal function is adequate. A dose of 2 to 4 meq per kg is given over a 2-hour period.

Prognosis The prognosis depends on the rapidity with which treatment is instituted. In general, the prognosis for recovery from coma is good.

INFANTS BORN TO DIABETIC MOTHERS

Fetal loss and neonatal fatality are several times higher in women with diabetes than in normal women. Almost all infants born before the completion of the twenty-eighth week of gestation die. Diabetic mothers should probably be delivered between the thirty-sixth and thirty-seventh weeks of gestation. The causation and pathogenesis of this increased morbidity and mortality are obscure.

Clinical features

1. Increased birth weight and size; generalized nonpitting edema.
2. Respiratory distress syndrome (including hyaline membrane disease) : accounts for more than half of the deaths.
3. Visceromegaly: cardiomegaly, hepatosplenomegaly.
4. Signs of hypoglycemia during first 48 hours. (Neonatal tetany has a number of features in common with symptomatic hypoglycemia. It is more common in males and premature infants and following complications of labor.)
5. Hyperbilirubinemia.
6. Increased incidence of congenital anomalies.

Treatment

1. Place infant in Isolette.
2. Antibiotics are indicated if infection is suspected.
3. Glucose 5 percent in 0.25 N saline solution orally beginning at 4 hours of age. This may reduce the incidence of hyperbilirubinemia.

TRANSIENT SYMPTOMATIC HYPOGLYCEMIA IN THE NEWBORN INFANT

During the first week of life newborn infants may manifest episodes of tremors, convulsions, difficulty in feeding, apathy, or respiratory distress. Extremely low values of blood glucose do not occur in normal infants during this period.

Abnormally low levels of blood sugar during the first week of life are:

1. Under 20 mg per 100 ml in the low-birth-weight infant
2. Under 30 mg per 100 ml from birth to 72 hours of age in the full-sized infant and under 40 mg percent thereafter.

Treatment

1. Glucose 50% in water intravenously—1 to 2 ml per kg.
2. Followed by continuous intravenous drip of glucose 15% in water —75 to 100 ml per kg per day until 48 hours of age.
3. Followed by glucose 10% in 0.25 N saline—100 to 110 ml per kg per day.
4. Oral feeding is introduced when symptoms disappear.
5. After 6 to 12 hours of intravenous glucose, if symptoms persist and hypoglycemia remains below 30 mg percent, hydrocortisone should be given—5 mg per kg per day by mouth at 12-hour intervals or ACTH—4 units per kg per day intramuscularly every 12 hours.

Treatment should be continued until blood glucose remains normal for 48 hours. Then glucose 5% is given intravenously for about 6 hours as oral feedings are given. Reactive hypoglycemia may occur if intravenous glucose is stopped suddenly.

GLYCOSURIA*

Several conditions that cause glycosuria must be differentiated from diabetes mellitus. Other forms of diabetes may result from hyperplasia of the pituitary (acromegaly) or adrenal (Cushing's syndrome) glands and hypersecretion of the alpha cells of the pancreas or the argentophil cells of the gastrointestinal mucosa (increased glucagon). Renal (orthoglycemic) glucosuria results from a lowered renal threshold for glucose and is characterized by symptomless glucosuria with a normal blood-sugar curve. Alimentary glucosuria, probably due to rapid glucose absorption, is of no clinical importance. It occurs in some persons following the ingestion of a high-carbohydrate meal. Pentosuria, fructosuria (fructokinase defect), lactosuria, mannoheptulosuria, sucrosuria, and galactosuria result from inborn errors of carbohydrate metabolism. These conditions are differentiated from glucosuria by the identification of the specific sugar in the urine. This is best done by paper chromatography. A positive glucose oxidase test (Clinistix, Tes-Tape) establishes the presence of glucose.

HYPOGLYCEMIA

A low blood-sugar level with symptoms of hypoglycemia may result from:

1. Hyperinsulinism: beta-cell hyperplasia or tumor.
2. Functional: of unknown causation, e.g., transient hypoglycemia in infants of diabetic mothers or in low-birth-weight infants. Strenuous exercise may cause hypoglycemia.
3. Glucagon deficiency: absence of alpha cells.
4. Specific enzyme defects—glycogen-storage diseases, galactosemia, hereditary fructose intolerance.
5. Decreased adrenal cortical (Addison's disease) or medullary hormones.
6. Decreased pituitary function: pituitary dwarfism or Simmonds' disease; lack of growth hormone.
7. Hepatic dysfunction: cirrhosis, infections, and severe intoxications.

---

* Glucosuria is used here to denote the presence of glucose in the urine; glycosuria is used to denote the presence of any sugar.

8. Leucine sensitivity: hypoglycemia follows a large protein intake.
9. Insulin overmedication (insulin shock) of diabetic patients.
10. Defective intestinal absorption: chronic diarrhea, celiac syndrome.

A low blood-sugar level does not necessarily produce symptoms; the level of hypoglycemia at which symptoms appear shows considerable individual variation (it may even appear at normal levels following a precipitous fall).

Clinical features   Early there are pallor, hunger, tingling sensations, increased perspiration, and irritability, followed by vomiting, behavior disorders, and tremors. If the condition is untreated, there may be convulsions and death.

Laboratory findings

1. Fasting blood-sugar level and glucose-tolerance test: constant FBS of less than 50 mg per 100 ml is found in the hypoglycemia of pancreatic tumors. Hypoglycemia of hepatic origin and glycogen-storage disease also reveals a low FBS.
2. Insulin-sensitivity test: Increased sensitivity to insulin is found in persons who have deficiency of insulin antagonist hormones, e.g., growth hormone (hypoglycemia of pituitary origin), adrenal corticosteroids (Addison's disease), epinephrine, or glucagon. Insulin, 0.05–0.1 unit per kg is given before breakfast. Normally the blood-glucose level falls about 50 percent in 15 minutes and begins to rise by 30 to 45 minutes. When one of the above disorders is present, the blood-sugar level may fall to critical levels. This is a dangerous test and should not be used indiscriminately.
3. Glucagon-tolerance test: If sufficient glycogen is present, the hepatic phosphorylase system produces glycogenolysis and the subsequent release of glucose. After a 4- to 12-hour fast glucagon 0.03 mg per kg (maximum dose 1 mg) is injected intramuscularly or intravenously. Normally the blood glucose should rise at least 50 mg per 100 ml within 15 to 45 minutes and return to fasting levels at 60 to 90 minutes.
4. Serum insulin assays: Elevated levels of insulin in peripheral blood are found in only two-thirds of patients with islet-cell tumors.
5. Catecholamines of urine and blood: measures epinephrine-like activity of blood—low levels are found in epinephrine-deficient persons.
6. Urinary or blood 17-hydroxycorticosteroids: decreased in Addison's disease.
7. Leucine-tolerance test: Leucine can be administered either orally 150 mg per kg or intravenously 75 mg per kg. Blood samples for

glucose and insulin determinations are taken at fasting and at 15-minute intervals for 1 hour than at 1½ and 2 hours after oral leucine. Leucine sensitivity causes the blood glucose to decrease to at least 50 percent of the fasting level within 45 minutes. Serum insulin rises at the same time.

8. Tolbutamide-tolerance test: 20 mg per kg is given intravenously, not to exceed 1 gm. Normally the blood glucose falls to 20 to 40 percent of the fasting value within 20 to 30 minutes, with a return to the initial level by 120 minutes.

9. Carbohydrate-withdrawal test (a guide to the usefulness of a high-protein diet): in organic hyperinsulinism or in impaired gluconeogenesis, hypoglycemia develops in 24 hours following withdrawal.

Treatment

1. Specific: e.g., glycogen-storage disease, leucine sensitivity—see descriptions under primary disease.

2. For an acute episode glucose 50% in water should be given intravenously (1 to 2 ml per kg). As an emergency measure, glucagon (0.3 mg per kg intravenously or intramuscularly, not to exceed 1 mg) or epinephrine (1:1000, 0.03 mg per kg intramuscularly, not to exceed 0.3 mg) may be used but must be followed by parenteral glucose or an orally administered high-carbohydrate diet.

3. For patients with tumors and severe cases (due to hyperplasia): partial pancreatectomy.

4. Adrenal corticosteroid treatment: in idiopathic type.

5. Ephedrine sulfate for epinephrine-deficient persons.

6. Leucine-induced hypoglycemia is treated by a diet containing adequate calories but low in leucine. High-carbohydrate feedings are given a half-hour after meals.

REVIEW QUESTIONS

1. Gigantism is produced by (a) eosinophilic adenoma; (b) basophilic adenoma; (c) chromophobe adenoma; (d) craniopharyngioma.

2. Pineal tumors usually occur (a) in males; (b) in females; (c) with equal frequency in both sexes; (d) in pseudohermaphrodites.

3. The most common endocrine disorder observed in early childhood is (a) hypothyroidism; (b) hyperthyroidism; (c) diabetes mellitus; (d) Cushing's disease.

4. The following statements are true of acquired hypothyroidism except for one: (a) there is retarded growth; (b) it usually becomes apparent clinically at 2 to 3 months of age; (c) there are low serum-cholesterol levels; (d) there are low BEI levels.

5. The clinical features of primordial dwarfism include all the following except for one: (a) infants are small at birth; (b) growth is slow from infancy; (c) facial features are immature; (d) skeletal proportions are normal.

6. The following items are associated with Turner's syndrome (gonadal dysgenesis) except for one: (a) FSH excretion in the urine is high before puberty;

(*b*) the majority of patients have chromatin-negative nuclear pattern; (*c*) dwarfism; (*d*) infertility.

7. The following are associated with acute adrenal insufficiency in children except for one: (*a*) increased serum-sodium and chloride levels; (*b*) increased serum-potassium level; (*c*) hypoglycemia; (*d*) purpura.

The following questions are of the matching type. On the blank next to the item in column I put the letter of the item in column II with which it is most closely associated:

I	II
8. Adrenal hyperplasia _____	(*a*) Moderately increased excretion of urinary 17-ketosteroids
9. Adrenal adenoma _____	(*b*) Markedly increased excretion of urinary 17-ketosteroids
10. Adrenal carcinoma _____	(*c*) Low excretion of urinary 17-keto-steroids

11. The following are associated with pheochromocytoma except for one: (*a*) hypertension; (*b*) glucose tolerance is decreased; (*c*) urinary excretion of VMA is increased; (*d*) this is a tumor of the cortex of the adrenal gland.

12. The following are associated with hypoparathyroidism except for one: (*a*) tetany; (*b*) low serum phosphorus; (*c*) Ellsworth-Howard test; (*d*) abnormal EEG and ECG findings.

13. Diabetes mellitus occurs before the age of 15 years in: (*a*) 1 percent; (*b*) 5 percent; (*c*) 10 percent; (*d*) 20 percent of patients with the disease.

14. A 2-hour postprandial level of blood glucose of more than (*a*) 110 mg percent; (*b*) 120 mg percent; (*c*) 140 mg percent; (*d*) 160 mg percent is presumptive evidence of diabetes mellitus.

15. The following statements related to infants born to diabetic mothers are true except for one: (*a*) visceromegaly; (*b*) hyperbilirubinemia; (*c*) increased incidence of congenital anomalies; (*d*) diabetic mothers should be delivered between the thirty-eighth and fortieth week.

16. All the following are characteristics of Cushing's disease except (*a*) osteoporosis; (*b*) polycythemia; (*c*) increased blood volume and plethora; (*d*) diabetic glucose-tolerance curve; (*e*) eosinophilia.

17. A 10-year-old child presents with a round, firm thyroid nodule. The best management of this patient is (*a*) excisional biopsy; (*b*) thiouracil; (*c*) iodides; (*d*) radioactive iodine; (*e*) observation until adolescence is completed.

The following questions are the matching type. In each blank in column I, insert the letter corresponding to the word or phrase in column II which is associated most appropriately.

I	II
18. Sexual precocity _____	(*a*) Birth weight normal; epiphyseal os-
19. Delayed adolescence _____	sification and fusion markedly re-
20. Pituitary dwarfism _____	tarded; infantile skeletal propor-
21. Hypothyroidism _____	tions; sexual development late.
22. Progeria _____	(*b*) Mature skeletal proportions; slen-

der, emaciated, birdlike features; arteriosclerosis.

(c) Birth weight normal; lower segment of skeletal proportion often short; FSH normal; premature epiphyseal fusion.

(d) Birth weight normal; moderate retardation of epiphyseal ossification and fusion; skeletal proportions normal.

(e) Retarded epiphyseal ossification; FSH low; prolonged hypoglycemia with insulin; sexual development infantile; normal skeletal proportions.

25 ALLERGY

Allergy is a biologic state of specific altered capacity to react (hypersensitivity) to a foreign substance (antigen) which, when it causes symptoms, is designated as an "allergen." It is estimated that 15 percent of Americans are subject to some form of allergic disease, including over 8 million who have asthma. Asthma is the leading cause of limitation of activity in the age group under 17. These children and adolescents lose about 7 million days of school each year.

There are various types of allergic reactions causing different diseases (see Table 25-1).

The clinical heterogeneity of allergic diseases requires that every attempt be made to distinguish between allergic conditions and idiosyncrasy and other diseases of intolerance, e.g., milk allergy and lactase deficiency.

Table 25-1

Types of reaction	Name of disease	Characteristics

A. Immediate-type hypersensitivity
Manifests in minutes or days mediated by histamine, humoral antibodies can be transferred with serum
	1. Atopic diseases
	    Hay fever
	    Asthma
	    Eczema
	    Urticaria
	2. Anaphylaxis
	    Shock from insect bite or penicillin
	3. Serum sickness
		Heredity important, sensitization necessary, type of antibody—IgE

B. Delayed-type hypersensitivity Manifests after many hours or days, no chemical mediators, can be transferred by lymphocytes (thymus–dependent)	1. Contact dermatitis Poison ivy, nickel, cosmetics dye 2. Allergy to microorganisms, e.g., skin tests for tuberculosis, *Candida albicans*, mumps	Heredity not important Contact sensitization Heredity not important

The hallmarks of the immediate type of allergic reaction are the wheal and flare in the skin, edema, spasm of smooth muscle, and increased secretion of involved membranes of the respiratory or gastrointestinal tract. The result of the antigen reacting with antibody is the release of chemical mediators, histamine being the most important.

Allergens, usually proteins, can be inhaled or ingested. Haptens or drugs can induce an allergic reaction through skin contact. Among the most common allergen offenders are plant pollens (ragweed, trees, grasses), mold spores, house dust, animal danders, feathers, wool or silk fabrics, vegetable seeds, vegetable gums, insects, foods, and drugs. Foods play a particularly important role as allergens during the first year of life.

FOOD ALLERGY

The diagnosis of food allergy can usually be made by a careful history, and the elimination of the suspected food followed by the reproducing of symptoms by challenging with the offending food.

The manifestations of food allergy are different in infants than in older children. During the first few months of life, the gastrointestinal mucosa is permeable to large antigenic protein fragments; and frequently if one or both parents has a major allergy, the infant will show manifestations of allergic gastroenteropathy early in life.

Clinical features in infants

1. The first major offender is cow's milk. Symptoms may appear at 2 to 4 weeks of age. Milk allergy is suspected to occur in about 5 percent of infants.
2. Gastrointestinal—abdominal discomfort and colic, regurgitation or vomiting, and diarrhea may contribute to irritability.
3. Atopic dermatitis may occur, extending from the intergluteal folds to the perianal region.

Clinical features in children
Egg white, nuts, milk, cereals (e.g., wheat), oranges, strawberries, peanuts, chocolate, and fish are among the most common offenders.

1. The symptoms can occur within minutes after ingestion or after hours or days.
2. Gastrointestinal—abdominal distension and discomfort, vomiting, diarrhea or constipation, or celiac syndrome.
3. Skin—atopic dermatitis and hives.
4. Behavioral—irritability, fatigue, and insomnia.
5. In children, it is not unusual to find food to be the cause of perennial allergic rhinitis or bronchial asthma.

Differential diagnosis

1. Hypertrophic pyloric stenosis (see p. 454).
2. Gastroenteritis—infection usually lacks the chronicity or recurrence of symptoms characteristic of allergy.
3. Cyclic vomiting (see p. 413).
4. Enzyme-deficiency diseases, e.g., disaccharidase—suspicion of allergy may appear to be confirmed by disappearance of symptoms when cow's milk is replaced by soybean formula; however, improvement may be due to the change in sugar and not protein.
5. Celiac disease or other causes of celiac syndrome.
6. Ulcerative colitis.

Prophylaxis

1. In families having a history of major allergic disorders, breast-feeding should be encouraged. If this is not possible, a milk substitute, e.g., soybean, meat base, should be the initial formula.
2. During infancy, foods should be introduced singly, in small amounts, and in a hypoallergic, heat-denatured form, e.g., evaporated milk, well-cooked cereal, hard-boiled egg, well-cooked meat.

Treatment

1. Elimination diet is the best method to identify the offender. A quick symptomatic response usually follows the removal of the allergenic food. A simple diet derived of specific hypoallergenic foods must be continued for at least 1 week, and symptoms must be reproduced by challenging with the offending food before it can be considered as a definite allergen.
   The success of an elimination diet can be impaired by several factors, such as failure to adhere to the restrictions imposed or use of by-products of the offending food (cheese, butter, or ice cream in patients sensitive to milk). Preservatives or tenderizers can also cause allergic symptoms.
2. Boiling can reduce the allergenicity of certain foods (grains and milk). Evaporated milk is better tolerated when cow's milk is given again. Suitable substitutes for cow milk are soybean, Nutramigen, and meat-base milks.

HAY FEVER AND ALLERGIC RHINITIS

Allergic rhinitis is caused by mucous membrane exposure to inhaled allergenic materials and mediated by a specific immunologic mechanism. In the first year of life allergic rhinitis most often is caused by food, with cow's milk being the important offender. Usually, these are children whose parents have suffered major allergic diseases.

Later in childhood symptoms recur most often in a particular season, e.g., hay fever. In the majority of affected children, hay fever is caused by a sensitivity to ragweed pollen, but other pollens of trees and grasses can be involved. Pollen may be windborne for several hundred miles.

Clinical features

1. Symptoms include sneezing (frequently in paroxysms), nasal congestion and watery discharge, conjunctival itching, and often cough.
2. Children characteristically perform the "allergic salute" by rubbing and pushing the tip of the nose upward with the palm of the hand.
3. Allergic "shiners" are due to infraorbital venous stasis secondary to edema of the nasal mucosa.
4. Annual recurrence corresponds to the season of pollination of the causative plant. Therefore, symptoms will be related to various pollen seasons, e.g., trees from April to June, grasses from May to July, and weeds from August until the first frost. Clinically, hay fever is distinguished from perennial allergic rhinitis or vasomotor rhinitis by its periodicity and seasonal recurrence.

A biopsy of the nasal mucosa during an allergic reaction shows profound edema of the submucosal tissue and infiltration by eosinophils, but even in long-standing situations the mucosa is intact with no evidence of tissue destruction. Further changes occur only when there is secondary infection.

When no special seasonal pattern and plant pollen can be implicated and symptoms occur all year, suggestive of "frequent colds," the diagnosis of perennial allergic rhinitis is made.

House dust is then the major offender, followed by animal danders and feathers. This continuous exposure is often aggravated by nonspecific irritants, e.g., chemical fumes, fresh paint, tobacco smoke, air pollutants, changes in temperature, or infections.

Diagnostic tests

1. Skin tests: All commonly used tests depend upon reproducing the allergic reaction on a small scale by exposing the patient to a minute amount of the suspected allergen. A good correlation of the positive skin tests with the clinical pattern of the specific offender will confirm the diagnosis. Failure to reveal positive skin tests does not exclude the allergic condition.
2. Eosinophilia: The presence of more than 5 percent of eosinophils in the mucoid nasal discharge is suggestive of allergy. Secondary infection causes the eosinophils to disappear, consequently their absence does not exclude allergy.
3. Roentgenograms: Excess adenoid tissue, polyps, or sinus involvement may be seen.

Treatment

1. Symptomatic: Antihistamines may provide considerable relief. Nose drops to provide vasoconstriction generally should not be used because of the tendency to make them a form of chronic treatment which may result in vasomotor rhinitis.
2. Environmental control: Many times the elimination of an offender, e.g., dog, may solve the problem.
3. Control of infection: When infection appears to play a significant role, appropriate antibiotics should be administered to interrupt the cycle of infection and allergic reactivity. Some children have benefited from desensitization injections with bacterial vaccines.
4. Surgery: Nasal polyps are frequently associated with allergic rhinitis, and if they are the primary cause of nasal obstruction, surgical removal is indicated. This should be followed by treatment with desensitization in order to lessen the tendency of recurrence.
5. Desensitization: Skin testing and desensitization may be necessary.

Prognosis   The reduced resistance of the allergic mucosa to infection results in an excessive number of upper respiratory tract infections. Such children are exceedingly prone to otitis media and later to sinus infections. More importantly, they have a high incidence of bronchial asthma (estimated at 30 percent) if untreated.

BRONCHIAL ASTHMA

Bronchial asthma is characterized by recurrent episodic attacks brought about by spasm of the bronchiolar smooth muscle. Mucosal edema, with excessive secretion of thick, tenacious mucus further contributes to bronchial obstruction.

Any child with intermittent asthma or who has more than three attacks in 1 year deserves a comprehensive work-up. A hereditary predisposition is thought to exist. Bronchial asthma is considered to be a hypersensitivity of the bronchial tree which can react to multiple stimuli: specific allergens, e.g., plant pollens, molds, house dust, animal dander (extrinsic asthma), or respiratory infections (intrinsic asthma). Infectious asthma occurs more often in infants. Many nonspecific stimuli, e.g., cold, chemicals, exercise, emotions, can act as triggering or aggravating factors.

An acute attack of asthma can start with a cough or sensation of hunger for air. Expiration is prolonged, and wheezing occurs throughout the chest. The attack will not subside spontaneously or promptly if infection is the cause or if the child is continuously exposed to the offender. During a prolonged attack, when all accessory muscles of respiration are used to improve ventilation, fatigue will occur accompanied by biochemical derangements.

Laboratory features

1. Respiratory alkalosis occurs very early during an attack due to hyperventilation.
2. Respiratory acidosis follows shortly due to a fall in PaO_2 and retention of CO_2.
3. Metabolic acidosis (falling blood pH and accumulation of lactic acid) will develop, in time leading to status asthmaticus.

Treatment   The principles of symptomatic treatment are bronchodilation, hydration, and relaxation.

1. Bronchodilation—the drug of choice is aqueous epinephrine 1:1,000 solution, 0.01 ml per kg subcutaneously, with a single maximum dose of 0.2 ml. This dose may be repeated twice at 20-minute intervals, while oral hydration is begun. Following adequate response, the bronchodilatory effect can be sustained for 8 to 12 hours by administration of Sus-Phrine (long-acting suspension) at half the dose of the aqueous epinephrine.

   Oral bronchodilator preparations may also be given for continued effect (Marax, Tedral, and Quadrinal are used commonly). (Antihistaminic drugs are contraindicated in asthma due to their drying activity.)

   In unresponsive cases, more potent bronchodilators (xanthine alkaloids) such as aminophylline can be given intravenously, 4 mg per kg over a 15-minute period. This should not be repeated before 6 hours.
2. Hydration: Oral hydration should be begun promptly. Humidification (cool vaporizer) of inspired air is helpful. Potassium iodide (1 drop per year, up to 10 drops) is given 3 to 4 times per day to liquefy bronchial secretions.
3. Antibiotics: If infection is suspected, antibiotic therapy should be instituted.
4. Aarane (cromolyn sodium) is a new drug which may be useful in the treatment of severe bronchial asthma. It is indicated in extrinsic asthma. Children receiving adrenal corticosteroids may tolerate a reduction or elimination of adrenal corticosteroids when Aarane is administered. This drug should not be used during an acute attack nor in status asthmaticus. If improvement occurs, it will take 2 to 4 weeks. The dose for children 5 years and over is one Aarane capsule (20 mg cromolyn sodium) administered with a special inhaler four times daily.
5. Environmental control: An appropriate home environment can effectively reduce the allergenic hazards. Wool and deep-piled carpeting should be avoided. The child's pillow and mattress should be of foam rubber or synthetic fillers or encased in plastic covers. Wall and window decorations should allow for easy dusting. Avoid dust collectors, e.g., venetian blinds and storage closets in the

child's bedroom. Stuffed, woolly, or furry toys should be removed. No pets (especially cats or dogs) should be in the home. Over-stuffed upholstered furniture should be replaced by simple furniture with foam-rubber padding or covered with plastic. Frequent vacuuming and washing of the floor will reduce the amount of dust. Hot-air furnace ducts are undesirable because they may provide allergenic offenders such as dust or thermophilic molds. Parental occupation may involve allergic hazards; for example, bakers or flour-mill workers can carry flour dust, molds, mites; furriers introduce animal hair, dyes, or insecticides.

Treatment of status asthmaticus If the acute attack does not respond to the preceding treatment, the child should be hospitalized.

1. Laboratory tests: Chest x-ray and blood count should be made. Blood electrolyte levels, pH, $PaCO_2$ and PaO_2 should be obtained and monitored. Cultures and sensitivity tests are made from the tracheal secretions.
2. Humidification: The child should be placed in a tent with ultrasonic fog, vaporizing 4 to 6 ml per minute and having an oxygen concentration of 30 to 40 percent.
3. Hydration and correction of electrolyte imbalance: Fluids are administered intravenously, and acidosis is corrected with sodium bicarbonate (see Chapter 7).
4. Sedation: Mild sedation may be helpful. Chloral hydrate, 15 mg per kg, every 8 hours is given orally or rectally. (Drugs, e.g., barbiturates, that depress the respiratory center are contraindicated.)
5. Antibiotics: If possible, antibiotics should be given orally to lessen the chance of an allergic reaction.
6. Adrenal corticosteroids: Steroid-dependent patients should be started immediately on hydrocortisone, intravenously. Any other child who does not respond to all the measures described above in 12 to 24 hours—and before showing the signs of life-threatening respiratory failure—should be started on hydrocortisone, intravenously (5 mg per kg every 6 hours). If this regimen brings improvement, it can be discontinued promptly when used only for several days.

Differential diagnosis Wheezing respirations and expiratory dyspnea may be due to various conditions that produce obstruction in the respiratory tract, and bronchial asthma may therefore be confused with any of the following:

1. Bronchiolitis—during infancy it may be very difficult to distinguish from the first episode of asthma.
2. Cystic fibrosis of the pancreas.
3. Croup—wheezing and dyspnea mostly inspiratory.
4. Pertussis and pertussis-like disease.

5. Chronic bronchopulmonary disease associated with bronchiectasis.
6. Aspirated foreign body.
7. Loeffler's syndrome is characterized by widespread, transitory pulmonary infiltrations and eosinophilia. It may be precipitated by various antigens but most commonly by roundworms.
8. Tuberculosis—the onset of miliary type, due to endobronchial infection, or due to bronchial compression from tuberculous lymphadenopathy.
9. Salicylate poisoning—the early tachypnea may simulate asthma.
10. Polyarteritis nodosa—pulmonary involvement may be associated with wheezing and eosinophilia.
11. Miscellaneous conditions, e.g., atelectasis, tumors of the lung, cysts, substernal goiter, and congenital heart disease.
12. Hysteria.

Prognosis With proper treatment, asthma can be controlled and acute attacks can be prevented. Alleviation of anxiety in both the child and the parents is paramount. Identification of offending allergens, desensitization, and environmental control are necessary. About 20 percent of children treated only symptomatically will develop chronic pulmonary disease.

ATOPIC DERMATITIS

Infantile eczema, also known as "atopic dermatitis" or "allergic eczema," is one of the most common allergic manifestations of infancy and usually the first to reveal the allergic constitution of the young infant.

One hypothesis is that the immature gastrointestinal barrier of the infant will permit large foreign proteins from allergenic foods, e.g., cow's milk or eggs, to pass and sensitize an individual with allergic diathesis. Atopic dermatitis involves more than an allergy to foods. These children's skin usually also react to house dust, feathers, animal danders, pollens, and molds. Clinical correlation is difficult to establish, but experience indicates that a variety of factors aggravate or influence the evolution of eczema. Irritating contactants, e.g., wool or chemicals, scratching caused by the intense itch, infection, and emotional factors complicate the disease and are to be coped with in treatment.

In the young infant, eczema usually starts on cheeks and face as an erythematous eruption followed by vesicles. Differentiation from seborrheic dermatitis is most important (see Table 25-2).

Differential diagnosis

1. Seborrheic dermatitis
2. Leiner's disease (erythroderma desquamativum)—the most severe form of seborrheic dermatitis

Table 25-2.   Comparison of atopic and seborrheic dermatitides

	Atopic dermatitis	Seborrheic dermatitis
Clinical aspect		
Young infant	Starts on cheeks as erythema with vesicles which can become infected and show crusts covering pus	Scalp: "cradle cap" and upper face, eyebrows; yellowish, waxy plaques continues in intertriginous areas
Preschool child	Lesions on flexural aspect of arms, popliteal spaces, inguinal creases become lichenified	
Other characteristics	Extremely pruriginous, eosinophilia present; depigmentation can follow; allergic background, skin tests positive	Seldom pruriginous; no eosinophilia; no depigmentation, no heredity factor, skin tests negative
Prognosis	25% clear by age 3; 50% develop other allergies (hay fever, asthma); can continue in adulthood	May have no allergies Good prognosis

3. Ritter's disease (dermatitis exfoliativa neonatorum)—a severe bacterial infection occurring in the first 2 weeks of life
4. Acrodermatitis enteropatica
5. Reticuloendotheliosis (Letterer-Siwe disease)
6. Metabolic-deficiency group (phenylketonuria, gluten-sensitive enteropathy)
7. Immunologic-deficiency group (Aldrich-Wiscott syndrome, ataxia-telangiectasia)

Treatment   The comprehensive but individualized approach with continuous observation is the only key to success. The main principles of treatment include elimination of suspected offenders, e.g., allergenic foods; local irritants, e.g., wool; contact with animals; and irritating soaps. Alleviation of itching, local care and treatment of infections, and management of emotional problems are equally important. In the acute phase infected vesicles soon become covered by crusts. Burow's solution compresses for only 1 to 2 days to relieve the inflammation and remove the crusts should be followed by a hydrophilic or corticosteroid cream. Bathing should be with soothing, anti-inflammatory colloidal Aveeno products.

Itching, scratching, inflammation, and infection produce a vicious circle and should be interrupted. Oral antihistamines and tranquilizers of the Atarax type are useful. Proper systemic antibiotics should be given for infections.

Adrenal corticosteroids will give the best improvement, but this is a long-term disease and should not be treated with steroids for prolonged periods.

If the condition is very severe and clearing of the skin is mandatory, a short treatment with prednisone on alternate-day therapy is most satisfactory.

Precautions The infant with eczema should not be vaccinated or exposed to individuals who received fresh vaccinations; they can develop eczema vaccinatum. Herpes infection, too, is a danger. As a prophylactic measure, these infants should be breast-fed if possible; breast-fed babies have less eczema and later in life a lesser percentage of other allergic diseases. Hospitalization, too, may pose a serious problem because of exposure to serious infection. Reverse isolation should be provided.

URTICARIA

A common condition in children, urticaria, or hives, is easily recognized as papular, erythematous, irregular wheals accompanied by itching. It is difficult often to determine the cause. When of allergic origin, urticaria can be caused by drugs, focal infection, helminthic infection, and foods. Characterized by its rapid change in shape and location, urticaria can disappear in several hours or in some cases persists and is regarded as chronic after 6 weeks duration. The chemical mediator is histamine or bradykinin.

Clinical syndromes manifesting urticaria

1. Systemic anaphylactic shock.
2. Serum sickness.
3. Contact dermatitis, e.g., poison ivy, can penetrate the skin and cause urticaria.
4. Dermatitis due to physical agents, e.g., cold, heat, sunlight, exertion, or mechanical stimulation (in dermatographism).
5. Emotional upsets.
6. Miscellaneous conditions, e.g., systemic lupus erythematosus, lymphoma, and urticaria pigmentosa.
7. Angioneurotic edema—giant, firm urticaria, known as angioneurotic edema, can be caused by a lack in the serum of the inhibitory activity against the first component of complement (C'1); this is hereditary angioedema. Another form of angioneurotic edema occurs in patients with rhinitis, nasal polyps, or bronchial asthma and is due to a special sensitivity to aspirin.

Treatment

1. Allergic urticaria: Elimination of the offender is essential. (If penicillin is implicated, milk which contains the antibiotic may have to be eliminated.)
2. Symptomatic: During the acute phase (*a*) epinephrine 1:1,000 solution, 0.1 to 0.2 ml subcutaneously, may be repeated two or three times; if successful, Sus-Phrine may then be administered; (*b*) antihistamines.
3. Tranquilizers, e.g., Atarax, are helpful to combat the emotional aspect.
4. Adrenal corticosteroids (orally—local use is of no value) may be of value if all other treatments fail.

STINGING INSECT ALLERGY

The most common offender insects are bees, wasps, yellow jackets, and hornets.

If an allergic state has been induced, the simple local reaction of swelling, itching, and burning takes other more serious clinical forms.

The systemic reaction varies from mild (generalized urticaria) to anaphylactic shock (hypotension, cyanosis, unconsciousness). Other symptoms of varying degrees of severity are wheezing, dyspnea, laryngeal edema with hoarseness, abdominal pain, vomiting, and angioedema.

Treatment

Mild reaction (local) Remove honeybee stinger and apply ice pack. Analgesics and antihistamines provide relief from local discomfort.

Generalized reaction Apply a tourniquet proximal to the sting (if possible) and release it slowly after all treatment has been given. Epinephrine, 1:1,000 solution 0.2 to 0.3 ml subcutaneously, is given proximal to the sting, followed by parenteral antihistamine, e.g., Benadryl 0.5 to 1 ml of a 50 mg per ml solution, and corticosteroids, e.g., Decadron 4 to 8 mg, intramuscularly to prevent delayed reactions. The sensitized patient is instructed to carry an emergency kit containing a tablet of ephedrine sulfate and an antihistamine for use when a physician is not available.

Anaphylactic shock (a medical emergency) A mixture of the following drugs is given intravenously: (1) Levophed, 0.2%, 2 ml, or epinephrine, 1:1,000 solution, 0.5 ml; (2) aminophylline; (3) an antihistamine; (4) hydrocortisone (Solu-Cortef), 100 mg. Oxygen should be administered, and assisted ventilation may be necessary. Laryngospasm and laryngeal edema may necessitate a tracheotomy.

Prophylaxis

1. Avoid area known to attract insects, e.g., flowers, shrubs.
2. Light-colored clothes purportedly attract fewer insects.
3. Wear appropriate attire, e.g., long sleeves, hat, socks, and shoes.
4. Desensitization therapy should be administered to any child who has experienced a systemic reaction. The reactions after subsequent stingings have been markedly reduced in 90 percent of hyposensitized individuals.

DRUG ALLERGY

Allergic reactions to drugs must be differentiated from other drug reactions, e.g., overdose, intolerance, idiosyncrasy, side effects, and secondary effects.

Hypersensitivity to a drug is the result of an immune response resulting in the formation of specific antibodies and/or of sensitized lymphocytes. Therefore, the drug inducing an allergic reaction has to be either an antigen (a protein) or a haptene (certain chemicals will combine with serum protein and become antigens).

Since in vitro demonstration of antibodies against a particular drug is sometimes very difficult, or impossible, the diagnosis of drug allergy is usually a clinical decision rather than one based on a laboratory procedure.

Clinical criteria helpful in identifying an allergic reaction due to a drug include:

1. Very small amounts of the drug can induce an allergic reaction.
2. The reaction is different from the drug's pharmacologic action.
3. Sensitization to the drug is necessary (the allergic reaction will appear after 5 to 7 days).
4. The symptoms are allergic in type, e.g., rash, urticaria, asthma, serum sickness, anaphylactic reaction.
5. The symptoms can be reproduced by the same drug on different occasions or sometimes by cross-reacting drugs.

Factors influencing the development of drug allergy

1. Age of patient. Statistically, adults have more drug reactions than children, but anaphylactic shock after penicillin can occur in infants.
2. Allergic individuals are more prone to develop drug reactions.
3. Route of administration, e.g., oral, is the least sensitizing and intravenous the most allergenic. Topical application, especially with penicillin, to injured skin is very sensitizing.
4. Repeated exposure to the drug increases occurrence of reactions.
5. The sensitizing capacity of specific drugs varies.

Clinical features Features are numerous and sometimes difficult to differentiate from the underlying disease. The most fearful is, of course, anaphylactic shock (usually occurring after injection of foreign sera, penicillin, and less frequently, after radiopaque organic iodides (Renografin), local anesthetics, streptomycin, vitamin B_{12}, iron-dextran. Serum sickness-like syndrome can occur following administration of antibiotics and penicillins and is characterized by any one or more of the following: fever, arthralgia, lymphadenopathy, urticaria with pruritus, leukopenia, and proteinuria occurring in succession or concurrently.

A number of cutaneous reactions are seen in drug reactions. The following list contains the morphologic patterns of skin lesions and their main causative agents:

1. Erythema multiforme-like eruption: penicillin, antipyrine, sulfonamides, bromides, iodides, salicylates.
2. Stevens-Johnson syndrome: sulfonamides, barbiturates.
3. Morbiliform eruptions: antibiotics, bromides, barbiturates.
4. Eczematous eruptions: neomycin, local anesthetics, antihistamine creams, mercurials.
5. Acneiform eruptions: bromides, iodides, glucocorticoides.
6. Fixed eruption: phenolphthalein, barbiturates, salicylates, sulfonamides, tetracyclines.
7. Photosensitization: chlorpromazine, tetracyclines, sulfonamides.
8. Purpuric eruptions: sulfonamide, quinidine, penicillin, thiazides.
9. Urticaria, the most common, can be caused by an infinite variety of drugs.

Other clinical manifestations of drug reactions are

1. "Drug fever": antibiotics, mercurial diuretics, sulfonamides
2. Lymphadenopathy: hydantoin
3. Hematologic:
    a. Agranulocytosis: chloramphenicol, aminopyrine, phenothiazines
    b. Aplastic anemia: chloramphenicol, phenylbutazone, sulfonamides
    c. Hemolytic anemia: antimalarials, primaquine, sulfonamides, penicillin, paraaminosalicylic acid
    d. Thrombocytopenia: quinine, sulfonamides, chloramphenicol, phenylbutazone
4. Hepatic damage: sulfonamides, chlorpromazine, paraaminosalicylic acid, chloroform
5. Vasculitis: procainamide, sulfonamides
6. Nephropathy: polymyxins, phenacetin, salicylates

PENICILLIN ALLERGY

Penicillin allergy, one of the most common drug allergies, is responsible for most of the anaphylactic shock reactions occurring in man.

The clinical aspect of penicillin allergy is classified as

1. Immediate systemic reaction with anaphylactic shock
2. Accelerated diffuse urticaria occurring after 2 to 24 hours
3. Late urticaria appearing 2 to 3 weeks after exposure, with diffuse erythema, fever, arthralgia, proteinuria, and lymphadenopathy

Other reactions have been listed above.
Two penicillin derivatives act as sensitizers:

1. "Major" haptenic group—benzylpenicilloyl (BPO).
2. "Minor" haptenic group, including benzylpenicilloate and other degradation products of benzylpenicillin. These "minor" haptenic groups have significant clinical importance, since they give rise to the reaginic antibody (IgE) responsible for the immediate-type hypersensitivity reactions.

(These products are available only for research purposes and not for routine skin testing or other routine laboratory procedures to identify potential reactors.)

Since discrepancies are found often between histories of penicillin allergy, documented clinical reactivity, and skin tests to different products of penicillin, the practicing pediatrician has no reliable method to identify the sensitized individual. Skin tests to penicillin should be performed only by the pediatric allergist, since severe reactions due to intradermal skin testing have been reported. Furthermore, a negative skin test does not exclude the possibility of a severe hypersensitivity reaction.

Treatment Prophylactic: Restrict potential allergenic drugs to serious indications. Keep in mind that allergic patients carry a special risk. Discontinue the suspected drug at the first manifestation of an allergic reaction and make an attempt to document this correlation. (In case of penicillin allergy, the tests should be performed by an allergist 1 to 3 months after the suspected clinical reaction.) Patients should be told about their hypersensitivity so that the same drug will not be given to them in the future.

In case of minor drug reactions (urticaria, pruritus, morbilliform rash) one can use antihistamines, ephedrine, and in recurrent urticaria due to penicillin, corticosteroids. Generalized reaction with anaphylactic shock requires emergency treatment.

REVIEW QUESTIONS

1. What percentage of children experience allergic conditions: (a) 5 to 10 percent; (b) 15 to 20 percent; (c) 25 to 30 percent; (d) 40 to 50 percent.
2. Edema and spasm of smooth muscle of the bronchioles are hallmarks of (a)

delayed-type allergic reaction; (*b*) immediate-type allergic reaction; (*c*) intermediate-type allergic reaction.

3. In allergic infants, food allergy usually appears at the following age: (*a*) 2 to 4 days; (*b*) 2 to 4 weeks; (*c*) 2 to 4 months; (*d*) 10 to 12 months.

4. Mild allergy is suspected to occur in about (*a*) 1 percent; (*b*) 3 percent; (*c*) 5 percent; (*d*) 10 percent of infants.

5. The most common cause of perennial allergic rhinitis is (*a*) ragweed pollen; (*b*) chocolate; (*c*) house dust; (*d*) fish.

6. Children allergic to whole cow's milk frequently tolerate all but one of the following: (*a*) soybean products; (*b*) evaporated cow's milk; (*c*) skimmed milk; (*d*) heated cow's milk.

7. It is estimated that the following percentage of unsuccessfully treated children with hay fever and allergic rhinitis will develop bronchial asthma: (*a*) 10; (*b*) 20; (*c*) 30; (*d*) 40.

8. All of the following apply to bronchial asthma except for one: (*a*) early hypoventilation with respiratory alkalosis; (*b*) retention of CO_2 and rise of PCO_2; (*c*) metabolic acidosis with falling blood pH and accumulation of lactic acid; (*d*) antihistaminic drugs are useful in treatment.

9. The maximum single dose of aqueous epinephrine, 1:1,000 solution, to be administered subcutaneously to a child is (*a*) 0.01 ml; (*b*) 0.02 ml; (*c*) 0.2 ml; (*d*) 0.5 ml.

10. Intravenous aminophylline administration should not be repeated before (*a*) 1 hour; (*b*) 2 hours; (*c*) 4 hours; (*d*) 6 hours.

11. The recommended intravenous dose of hydrocortisone in the treatment of severe asthma is (*a*) 2 mg per kg every 4 hours; (*b*) 5 mg per kg every 4 hours; (*c*) 2 mg per kg every 6 hours; (*d*) 5 mg per kg every 6 hours.

12. In the young infant, eczema usually starts in (*a*) the anticubital fossa; (*b*) scalp; (*c*) cheeks and face; (*d*) buttocks.

13. If an allergic child is to be given a dog as a pet, the best procedure to follow is to (*a*) skin test for dog-dander sensitivity; (*b*) observe his reaction while with a friend's dog; (*c*) give him antihistamines if symptomatic; (*d*) get a short-haired dog.

26

SKIN DISORDERS

There is an appreciable physical and functional difference between the skin of the child and that of the adult. The physical dimensions of the skin at birth are 0.21 sq meters area and 0.20 kg weight. During adult life it covers 1.8 sq meters and weighs 4.2 kg. At birth and throughout childhood the epidermis is just 1 mm thick in most areas. The adult epidermis thickens to 2 mm and in addition creates fully developed adnexa, i.e., nails, hair, and sebaceous, apocrine, and exocrine glands. The functional differences are ones of degree normally, but these differences are reflected more clearly in the diseased skin.

Skin disorders are quite distinctive because most dermatoses produce visible structural alterations. In many diseases, the pathologic processes occurring in the skin are similar to those seen in other organs of the body. For example, inflammation, hyperemia, hypertrophy, atrophy, degeneration, and neoplasia are found. Some diseases, such as toxic erythema and generalized pruritus, are merely cutaneous manifestations of an internal condition. In dermatology, histopathology is of great diagnostic value because pathologic responses of the skin to disease are unique. The epidermis (ectoderm) and dermis (mesoderm) are unlike in development and structure and therefore undergo different pathologic changes. Careful attention to the relative proportion and the varied types of changes in the epidermis and dermis often permits a definitive diagnosis to be made microscopically when the clinical diagnosis is in doubt.

Certain skin diseases occur only in childhood, others are more prevalent during this period, while many occur rarely at this time. Because of the more tender and delicate nature of the skin of infants and children, as well as the almost constant exposure to trauma, most skin diseases during childhood are attributable to physical causes, infection, or allergy. To these one must add the genodermatoses, or hereditary, congenital, and nevoid anomalies, which usually are first seen during childhood. Numerous dominant or recessive hereditary skin disorders are known, and although each is relatively rare, the total incidence is considerable. The conditions seen in each age group vary to some extent, and so they are presented in these categories in the following text.

SKIN DISORDERS OF THE NEWBORN

MILIA

These are elevated, pinhead-sized papules, usually located on the nose and chin, resulting from retained sebaceous or keratinous material. They usually clear spontaneously within a few days to a week, although they may persist or recur until early adulthood. As there is no communication with the skin surface, removal must be by incision.

LIVIDOSUS ANNULARIS

This is a blotchy ringlike pattern of the skin due to vasomotor instability. It disappears spontaneously during the first year of life.

ERYTHEMA TOXICUM OF THE NEWBORN

Erythema toxicum, a generalized erythematous blotchy eruption, with or without wheals, is found during the first few days of life. It appears in approximately 30 percent of infants between the first and third days after birth. The eruption is characterized by erythema, pustules, and papules and is predominantly distributed over the chest, back, face, and extremities. Pustules occur in 10 percent of the cases; these are sterile and contain large numbers of eosinophils. It may be due to a sensitivity to a contactant, e.g., soap, oil, although a number of cases have been observed at the time of birth suggesting other causation. No treatment is necessary, and the eruption disappears spontaneously by the end of the first week.

TRAUMATIC SUBCUTANEOUS FAT NECROSIS

This is an uncommon condition which is usually due to trauma of delivery, e.g., trauma from forceps, and is seen most often on the cheeks, shoulders, or buttocks. It is characterized by sharply demarcated indurated areas that gradually disappear in several weeks with no treatment.

SCLEREMA NEONATORUM (Sclerema Adiposum)

This condition occurs at birth or before the tenth day, although in some cases it may appear several months after birth. Premature and debilitated infants are affected. The lesions first appear on the buttocks as waxy white indurations. The skin is cold and does not pit on pressure. These skin changes then appear over the body, sparing the palms, soles, and the scrotum. Immobility of the joints is quite frequent, and the infant is unable to take feedings in the normal manner. The body temperature is reduced.

The causation is unknown. It is thought, however, that the reduction of unsaturation of fatty acids, normally found in the subcutaneous tissues of the neonate, plays a role by raising the melting point of the fat, with subsequent solidification at reduced temperatures.

Treatment is directed at maintaining fluid and electrolyte balance and nutrition. The primary disease should be combated, and adrenal corticosteroids may be of value.

The prognosis is grave and depends to a great extent on control of the primary disease. Death usually occurs in 3 to 4 days.

SCLEREMA EDEMATOSUM (Scleredema)

This condition occurs at birth in premature and debilitated infants. The lesions appear first as white waxy swellings of the lower extremities. Early in the disease, the lesions pit on pressure. As the disease progresses, it involves the dependent areas of the body and ultimately the other areas of the body. Late lesions do not pit on pressure. This condition is readily confused with sclerema neonatorum. There is reduced body temperature but no immobilization of the joints. The pathologic change is in the corium and consists of edema, whereas in sclerema neonatorum there is solidification of the fat. The prognosis is better in sclerema edematosum than in sclerema neonatorum; the children usually recover if attention is given to elevating the body temperature, feeding, and fluid balance. Adrenal corticosteroids are also very helpful. Broad-spectrum antibiotics should be given to protect against secondary infection.

IMPETIGO NEONATORUM

This is caused by staphylococcal, streptococcal, or viral infection and is characterized by superficial vesicles and pustules on an erythematous base. They are usually located in the folds and creases of the skin, especially in the diaper area and on the neck. It may appear as early as the second day. In the nursery, impetigo neonatorum may assume epidemic proportions.

Prophylaxis   It is most important to have aseptic technique in the nursery and to isolate all diagnosed cases.

Treatment   Treatment is discussed under Impetigo Contagiosa, later in this chapter.

PEMPHIGUS NEONATORUM

This is a condition characterized by bullous lesions over the entire body except the palms and soles, with mild to severe constitutional symptoms. It is probably a very severe form of bullous impetigo neonatorum and is a different entity from any of the pemphigus conditions that are described in adults. The condition may simulate the skin manifestations of congenital syphilis.

Treatment   Chemotherapy and antibiotics are administered for the infection. Dehydration and electrolyte imbalance should be corrected, and blood transfusion will replace serum lost via the skin.

Prognosis   The prognosis is guarded.

DERMATITIS EXFOLIATIVA NEONATORUM

This rare disease is a serious acute bacterial infection of the skin. It occurs during the first month of life. It often begins as an erythema on the face with rapid spread over the entire body, followed by severe generalized exfoliation. There is easy removal of the undenuded skin by friction (Nikolsky's sign). This disease must be differentiated from pemphigus neonatorum and congenital syphilis.

Treatment   The same as for pemphigus neonatorum, above.

Prognosis   The prognosis is guarded.

MONILIA OF THE SKIN

This is discussed under oral moniliasis in Chapter 12, "Diseases of the Newborn."

SYPHILITIC ERUPTION

This is discussed under Syphilis in Chapter 14, "Infectious Diseases."

HEMANGIOMA

Hemangiomas are common and may be present at birth. They may be divided clinically into:

1. Port-wine stains, which are flat and purplish. These should be differentiated from the common fetal hyperemia found in the new-born infant (over the bridge of the nose, eyelids, and back of the neck) which will disappear spontaneously by 1 to 2 years of age.
2. Capillary (strawberry) hemangiomas, small and usually elevated. Premature infants are prone to develop them. They are usually single but several may appear in the same patient. Commonly the lesions enlarge during the first 6 to 9 months, after which they tend to become quiescent and finally regress. Large capillary or cavernous hemangiomas may become the site of platelet agglutination leading to thrombocytopenic purpura and disseminated intra-vascular coagulation (see p. 597).
3. Cavernous hemangiomas, which are large, cystic, elevated, and extend deep into the skin, are composed of larger vessels than either of the above conditions. Extensive lesions of the skin may be associated with visceral or mucous membrane involvement: von Hippel-Lindau disease—hemangiomas of the retina, cerebellum, and spinal cord and cysts of the kidney, pancreas, and testes; Sturge-Weber syndrome (see Chapter 20, "Neurologic Conditions"); Osler-Rendu-Weber disease (see Chapter 22, "Blood Disorders"); Patou's syndrome (see Chapter 8, "Genetics").

Treatment Port-wine stains are handled best with "cover-mark" cosmetics. At a later age tattooing or plastic surgery may be considered. For capillary and cavernous hemangiomas, carbon dioxide snow, sclerosing solutions (sodium tetradecyl sulfate 3%), surgery, and radium are commonly employed, depending upon the type and location of the hemangioma. These hemangiomas (especially the capillary type) may sclerose spontaneously before 4 to 6 years of age. Cosmetic results are usually better without therapy. Therefore, unless complications occur, or the mass is in such a location as to interfere with function, no treatment is advisable. If the lesions are growing rapidly, treatment should not be delayed. All treatments may leave residual scars.

NEVI (Moles)

Nevi are generally recognized as more or less local, often well-defined lesions due to congenital anomalies of pigmentation or to faulty development of dermal, epidermal, or vascular structures. The "common moles," or intradermal nevi, are circumscribed areas of pigmentation in the skin. They vary in size from pinpoint lesions to those covering several square inches, and in color they range from cream to black. (Mongolian spots—irregular areas of pigmentation on the buttocks, trunk, or lower extremities—may occur in any race and usually disappear by 1 to 2 years of age.) Malignant degeneration of nevi is very infrequent and is said to occur only after puberty. Treatment is excision in the cases where the nevus is subject to irritation and trauma, or causes disfigurement.

CONGENITAL SKIN DEFECT

This is usually found in the midline of the scalp or over the spine and is about 5 mm in size. There is no hair or other epidermal structure over the involved part. Rarely there is an associated congenital dermal sinus, which ends blindly or has some connection to the meninges. This may become infected and may lead to repeated episodes of meningitis.

PILONIDAL CYSTS AND SINUSES

These are common congenital dermal sinuses that occur in the region of the coccyx and sacrum. Most often these sinuses end blindly; rarely, they may extend into the spinal canal. They infrequently become infected during childhood. If they remain asymptomatic, no treatment is necessary. Infected sinuses and cysts should be removed surgically.

SKIN DISORDERS DURING INFANCY

ECZEMA

This is discussed in Chapter 25, "Allergy."

SEBORRHEIC DERMATITIS

This common disease of infancy is a chronic inflammatory reaction of the skin characterized by an involvement primarily of the scalp and intertriginous areas. The cause is a disturbance of the sebaceous glands, but the specific mechanism is unknown. Allergy and secondary infection may be contributory or predisposing factors. The mildest and more frequent form is "cradle cap," which is characterized by the presence of greasy scales on the scalp. In the more severe forms, the seborrhea may involve the forehead, eyebrows, creases behind the ears, cheeks, genitocrural folds of the diaper area, and the entire trunk. There are redness, scaling, and sometimes oozing but very little itching. Recurrences are frequent, but the condition usually clears spontaneously by the end of the first year of life. Seborrhea is sometimes difficult or impossible to differentiate from an atopic dermatitis (eczema). The treatment of cradle cap consists of softening and removing the crusts by topical applications of a mild ointment or lotion followed by shampoos and brushing. For the severe forms ointments or lotions containing crude coal tar 2%, a mild antibacterial such as a quaternary compound, or salicylic acid in Aquaphor may be used. The dermatitis in other parts of the body responds well to the local application of a hydrocortisone-antibiotic preparation.

ERYTHRODERMA DESQUAMATIVA (Leiner's Disease)

This disease occurs most frequently in breast-fed infants. The cause is unknown, but it may be a severe form of seborrheic dermatitis. Diarrhea may be an associated symptom. The onset is between 1 and 3 months of age. The skin lesions are those of generalized seborrheic dermatitis: seborrhea of the scalp, intertrigo of the groins and axillae, and diffuse redness and scaling.

Although the disease is self-limiting (1 to 3 months) and there is no recurrence, the prognosis is guarded because occasionally death may occur.

Treatment

1. Antibiotics and chemotherapy to treat secondary infection
2. Use of milk substitute, e.g., soybean formula
3. Maintenance of fluid and electrolyte balance
4. Local therapy with 2 percent sulfur and salicylic acid or topical adrenocortical steroid-antibiotic ointment.

DIAPER DERMATITIS

This comprises a group of cutaneous reactions that involve the area covered by the diaper and which include ammonia dermatitis, perianal dermatitis, intertrigo, contact dermatitis, and moniliasis.

Ammonia dermatitis This condition is characterized by an erythematous, vesicular, or ulcerated eruption caused by liberation of ammonia from urine by urea-splitting organisms from the stool. Exposed areas are more severely involved than intertriginous areas. This condition frequently leads to an ulceration of the urethral meatus in a circumcised infant, which when healed may result in urethral stenosis due to scarring.

Treatment
1. Exposure of the involved skin area to air is helpful as well as more frequent changing of diapers.
2. Use of disposable diapers or a nonvolatile antiseptic as the last rinse of the diapers, e.g., quaternary ammonium compounds (Diaparene chloride 1 : 10,000 solution) ; these compounds are relatively nontoxic and excellent for this purpose.
3. A hydrophilic ointment with a mild germicidal action or a protective ointment may be applied to the skin over the diaper area.

Perianal dermatitis This condition is due to fecal irritation and characterized by an area of erythema, excoriation, desquamation, and superficial ulceration around the anus. The area involved may vary from 2 to 4 cm, severe at the anus and fading at the periphery. It is common in the newborn infant, in whom it is associated with transitional stools, and in infants and children with diarrhea and following oral antibiotics. Allergy may play a role as a cause of this condition.

Treatment   Exposure to the air, prompt diaper changes after bowel movements, and applications of an antibacterial water-repellent cream are indicated.

Intertrigo   This is a dermatitis occurring between two apposition surfaces of the skin. It is more common in obese infants who are not kept clean. It appears in the folds of the skin, such as the groin and the neck.

Treatment   Proper bathing and application of a dusting powder are helpful. Antibiotics may be used locally if secondary infection is present. The skin folds may be separated with cotton to permit free access of air.

Contact dermatitis   This condition is caused by skin reaction to chemicals used to wash diapers, e.g., detergents, harsh soaps, or bleaches.

Moniliasis   This condition is characterized by sharply circumscribed erythematous moist surfaces, often following oral moniliasis.

Treatment   Sponging of the involved area with 1:2,000 benzalkonium chloride several times daily and treatment of oral and intestinal moniliasis, e.g., Nystatin (Mycostatin), is the usual treatment.

MILIARIA RUBRA

This condition, known as prickly heat, is seen mostly in warm weather when there is excessive perspiration. It is a fine papular rash, usually over the shoulders and neck and in the skin folds due to occlusion of the pores of the sweat glands.

Treatment

1. The involved areas should be sponged or bathed frequently; the infant should be kept cool and dressed lightly.
2. A dusting powder applied lightly or calamine lotion is helpful.

ACRODYNIA (Dermatopolyneuritis)

This is a syndrome of unknown causation in infants and young children characterized by symptoms and signs of involvement of the skin and nervous system. Mercury hypersensitivity or poisoning has been implicated as the cause. Elevated levels of mercury are found in the urine. The onset is usually insidious, and there may be any or all of the following findings:

1. The hands and feet may take on a pink hue and desquamate.
2. The tip of the nose and cheeks may also be pink.
3. Ptyalism.
4. Photophobia.
5. Personality changes (peevishness).
6. Excessive perspiration and increased thirst.
7. Hypertension.
8. Hypotonia.
9. Loss of teeth, nails, and hair.
10. Rash which is inconstant and protean.

Treatment   BAL and EDTA (see Lead Intoxication, p. 115) as well as D-Penicillamine have beneficial effects.

Prognosis   There is a good prognosis. Spontaneous cure in several months is usual.

CONGENITAL ECTODERMAL DYSPLASIA

Various forms of this heredofamilial disease have been described. Chondroectodermal dysplasia (Ellis-van Creveld syndrome) is characterized by faulty development, deficiency, or absence of some or all of the epidermis and its derivatives, e.g., hair, teeth, sweat glands, and nails. Dyschondroplasia, polydactylism, and congenital heart defects are also present in addition to the ectodermal dysplasia.

In the hidrotic type, there are normal sweat glands but defective development of teeth, nails, and hair; it is inherited as an autosomal dominant trait. In the anhidrotic type, sweat glands are absent or defective, resulting in decreased heat tolerance and otherwise unexplained fever. The hair is sparse, thin, and fine; the eyelashes and eyebrows are sparse or lacking; there is partial or complete absence of the deciduous and permanent teeth. Other findings may be lack of nipples, everted lips, absence of senses of taste and smell, absence of lacrimation, and chronic laryngitis and pharyngitis. This type is inherited as a sex-linked recessive trait.

There is no specific treatment.

SKIN DISORDERS DURING CHILDHOOD

FURUNCULOSIS

This is a pyogenic infection of the skin, frequently involving the scalp. There are numerous boils that appear in crops. The most common etiologic organism is the staphylococcus. The predisposing factors are poor nutrition and uncleanliness.

Treatment   Antibiotics should be given systemically and locally. Stock vaccines and autogenous vaccines have been used in resistant cases. Incision and drainage should be used when necessary.

OTITIS EXTERNA

This involves the outer one-third of the external auditory canal, the external auditory meatus, and the lateral surface of the auricle. The eruption, which is usually bilateral, is characterized by the presence of erythema, edema, exudate, desquamation, and crust formation. It is intensely pruritic and painful; pain is aggravated by moving the pinna. The predominating causative organisms are *Pseudomonas aeruginosa* and staphylococcus. Occasionally it may be mycotic. The condition is to be differentiated from otitis media. The tympanic membrane is normal.

Treatment   Intermittent compresses with Burow's solution 1:10, followed by the topical application of antibiotics and hydrocortisone are used. External otitis due to fungous infections tends to be resistant to treatment and often becomes chronic.

IMPETIGO CONTAGIOSA

This skin disease is usually caused by staphylococci or streptococci and is characterized by the formation of vesicles and pustules on an erythematous base which later form yellowish crusts. Pruritus is common, and the impetigo spreads by autoinoculation. It is contagious, and epidemics may occur, especially during the summer.

Treatment

1. The skin should be washed twice daily with an antiseptic soap (pHisoHex) and all crusts gently removed.
2. An antibacterial ointment, bacitracin or neomycin, should be applied to the lesions several times a day.
3. The child's hands should be kept away from the lesions. The hands should be washed with an antibacterial soap.
4. Antibiotics (orally or parenterally) may be used in resistant cases.

ERYSIPELAS

This is a streptococcal infection of the skin, characterized by a painful erythematous induration with sharply demarcated borders. In infancy, the lesions are found most frequently about the umbilical cord stump and genitalia; hemolytic streptococci may be cultured from the blood. During childhood the face is most commonly involved. Erysipelas is to be differentiated from a diffuse cellulitis (edges not elevated and constitutional symptoms less severe).

Treatment   Antibiotics (penicillin) are effective.

Prognosis   The prognosis is good.

HERPES SIMPLEX

This disease is discussed in Chapters 12, "Diseases of the Newborn," and 14, "Infectious Diseases."

STEVENS–JOHNSON SYNDROME (Erythema Multiforme Exudativa)

This syndrome is a severe form of erythema multiforme of unknown etiology. It is thought by some to be due to a hypersensitivity reaction to infection or drugs. It is more common in males and is characterized by

1. Lesions on the mucous membrane, usually faucial or buccal
2. Erythematous, papular skin eruption with peripheral spread, developing into confluent and widespread vesicular-bullous lesions
3. Conjunctivitis and photophobia
4. Constitutional symptoms: high fever, malaise, anorexia, and generalized aches and pains

Treatment

1. Symptomatic: Maintain fluid and electrolyte balance. Antibiotics are of questionable value but may be administered to prevent secondary infection.
2. Adrenal corticosteroids may be of value.

Prognosis   The prognosis is guarded. There is a mortality rate of 10 percent during the early phase. Loss of vision due to corneal ulceration may occur.

VERRUCAE (Warts)

Verrucae are autoinoculable, small circumscribed growths of the epidermis. They are of viral origin. Several types are found, depending upon the site of development:

1. Verruca vulgaris: on the hands and fingers.
2. Verruca plantaris: on the palms and soles, often associated with considerable pain.
3. Verruca plana juvenilis: on the face, forehead, and dorsal surface of the hands.
4. Verruca filiformis: on the eyelids, neck, and bearded area in older adolescent boys.
5. Verruca acuminata: on mucosal areas. These are usually multiple, pinkish, and frequently confluent, occurring on moist areas around the genitalia, anus, and mouth.

Treatment Warts are resistant to therapy and have a tendency to recur. Treatment is individualized for the type of wart.

1. Verruca vulgaris: electrodesiccation and curettage is the most satisfactory procedure.
2. Verruca plantaris: preparation of the wart site with salicylic acid 40% followed by electrodesiccation and curettage; dry ice or cantharidin or podophyllum solution of acetone and flexible collodion may be applied to the wart for several weeks (this is also useful in periungual warts).
3. Verruca plana juvenilis: electrodesiccation and curettage should not be used for these lesions; such removal will produce scars. A desquamating agent, e.g., lotion of sulfur and resorcin, should be used. The condition is usually self-limiting.
4. Verruca filiformis: electrodesiccation without curettage is the method of choice.
5. Verruca acuminata: best removed by treatment with podophyllum 20% in compound tincture of benzoin.

Verruca vulgaris of children will often respond to suggestion or psychotherapy.

URTICARIA (Hives)

See Chapter 25, "Allergy."

MOLLUSCUM CONTAGIOSUM

This condition is caused by a virus and is characterized by small, umbilicated, elevated, waxy, pearl-like lesions. Pressure results in the expulsion of a cheesy material.

Treatment Removal of the molluscum body in each lesion by curettage and chemical cauterization of the base to prevent recurrence and control bleeding is effective.

PSORIASIS

Psoriasis is a chronic recurrent disease of unknown etiology characterized by erythematous plaques covered with silvery white scales that leave minute bleeding points when removed. These may become confluent, forming large patches. The extensor surfaces of the elbows and knees are most commonly involved, although the scalp, palms, soles, and nails may show the early lesions at first. Family incidence of diabetes is frequent.

Treatment No therapy is entirely satisfactory. A low-fat diet and ultraviolet irradiation have been recommended. Keratolytic ointments such as ammoniated mercury 5% or crude coal tar and salicylic acid have been used. In severe cases adrenal corticosteroids may be tried.

PITYRIASIS ROSEA

Pityriasis rosea is of unknown causation and is characterized by pruritic, erythematous, papulosquamous lesions appearing chiefly on the trunk, arms, and thighs, very seldom on the face. The lesions are at first pinpoint, then increase in size to 1 to 2 cm. The long axis of the lesion follows the lines of cleavage of the skin. A herald lesion—larger than the others, usually on the chest—appears several days before the more generalized eruption. The condition is self-limited (6 weeks). Ultraviolet irradiation may shorten the course of the disease. It is moderately contagious and is more frequently seen in girls.

IVY DERMATITIS (see p. 681)

TUBERCULOSIS OF THE SKIN

Tuberculosis of the skin is uncommon in the United States. The lesions may be due to tubercle bacillus infection in the skin (either primary or secondary) or to an allergic effect on tuberculin-sensitized tissues (tuberculids). Some of the tubercle bacillus infections are:

1. Scrofuloderma: an extension from tuberculous bones or glands. The cervical glands are commonly involved. The glands are enlarged, firm, and adherent to the skin. Later they may suppurate and become fluctuant. The overlying skin may ulcerate and a draining sinus may be established. This may heal spontaneously but more often tends to become chronic.
2. Lupus vulgaris: characterized by small reddish-brown (apple-jelly) papules. These papules coalesce to form patches that are irregular in size and shape. They occur most commonly on the face. Necrosis, ulceration, and fibrosis, over a period of years, is the usual course.
3. Primary complex, where the portal of entry is the skin: characterized by an ulcer, lymphangitis, and lymphadenitis.
4. Disseminated tuberculosis, where the skin may share the infection with other organs: the eruption is multiform; the prognosis is very poor.

Typical tuberculids are:

1. Lichen scrofulosorum: rosacea-like tuberculid and papulonecrotic tuberculid. All occur as crops or showers of small, discrete, pea-sized nodules, usually symmetric in distribution and most fre-

quently occurring on the chest, back, face, and the anterior surface of the extremities.

2.   Erythema induratum (Bazin's disease): characterized by symmetric indurated subcutaneous nodules, usually on the back of the leg or the thigh, which may ulcerate or heal by absorption.

Treatment   General measures to improve resistance are important in both forms of cutaneous tuberculosis. These include adequate diet and rest. Antibiotic therapy is indicated in all instances irrespective of apparent activity of other lesions. Surgical excision if possible may be indicated.

SCABIES

Scabies is a contagious parasitic disease of the skin caused by the itch mite (*Acarus scabiei*), which burrows into the skin. It is characterized by severe itching, particularly at night, and is often followed by secondary infection from scratching. The lesions are discrete, excoriated, small papulovesicles associated with linear scratch marks. Vesicular bullous lesions may be seen in infants. The most common locations are the lower part of the trunk, umbilicus, penis, thighs, legs, and interdigital webs. In infants the lesions are frequently located on the face and feet.

Treatment

1.   All intimate contacts should be treated at the same time.
2.   Infected clothes and bed linens should be sterilized.
3.   Benzyl benzoate 25% or a benzyl benzoate-DDT-benzocaine emulsion (Topocide) is applied after a warm, soaking bath, while the skin is still moist. Two more applications are made at 12-hour intervals. If there is still itching, the treatment can be repeated in 1 week. Insecticides such as the gamma isomer of hexachlorbenzene (Kwell) are also very effective.

RINGWORM OF THE SCALP (Tinea Capitis)

This is a fungous infection and is a common cause of loss of hair in children. It is characterized by a well-demarcated circular lesion or lesions of the scalp. It occurs most often in boys from 5 to 12 years of age. The hairs in the area are very brittle, lack luster, and often are broken off close to the scalp, so that the affected area appears bald. Occasionally boggy, encrusted lesions (kerions) will be the presenting lesions or will develop in response to therapy.

Diagnosis   Fluorescence with Wood's lamp will identify the infected hairs. If *Microsporum audouini* or *M. lanosum* is present, the spores appear green. Microscopic examination of hair and skin scrapings or cultures on Sabouraud's agar will identify the fungus.

Treatment Griseofulvin, 10 mg per lb per day, orally for 1 to 2 weeks, is the usual treatment. Rarely, 20 to 40 mg may be necessary. Antifungicidal ointments are of doubtful value. If not cured earlier, practically all cases clear spontaneously at puberty apparently because of a change in the pH of the skin which occurs at that time.

RINGWORM OF THE FEET

Ringworm of the feet (athlete's foot, dermatophytosis) is a very common disease, characterized by vesicles, fissures, maceration, and desquamation between the toes. There may be an associated hyperhidrosis. Pruritus, which is variable, will at times be the presenting symptom. There may be similar lesions of the fingers and the volar aspects of the hands. These lesions may be primarily mycotic, from which organisms are recoverable, or they may be the result of the id reaction, in which case organisms will not be found. The criteria of the id reaction are:

1. Primary inflammatory site, usually the toe webs, from which mycotic organisms are recoverable.
2. Secondary distant site with lesions characterized by symmetry, vesicle formation, pruritus, and from which mycotic organisms are not recoverable.
3. The trichophytin test is positive.
4. Treatment of the primary site will produce clearing of the secondary sites without any local therapy being applied to the secondary sites.

It has long been contended that dermatophytosis is disseminated via public shower baths; however, this tenet is no longer considered to be valid; rather, it is individual susceptibility (perspiration, poor foot hygiene, poor evaporation of moisture) that is now regarded as the primary predisposing factor in the occurrence of dermatophytosis.

Treatment

1. Acute lesions: potassium permanganate compresses, 1:5,000.
2. Subacute and chronic lesions: half-strength Whitfield's ointment. Ointment is applied only upon retiring.
3. Moist lesions: potassium permanganate 1:5,000 soaks may be used until the secondary infection has cleared.
4. Griseofulvin, 250 mg four times daily, orally, for 4 weeks or longer.

In infections of long duration, therapy may not be very effective.

ALOPECIA AREATA

Alopecia areata is characterized by a single area or several circumscribed areas of baldness. The etiology is unknown, and there is no specific treatment. Vitamin B complex has been recommended; locally, massage and ultraviolet rays may be helpful. In almost all cases, the prognosis is good and recovery will be complete; however, there may be recurrences. Foci of infection and emotional trauma have been incriminated. (Patchy alopecia may also occur as a manifestation of congenital syphilis, but this may be recognized by its "moth-eaten" appearance, and tinea capitis must always be ruled out with Wood's lamp examination.)

Treatment Adrenal corticosteroids parenterally, in intralesional injections, or locally may be effective in arresting the process.

ACNE VULGARIS

This is a disease of early adolescence consisting of an inflammation of the hair follicles and sebaceous glands, with seborrhea, hyperkeratinization, hyperplasia, and the production of papular and pustular lesions intermingled with comedos. Seborrhea is usually present. The comedo, which results from overproduction or poor elimination of sebum, is the primary lesion of acne. The most common locations are the face, shoulders, and back. Endocrine factors probably play a role in this condition. Treatment is often disappointing as to prompt relief, but the condition usually clears spontaneously in time.

Treatment

1. The face should be washed regularly with a cleanser such as Lowila, especially upon arising and at bedtime.
2. After washing at bedtime, a drying skin lotion containing sulfur and/or salicylic acid should be applied, e.g., lotio alba or Sulforcin.
3. Comedos should be removed as they appear.
4. Small doses of ultraviolet rays may be given weekly.
5. Estrogen therapy may be considered for females who have a severe exacerbation of the lesions during the premenstrual cycle. It is not advisable in males.
6. Tetracyclines in low dosage (250 mg per day) have been used successfully to treat the pustular and cystic types.

The essentials of acne therapy are to carry the patient through the psychologically trying time and to prevent disfiguring scar formation.

PEDICULOSIS

This condition is produced by lice in the hair of the scalp, pubis, and axillae. It is characterized by pruritus, with secondary dermatitis from scratching.

Treatment Kwell and Eurax lotions are effective. Topical application followed by a thorough shampoo in the morning will cure most cases. All possible contacts (family, schoolmates, etc.) must be examined and treated to prevent reinfection.

REVIEW QUESTIONS

1. The following facts are true of erythema toxicum except (a) erythema and papules appear; (b) distribution is usually over chest, back, face, and extremities; (c) it appears between the first and third day after birth; (d) it should be treated with antibiotics.

2. Column I lists some skin diseases seen in the neonatal period; column II contains some statements concerning these diseases. Match the two:

I		II	
A.	Erythema toxicum _____	(a)	Due to vasomotor instability
B.	Sclerema neonatorum _____	(b)	Superficial vesicles and pustules on an erythematous base
C.	Lividosus annularis _____		
D.	Impetigo neonatorum _____	(c)	May be due to reduction of unsaturated fatty acids
E.	Pemphigus neonatorum _____	(d)	May be due to sensitivity to contactants
		(e)	Bullous lesions over the entire body except for the palms and soles

3. Nikolsky's sign is commonly associated with (a) syphilitic eruption; (b) dermatitis exfoliativa neonatorum; (c) pemphigus neonatorum; (d) impetigo neonatorum.

4. Fetal hyperemia in the newborn infant usually will disappear spontaneously by (a) 6 months; (b) 1 to 2 years; (c) 5 years; (d) adulthood.

5. Port-wine stains are managed best with (a) cover-mark cosmetics; (b) carbon dioxide snow; (c) sclerosing solution; (d) radium.

6. "Cradle cap" is a mild form of (a) seborrheic dermatitis; (b) infantile eczema; (c) ringworm of the scalp; (d) impetigo contagiosa.

7. The following statements are true of Leiner's disease except (a) it occurs most frequently in breast-fed infants; (b) its onset is between 1 and 3 months of age; (c) a virus has been identified as the etiologic agent; (d) it is characterized by seborrhea of scalp, intertrigo of groins and axillae, and diffuse redness and scaling.

8. All the following statements concerning acrodynia are true except for (a) elevated mercury levels are found in the urine; (b) there is photophobia; (c) there is hypertonia; (d) treatment consists of BAL and EDTA.

9. The following facts concerning congenital ectodermal dysplasia are true except (a) sweat glands may be normal, but there may be defective development of teeth, nails, and hair in one form of this disease; (b) one form of this disease has sweat glands absent or defective with defective development of teeth, nails, and hair; (c) one form of the disease is sex-linked autosomal dominant, and the other type is sex-linked recessive; (d) polydactylism and congenital heart defects may be associated with the ectodermal dysplasia.

10. Otitis externa consists of all the following except (a) predominant causative organisms are *Pseudomonas aeruginosa* and staphylococcus; (b) tympanic membrane is normal; (c) involves outer one-third of the external auditory canal; (d) usually is unilateral.

11. The following questions are the matching type. In each blank in column I, insert the letter corresponding to the word or phrase in column II which is associated most appropriately.

	I			II
A.	Molluscum contagiosum _____		(*a*)	Benzyl benzoate used in treatment
B.	Psoriasis _____			
C.	Pityriasis rosea _____		(*b*)	No specific treatment; etiology unknown
D.	Ivy dermatitis _____			
E.	Scabies _____		(*c*)	Seen in early adolescence
F.	Ringworm of scalp _____		(*d*)	Griseofulvin
G.	Alopecia areata _____		(*e*)	Treatment with Kwell
H.	Acne vulgaris _____		(*f*)	Small, umbilicated, waxy, pearl-like lesions
I.	Pediculosis _____			
			(*g*)	Herald patch
			(*h*)	Desensitization available
			(*i*)	Extensor surfaces of elbows and knees are most commonly involved; family incidence of diabetes frequent

12. All the following statements concerning Stevens-Johnson syndrome are true except (*a*) it is a severe form of erythema multiforme; (*b*) it is more common in males; (*c*) nearly 100 percent of patients recover; (*d*) constitutional symptoms occur such as generalized aches and pains, high fever, and malaise.

13. Von Hippel-Lindau disease, Sturge-Weber syndrome, Osler-Rendu-Weber syndrome, and Patau's syndrome have in common one of the following: (*a*) abnormal karyotype; (*b*) hemangiomas; (*c*) hives; (*d*) ectodermal defects, mostly in the midline.

INDEX